NECK ACHE AND SHOULDER PAIN

NECK ACHE AND SHOULDER PAIN

Ian Macnab, M.B., ChB., F.R.C.S.C.

Former Chief, Division of Orthopaedic Surgery
The Wellesley Hospital
Emeritus Professor of Surgery
University of Toronto
Toronto, Ontario, Canada

John McCulloch, M.D., F.R.C.S.C.

Professor of Orthopaedics
Northeastern Ohio Universities
College of Medicine
Rootstown, Ohio

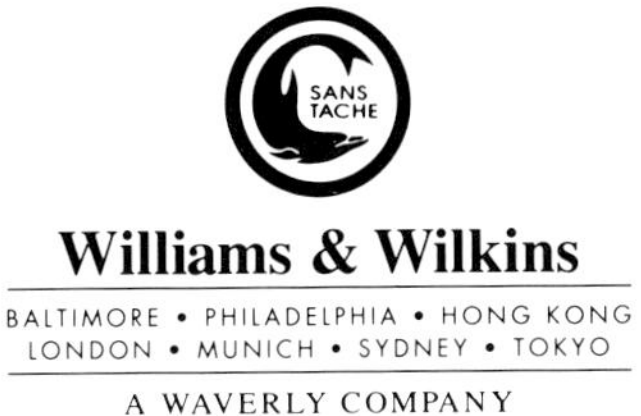

Williams & Wilkins

BALTIMORE • PHILADELPHIA • HONG KONG
LONDON • MUNICH • SYDNEY • TOKYO

A WAVERLY COMPANY

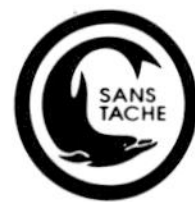

Editor: William M. Passano III
Project Manager: Victoria Rybicki Vaughn
Copy Editor: Robert Winkler
Designer: Norman W. Och
Illustration Planner: Ray Lowman

Copyright © 1994
Williams & Wilkins
428 East Preston St
Baltimore, Maryland 21202   USA

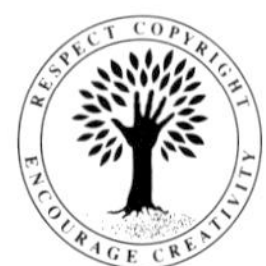

Accurate indications, adverse reaction, and dosage schedules for drugs are proved
in this book, but it is possible that they may change. The reader is urged to
review the package information data of the manufacturers of the medications
mentioned.

Printed in the United States of America

Library of Congress Cataloging-in-Publication Data

Macnab, Ian.
    Neck ache and should pain / Ian Macnab, John McCulloch.
       p.   cm.
    Includes bibliographical references and index.
    ISBN 0-683-05354-X
    1. Neck pain.   2. Should pain.   I. McCulloch, John A;
II. Title.
    [DNLM: 1. Neck.   2. Shoulder.   3. Shoulder Joint.   4. Pain.   WE
708 M169n 1993]
RC936.M24   1993
617.5′3—dc20
DNLM/DLC
for Library of Congress   93-26999
                                                                       CIP

        93 94 95 96 97 98
 1 2 3 4 5 6 7 8 9 10

DEDICATION

To the youth in medicine:

There are those who have gone before you: Dr. E.D. Codman, who in 1934 was the first to describe the pathology and pathogenesis of rotator cuff tendonitis.

There are those who are here now: Dr. J.W. Fielding and Dr. Ed Simmons, who have contributed so immensely to our knowledge of the cervical spine.

But the future belongs to the youth of medicine: you will contribute to an even better understanding of the neck and shoulder. You are our growth industry, our intellectual property that is so valuable. Let us hope that you are not overrun by a smothering bureaucracy.

To you this book is dedicated.

I.M.
J.M.

PREFACE

*"Knowledge is a process of piling up facts.
Wisdom lies in their simplification."*
                                        Martin A. Fisher

Without any pretension to be wise, we hope in this short book to simplify the problem of treating a patient who becomes progressively handicapped because of persistent pain in the neck, shoulder, or arm. Although the primary aim is to describe degenerative conditions, chapters have been included on fractures, inflammatory and infective disorders, and tumors. As a source of symptoms, the anatomical region of the neck and shoulder is clinically inseparable, so there is a large section on shoulder pain. In the end, we hope you, the developing medical care worker—whether you are a primary care physician, orthopaedic resident, therapist, or nurse—will have a somewhat better understanding of the patient with neck ache and shoulder pain.

When a patient complains of a grumbling pain in the shoulder, it is dangerously easy to attribute this symptom to a local lesion of the glenohumeral joint, with some vague pathological diagnosis such as "bursitis." Too often, the treatment suggested is empirical: prescription of anti-inflammatory drugs, reinforced on occasion by the injection of local steroids in, around, or relatively near the glenohumeral joint. Frequently, it is solely the failure of the patient to respond to such Brownian movements of therapy that induces the physician to probe more deeply into other possible sources of the patient's complaint.

Pain in the neck and shoulder is a symptom and not a disease; the source of the symptom may occasionally be obscurely remote from the site of discomfort. The pain may arise from one of the shoulder girdle neuritides, or it may be caused by an apical tumor of the lung. It is a common manifestation of cervical disc degeneration which, in turn, may be mimicked by one of the thoracic outlet syndromes. Although rotator cuff degeneration may be the most common cause of shoulder pain, this pathological lesion itself has many facets, each demanding a specific mode of therapy.

It is necessary, therefore, to have a very clear-cut concept of possible sources of pain when presented with the problem of a patient seeking relief from the irksome burden of a constantly painful neck or shoulder. In order to differentiate these lesions, the clinician must diligently elicit an accurate and lucid history of the onset and progress of the patient's complaints, and, guided by this history, conduct a routine examination seeking specific abnormalities. Treatment depends on identification of the pathological process; in order to suggest a logical line of treatment, it is necessary to preface each chapter of this book with the present-day concepts of the pathogenesis of symptoms. Only by attempting to localize accurately the site and nature of the pathology in every instance can treatment be conducted along rational lines.

The two most common causes of pain in the shoulder are degenerative changes in the soft tissues around the glenohumeral joint and cervical disc degeneration. The main body of the text is therefore devoted to a description of the symptom complexes that arise from these sources. At the end of this book is a short chapter describing diverse and sometimes misleadingly obscure causes of pain in the arm.

Although this book is not designed as a text of surgical techniques, the principles of common operative procedures are briefly described to serve as a guide for physicians informing their patients of the purpose of the proposed surgery, as basic information for physical therapists for their important role in postoperative rehabilitation, and as a launching pad for young physicians who will in the future improve the reconstructive procedures presently available.

No book is ever the work of just one author. As the senior author, I would like to acknowledge my indebtedness to the late V.H. Ellis, with whom I had the pleasure of working at the Royal National Orthopaedic Hospital in Great Portland Street, London. Mr. Ellis kindled my interest in the rotator cuff, the lesions to which it is susceptible, and their management.

When I came to Canada, I realized that shoulder lesions were the bane of the Worker's Compensation Board. This treatise could not have been completed without the generosity of the Worker's Compensation Board of Ontario, which undertook the funding of my clinical research fellows over a five-year period. The clinical fellows who carried out all the basic anatomical studies and the basic studies on the pathological changes that occur are: Dennis Weiner, Jim Rathbun, Bernard Nolan, Ted English, and Peter Welsh.

During this study, I was entirely dependent on the generosity of the late Dr. Bill Anderson, who made it possible for me to obtain specimens from the autopsy room at the Queen Elizabeth Hospital in Toronto, and who also acted as my advisor in regard to the significance of the histological findings.

Now I pass the torch to my junior colleague (J.M.). Along with his research staff (Nancy Vickroy and Russ Mounts), he has added new concepts to my original text in the hope of improving the product. The youth movement is alive and well in medicine! He would like to thank his colleagues for so much help: Dr. Peter Welsh, who helped with the shoulder section; Dr. Mark Leeson, who contributed to the tumor sections; and Dr. Dennis Weiner, who wrote the chapter on torticollis. Many other colleagues contributed time and effort to cover a busy practice while words were being put to paper. Those who made extra effort to round up illustrations included Dr. Mark Peterson and Dr. Jerry Lange (chief residents, orthopaedics, Akron City Hospital); Dr. Ed Bury, Dr. Bill Taylor, and Dr. Andy Kurman (neuroradiologists in Akron), Dr. Dave Bacha, Dr. Ray Federman, Dr. Andy Raynor, and Dr. Bill Wojno (rheumatologists in Akron); Dr. Godfrey Gaisie (chief of radiology at Childrens Medical Center of Akron); and orthopaedic colleagues Tim Meyer, Dan Bethem, Scott Weiner, John Biondi, Barry Greenberg, and Rick Brower. A special thank you to Leanne L. Seeger, ed., *Diagnostic Imaging of the Shoulder* (Williams & Wilkins 1992), for permission to use illustrations from her text. In the end, the person who had to see all the illustrations hit my desk running was Madeline Vincent, our wonderful x-ray technologist at Summit Orthopaedic Group.

No text can be written without reading texts that have gone before, perhaps the greatest of them being Grant's *Method of Anatomy* (Williams & Wilkins, 1989). Shoulder texts, such as Rockwood and Matsen's *The Shoulder* (W.B. Saunders, 1990); Post's *The Shoulder* (Lea & Febiger, 1988); Watson's *Surgical Disorders of the Shoulder* (Churchill Livingstone, 1991); and Campbell's *Operative Orthopaedics* (Mosby, 1992) were invaluable sources of information. Most importantly, J.M. would like to thank Dr. Paul Young, a St. Louis neurosurgeon who has taught him so much about the neck during the twice-yearly St. Louis microsurgical workshops, and who allowed him to borrow material from his text, *Microsurgery of the Cervical Spine* (Raven Press, 1991).

We would like to express our thanks to Jennifer Locking, Grace Wigley, Nancy Vickroy, Rose Fowler; to Isabel Coles for typing and retyping the text; to Maggie Littlefield for the art; to Katy Lipnicki and Tina Schoch for the photography. As always, the media center and Akron City Hospital performed under pressure and delivered the goods. Timothy Grayson and Vicki Vaughn at Williams & Wilkins used their remarkable skills in collecting a series of disjointed typewritten pages, diagrams, legends, and photographs—converting this collage into a simple and readable text.

Ian Macnab
John McCulloch
Summer, 1992

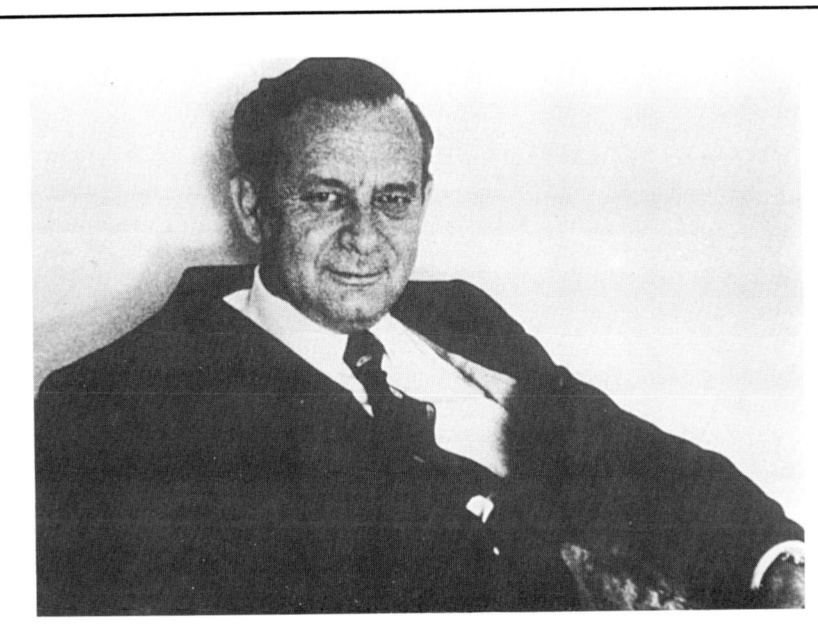

In Memory

DR. IAN MACNAB

1921–1992

It is with sadness and gratitude that I write this additional preface. Ian passed away November 25, 1992—the day I completed revisions for the appendix on exercises. It is hard to believe he is no longer with us. It is sad he will not see his last academic effort published. Although he had been retired for a number of years, he still was ahead of his time, a fact that became obvious when I asked Peter Welsh to review the shoulder section of the book (not one of my strengths), and he came back with very few changes.

It is with immense joy and gratification that I recall my years with Ian as student, resident, fellow, and colleague. At all times he was intensely loyal to me and to every young orthopaedic surgeon who came in contact with him. Any time you wanted to head in a new academic direction, he offered total support and jumped into the fray to question and prod. His enthusiasm for the growth and development of his young colleagues was legend and will continue to be a source of strength and guidance for all of us as we advance through our careers.

He leaves behind so many senior clinicians indebted to his genius: Dr. Ed Simmons, Sr., Dr. Carroll Laurin, and Dr. Bob Jackson. Most importantly, he leaves behind an inspired group of Macnab Club members: Dr. A. Beaupre (Quebec City, Canada), Dr. P. Benton (Atlanta, GA, USA), Dr. F. Boumphrey (Cleveland, OH, USA), Dr. Michael Bushik (Toronto, Canada), Dr. K.C. Chan (Joplin, MO, USA), Dr. Michael Chapman (Toronto, Canada), Dr. Gordon Crawford, (Barrie, Canada), Dr. Desmond Dall (Los Angeles, CA, USA), Dr. J. Robin De-Andrade, (Atlanta, GA, USA), Dr. William G. DeHaas (Victoria, Canada), Dr. John Dooley (Surrey, England), Dr. Dennis Drummond (Philadelphia, PA, USA), Dr. Edward English (Toronto, Canada), Dr. Stanley Grabias (West Reading, PA, USA), Dr. Robert Hercia (Oakville, Canada), Dr. Henry Hood (Lancaster, OH, USA), Dr. Kenneth Hughes (Richmond, Canada), Dr. Joseph B. Kornacki (Westmount, Canada), Dr. Stanley Leete (Campbell River, Canada), Dr. Lorenzo Marcolin (Washington, DC, USA), Dr. Robert McBroom (Toronto, Canada), Dr. John McCulloch (Akron, OH, USA), Dr. Graeme McIvor (Saskatoon, Canada), Dr. Paul Moreau (Riyadh, Saudi Arabia), Dr. Bernie Nolan (Lancaster, OH, USA), Dr. Chris Offierski (Niagara Falls, Canada), Dr. Talley Parrott (Columbia, SC, USA), Dr. H.F. Pompe VanMeerdervoor (Dayton, OH, USA), Dr. Calame Sammons (Huntsville, AL, USA), Dr. John P. Theo (Lubbock, TX, USA), Dr. Ensor Transfeld (Minneapolis, MN, USA), Dr. Douglas Wardlaw (Aberdeen, Scotland), Dr. Dennis Weiner (Akron, OH, USA), Dr. Peter Welsh (Toronto, Canada), Dr. David Wong (Denver, CO, USA), Dr. Charles Zaltz (El Paso, TX, USA).

John McCulloch

CONTENTS

One / Neckache

Two / Shoulder Pain

Three / The Bridge

Neck Ache

1

Anatomy and Biomechanics of the Cervical Spine

"Surgeons and anatomists see no beautiful women in their lives, but only a ghastly stack of bones with Latin names to them, and a network of nerves and muscles and tissues, inflamed by disease."

—Mark Twain

ANATOMICAL CONSIDERATIONS
Skeletal Anatomy

The seven cervical vertebrae have distinctive anatomical features (Fig. 1.1). The first and second vertebrae are morphologically unique and will be discussed separately. The spinous processes of the second to the sixth cervical vertebrae are bifid. The spinous process of the seventh cervical vertebra is much longer than those above, making it easy to palpate the vertebra prominens on clinical examination. The cervical vertebral bodies are about one-half the size, in all dimensions, of the lumbar vertebral bodies, and the disc space is less than one-half the height of a lumbar disc.

Almost everyone who writes about the neck will separate the region into the upper cervical (C1-C2) and the rest of the cervical spine (C3-C7). We are no exception.

C1-C2

The C1 (atlas) and C2 (axis) junction is like no other vertebral articulation in the body (Fig. 1.2). During development, the C1 vertebral level gave its body to C2, leaving C1 a ring and C2 a body (odontoid or dens) on a body.

The ring of the atlas is interrupted by the lateral masses that articulate with two occipital condyles of the skull. The ring is thus divided into a shallow anterior arch and a deeper posterior arch (Figs. 1.2 and 1.3). Lateral to the lateral masses sits the vertebral artery; posterior to the lateral masses passes the suboccipital nerve.

Within the ring of the atlas the odontoid occupies one-third of the space, one-third is filled by the spinal cord, and one-third is open space (Fig. 1.3). The ring of C1 rotates around the odontoid peg, the peg being married to the C1 anterior arch by a complex set of ligaments (Fig. 1.4).

The axis is a lot like the rest of the cervical vertebrae except: (*a*) the odontoid or dens sits on top, and (*b*) the superior facet is anterior so that it articulates with C1 (Fig. 1.2).

Biomechanics of C1-C2. A little less than 50% of cervical rotation occurs at the C1-C2 junction. The C1-C2 level allows very little flexion and approximately 25% of extension (8). All of these movements are rigidly controlled by a highly

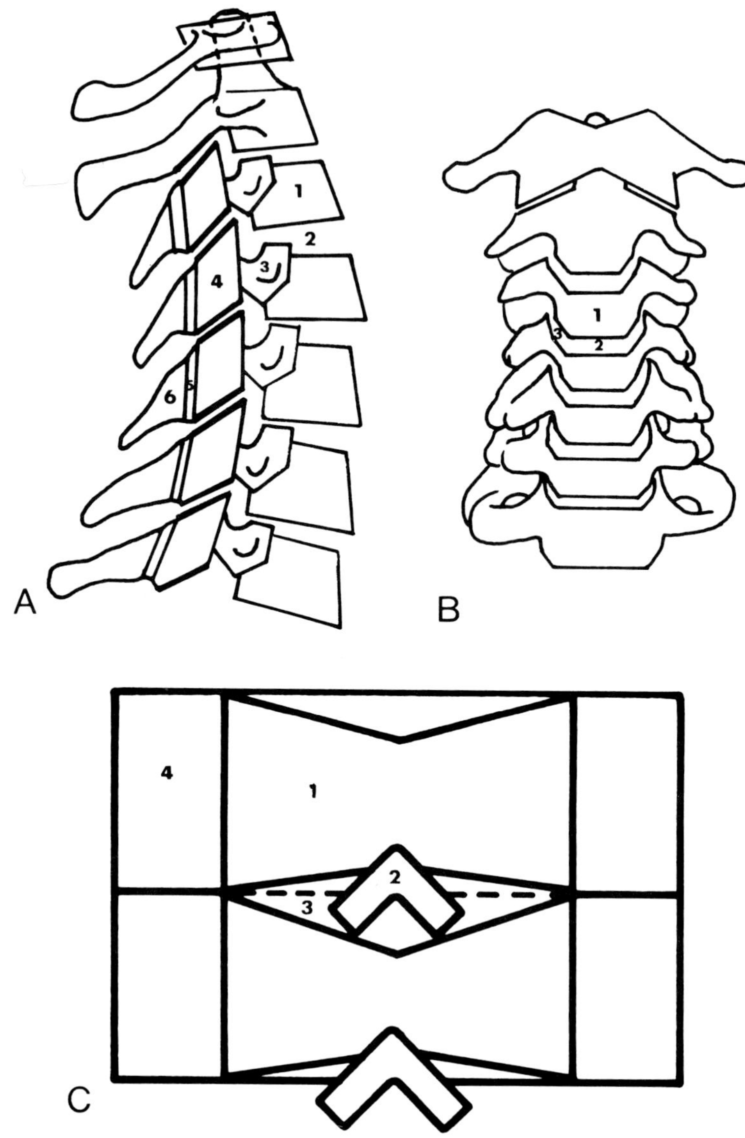

Figure 1.1. **A,** lateral schematic of the seven cervical vertebrae. Vertebral body (*1*), disc (*2*), nerve root canal (*3*), lateral mass (*4*), lamina (*5*), and spinous process (*6*). **B,** anterior schematic of the seven cervical vertebrae. Vertebral body (*1*), disc (*2*), neurocentral joints (*3*). **C,** posterior schematic of two cervical vertebrae. Lamina (*1*), bifid spinous process (*2*), interlaminar space (*3*), lateral mass (*4*). The *broken line* through the interlaminar space represents the superior border of the vertebral body.

innervated group of suboccipital muscles, the names of which we quickly learned, and just as quickly forgot, in medical school.

Instability of C1-C2.   The normal relationship between C1 and C2 allows for less than 3 mm separation between the dens and the anterior arch of the atlas. Above 3 mm, the C1-C2 junction is considered unstable in flexion and extension (Fig. 1.5) (15).

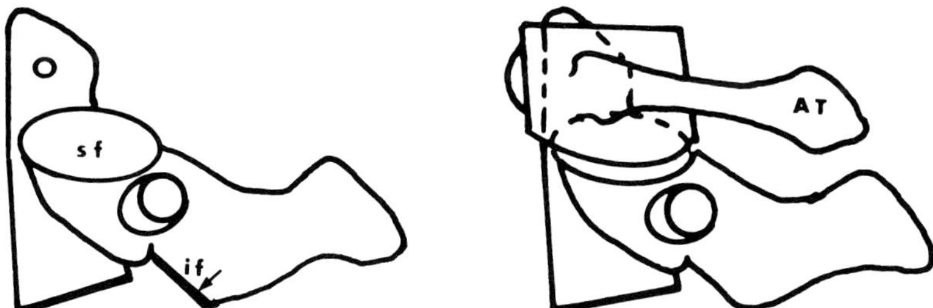

Figure 1.2.   Atlantoaxial junction. *Left.* C2 showing the odontoid (*o*), superior facet (*sf*), and inferior facet (*if*). *Right.* Atlas (*AT*) superimposed on axis (*C2*).

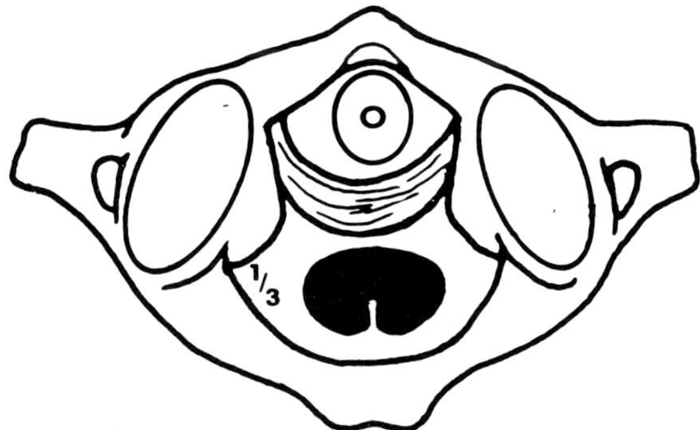

Figure 1.3.   Axial schematic of C1 showing odontoid (*o*) and cord, with one-third more space available. Note the transverse ligament behind the odontoid.

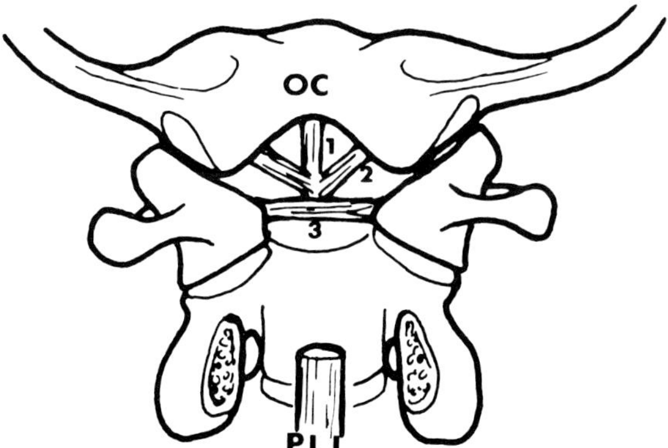

Figure 1.4.   Posterior view of some of the complex sets of ligaments that stabilize the odontoid in the ring of C1. The lamina of C1 (posterior ring) and of C2 have been removed, as well as the odontoid (*PLL* = posterior longitudinal ligament, *OC* = occiput). Apical ligament (*1*), alar ligament (*2*), and transverse ligament (*3*).

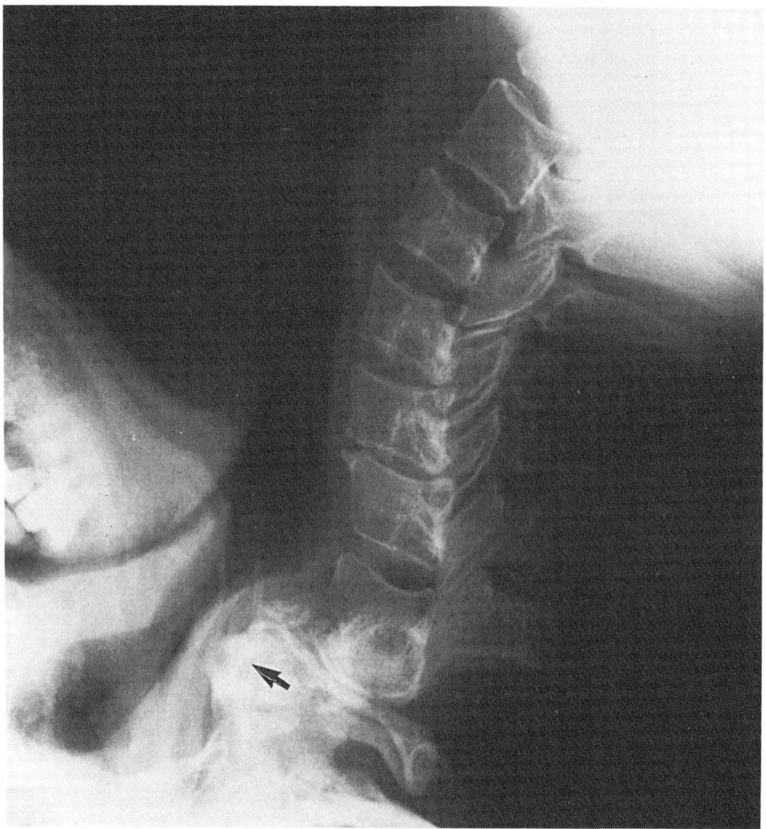

Figure 1.5.   A lateral x-ray showing the odontoid and C1 moving forward more than 3 mm on the axis.

Through erosion of ligamentous support by inflammatory conditions, such as rheumatoid arthritis, the peg of the odontoid may shift upward or cephalad (Fig. 1.6), which is another form of C1-C2 instability.

The last form of subluxation or instability of the C1-C2 junction can occur with congenital abnormalities such as os odontoideum (Fig. 1.7).

C3-C7

Anatomy dictates that we should look at this portion of the cervical spine as two columns—the anterior disc/vertebral column and the posterior elements (Fig. 1.8).

The disc/vertebral column C3-C7 contains five vertebral blocks and four intervertebral discs. The cervical vertebral bodies are ovoid, with their longest diameter transversely in the coronal plane. The superior and inferior surfaces are saddle-shaped due to the laterally placed uncovertebral joints, also known as the joints of Luschka (14) or neurocentral joints (Fig. 1.9). These joints, which form towards the end of the first decade, are notable for two reasons:

1. During midlife they are in a position that prevents a disc rupture from directly pressing on the nerve root (Fig. 1.9).

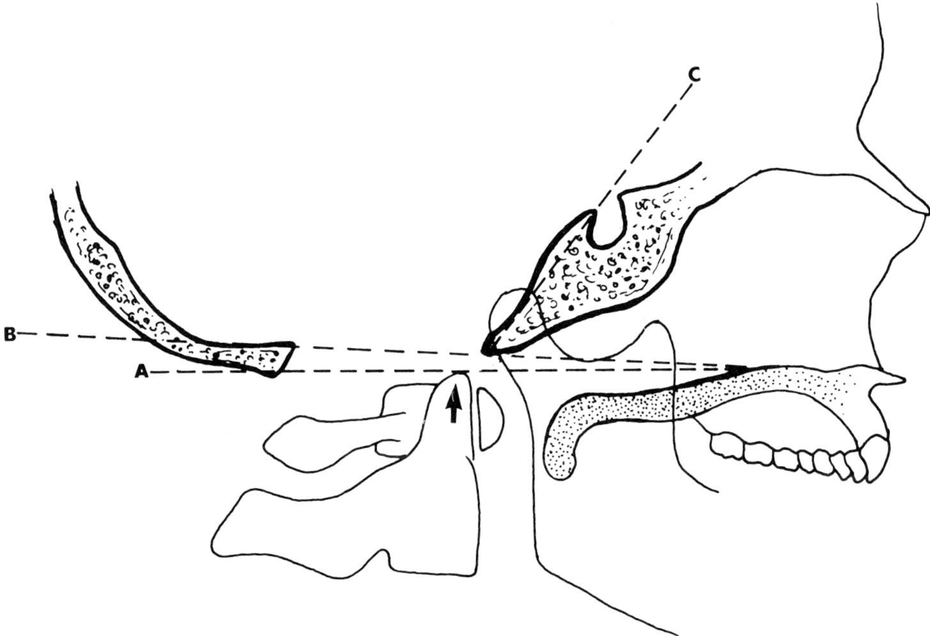

Figure 1.6.   A second form of C1-C2 instability is upward migration of the odontoid process (*peg*) into the foramen magnum (*arrow*). If the tip of the odontoid is more than a few millimeters above Chamberlain's line (**B**) or McGregor's line (**A**), basilar invagination of the odontoid is present. This is most likely to occur in rheumatoid arthritis. McRae's line (**C**) is used to measure platybasia, flattening of the base of the skull. (It's a useless measurement for an unimportant condition!)

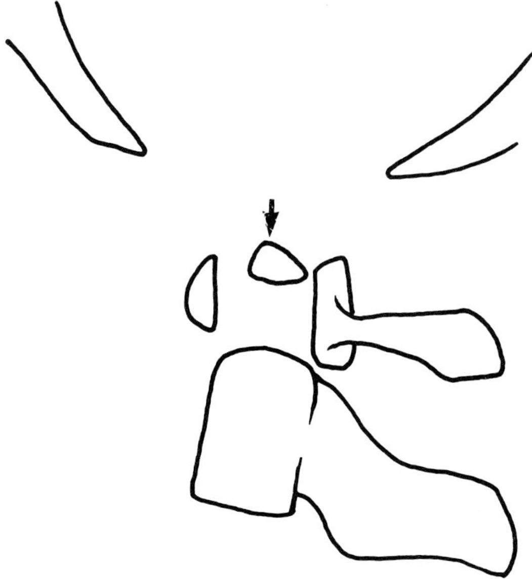

Figure 1.7.   Lateral schematic showing os odontoideum (*arrow*). This incomplete formation of the odontoid peg is often associated with instability.

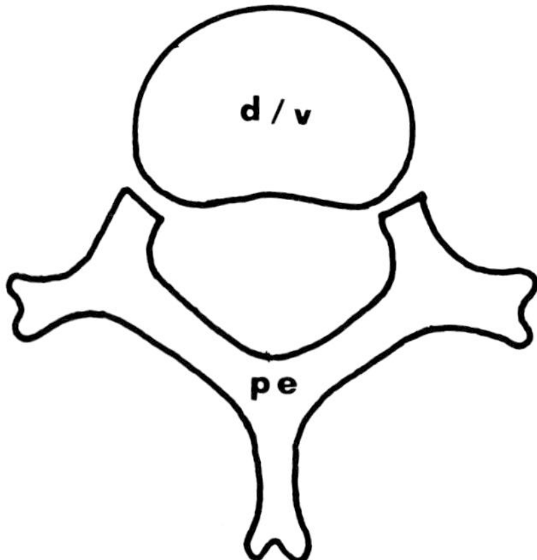

Figure 1.8.   Axial schematic showing the disc/vertebral column (*d/v*) and the posterior elements (*pe*).

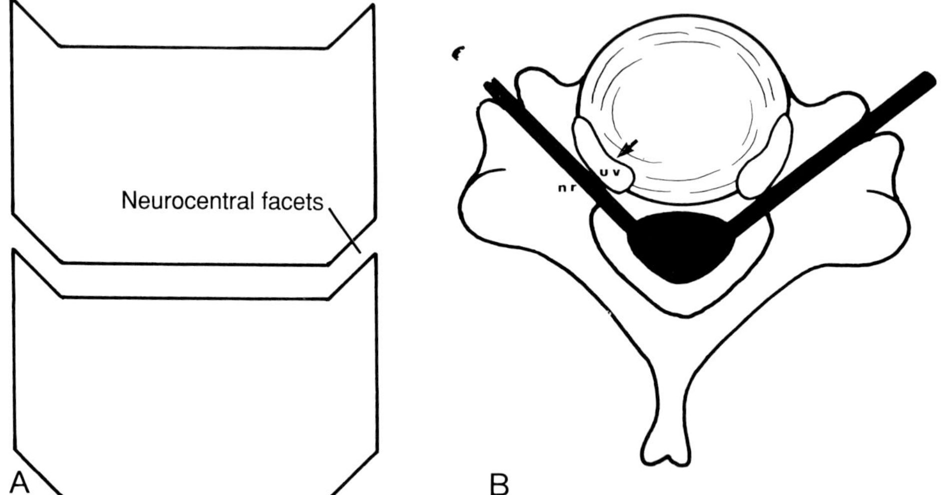

Figure 1.9.   **A,** an anterior schematic view of neurocentral joints. **B,** axial schematic showing how the neurocentral joints—uncovertebral joints (*uv*)—are in a position to protect the nerve root (*nr*) from a disc herniation (*arrow*).

2. Because they are synovial-like joints they are capable of osteophytic formation that interferes with root function later in life (Fig. 1.10).

The intervertebral discs in the neck serve the same function as in the lumbar spine:

- They hold the vertebral bodies together.
- They allow for movement.
- They absorb shock.

The shock absorber is the nucleus pulposus, a gel-like substance that obtains its physical characteristics from the combination of proteoglycans and water. The nucleus is contained by the cartilaginous end plates superiorly and inferiorly, and

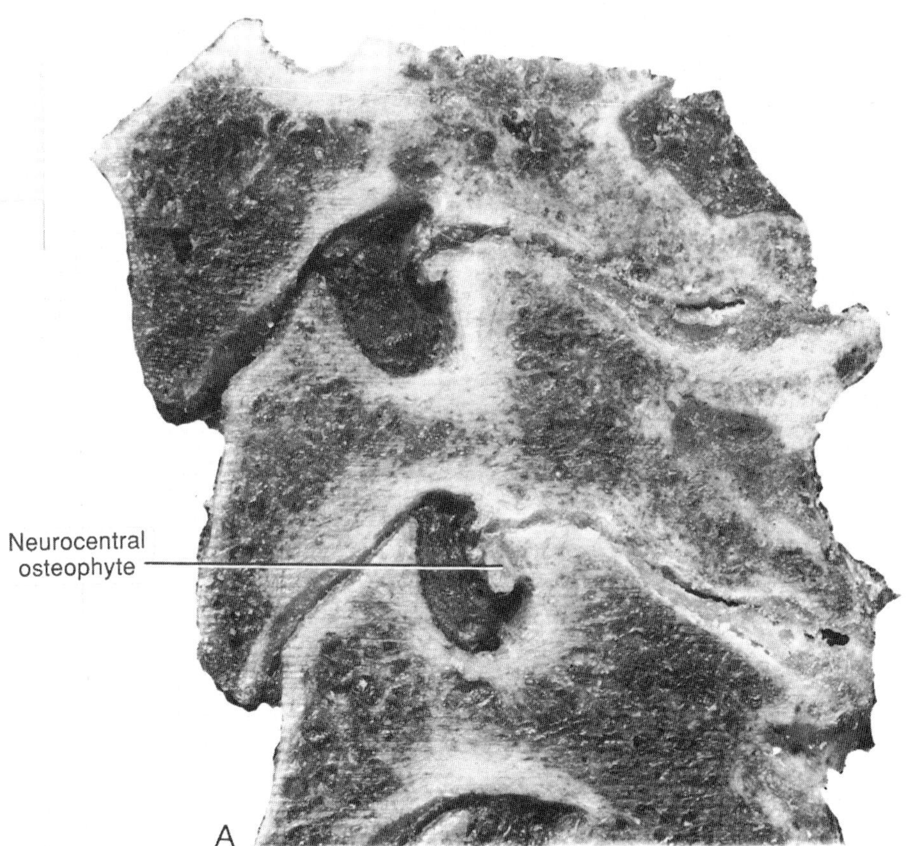

Figure 1.10.   **A,** sagittal autopsy specimen, showing a neurocentral osteophyte protruding into the nerve root foramen.

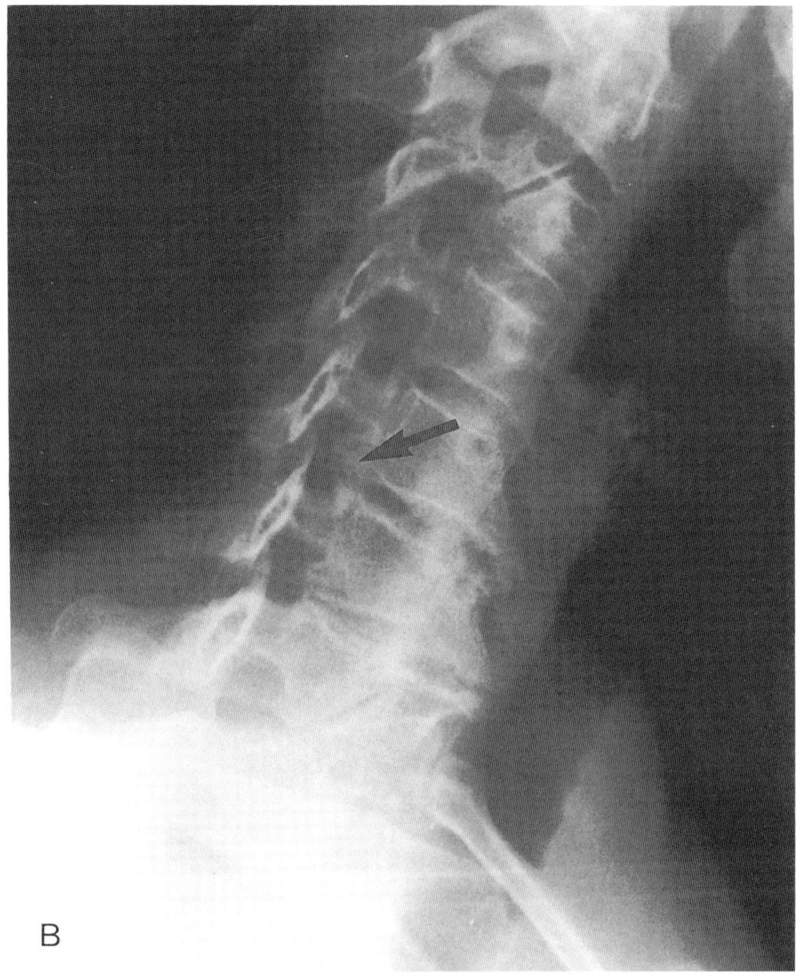

Figure 1.10.   **B,** an oblique x-ray showing the osteophyte (*arrow*).

is surrounded by the annulus fibrosus. After absorbing the force, the nucleus transfers the force to the annulus fibrosus. The annular collagen and its arrangement, along with its Sharpey fiber insertion into the osseous epiphyseal ring and vertebral bodies, makes it well suited to absorb this force transfer (Fig. 1.11).

The shape of the intervertebral disc, wide anteriorly and narrow posteriorly gives the cervical spine its lordosis (Fig. 1.1*A*). Although the disc is avascular, it is biologically active, absorbing its nutrients through diffusion.

The posterior elements include the paired pedicles, the paired transverse processes, the paired lamina, and the single spinous process (Fig. 1.12). Bony outriggers for the attachment of muscles appear everywhere!

As in the lumbar spine, the cervical pedicles attach to the upper half of the vertebral body. Unlike the lumbar spine, the pedicles of the cervical spine project posterolaterally. This has great bearing on the dimension of the cervical spinal canal (Fig. 1.13).

Each vertebral segment has paired superior and inferior facet joint surfaces bridged by a large mass of bone known as the lateral mass or articular pillar (Fig. 1.14). The lateral mass is truly a mass, having the same height as a vertebral body. Attaching to each lateral mass is the lamina, which meets in the midline at a bifid spinous process (C7 is not usually bifid).

Although ligamentum flavum is present in the cervical spine and attaches to the lamina just as in the lumbar spine (Fig. 1.15), there is very little interlaminar space in the neck. From behind, the cervical spinal cord is almost completely covered by bone (Fig. 1.1*C*).

The transverse processes are formed by a rudimentary costal process anteriorly and by a true transverse process posteriorly. These are joined by a bridge of bone—the costotransverse bar—to form the vertebral artery foramen (Fig. 1.12). The third, fourth, fifth, and sixth vertebrae present prominent tubercles at the termination of their costal processes. These are points of muscular attachment. The anterior tubercle of the sixth cervical vertebra has the eponym, Chassaignac's tubercle, but is better known as the carotid tubercle. It is readily palpated deep to the inferomedial border of the sternomastoid muscle and provides a useful surface landmark (Fig. 1.16).

The presence of the anterior and posterior tubercles gives a grooved configuration to the transverse processes. The cervical nerve roots, after emerging from the intervertebral foramina, run anterolaterally in this bony canal and emerge behind the vertebral artery (Fig. 1.17).

The anterior element of the seventh cervical vertebra is usually very small, thereby affording room for the vertebral artery to reach the vertebral artery foramen in the sixth transverse process. However, it must be remembered that an anomalous cervical rib of varying size may be present at this level and may, at times, be the source of compression of the neurovascular bundle.

Joints of Luschka.   The morphology of the articulation between the cervical vertebrae is of great significance. The lumbar vertebral segments are connected by three joints: the intervertebral disc anteriorly and two zygapophyseal joints posteriorly. The lower five cervical vertebrae are connected by five joints: the intervertebral disc anteriorly, the two zygapophyseal joints posteriorly, and in addition to these, the neurocentral joints (Figs. 1.9 and 1.18).

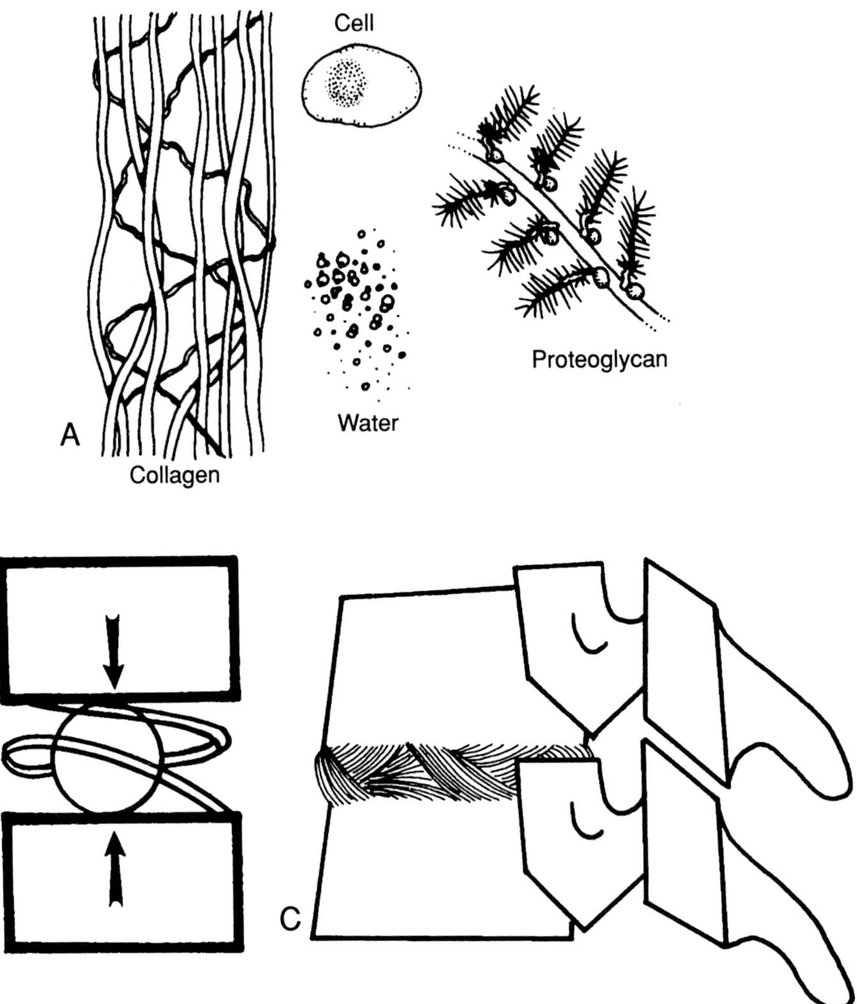

Figure 1.11. **A**, biochemistry of the disc. Cellular elements build noncellular components of proteoglycan (which binds water). This forms the liquid cement of the annulus and nucleus in which is embedded the reinforcing bars of collagen. There is very little collagen in a nucleus and very little proteoglycan in the annulus. **B**, the annular/nuclear complex is in a fluid state such that forces (*arrows*) are absorbed by the nucleus (*circle*) and transferred to the annulus. **C**, the annulus, in turn, can absorb tremendous force because of its crisscross or chinese-fingers structure. The absorbed force is transferred to the vertebral bodies, muscles, and ligaments.

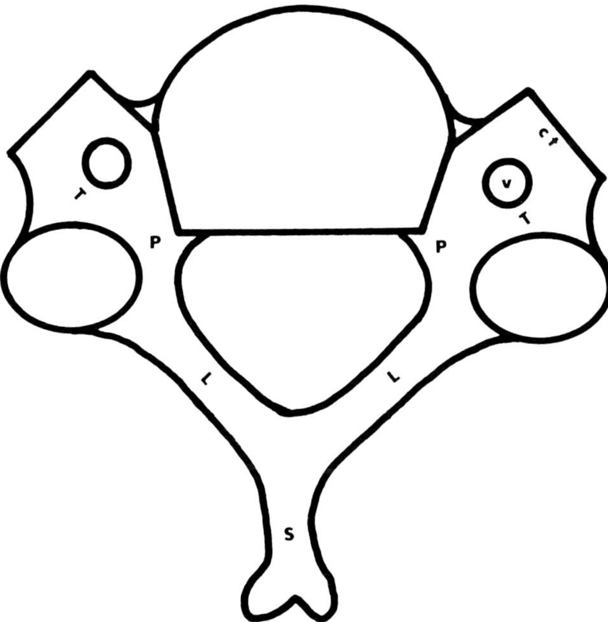

Figure 1.12.   Axial schematic showing the paired pedicles (*P*), paired transverse processes (*T*), paired lamina (*L*), and single spinous process (*S*). The costotransverse bar (*ct*) completes the bony foramen for the vertebral artery (*v*).

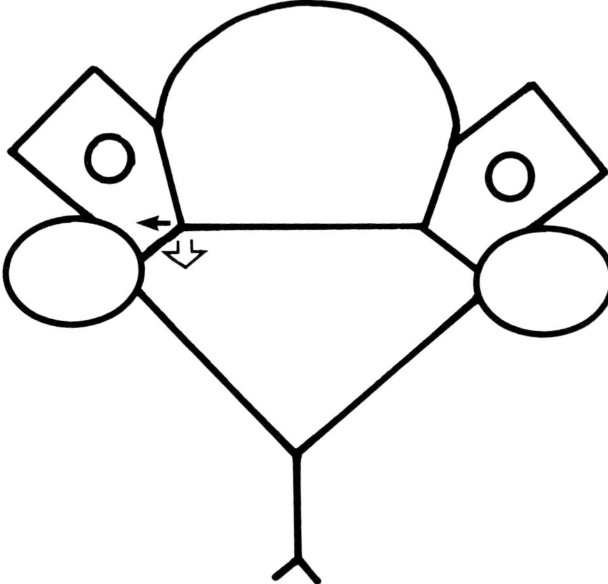

Figure 1.13.   Axial schematic to show the pedicle orientation to the vertebral body. If the pedicle were directed more posteriorly (*open arrow*) the spinal canal would be larger. Direct the pedicle more laterally (*closed arrow*) and the canal would be smaller.

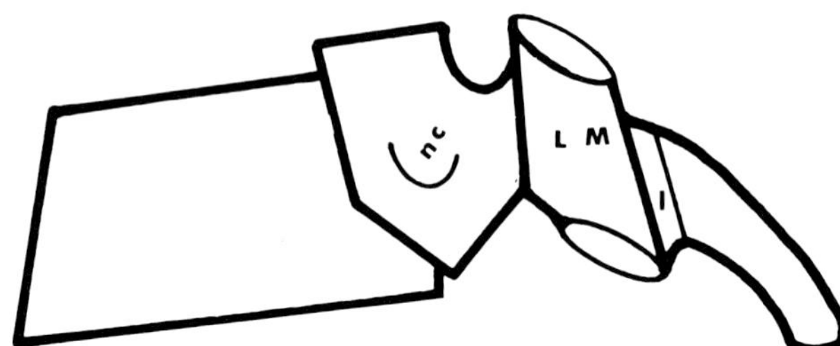

Figure 1.14.   A lateral schematic showing the lateral mass (*LM*). In front is the neural canal (*nc*), behind is the lamina (*l*).

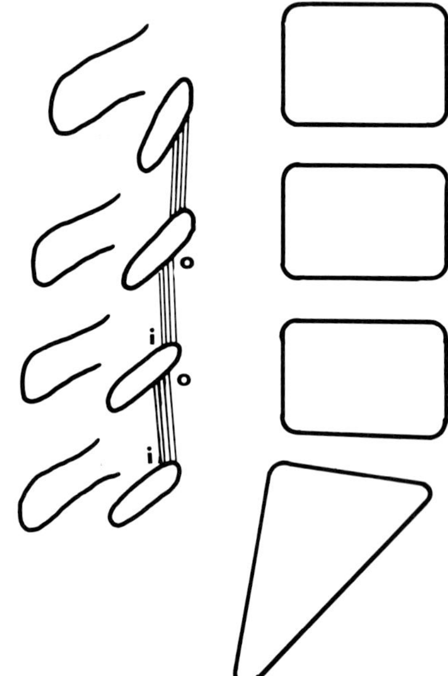

Figure 1.15.   The origin (*o*) on the anterior surface of the cephalad lamina and the insertion (*i*) on the posterior edge of the caudal vertebrae as in the lumbar spine. The arrangement is the same in the cervical spine.

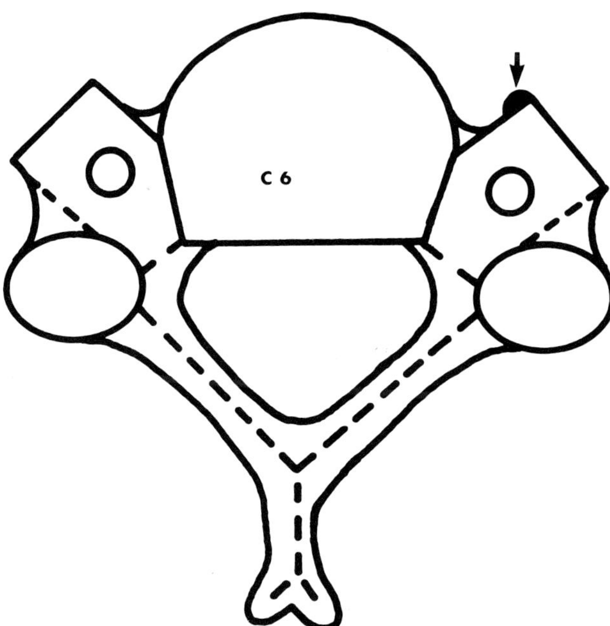

Figure 1.16.   Location of the carotid tubercle (Chassaignac's tubercle), which is a prominent bone palpable at the inferomedial border of the sternomastoid muscle. (The *broken lines* are there to show you how easy it is to do an axial line drawing.)

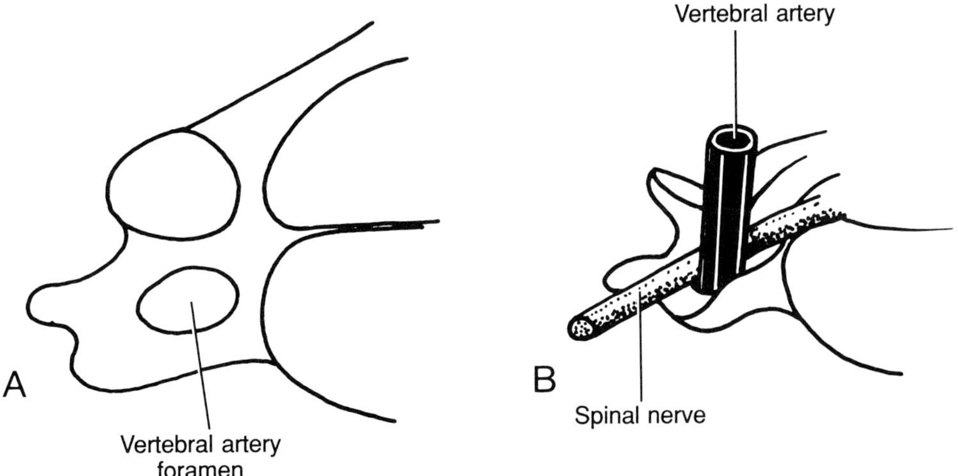

Figure 1.17.   The vertebral artery foramen with the nerve root posteriorly.

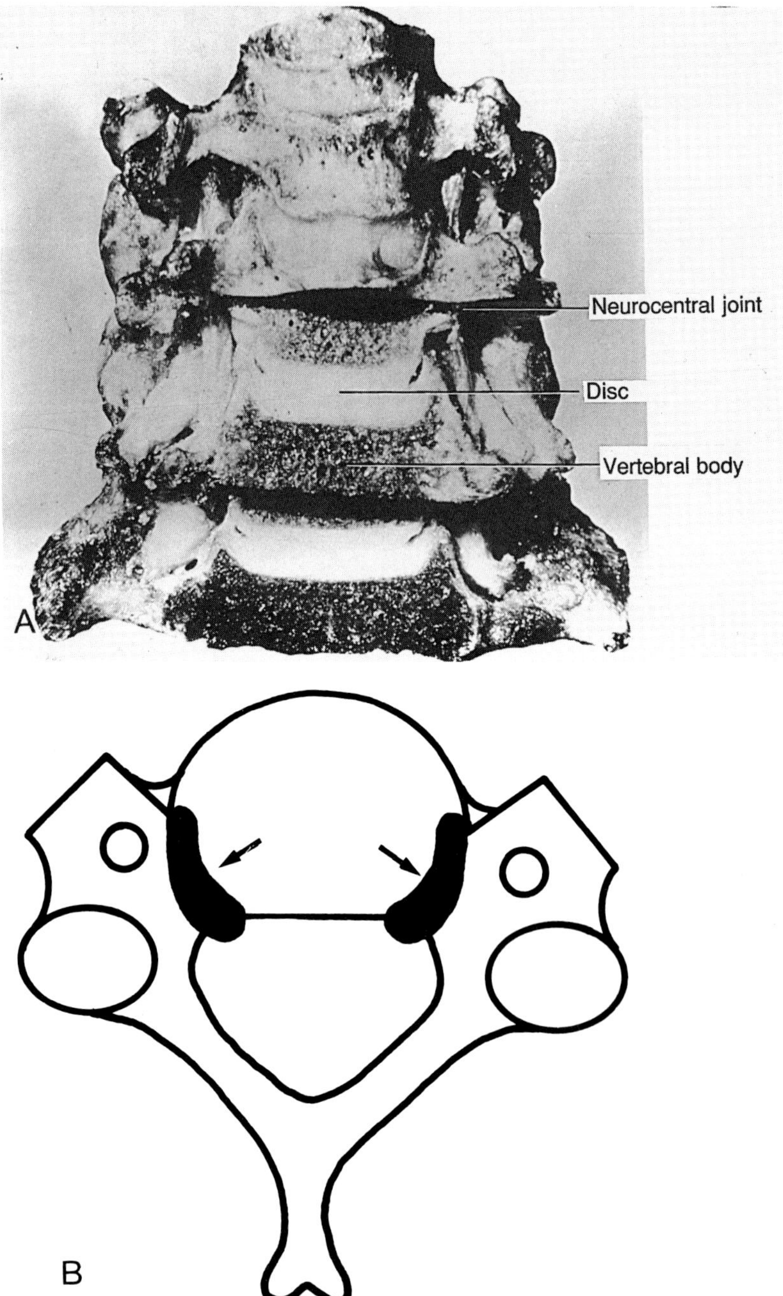

Figure 1.18. **A,** anterior section to show tip of neurocentral joint. **B,** the uncovertebral or neurocentral processes (*arrows*) on axial schematic.

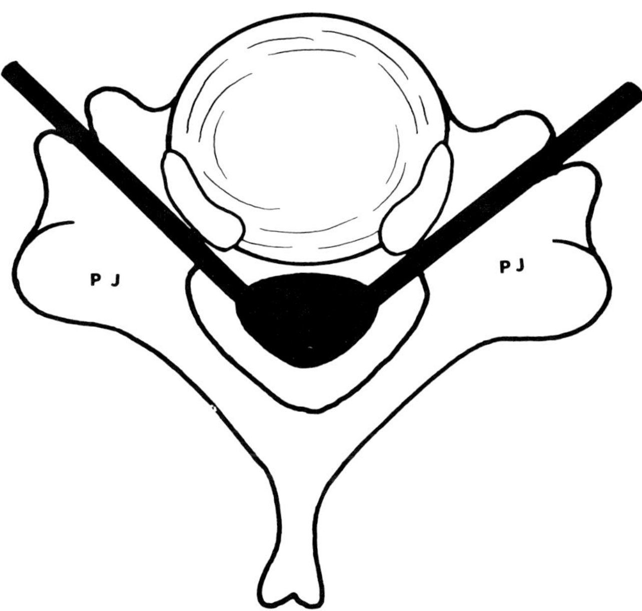

Figure 1.19.   The neurocentral joint lies in front of the nerve root and the posterior joint (*pj*) surface lies posteriorly.

The neurocentral joints consist of two projections of bone arising from the posterolateral portion of the vertebral body, articulating with the vertebra above (Fig. 1.18). They lie between the disc and the nerve root canal (Fig. 1.19). Vesalius illustrated these joints very accurately in his book, *De fabrica corporis humani,* and they were subsequently described in detail by Luschka (14), whose name they commonly bear. Although Luschka described them as synovial joints, on careful dissection no evidence of a synovial lining can be found, regardless of the age of the patient.

The morphology of these "joints" is interesting. They lie at the junction of the neural arch and the centrum of the vertebral body, hence the name, neurocentral joint. In the lower cervical segments, the nerve root escapes from the intervertebral foramen and passes anterior to the zygapophyseal joints and posterior to the neurocentral joints (Fig. 1.19). At the first and second cervical segments, it can be seen that the nerve root emerges posterior to the zygapophyseal joints. The fact that the nerve roots pass behind the apophyseal joints at the first and second vertebrae, and behind the neurocentral joints of the vertebrae below this level, suggests that the apophyseal joints of the first two cervical vertebrae represent enlarged neurocentral joints.

One other observation helps one to understand this strange anatomical phenomenon. The transverse process of a cervical vertebra represents a "true" transverse process derived from the neural arch, and the costal element represents a rudimentary rib. The neurocentral joint is formed at the base of the fused costal and transverse elements. In the thoracic region, the rib articulates with two adjacent vertebral bodies. In the cervical region, the costal element of the transverse processes is fused to the vertebra below, and it is possible that

Luschka's joint represents a rudimentary superior costovertebral articulation (Fig. 1.20).

Biomechanics of the Cervical Spine (C3-C7).   The spine, in general, and the cervical spine in particular, is a remarkable structure. It is capable of flexion, extension, lateral flexion, and rotation to help us see and hear; at the same time, it supports the head above the shoulders and provides a conduit for the spinal cord.

Most cervical flexion is in the subaxial region, approximately 10° per segment (8, 13). Total flexion is limited more by the fact that the chin bumps into the chest, than by the guy wires of the ligaments and muscles. During flexion, the disc narrows in front and widens behind; some even believe the nucleus shifts posteriorly, but we have our doubts. Some flexion occurs because the upper vertebral body subluxates forward on its lower mate, a normal condition that can unnecessarily alarm the unwary (Fig. 1.21). The greatest amount of flexion occurs at C4-C5 and C5-C6, which partly explains why degenerative disc disease is naturally greater at these two levels (13).

Extension is less than flexion because the spinous processes bump into each other (Fig. 1.22). It is interesting that they are bifid to allow for just a few more degrees of extension (Fig. 1.1*C*). There is about 60° of rotation to each side, passively limited by the structure of the vertebrae, discs, facets, and attaching ligaments. Lateral flexion is the least range of movement in the cervical spine, with a good proportion of that movement coming about only because of rotation.

The first disc in the body is at C2-C3. Unlike the thoracic and lumbar spines, the cervical disc is relatively thicker or higher, to form 25% of the relative height of the vertebrae (Fig. 1.1). The fact that it is much thicker or higher anteriorly gives the cervical spine its lordotic curve. In addition the discs serve as spacers to keep the neural foramina open.

Instability of the vertebral structure of the cervical spine has been studied by White and Panjabi (15) in their classic article and subsequent text. They destroyed ligaments and facets of the cervical spine below C2 and loaded the spine to determine degrees of instability. They defined stability as "the ability of the spine to limit its pattern of displacement under physiologic loads so as not to damage or irritate the spinal cord or nerve roots." They concluded that:

1. Horizontal displacement greater than 3.5 mm constitutes instability (Fig. 1.23).
2. Angular deformity greater than 11° on either resting lateral or flexion-extension films constitutes instability (Fig. 1.24).
3. On stretching a cervical spine with traction, more than 1 cm of separation between adjacent vertebral segments constitutes instability (Fig. 1.25).

The spinal cord is approximately 10 mm in size and the cervical bony canal has an average sagittal diameter of 17 mm. That leaves some room for contraction and expansion of the cervical portion of the cord during neck movements. The cord lies suspended in its cerebrospinal fluid (CSF) water bath, through intimate attachments of its surrounding pia, arachnoid, and dural membranes. Laterally, the cord is fixed to the dura by the dentate ligaments (Fig. 1.26), which hold the cord in a relative position to the vertebral elements.

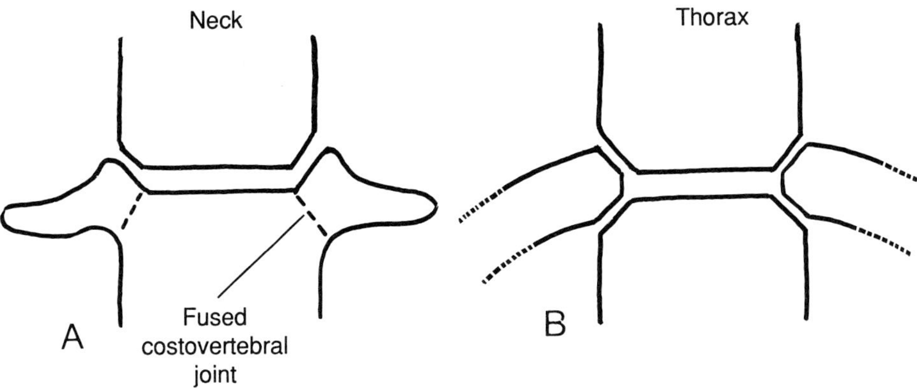

Figure 1.20.   The neurocentral joint may be a rudimentary superior costovertebral articulation.

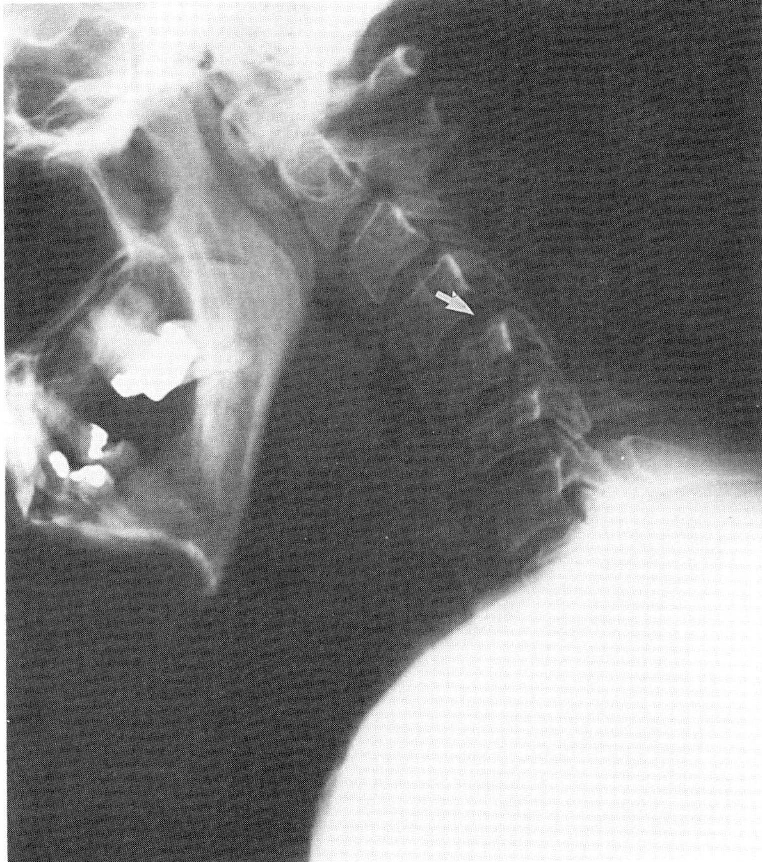

Figure 1.21.   There is normally some subluxation of vertebrae when the normal neck is flexed (*arrow*).

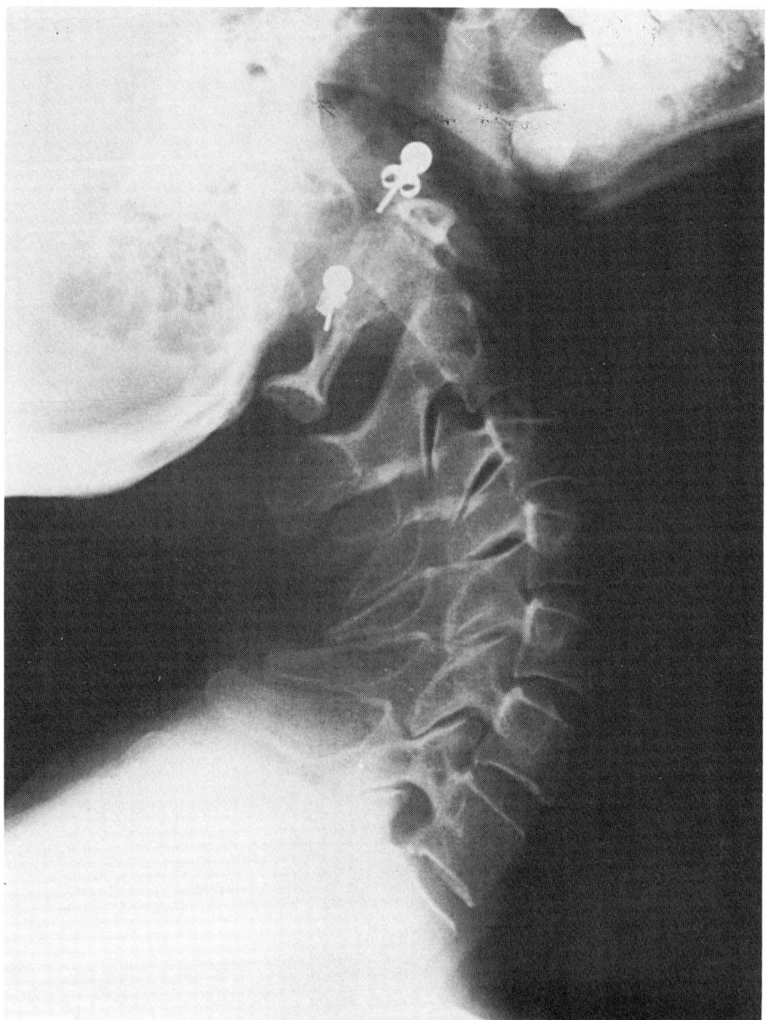

Figure 1.22.   Extension ends when the spinous processes bump into each other (*arrow*).

The cord lies posterior to the center of sagittal rotation of the cervical spine, and thus has to stretch during flexion and buckle during extension. This is allowed by the slack in the canal (17 mm canal vs. 10 mm cord). But narrow the canal congenitally and/or with degenerative changes (5, 7), and the buffer space disappears. Then, in flexion, the cord may be pulled over the pathology (Fig. 1.27) to cause a sudden, temporary electric-like shock to radiate down the body and into the arms and legs (Lhermitte's sign) (3).

Vascular Anatomy

The two major vascular trunks in the neck are the vertebral artery and its surrounding venous plexus, and the carotid sheath containing the carotid artery and internal jugular vein (and the vagus nerve). The vertebral artery is the first branch of the subclavian (Fig. 1.28). Although variations are common, the verte-

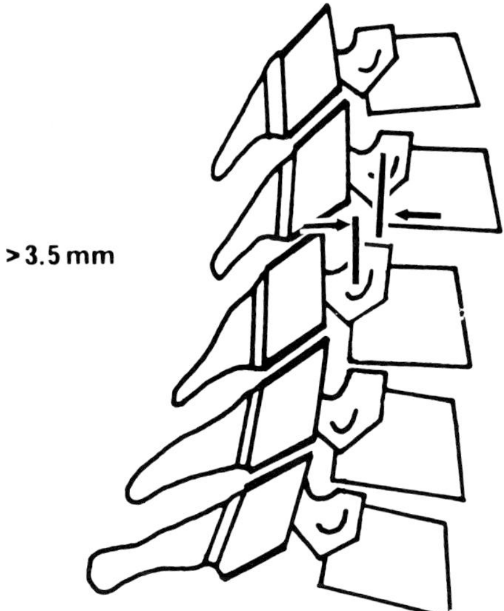

Figure 1.23.   Schematic lateral showing subluxation between C3 and C4 (*arrows*). If it exceeds 3.5 mm, the segment is considered unstable. The distance between the two lines in millimeters is the extent of subluxation.

bral artery usually enters the transverse process of the sixth cervical vertebra, ascending through the vertebral foramina until it leaves the foramen in the second cervical vertebra; at this point it angles posteriorly to course around the lateral surface of the superior articular facets before piercing the atlantooccipital membrane. Within the skull, it joins the opposite vertebral artery to form the basilar artery, supplying the contents of the posterior cranial fossa. The first large branch from the vertebral artery after it enters the foramen magnum is the posterior inferior cerebellar artery. It is thrombosis of this vessel that gives rise to the Wallenberg syndrome (9). In the neck, the vertebral artery supplies the vertebrae, the attached ligaments and muscles, the facet joints (zygapophyseal joints), as well as the spinal cord, its surrounding meninges, and the nerve roots.

The common carotid artery ascends deeply through the anterior triangle of the neck at the medial border of the sternomastoid (Fig. 1.29). At the superior border of the thyroid, it bifurcates into the internal and external carotid artery. The internal carotid will be branchless until it enters the skull to supply the brain. The external carotid supplies the external neck. Its collateral branches include the superior thyroid, lingual, facial, and three minor branches that will remain nameless. The only collateral branch of importance is the superior thyroid artery, which has to be mobilized, along with the superior laryngeal nerve, to get at the C3-C4 disc space through the anterior triangle.

Neuroanatomy

It is best to think of neuroanatomy as the content of the spinal canal (spinal cord), the projections of the spinal cord (roots), and the terminal branches of the roots.

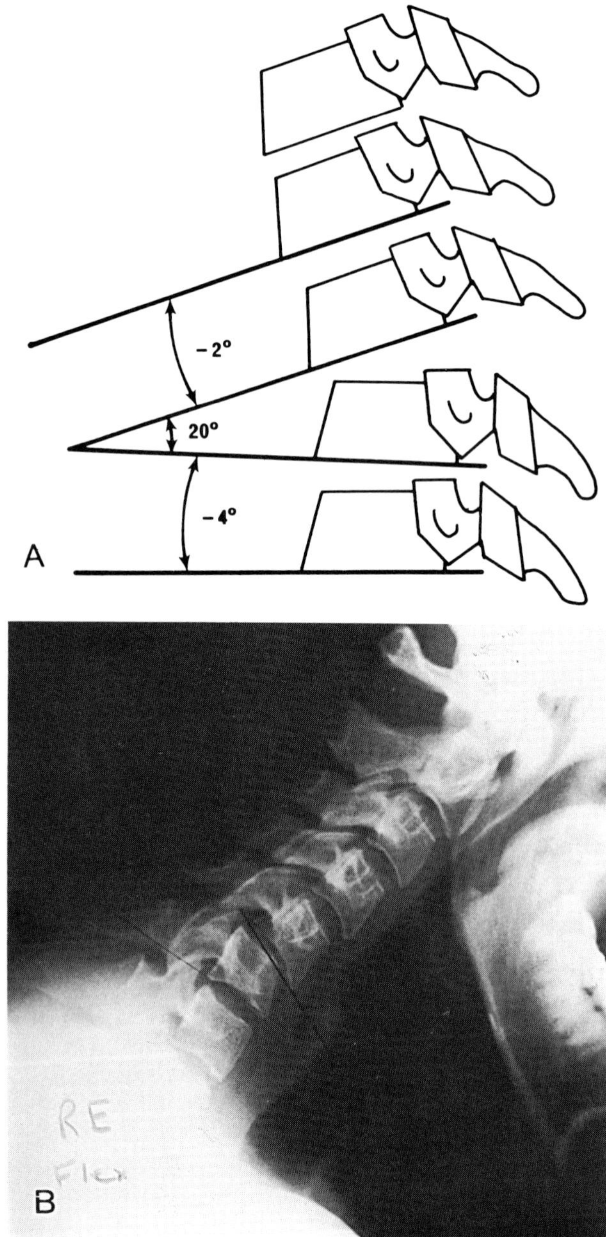

Figure 1.24. **A,** measurement of angulation is shown (15). If it exceeds similar angle measurements of segments above and below by more than 11°, the segment is considered unstable. In this example, the minimum difference is 16°. **B,** measure the angle. Is it unstable?

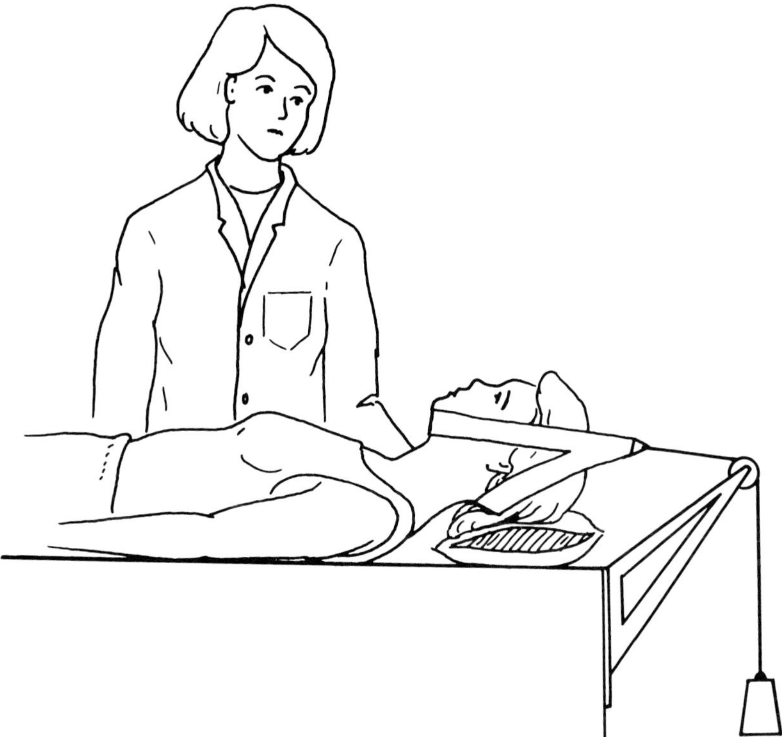

Figure 1.25.   The traction or stretch test must be done very carefully. Add increments of weights up to 30% of body weight (up to 65 lb). Each time weight is added a neurological exam is completed. If one vertebrae separates from another by any degree, or the patient develops neurological symptoms or signs, the test is positive for instability.

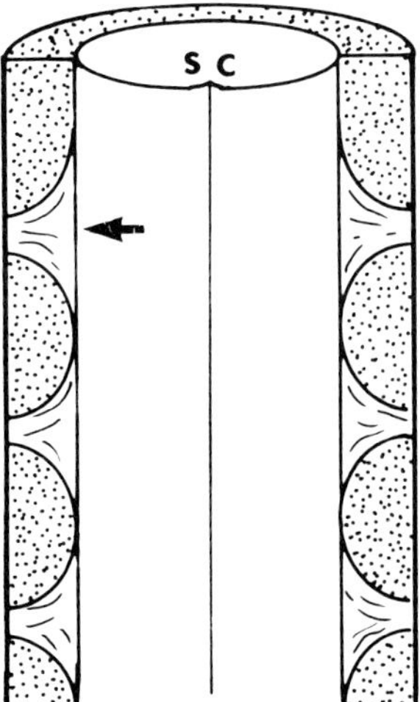

Figure 1.26.   The dentate ligaments anchor the spinal cord (*sc*) to the dura (*arrow*).

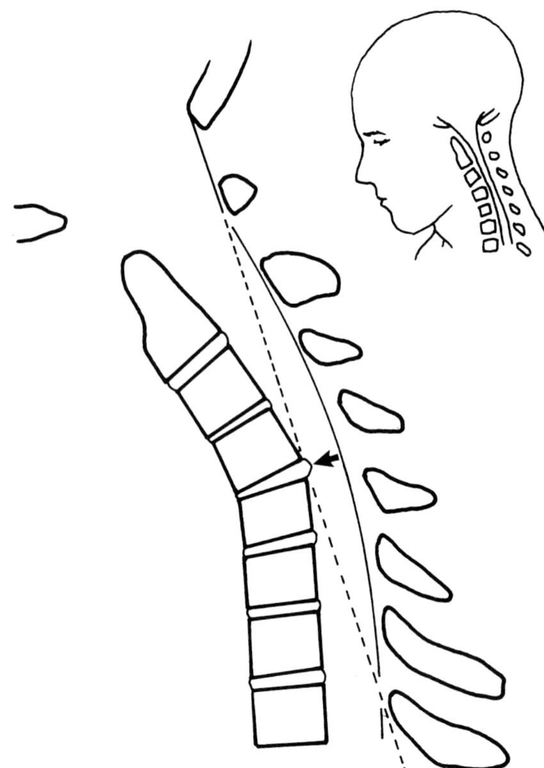

Figure 1.27. The *arrow* shows how on flexion the cord may be pulled over pathology (a bulging disc at C3-C4).

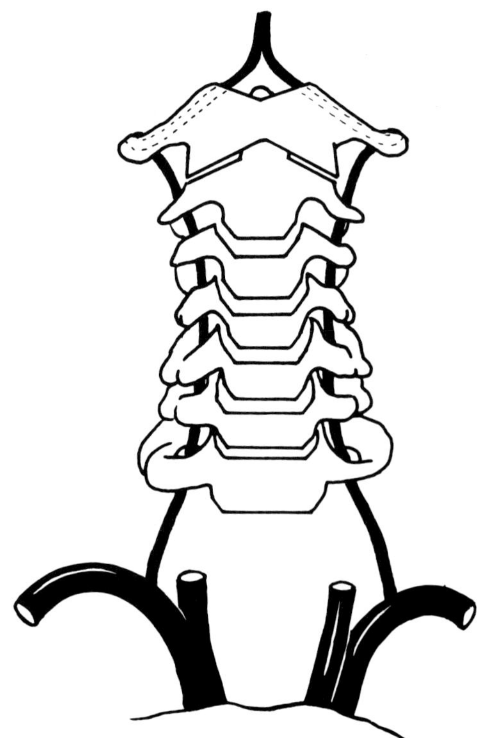

Figure 1.28. The vertebral artery is shown as a branch of the subclavian. Do you see anything wrong? (The vertebral artery enters its first foramen at C6, not C7 as shown here!)

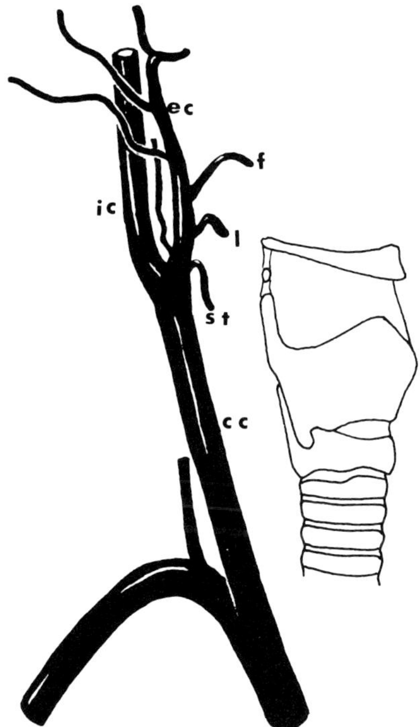

Figure 1.29.   The common carotid artery (*cc*) with the branchless internal carotid (*ic*) and the external carotid (*ec*). The important branches of the external carotid are the superior thyroid (*st*), lingual (*l*), and facial (*f*).

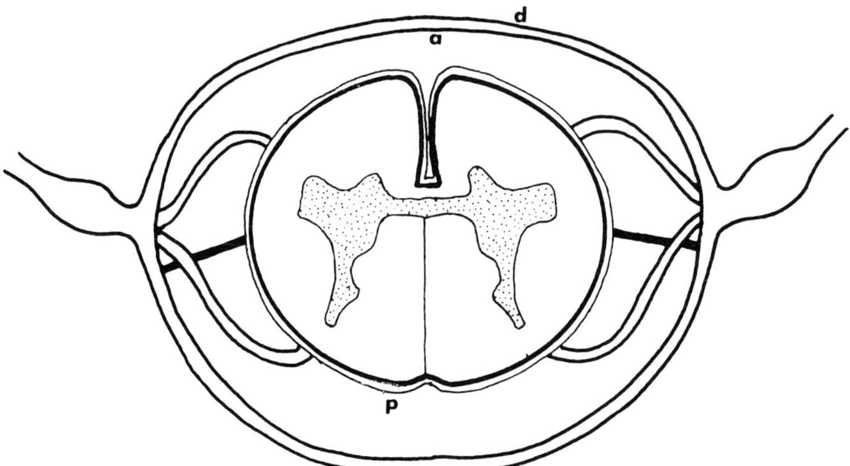

Figure 1.30.   The coverings of the spinal cord. The pia (*p*), arachnoid (*a*), and dura (*d*) with the dentate ligaments.

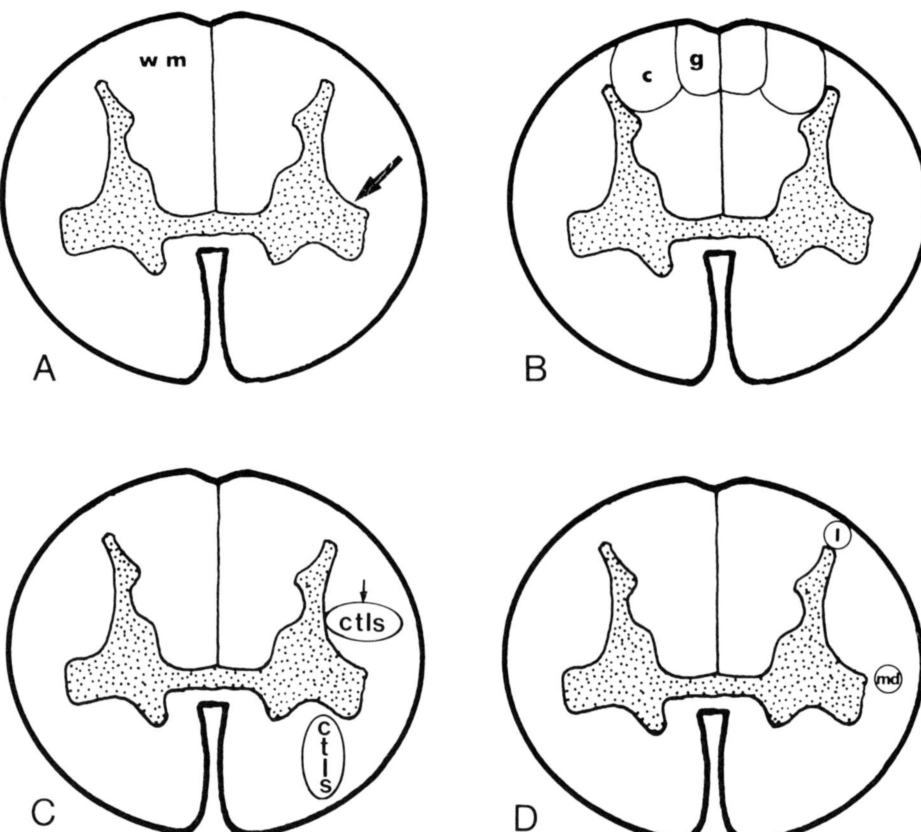

Figure 1.31.   **A,** the spinal cord on cross section. White matter (*wm*) and gray matter (*arrow*). **B,** the posterior columns; the gracile (*g*) medially and the cuneate (*c*) tract laterally. **C,** the descending corticospinal tract posteriorly and the ascending spinothalamic tract anterolateral (*arrow*). Note how the cervical, thoracic, lumbar, and sacral fibers (*ctls*) are arranged. **D,** the smaller collection of fibers in the micturition tract (*md*) and the tract of Lissauer (*l*).

Spinal Cord

The medulla oblongata ends at the foramen magnum to become the cervical spinal cord. Like the brain, the spinal cord is encased in membranes or coverings (Fig. 1.30).

The cervical spinal cord has a fairly constant anteroposterior (AP) diameter of 10 mm and a variable transverse diameter that is largest (20 mm) at the cervical enlargement (C4-T1, for the brachial plexus exit).

On cross section the cord has the H-shaped internal gray matter surrounded by white matter. The white matter is constituted by ascending and descending spinal cord tracts (Fig. 1.31*A*).

Posterior (Dorsal Column) Funiculus

Medially lies the gracile tract and laterally the cuneate tract (Fig. 1.31*B*). Both convey discriminative general sensations of vibratory, joint position, tactile, two-point discrimination, and stereognosis. The sacral, lumbar, and lower thoracic tracts are in the gracile tract, and the fibers from T6-C1 are more lateral in the cuneate tract. Interruption of these tracts results in loss of these discriminative sensations on the same side of the body.

Lateral Funiculus

The lateral funiculus is roughly divided into an anterior half and a posterior half. Posteriorly lies the descending corticospinal (motor) tract. These descending tracts have already crossed from one side to the other in the medulla oblongata so that a lesion in the left corticospinal tract produces changes on the same (left) side of the body. Note that a lesion in the brain (stroke) above this decussation will cause motor changes on the opposite side of the body. Changes caused by both lesions include spastic weakness, increased tone, exaggerated tendon reflexes and an extensor plantar response.

Towards the front of the lateral funiculus lie the ascending spinothalamic tracts that conduct pain and temperature sensation. These tracts have also crossed before arriving in the cervical spinal cord, but this crossing has occurred distally at the level of entry of the fibers into the cord. Thus, a lesion in the left fiber tract will cause loss of pain and thermal sensation on the opposite right side below the lesion. The topography of the fibers in this tract are also important and shown in Figure 1.31C.

Anterior Funiculus

The anterior columns contain the relatively unimportant medial vestibulospinal and reticulospinal tracts.

Miscellaneous Tracts.   Two tracts merit mention (Fig. 1.31D).

1. The descending and ascending tracts for micturition, defecation, and erection. They convey impulses bilaterally and thus a unilateral lesion does not affect actions of the organs associated with the elimination of waste or reproductive products.
2. The tract of Lissauer, which transmits uncrossed pain and thermal sensation. The uncrossed nature of this tract accounts for some persistence in pain and temperature sensation with a lesion in the opposite spinothalamic tract.

Gray Matter

The gray matter has appeared in the past few diagrams as an H-shaped structure. It is divided into dorsal (posterior) horns, an intermediate zone, and anterior (ventral) horns. The gray matter has been mapped into layers or lamina, six of which are posterior, one of which is intermediate, and three of which are ventral. Various tracts ascend/descend and synapse in the various layers. In the ventral horn, the arrangement is such that the more medial motor neurons innervate the more proximal muscles.

Blood Supply to the Spinal Cord

Like everything else in the body, the spinal cord cannot exist without nutrients, which it obtains through the blood stream. The arterial supply of the spinal cord arrives from three sources (Fig. 1.32) (4, 6, 10, 11):

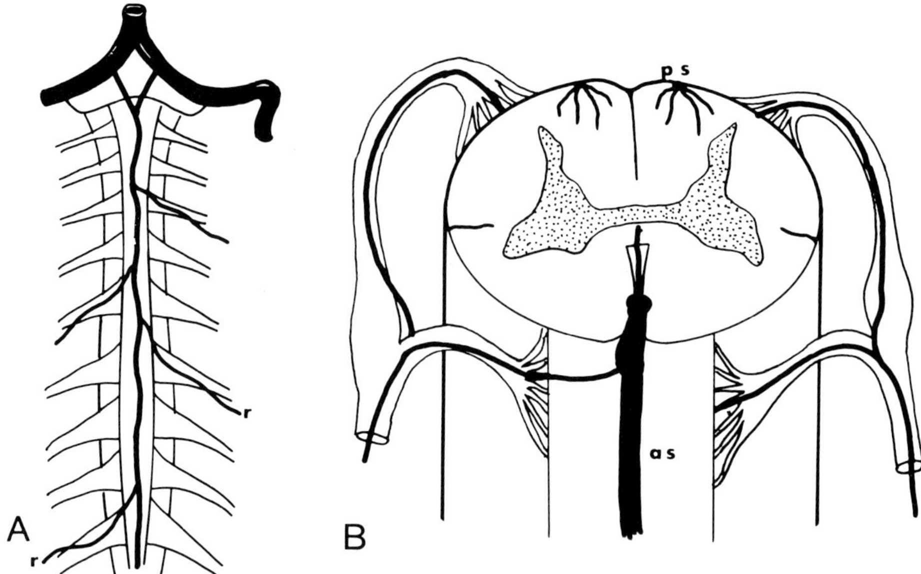

Figure 1.32.   **A,** the anterior spinal artery lies in the anterior sulcus of the spinal cord where it receives contributions from the radicular arteries (*r*). **B,** the anterior spinal artery (*as*) in the anterior sulcus and the paired posterior spinal arteries (*ps*).

1. The anterior (median) spinal artery, which is a descending arterial branch from the vertebral basilar system. It is the dominant blood supply to the cord serving the anterior two-thirds of the white and gray matter.
2. The bilaterally paired posterior spinal arteries, which also originate from the vertebral-basilar system via the posterior cerebellar artery. These smaller arteries supply the posterior one-third of the cord (Fig. 1.32).
3. The radicular arteries, which arise from the vertebral arteries, reinforce the anterior spinal artery. Note that:
   a. Not every cervical level has radicular branches.
   b. Radiculars may be anterior or posterior, together or separate (the most common radicular artery and the most common anterior-posterior combination is usually on the C6 root).
   c. Filling of the anterior spinal artery depends on at least one major radicular branch.

Nerve Roots

Each cervical anatomical level has a motor (ventral) and sensory (dorsal) nerve root (Fig. 1.33). The C1 level is the exception, having no sensory branch. The cervical nerve roots are approximately 2 mm in diameter and, on leaving the cervical cord, head slightly inferiorly and anteriorly, exiting through the neural foramen (Fig. 1.1*B*). Each root sends fibers to the cervical and/or the brachial plexus. The fiber innervation (and thus the neurological deficit) of the nerve roots most commonly affected by cervical disc disease (1) are summarized in Table 1.1.

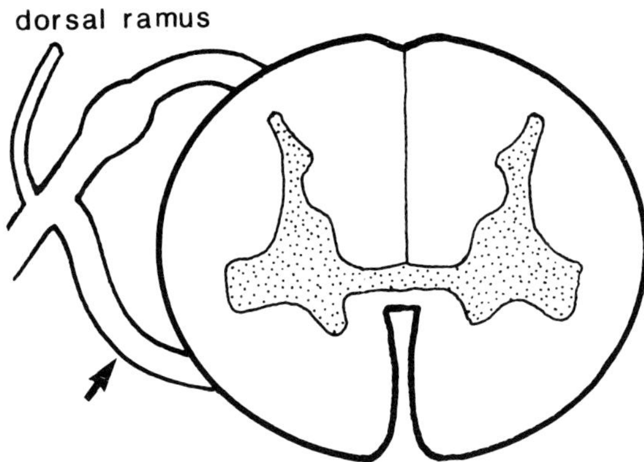

Figure 1.33.   The dorsal (*sensory*) root and ganglion, and the ventral (*motor*) root (*arrow*).

Table 1.1.   Neurological Deficits Possible in Cervical Disc Disease

Root	Motor	Sensory Loss	Reflex
C5	Abduction-shoulder Ext. rotation-shoulder Flexion-elbow	Upper arm and proximal forearm	Deltoid Biceps Brachioradialis
C6	Flexion-elbow Extension-wrist Int. rotation-shoulder Pronation forearm	Thumb and index finger	Biceps Brachioradialis
C7	Extension-elbow Flexion-wrist Supination-forearm	Middle finger	Triceps

It would be nice if the neuroanatomy in Table 1.1 held true all the time so the clinician would have no trouble determining the anatomical level in cervical disc disease. Unfortunately, life is not so simple in the brachial plexus because of significant variations in innervations:

1. There is often a variation in what rootlet fibers join which root (i.e., some rootlets that should be in C6 may exit in the C7 root).
2. Roots may be prefixed or postfixed (i.e., higher or lower by one segment).
3. Additional clinical reasons will be explained in Chapter 3.

Brachial Plexus

As mentioned earlier, the neuroanatomy of the cervical region is tremendously variable, but standard anatomic texts generally consider the brachial plexus as the recipient of contributions from the spinal roots C5-T1 (Fig. 1.34).

The clavicle divides the brachial plexus into the proximal supraclavicular region in the neck and the distal infraclavicular region in the axilla and arm. Note the three collateral branches of the supraclavicular portion of the brachial plexus (Fig. 1.35 and Table 1.2). Lesions of the supraclavicular portions of the brachial plexus will present with winging of the scapula and weakness of external rotation of the shoulder. Injuries below this level will leave these functions intact. Injuries to the T1 root will disrupt sympathetic preganglionic fibers destined for

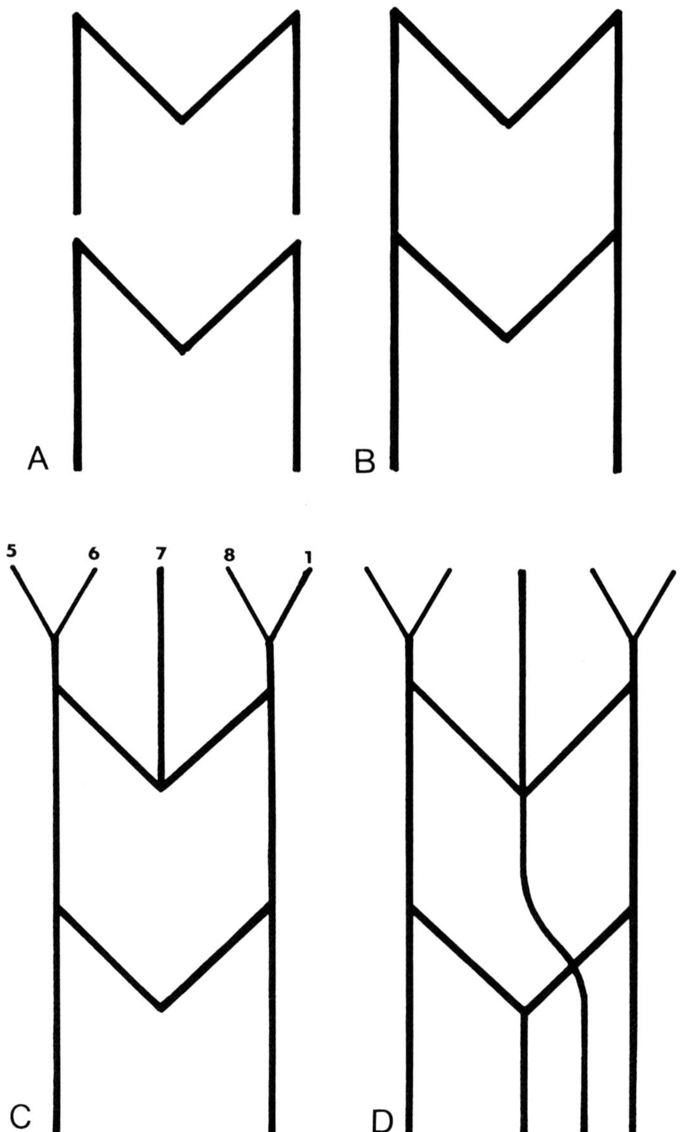

Figure 1.34. So you want to draw the brachial plexus.
A. Start with two Ms (Macnab and McCulloch).
B. Join them.
C. Add the roots (5,6,7,8,1).
D. Extend the stems of the Ms.
Now you have the beginning of the brachial plexus.

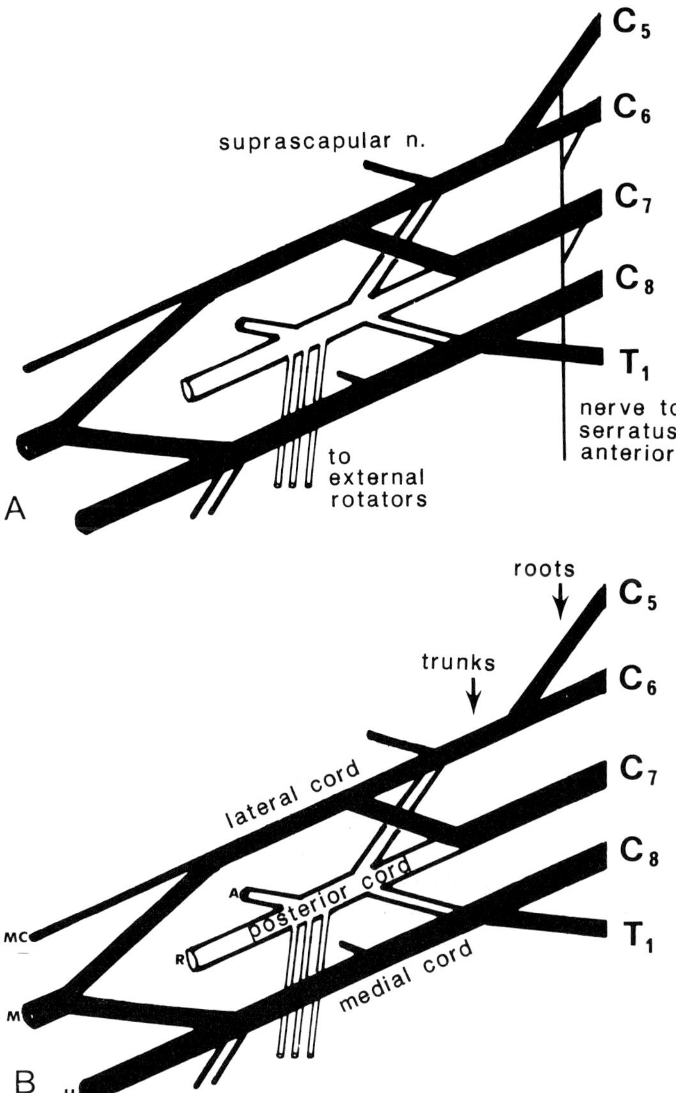

Figure 1.35. **A,** the collateral branches of the supraclavicular portion of the brachial plexus. The long thoracic and suprascapular are labeled. **B,** the posterior, lateral, and medial cords. The posterior cord terminates as the radial (*R*) and axillary (*A*) nerves. The medial cord as a branch to the median (*m*) nerve and ulnar (*u*) nerve, and the lateral cord as a branch to the median nerve and the musculocutaneous (*mc*) nerve.

the oculomotor nerve and produce Horner's syndrome—anhidrosis, miosis, enophthalmus, and ptosis (2).

Infraclavicular Regions of the Brachial Plexus

Injuries to this region are more common than supraclavicular root avulsions, simply because fractures and dislocations of the shoulder region are more common. Think of this portion of the brachial plexus in three sections:

Table 1.2.   Collateral Branches of the Supraclavicular Portion of the Brachial Plexus

Branch (Root)	Muscle Supply	Lesion
Dorsal scapular (C5)	Levator scapulae Rhomboids	Winging of scapula
Suprascapular (C5,6)	Supraspinatus Infraspinatus	Loss of external rotation of shoulder
Long Thoracic	Serratus anterior	Winging of scapula

Table 1.3.   Collateral Branches of the Infraclavicular Portion of the Brachial Plexus

Cord	Branch (nerve)	Supply
Lateral	1. Lateral pectoral n.	Upper portion pectoralis major
Medial	1. Medial pectoral n.	Pectoralis minor and lower portion pectoralis major
Posterior	1. Upper subscapular n. 2. Thoracodorsal 3. Lower subscapular n.	Subscapularis latissimus dorsi Subscapularis teres major

- Cords
- Collateral branches
- Terminal branches

Cords.   The cords (medial, lateral, and posterior) are named relative to their position around the axillary artery. The posterior cord will receive fibers from all roots (Fig. 1.35) and terminate as the radial and axillary nerves. The lateral cord will receive fibers from the upper cervical roots (C5-C7); the medial cord will receive fibers from the lower cervical roots (C8, T1). The cords give off collateral nerve branches as they travel through the axilla and will end as terminal branches of the brachial plexus.

Collateral Branches.   The collateral branches are shown in Figure 1.35 and Table 1.3.

Terminal Branches.   There are six terminal branches to the cords of the brachial plexus—two for each cord (Fig. 1.35 and Table 1.4).

Cervical Plexus

The cervical plexus (Fig. 1.36) is formed by the anterior (ventral) primary rami of C1-C4 (the brachial plexus is C5-C8 and T1). Ramus C4 communicates with the brachial plexus and is common to both the cervical and brachial plexus. The posterior primary rami are motor only and innervate the suboccipital muscles. The sinuvertebral nerve is considered a branch of the posterior primary rami (Fig. 1.36*B*).

At its origin, the cervical plexus is hidden behind the sternomastoid (Fig. 1.36*C*). Its motor branches supply the anterior strap muscles and contribute branches to the sternomastoid and trapezius. The sensory branches are shown in Figure 1.36.

Table 1.4.   Terminal Branches of the Brachial Plexus

Cord	Branches
Lateral	1. Musculocutaneous nerve 2. Branch to median nerve
Medial	1. Branch to median nerve 2. Ulnar nerve
Posterior	1. Radial nerve 2. Axillary nerve

The most important nerve of the cervical plexus is the phrenic nerve (C3-C5) that traverses the neck to innervate the diaphragm (sensory and motor).

Autonomic Nervous System

Are you ready for a test? Did you feel your heart suddenly pick up speed? That's the autonomic nervous system kicking in. This system stimulates and controls all structures not under conscious control. This includes:

- Cardiac muscle
- Most glands
- All smooth muscle

The autonomic nervous system is divided into two parts:

- The sympathetic nervous system
- The parasympathetic nervous system

By and large, each target is supplied by both systems—the sympathetic to stimulate for fight or flight, the parasympathetic to cool things down.

Sympathetic Nervous System

There are two neurons in the sympathetic nervous system. The cell bodies of the first neuron (preganglionic) are located in the lateral gray horn of the spinal cord between T1 and L3 (Figs. 1.36*B* and 1.37). The axons leave the cord via the ventral roots of T1-L3 and enter the sympathetic trunk. The sympathetic trunk is a series of ganglia extending from the neck to the sacrum.

In the neck, the cervical sympathetic trunk consists of three ganglia (superior, middle, and inferior) lying loosely on the longus colli muscles laterally.

The inferior cervical sympathetic ganglia and the first thoracic ganglion are usually fused and known as the stellate ganglion.

The first order neurons synapse in these ganglia to branch to the glands of the head and neck, and the structures in the arm.

The first order neurons are myelinated (white) and are known as the preganglionic fibers and white ramus (Fig. 1.36*B*). The postganglionic second order neurons are nonmyelinated and gray.

Parasympathetic Nervous System

This system is also two-neuron-structured; a preganglionic and postganglionic neuron. The cell bodies of the preganglionic fibers are located in the brain stem

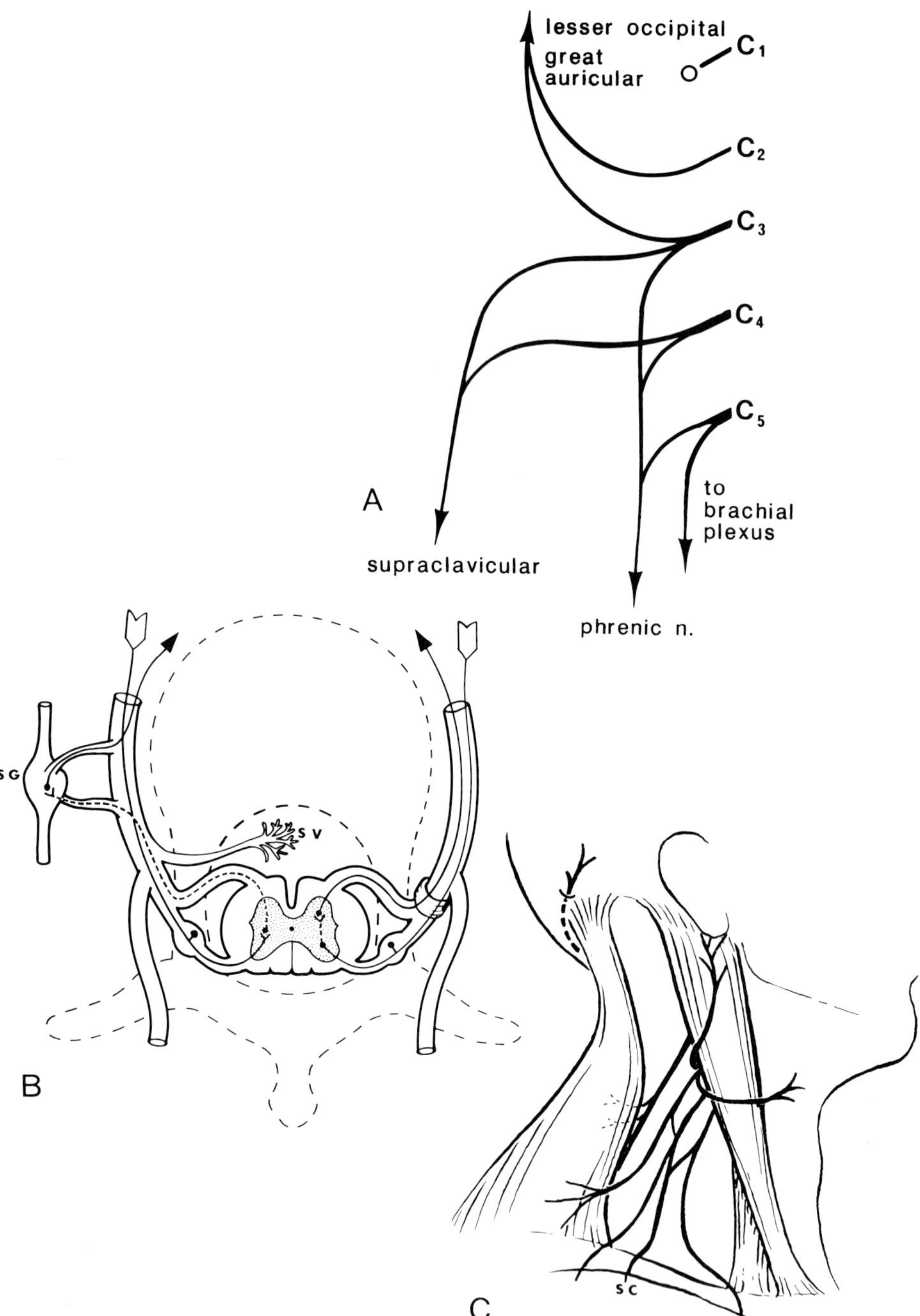

Figure 1.36.   A, the cervical plexus. **B,** the sinuvertebral nerve (*sv*) and sympathetic ganglion (*SG*). **C,** the origin of the cervical plexus hides deep to the sternocleidomastoid muscle (*sc* = supraclavicular nerves).

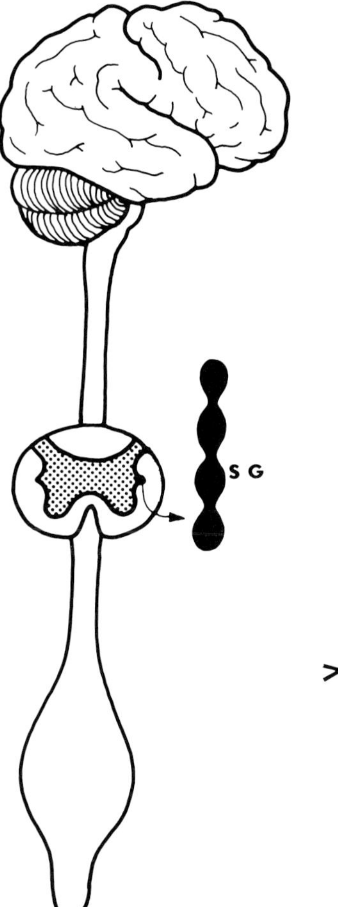

Figure 1.37.   The sympathetic preganglionic fibers originate in the lateral gray matter and leave in the ventral root to synapse in the sympathetic ganglion (*SG*). (Also see Fig. 1.36*B*.)

and the sacral cord. The ganglions of the parasympathetic nervous system are located near their target organs. From here, first-order neurons synapse and then innervate the target organ or structure (Fig. 1.38).

Physiology of the Autonomic Nervous System

The sympathetic nervous system stimulates for fight or flight. It speeds the heart, dilates the bronchi, and dilates the pupils, among other things. Drugs that stimulate sympathetic activities are known as adrenergic drugs, the most well-known being adrenaline. Drugs that block the sympathetic nervous system are commonly used to treat hypertension.

The parasympathetic nervous system calms troubled waters—it slows the heart and prepares the GI tract for intake and output. Cholinergic drugs stimulate the parasympathetic nervous system and are not routinely used. Agents that block the parasympathetic nervous system (atropine) are used to dilate the eyes and speed up the heart.

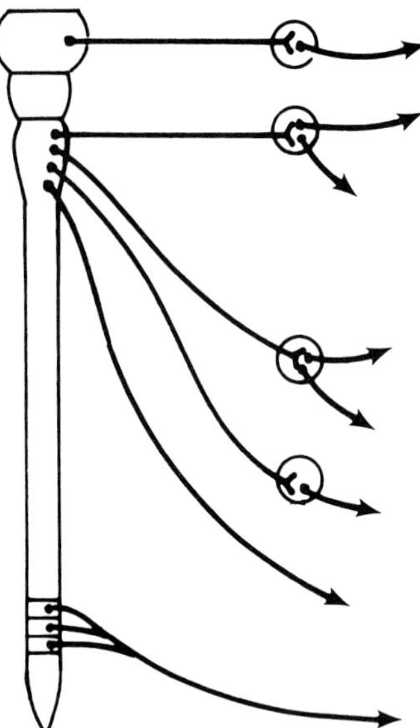

Figure 1.38.   The parasympathetic fibers originate in the brain stem and sacral cord, and travel long distances as preganglionic fibers to synapse near the target organs.

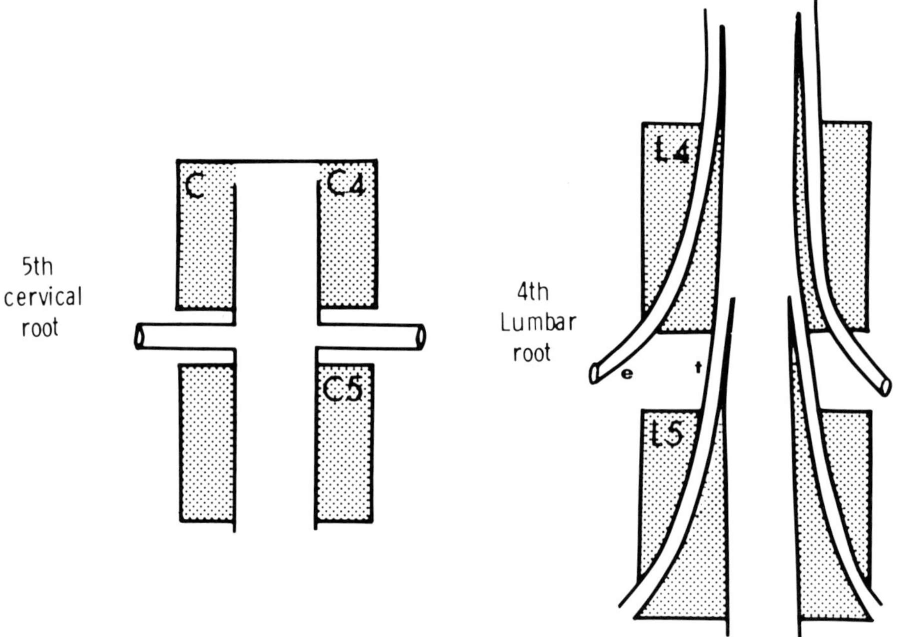

Figure 1.39.   The cervical nerve roots exit horizontally so that medial and lateral pathology catches the same root. In the lumbar spine, medial pathology catches the traversing root (*t*) and lateral pathology catches the exiting root (*e*).

Surgical Anatomy of the Cervical Nerve Roots

The course taken by the nerve roots in the cervical spine differs greatly from that taken by the lumbar nerve roots. In the lumbar spine, the roots run obliquely, passing over an intervertebral disc before emerging through the foramen below (Fig. 1.39). For example, the fourth lumbar nerve root crosses over the L3-L4 disc and emerges through the intervertebral foramen of L4-L5. In the cervical spine, the roots run a more transverse course with the fifth cervical root emerging through the C4-C5 foramen (Fig. 1.39). This anatomical variance can be summarized this way: in the cervical spine, the root emerges above the pedicle whose segmental number it bears.

A foraminal stenosis at the L4-L5 segment in the lumbar spine will compress the exiting fourth lumbar root; a disc herniation will compress the traversing fifth lumbar root. Foraminal stenosis and a disc herniation at C5-C6 in the cervical spine will compress the sixth cervical root only. This anatomical relationship becomes especially important when employing diagnostic nerve root infiltration (12).

As they leave the spinal cord, the nerve roots are encased in a funnel-shaped prolongation of the dura. As they approach the intervertebral foramen, the motor and sensory components are separated, enclosed in an arachnoid and dural sleeve with the two sleeves being separated by the so-called interradicular septum. Beyond the foramen in the transverse gutter, the arachnoid sleeve ends just proximal to the dorsal root ganglion (Fig. 1.40). From here, the dura blends

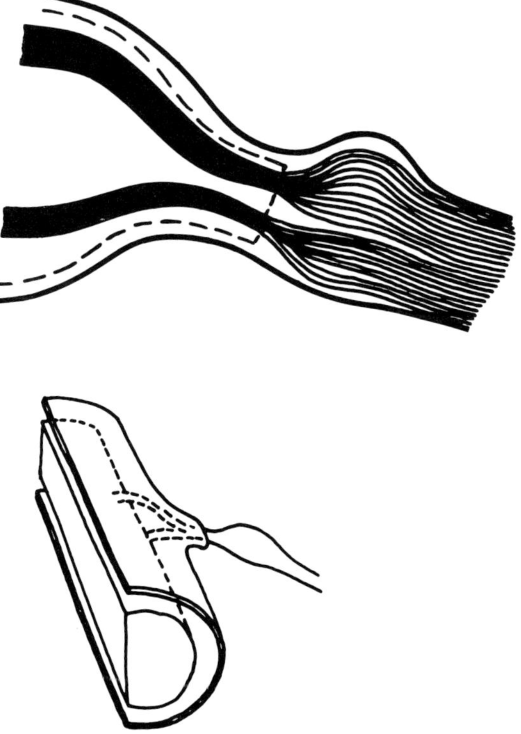

Figure 1.40.   Beyond the foramen, the arachnoid sleeve (*broken line*) ends just before the ganglion.

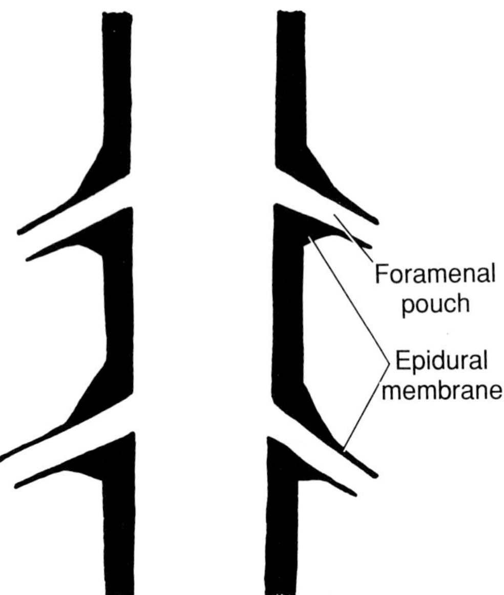

Figure 1.41.   The arachnoid sleeve forms a foraminal pouch as seen in Figure 1.42 (*left*). The foraminal pouch is evident at C4-C5 but is obliterated at C5-C6 bilaterally.

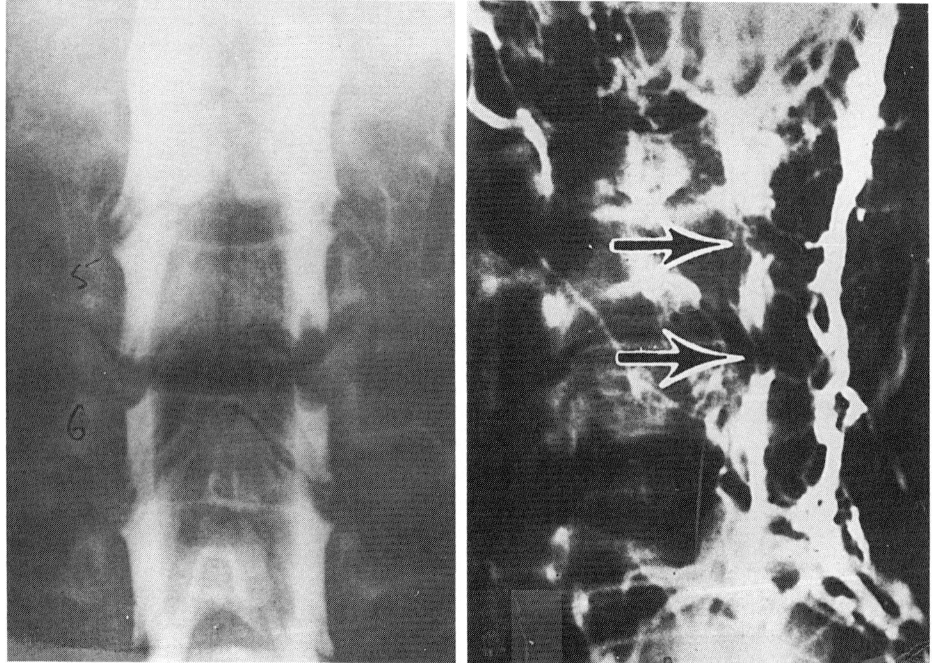

Figure 1.42.   *Right*. Epidural contrast with defects (*arrows*). *Left*. Subdural contrast (cervical myelogram).

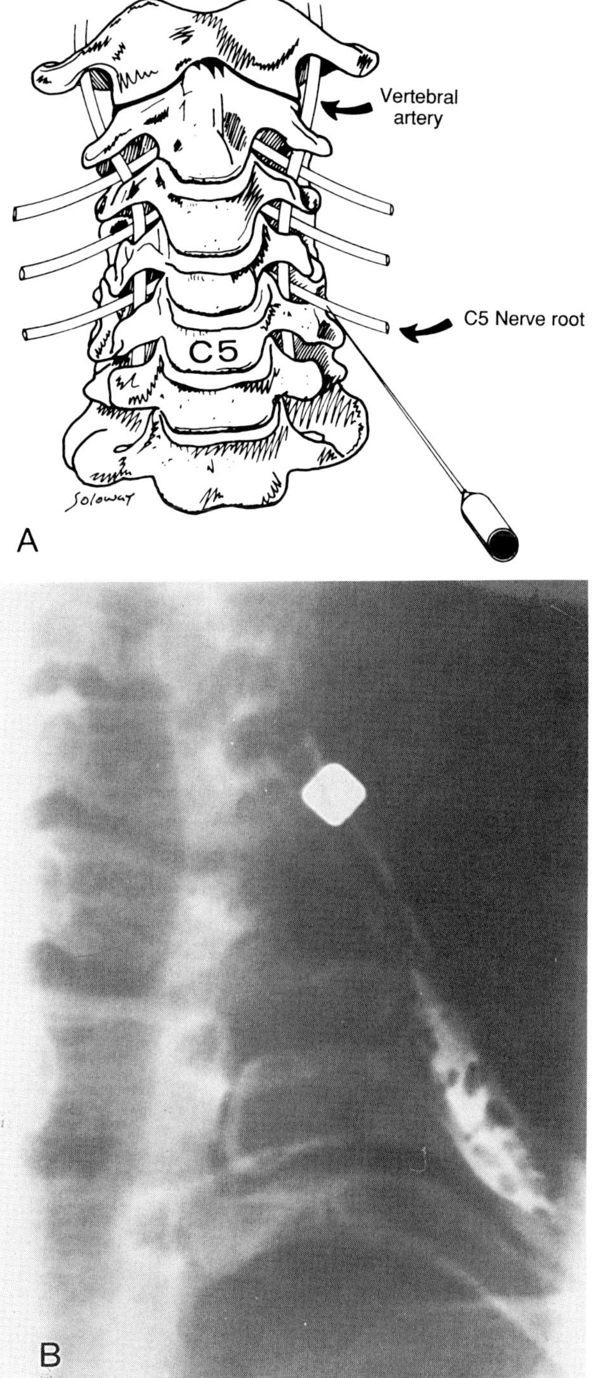

Figure 1.43.   Technique of root sheath block (*upper*) and contrast in a root sheath (*lower*).

intimately with the emerging nerve roots. The recognition of this foraminal pouch is important in interpreting myelograms (Fig. 1.41). Surrounding the dura, a thin vascular membrane called the epidural membrane is thickened around the nerve roots. In the spinal canal, the epidural membrane is firmly attached to the ligamentum flavum, the laminae, the posterior longitudinal ligament, and the disc. Outside the foramen, the epidural membrane becomes continuous with the periradicular sheath. The periradicular sheath has a loose attachment to the nerve root but is firmly attached to the periosteum of the transverse process and the scalene muscles. This sheath continues as a loose connective tissue surrounding the peripheral nerves, forming the epineural sheath of the cervical plexus.

The epidural membrane is an important anatomical entity in the radiological assessment of root lesions using the technique of epidural myelography and nerve root infiltration (12). When radiopaque dye is inserted into the epidural space, it will flow out of the intervertebral foramen into the epidural tunnel around the nerve root. The flow of dye will be impeded by any obstruction (Fig. 1.42).

In the technique of nerve root infiltration, an attempt is made to place the tip of the needle within the periradicular sheath (12). With successful placement, contrast material will run along the course of the nerve root, giving rise to tubular configuration (Fig. 1.43). With the position of the needle confirmed in this manner, 1 ml of local anesthetic is injected. Temporary abolition of the arm pain indicates that the symptomatic segment has been localized and the site of the involved nerve root demonstrated.

CONCLUSION

From the knowledge of anatomy flows an understanding of clinical syndromes and a foundation for surgical intervention. This short summary of anatomy was presented in the hope of stimulating your desire to read more and gain an even greater understanding.

REFERENCES

1. Arnold JG Jr: The clinical manifestations of spondylochondrosis (spondylosis) of the cervical spine. Ann Surg 141:872–889 (1955).
2. Barre JM: Sur un syndrome sympathetique cervical posterior et sa causa frequente, arthrite cervical. Rev Neural (Paris) 1:1246–1248 (1926).
3. Burrows EH: The sagittal diameter of the spinal canal in cervical spondylosis. Clin Radiol 14:77–85 (1963).
4. Chakravorty BG: Arterial supply of the cervical spinal cord (with special reference to the radicular arteries). Anat Rec 170:311–330 (1972).
5. Crispin AR and Lees F: The spinal canal in cervical spondylosis. J Neurol Neurosurg Psychiatry 26:166–170 (1963).
6. Crock HV and Yoshizawa H: The Blood Supply of the Vertebral Column and Spinal Cord in Man. Springer-Verlag, New York (1977).
7. Edwards WC and LaRocca H: The developmental segmental sagittal diameter of the cervical spinal canal in patients with cervical spondylosis. Spine 8:20–27 (1983).
8. Fielding JW: Cineroentgenography of the normal cervical spine. J Bone Joint Surg 39A:1280–1288 (1957).
9. Ford F and Clarke D: Thrombosis of the basilar artery. Bull Johns Hopkins Hosp 98:37 (1936).

10. Hassler O: Blood supply to the human spinal cord: a microanagiographic study. Arch Neurol 15: 302–307 (1966).

11. Herren RY and Alexander L: Sulcal and intrinsic blood vessels of human spinal cord. Arch Neural Psych 41:686–687 (1939).

12. Kikuchi S, Macnab I, and Moreau P: Localization of level of symptomatic cervical disc degeneration. J Bone Joint Surg 63B:272–277 (1981).

13. Lind B, Schlbom H, Nordwall A, and Malchau H: Normal range of motion in cervical spine. Arch Phys Med Rehabil 70:692–695 (1989).

14. Luschka H: Ent wickel ung squeschickle de Formbestanadtheite des Eiter uund den granulationen. Vol 7, 54 A Emmerling Frieberg in Bresqua (1845).

15. White AA and Panjabi MM: Update on the evaluation on instability of the lower cervical spine. In: AAOS Instruction Course Lectures, XXXVI, pp 513–520. CV Mosby, St. Louis (1987).

2

Cervical Disc Degeneration— Pathogenesis of Symptoms

"An adult is one who has ceased to grow vertically but not horizontally."

—Anonymous

INTRODUCTION

We are all getting older, and in doing so we are simply "wearing out." Some call it degeneration, but it is difficult to tell a patient he or she is becoming a degenerate! It is best to understand the changes below simply as part of the aging system, no different than graying of the hair or wrinkling of the skin. Just because the cervical spine is showing signs of the aging process, it does not mean the patient must have symptoms. Just because the patient has normal cervical spine x-rays, it does not mean the patient cannot have a soft disc rupture causing severe arm pain.

What is more important in cervical disc disease is the combination of events. The best example of this is in cervical myelopathy where degenerative changes encroach on a congenitally narrow canal and progressive disability develops because of abnormal mobility (from the degeneration). Take a wide cervical spinal canal, add significant degenerative changes (terrible-looking x-rays) but have the osteophytes bridge the disc space so that it is a nonmobile segment, and the patient may not have symptoms at all.

The message is simple. Don't try to understand cervical disc disease by looking at x-rays; above all, don't treat the x-rays—treat the patient.

The aging process starts at age 25 and progresses. Genetic codes and occupational and leisure activities combine to determine the final outcome. Some patients come from families with significant degenerative disc disease codes; some patients pursue occupations (truck drivers) that may accelerate the process, and some patients do bad things that advance the process of degeneration, such as smoke or play contact sports like tackle football. It takes the right combination of events to convert the universal aging process into symptomatic cervical disc disease.

CLASSIFICATION

When you read Chapter 3 on clinical assessment, you will note that we have divided the clinical syndromes into:

* Neck ache
* Radiculopathy
* Myelopathy
* Miscellaneous syndromes

42

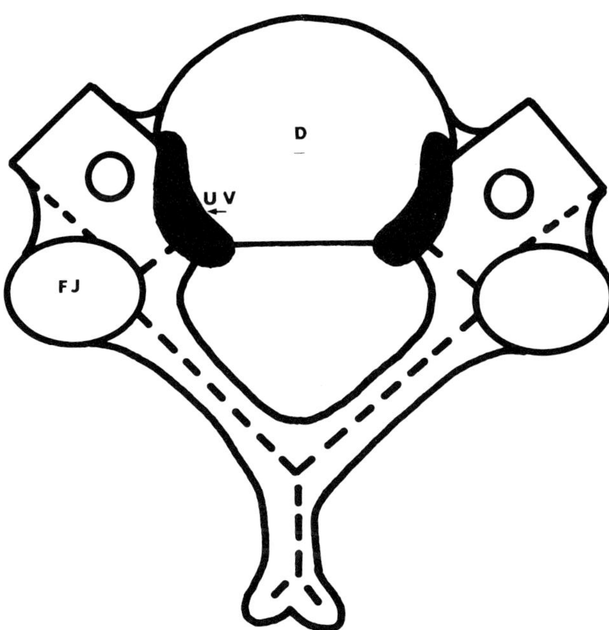

Figure 2.1.   Three of the four big players in motion segment degeneration: the disc (*D*), the facet joints (*FJ*) and the neurocentral joints (uncovertebral joints—*UV*). The fourth player, ligamentum flavum, is shown in Figure 2.5.

They all occur secondarily to the degeneration in the structures of the cervical spine. Why one syndrome occurs in one patient and not another is unknown. Accept it that, in cervical disc disease, multiple factors may cause one or more of these syndromes, or one factor (e.g., a disc rupture) can cause one (e.g., acute radicular pain) or more (e.g., acute radicular pain and myelopathy) of these syndromes (12).

PATHOGENIC FACTORS IN CERVICAL DISC DISEASE

It is best to think of all the structure in a segment that can wear out and contribute to symptomatic cervical disc disease (Fig. 2.1).

Disc

"What comes first, the chicken or the egg?"

What comes first, degeneration in the disc with secondary changes elsewhere, or primary changes in the facet joints leading to secondary changes in other parts of the segment? The question remains unanswered, but most would suggest the "beginning of the end" in a spinal motion segment starts in the disc.

Disc degeneration is a gradual process that has been staged by Kirkaldy-Willis (8). The nuclear-annular complex of the disc degenerates in concert as outlined in Table 2.1.

The disc, as a relatively noncompressible gel, depends on its proteoglycan-water complex for its physical ability to absorb loads. As the nucleus loses its water-binding capacity (1), it becomes compressible and less able to absorb and transfer forces to the annulus (7). In turn, the annular collagen fibers break

Table 2.1.   Stages of Disc Degeneration[a]

	Nucleus Pulposus	Annulus Fibrosus	Facet Joint	Result
Normal	Proteoglycan/ water Noncompress-ible gel	Fibrous structure with high tensile strength	Smooth gliding	Nucleus absorbs forces Force transfers to annulus Smooth pain-free movement
Stage I— dysfunction	Loss of water, breakdown of proteoglycan	Fissuring and tearing of fibers	Synovitis hypomobility	Intermittent axial pain
Stage II— instability	Nuclear protusion	Fissuring, disc resorption	Capsular laxity and subluxation	Axial pain and/ or acute radicular pain from HNP
Stage III— stability	Desiccation and narrowing	Osteophyte formation	Osteophyte formation	Minor axial pain, neurological compromise

[a]After Kirkaldy-Willis (8).

down and cease to function as force absorbers. The result is desiccation of the nucleus with fragmentation and tears or fissuring of the annulus (9, 11). The disc height decreases, the annular fibers bulge into nerve root, and cord territory and abnormal movements (instability) occur in the motion segment. In an attempt at repair and stabilization, fibrotic changes occur in the nucleus—it takes on the histological appearance of the annulus—and stabilizing osteophytes appear at the margins of the disc space (8) (Fig. 2.2). During this degenerative process, nuclear material may or may not rupture through a tear in the annulus to cause nerve root and/or cord pressure (Fig. 2.3).

Neurocentral Joints of Luschka

With narrowing of the disc space, the joint space of Luschka disappears and spurs form, another source of root encroachment (Fig. 2.4).

Ligamentum Flavum

The aging process does not spare the ligamentum flavum. With degeneration, the ligamentum flavum loses its elastic fibers (normally 80% of its makeup), breaks down and hypertrophies its collagen bundles, and becomes edematous. The ligamentum flavum no longer serves as a taut protective membrane but rather hypertrophies and buckles into the spinal canal (Fig. 2.5).

The four big players in motion segment degeneration and the production of abnormal motion segment pain and neurological compromise are:

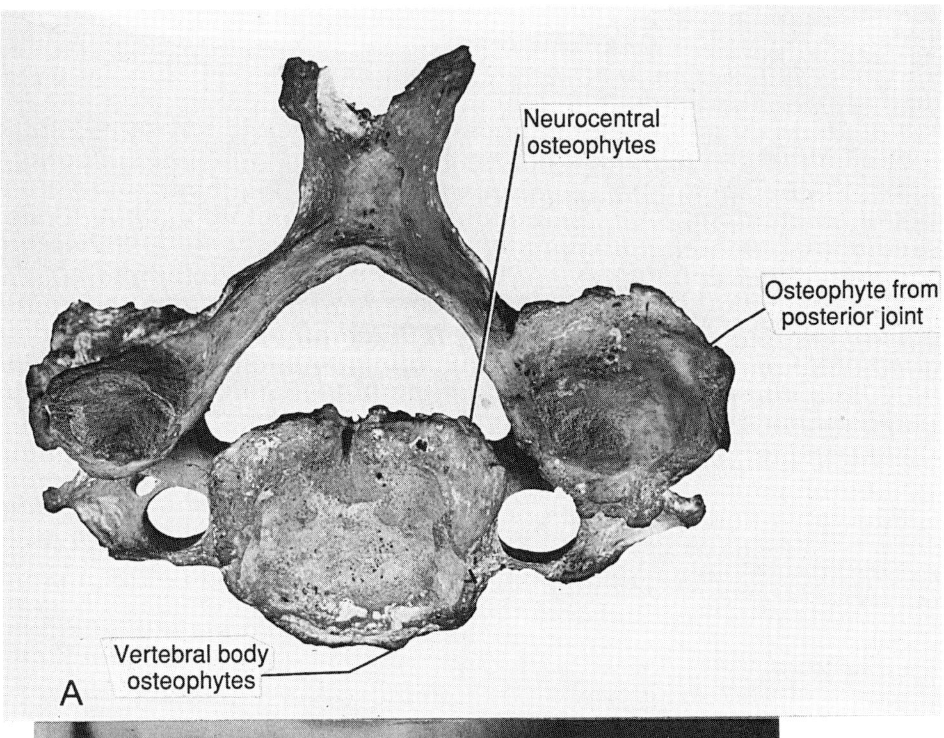

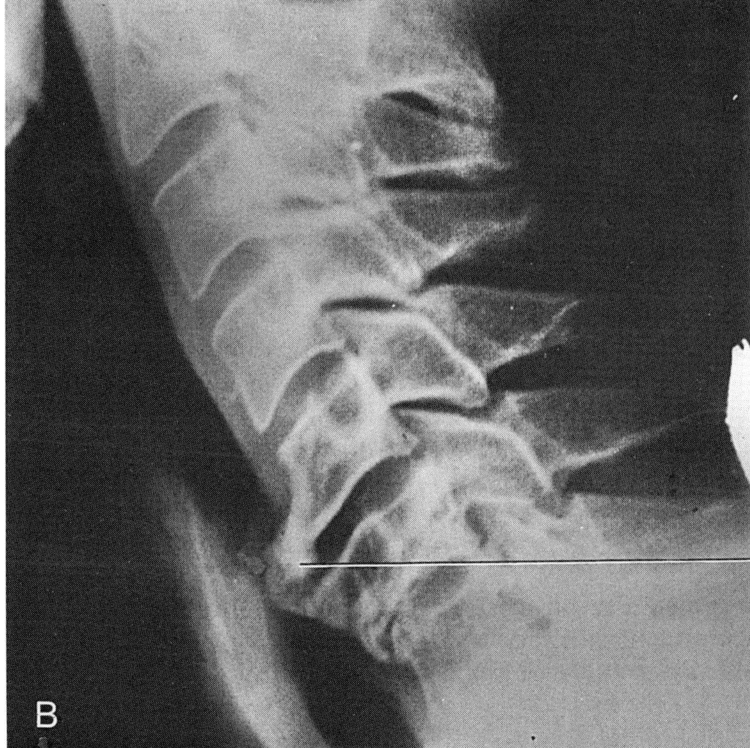

Figure 2.2. **A,** in an attempt to naturally stabilize the motion segment, three sources for osteophytes mobilize. Stabilizing osteophytes may form around the edge of the vertebral body, the facet joint, and the neurocentral joint. **B,** vertebral body osteophyte. They are large and they meet (kissing osteophytes)—the ultimate stability!

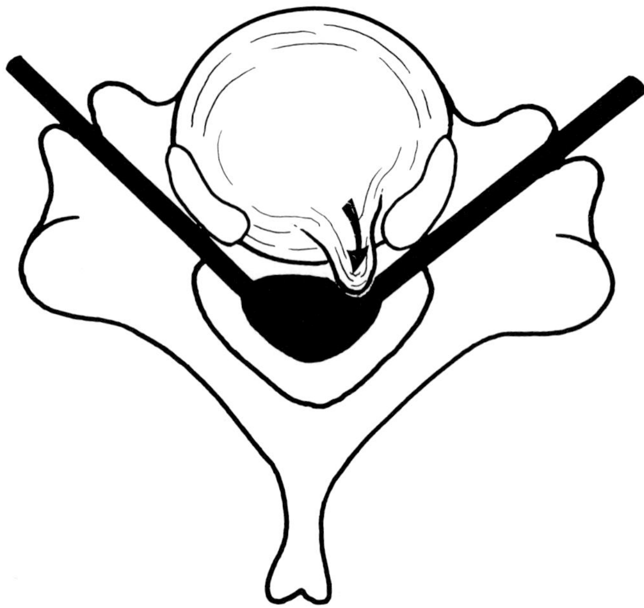

Figure 2.3.   During the degenerative process, nuclear material may rupture through a tear in the annulus (*arrow*) to cause nerve root or cord compression.

- The disc space
- The facet joints
- The joints of Luschka
- The ligamentum flavum

Lesser players are the posterior longitudinal ligament (PLL), which fibroses and in some individuals ossifies (2) (Fig. 2.6); the supporting ligaments, such as the interspinous/supraspinous (ligamentum nuchae) ligaments, which also show collagen degeneration (breaking of both main chain and side chain fibers); and end plate sclerosis and loss of some nutrient channels to the disc. Unknown players in this process are the dentate ligaments that anchor the spinal cord to the dura (Fig. 1.26). It has been postulated by some that the dentate ligaments hold the cord down, while the degenerative changes and abnormal segment mobility "beat up" on the spinal cord (a concept fast losing support).

What Is the Effect of These Degenerative Changes?

Figure 2.7 tells all. No single event determines whether cervical disc degeneration will become symptomatic cervical degenerative disc disease. The size of the spinal canal is of vital importance (5).

Spinal Canal Size

The normal canal diameters are shown in Figure 2.8. The average sagittal diameter of the *spinal canal* is 17 mm, larger at the foramen magnum C1-C2 junction (Chapter 1) and smallest at C4, the beginning of the cervical cord enlargement. The average sagittal diameter of the cervical *spinal cord* is 10 mm, with the cervical cord enlargement (C4-T1) affecting predominantly the trans-

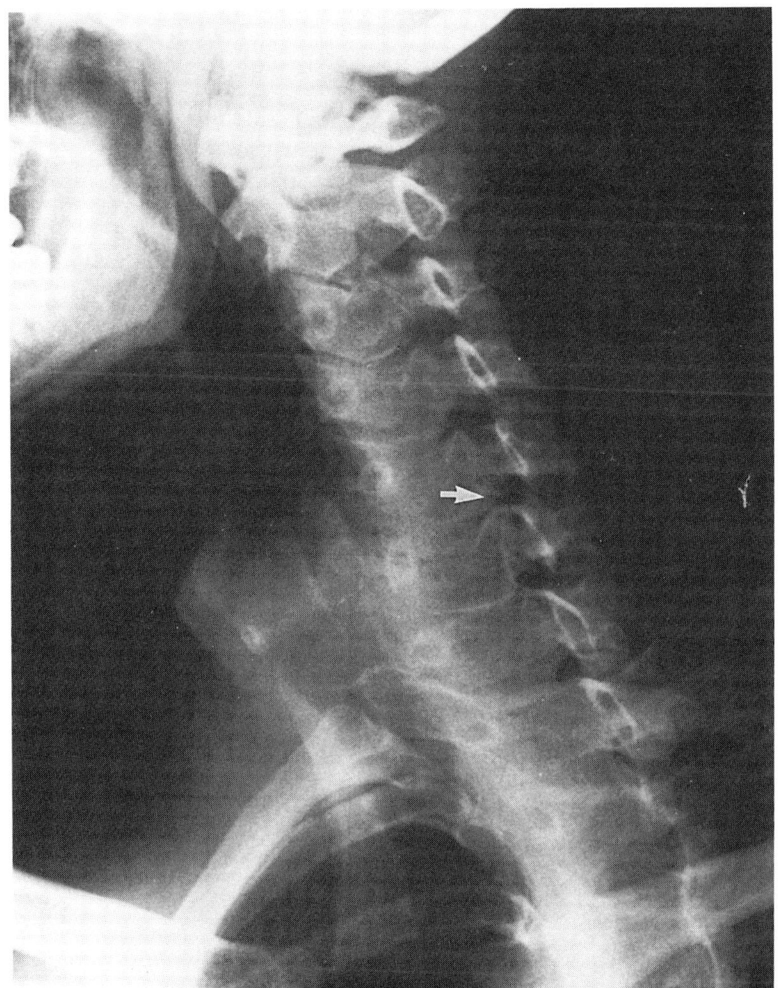

Figure 2.4.   An osteophyte from the neurocentral joint projects into the nerve root foramen (*arrow*).

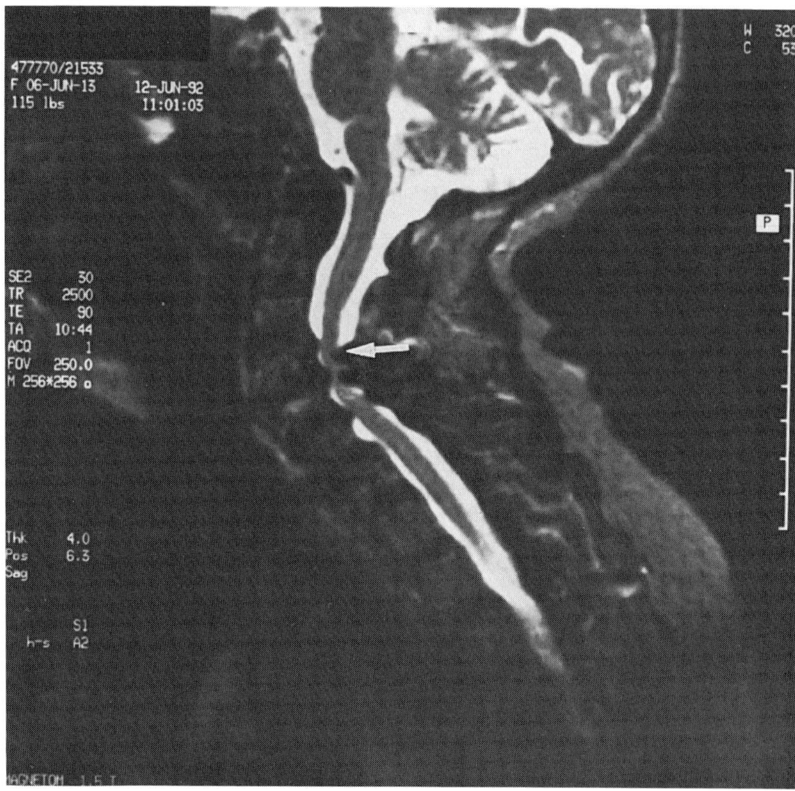

Figure 2.5.   A T1-weighted sagittal MRI showing ligamentum flavum bucking into and narrowing the spinal canal (*arrow*).

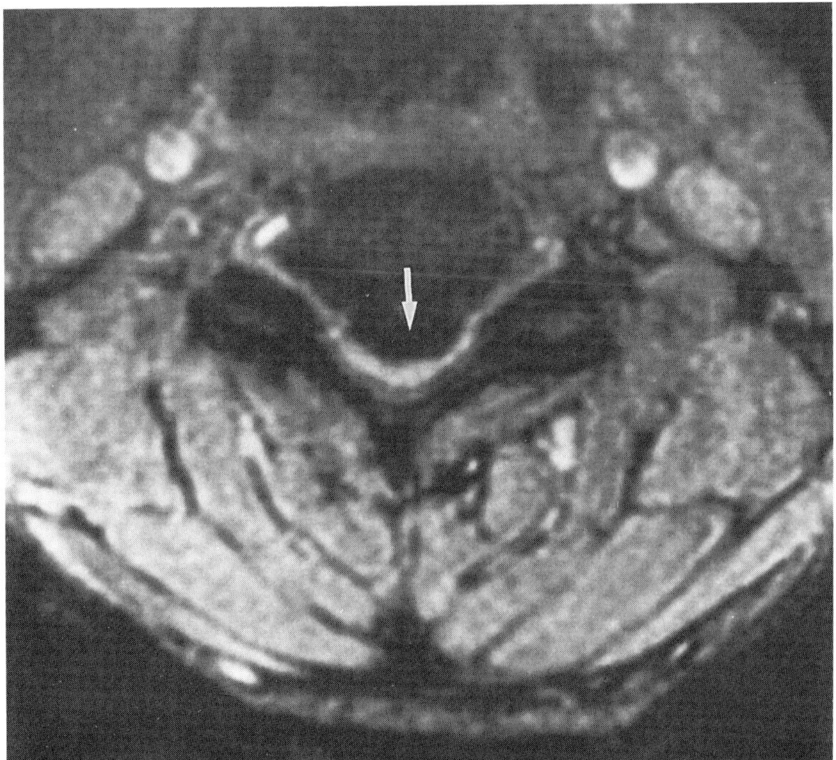

Figure 2.6.   The posterior longitudinal ligament (*PLL*) has ossified (*OPLL*) (*arrow*) to narrow the spinal canal (T1 axial MRI).

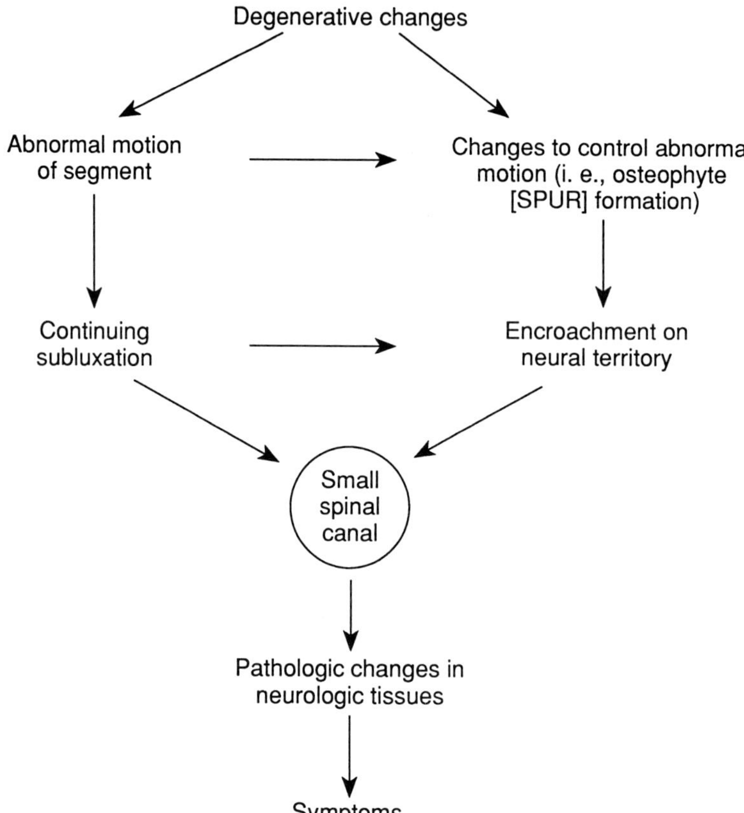

Figure 2.7.   The pathogenesis of symptoms in cervical motion segment disorders.

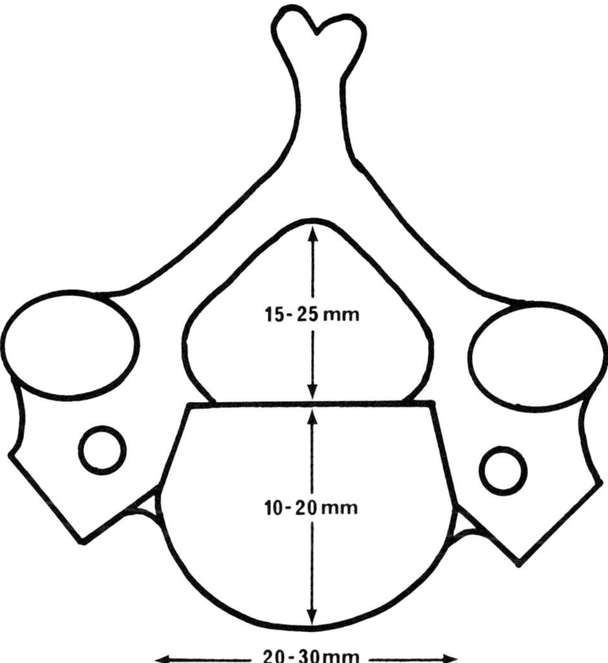

Figure 2.8.   A summary of cervical segment dimensions (rounded off to make them easy to remember).

verse dimension of the spinal cord. A 10-mm spinal cord and a 17-mm spinal canal appear to leave a lot of room.

There are two ways to reduce canal size:

1. Start with a congenitally small canal. Any canal below 13–14 mm in sagittal diameter is considered a congenitally small canal (Fig. 2.9).
2. Narrow the canal even further with degenerative changes (6). As outlined in Figure 2.8, it is likely both factors play a role in narrowing of the space available for neurological structures (3).

Pathological Changes

Within the skeletal system, degeneration of the disc and facet joints allows for abnormal movement in the motion segment. This will cause axial neck pain in some but not all patients.

More importantly, the pathological changes described above encroach on neurological tissues to cause varying degrees of compression and tension. As long as motion persists in such a segment, repeated trauma to the nerve roots and cord eventually results in permanent changes in these neurological structures.

Cord Changes

The range of spinal cord changes goes from a block of axoplasmic flow, to demyelination of compressed axons, to scarring (gliosis) in the white matter tracts. Within the gray matter, cellular loss and gliosis become evident. The end stage is cystic degeneration and cavitation of central gray matter.

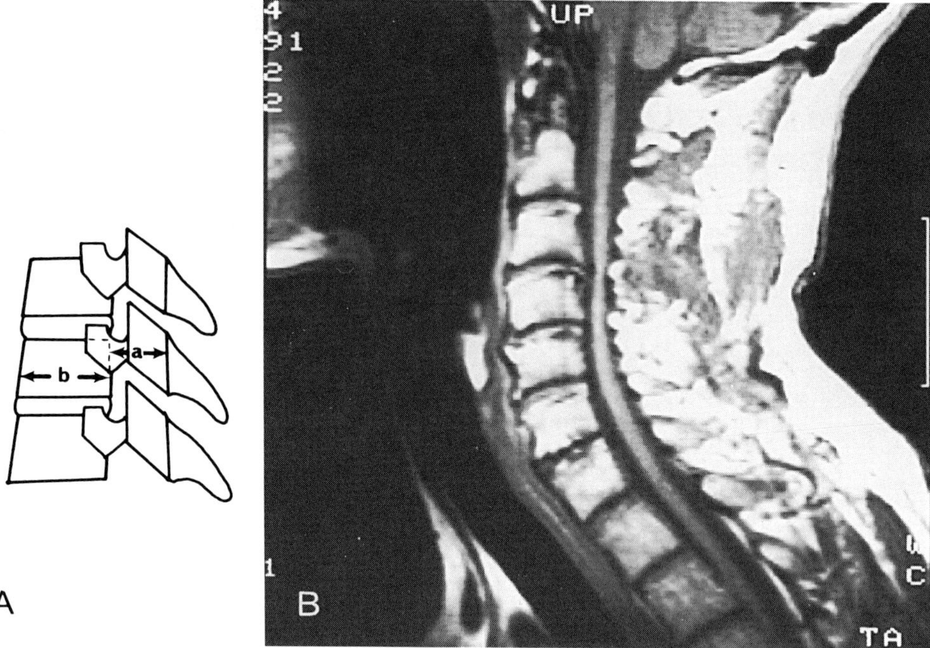

A   B

Figure 2.9.   **A,** schematic to show how canal size is measured. Pavlov's ratio is the canal diameter, *a*, divided by the vertebral body breadth, *b*. A ratio of less than 1:1 is considered a small canal. **B,** a congenitally small canal on MRI.

Nerve Roots

Arachnoiditis and end stage scarring occur within the pial layer of both the cord and the root. This scarring in the nerve root sheath binds the nerve root to its dural pouch, causing further root irritation.

Ossification of the Posterior Longitudinal Ligament (OPLL)

Brief mention needs to be made of ossification of the posterior longitudinal ligament (OPLL) (2, 10). Originally thought to be a disease confined to Asians, more cases are being seen in Europe and America. For some unknown reason, the posterior longitudinal ligament becomes ossified and significantly narrows the spinal canal (Fig. 2.6). It tends to be multisegmental, continuous, or interrupted and affects higher levels than degenerative disc disease. It is more common in Asian males and has a typical CT appearance.

If it becomes symptomatic, it is in the form of myelopathy. The only treatment is surgical decompression.

Incidence of Cervical Degenerative Disc Disease

Cervical disc degeneration is very common. In the 50-year-old patient population, 50% will have x-ray evidence of disc space narrowing and/or osteophyte formation. This is approximately the same incidence as gray hair and wrinkled skin!

Individuals who smoke, work with vibrating equipment (such as highway truck drivers), do heavy manual labor, and pursue unusual leisure activity (such as high diving) will have a higher incidence of degenerative changes on x-ray.

The levels involved are C5-C6 > C6-C7 > C4-C5 with 95% of symptomatic patients having symptoms arising from one or more of these levels. Although apophyseal joint changes occur at all levels, there is a tendency for more advanced changes in the apophyseal joints to occur at C2-C3 and C3-C4.

In the 65-year-old population, 75% of patients will have degenerative changes on x-ray, but obviously not all will be symptomatic. Don't tell them they have arthritis!

CONCLUSION

It is evident that the conversion of cervical disc degeneration into symptomatic cervical disc disease (4) is a complex process. As we age, we all degenerate our cervical spine, but for symptoms to appear, abnormal motion segment mobility must occur. The presence of a small spinal canal adds to the misery.

REFERENCES

1. Adams P, Eyre DR, and Muir H: Biochemical aspects of development and aging of human intervertebral discs. Rheumatol Rehabil 16:22–29 (1977).
2. Bakay L: Ossification of the posterior longitudinal ligament. Neurosurgery 288:2243–2244 (1985).
3. Bohlman HH and Emery SE: The pathophysiology of cervical spondylosis and myelopathy. Spine 13:843–846 (1988).
4. Dillin W, Booth R, Cuckler J, Balderston R, Simeone F, and Rothman R: Cervical radiculopathy: a review. Spine 11:988–991 (1986).
5. Edwards WC and LaRocca H: The development of segmented sagittal diameter of the cervical spinal canal in patients with cervical spondylosis. Spine 8:20–27 (1983).
6. Epstein JA, Carras R, Hyman RA, and Costa S: Cervical myelopathy caused by developmental stenosis of the spinal canal. J Neurosurg 51:362–367 (1979).
7. Hickey SD and Huckins DW: Relation between the structure of the annulus fibrosis and the function and failure of the intervertebral disc. Spine 5:106–116 (1980).
8. Kirkaldy-Willis WH: Managing Low Back Pain, 2nd ed. Churchill Livingstone, New York (1988).
9. Lipson SJ and Muir H: Experimental intervertebral disc degeneration: morphological and proteoglycan changes over time. Arthritis Rheum 24:12–21 (1981).
10. Nagashima C: Cervical myelopathy due to ossification of the posterior longitudinal ligament. J Neurosurg 37:653–660 (1972).
11. Oda J, Tanaka H, and Tsuzuki N: Intervertebral disc changes with aging of human cervical vertebra from the neonate to the 80s. Spine 13:1205–1211 (1988).
12. Wilkinson M: Cervical Spondylosis, 2nd ed, pp 1–9. WB Saunders, Philadelphia (1971).

3

Cervical Disc Disease: Clinical Assessment

*"Although I know that pain isn't real, I certainly dislike what
I fancy I feel."*

—Ogden Nash

INTRODUCTION

There are so many symptoms, and so many personalities, that evaluating a patient with neck and arm pain can be exasperating. Understanding the patient is just as important as diagnosing his or her disease. This chapter will attempt to clarify organic or physical disease processes in the neck, and Chapter 5 will delve into the nature of the patient.

CLASSIFICATION

Excluding shoulder conditions, symptoms affecting the neck can be classified into:

1. Mechanical neck (axial) pain
2. Radiculopathy
3. Myelopathy
4. Miscellaneous
   a. Vertebral basilar insufficiency
   b. Dysphagia

In trying to package syndromes into neck pain, arm pain, and so on, you must accept that, in addition to these "pure" syndromes, there will be many patients with a combination of syndromes. The two most common associations are patients with neck ache and radicular pain. An interesting rarity is the patient who exhibits neck and arm pain, and goes on to develop myelopathy.

Mechanical Neck (Axial) Pain

Axial pain comes in three forms:

1. Myofascial pain (see Chapter 5)
2. Intermittent acute episodes of significant neck pain that are the prodromal symptoms of subsequent radicular pain
3. Mechanical neck pain from degenerative disc disease

Intermittent Acute Neck Pain (Prodrome)

These patients are more commonly men, 35–45 years of age. They have virtually normal neck function until they pursue vigorous activity such as sports (es-

54

pecially basketball), overhead activity, or a long car ride. They go to bed with neck stiffness and awaken with significant neck pain, often associated with a twisted neck.

On physical examination they will appear with a head tilted in various directions and allow very little neck movement, especially in a direction opposite to the tilt of the head.

In the absence of radiating arm pain, one would not expect to find neurological changes in the arms. On x-ray the cervical lordosis will be absent and a scoliosis will be apparent.

With or without treatment the acuteness quickly resolves, and after a few weeks to a few months of chronic neck discomfort, normal neck function prevails until the next episode—weeks, months, or years later.

After a few of these episodes of acute axial pain, the patient will self-stabilize the motion segment, develop the syndrome of degenerative disc disease, or rupture a disc and exhibit acute radicular syndrome.

Mechanical Neck Pain From Degenerative Disc Disease

Mechanical neck pain is a pain in the neck that is aggravated by activity and relieved by rest. It is important to distinguish this mechanical component from neck ache that doesn't disappear with rest and is not significantly altered by activity. The latter case should alert you to the potential for more serious problems such as tumors or infections (Chapter 9).

The pain of cervical disc degeneration is frequently precipitated, aggravated, and perpetuated by any activity that maintains the neck in extension. Some activities, such as painting the ceiling, obviously hold the neck fully extended, but most patients are not aware of other common daily activities that also place an extension strain on the neck. These extension strains start as soon as the patient arises in the morning. The neck is commonly extended while shaving, putting on shoes and socks, knitting, reading with bifocals or half-moon glasses, and by incorrect posture while driving, using the telephone, or even excitedly watching a football game on TV. During housework, extension strains are applied to the neck while making beds, vacuuming, reaching for high shelves, and carrying a clothes basket.

It is only when pointedly asked that the patient will remember these events; learning about them is not only important for a diagnosis but for therapeutically guiding the patient.

Stress and tension play an important role in the production and perpetuation of many discomforts derived from musculoskeletal disorders. This is particularly true with cervical disc degeneration. Stress and tension play such a prominent role in the symptom complex that the clinician may overlook underlying cervical disc degeneration. Under certain stressful situations or states, the patient may assume the "fight" position, with the neck muscles held taut and the chin thrust forward. In the presence of cervical disc degeneration, this posture will cause pain. The increased discomfort will understandably increase the patient's frustration and initiate a vicious circle.

Listen carefully to every detail of the story that the patient discloses. What may appear trivial to you may be painfully important to the patient. "I get this terrible grinding sensation in my neck" is a fairly common, unpleasant experience noted by many patients. There is nothing you can do about this from a physical point of view, but there is a lot you can do by discussing the problem in detail with the patient. You must examine the neck specifically for this one symptom. Take an x-ray. Your obvious interest and your thorough examination will encourage the patient to accept what you know is true—namely, that the clicking or grinding, though unpleasant, does not mean something terrible or irreversible is going to happen to the neck and that, without specific treatment, this noise will settle down with the passage of time.

The pain can aptly be classified as a severe constant nuisance, preventing the patient from easily accomplishing the ordinary activities of daily living. It is only infrequently that a cervical disc degeneration without root irritation will exhibit pain of immobilizing intensity. The pain of cervical disc degeneration is difficult to bear, and these patients are frequently dejected.

They frequently sit with the neck slightly flexed, looking up at you as though they are peering through the top of bifocal glasses. The slightly flexed position of the neck is the position of comfort. On examination, the movements of the cervical spine are restricted to a varying degree—sometimes grossly, sometimes hardly at all.

Normally, when one flexes the neck the chin touches the chest. Rotation is permitted through a range of 80° to either side. Lateral flexion permits the ear to come within two finger breadths of the shoulder, and on full extension the occipitomental line is 30° above the horizontal.

A decrease in all these movements is to be expected over the age of 45, but this decreased range is not associated with pain at the limit of movement. The first movement to be lost is extension. Often, the permitted range of painless movement will only bring the occipitomental line to 10° below the horizontal line. Although lateral flexion may be markedly limited in the erect position, when the patient lies down with the head resting on the bed, the range of movement is greatly increased. This is an important observation; when there is a marked functional overlay, the patient does not demonstrate the increase in range of lateral flexion when the head is lying on the bed. This permitted increase in range of lateral flexion is probably because the weight of the head—14 lb—is supported by the bed when the patient is lying down.

Patients with cervical disc degeneration will note discomfort when pressure is applied to the spinous processes posteriorly, but the discomfort is never very marked. Gross tenderness during this phase of examination generally denotes a significant emotional or functional component in a patient's disability.

Anterior cervical tenderness may be specific and of localizing value. With the patient relaxed and the head supported with a soft pillow, the examiner's fingers, placed anterior to the sternomastoid, are pressed gently into the sulcus between the sternomastoid and the trachea. The trachea is displaced by the tips of the examiner's fingers and the pulps of the fingers can palpate the anterior surface of the vertebral bodies. Although this form of examination is not pleasant for anybody, when a patient is suffering from cervical disc degeneration, pressure over the involved segment gives rise to an acute discomfort, and on occasion may reproduce the radiation of pain complained of clinically. If the sternomastoids are tender, any pressure over the front of the neck is painful, and nothing can be learned from this form of anterior palpation.

Associated Symptoms

It is not unusual for patients with axial neck pain to have headache discomfort and radiation of pain across the back of both shoulders. A rare associated symptom is dysphagia, which is thought to be due to anterior osteophytes interfering with esophageal function.

Other unusual symptoms such as blurring of vision or tinnitus should lead you to consider vertebral basilar insufficiency or other neurological disorders.

Radiographic Assessment

Plain X-rays. Usually all that is needed to establish the diagnosis is plain x-ray (Fig. 3.1). Exclusive of the open mouth view for the C1-C2 junction, plain films should include a standard AP and lateral views with obliques. In a heavyset, bullnecked patient the C7-T1 junction will only be seen on a swimmer's view (Fig. 3.2). Cervical vertebral subluxation will be aggravated by flexion views (Fig. 3.3).

Bone Scan. In the face of persistent pain in spite of conservative treatment intervention, a bone scan is a useful investigation (Fig. 3.4).

CT/MRI. In mechanical neck pain, CT and MRI are rarely helpful and ordering such expensive tests is to be discouraged.

Radiculopathy

There are two basic patterns to radiculopathy in cervical disc disease (7):

1. Acute radiculopathy
2. Chronic radiculopathy

Acute Radiculopathy

This patient is the extension of the syndrome described under axial pain. A middle-aged male (usually), after experiencing one or a number of episodes of acute neck spasms, has shoulder and arm pain. The extremity discomfort so dominates that patients will often comment that they now have very little neck pain.

Characteristics of the pain are:

1. Location—the pain is parascapular (especially in a C6 or C7 root lesion) across the back of the shoulder girdle and down the arm.
2. Radiation—the distribution of the arm pain for the most common root lesions is outlined in Table 3.1. The actual location of the pain is not useful for distinguishing C6 or C7 root lesions.
3. Aggravation—the arm pain is aggravated by neck movements, especially flexion. The pain is often aggravated by coughing and sneezing (Valsalva test).
4. Relief of pain—the arm pain is relieved by abducting the shoulder (Fig. 3.5) and by traction on the head.
5. Associated neurological symptoms—these are largely sensory paresthetic symptoms, which may include whole-hand tingling or tingling confined to a specific finger. Table 3.2 summarizes the localizing value of these symptoms.

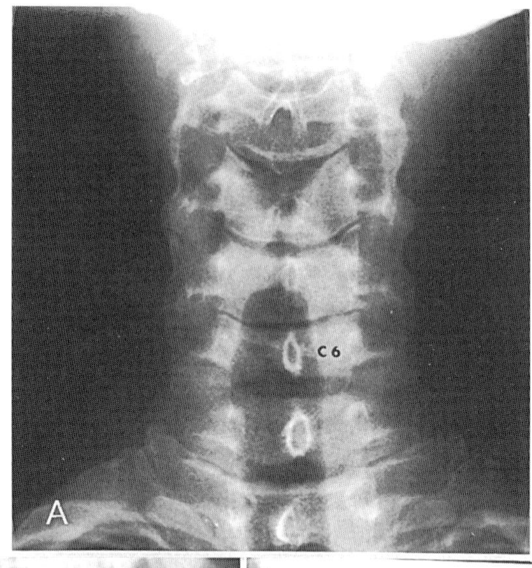

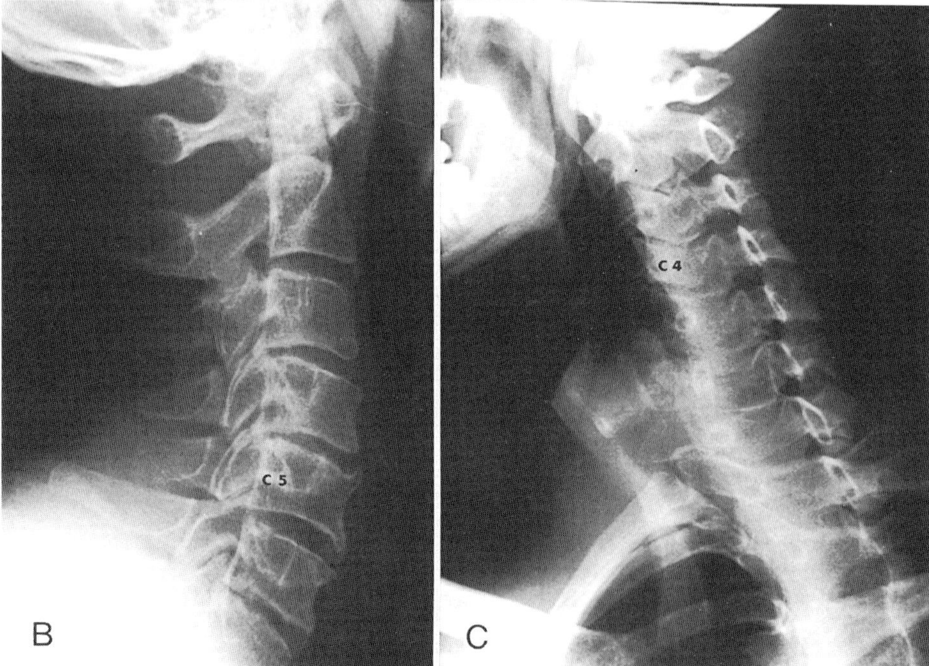

Figure 3.1.   Routine subaxial cervical spine x-rays should include an AP (**A**), lateral (**B**), and obliques (**C**).

6. Neurological signs—the weakness, sensory loss, and reflex alteration that may occur in acute cervical disc ruptures are summarized in Table 3.3 (4). The neurological changes in the acute radicular syndrome are more obvious than in chronic syndromes. Still, the neurological lesion may not obviously point to the level of the lesion and further investigation may be needed (see *Investigation of the Patient With Radiculopathy* below).

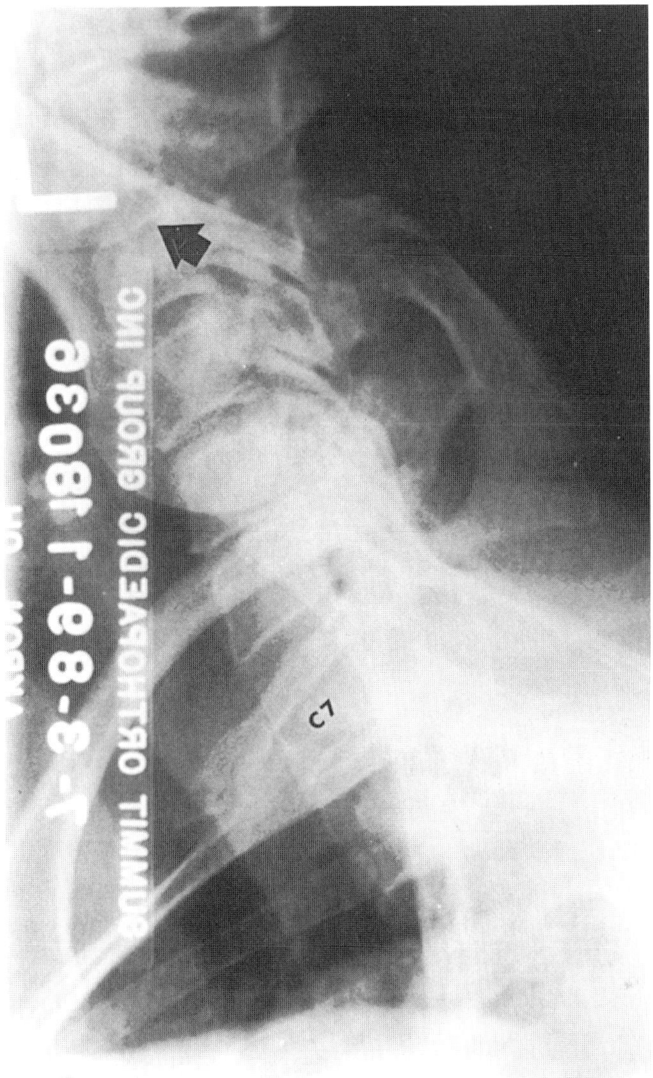

Figure 3.2. In heavyset, bullnecked individuals the C7-T1 junction is not easily seen on routine lateral x-rays and a swimmer's view is required. Note the elevated shoulder (*arrow on humerus*) such that the arm is in the overhead "swimmer's" position.

7. Muscle tenderness—depending on the root involved, specific muscles may be tender (e.g., for a C6 root, the biceps muscle may be tender; for a C7 root lesion, the triceps muscle may be tender).
8. Miscellaneous symptoms—on one occasion a patient may present with Lhermitte's sign: sudden radiating discomfort down the arms and legs with neck flexion or extension that immediately disappears when the movement is stopped. Headache is rarely an accompanying symptom in such a patient.

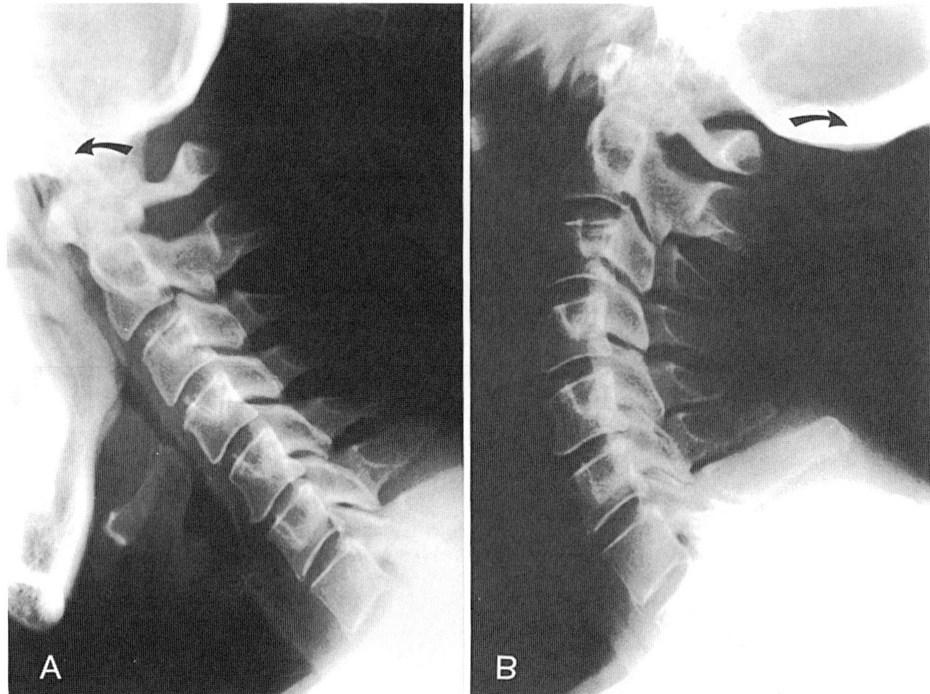

Figure 3.3.   The addition of flexion/extension views is helpful in assessing subluxation. In this individual, little flexion is allowed (**A**) because of muscle spasm.

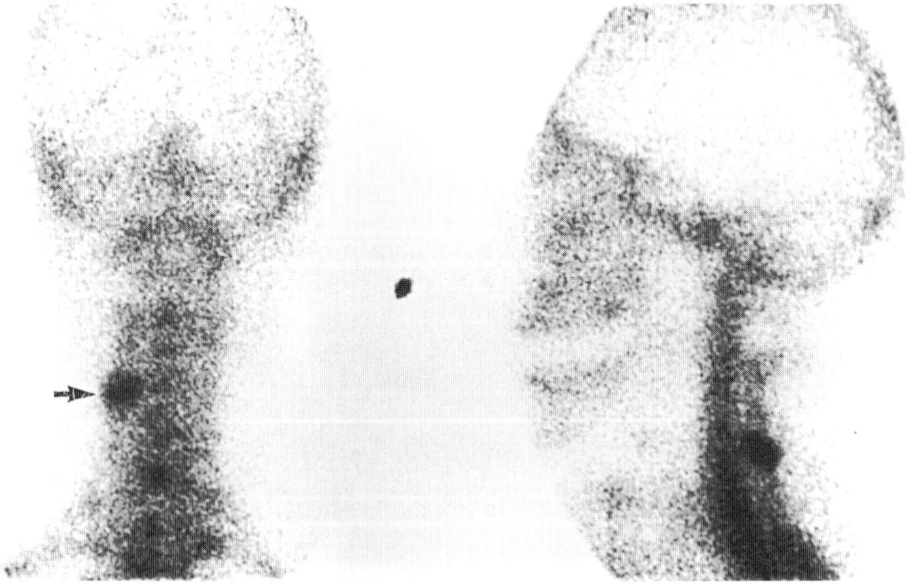

Figure 3.4.   A bone scan showing single focus of increased tracer uptake in inflamed facet joint (*arrow*).

Table 3.1.   Root Localization Value of Radiating Arm Pain

C5 root—pain localized to cap of shoulder and deltoid region
C6-C7—Pain down lateral aspect of arm and extensor surface of forearm

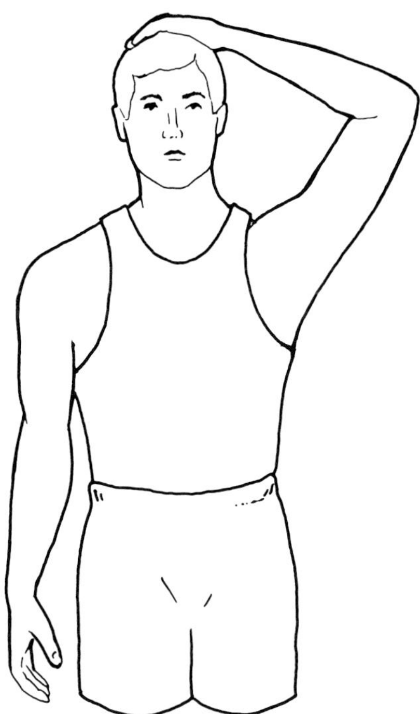

Figure 3.5.   Relief from arm pain is sometimes achieved by shoulder abduction and resting the hand on top of the head.

*Table 3.2.   Root Localization Value of Paresthesia**

C5   Over deltoid
C6   Thumb (index)
C7   Middle (index)

*Whole hand numbness may appear in isolated C5, C6, or C7 root lesions.

Table 3.3.   Neurological Findings in Acute Radicular Syndrome

Root	Motor	Sensory Loss	Reflex
C5	Abduction-shoulder Ext. rotation-shoulder Flexion-elbow	Upper arm and proximal forearm	Deltoid Biceps Brachioradialis
C6	Flexion-elbow Extension-wrist Int. rotation-shoulder Pronation-forearm	Thumb and index finger	Biceps Brachioradialis
C7	Extension-elbow Flexion-wrist Supination-forearm	Middle finger	Triceps

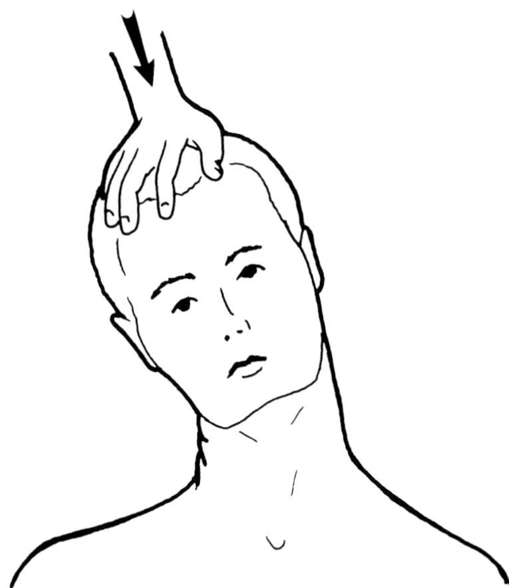

Figure 3.6.   The Spurling test. With the neck extended slightly and tilted to the symptomatic side, axial pressure is applied to the top of the head. This is thought to further narrow the foramen and is considered positive if pain radiates down the arm.

Chronic Radiculopathy

Chronic radiculopathy is far more common than the acute syndromes, occurs in an older age group (usually above 50), and is equally distributed between the sexes. Reasons why chronic radiculopathies are more common than acute:

- The uncovertebral joint protects the nerve root from an acute disc rupture.
- Acute radiculopathies more readily improve with conservative care, whereas chronic radiculopathies tend to persist in spite of conservative care. This is easy to understand considering how a soft-disc herniation, with time and treatment, can shrink and disappear but an osteophyte pressing on a nerve root will not disappear as long as movement continues at that segment.

The nature of the pain, aggravating and relieving characteristics, and neurological symptoms and signs may all be the same as in acute radiculopathies, with the following modifications. In chronic radiculopathy:

- Neck pain is more common.
- Arm pain is less acute and more persistent.
- The movements that close the foramen and aggravate symptoms are extension, lateral flexion, and compression to the symptomatic side (Spurling's test) (Fig. 3.6).
- The movement that opens the foramen and thus relieves symptoms is flexion.
- The neurological symptoms and signs are much less obvious, necessitating more in the way of investigation to establish a diagnosis.

The reasons neurological symptoms and signs are of less localizing value in chronic radiculopathies are:

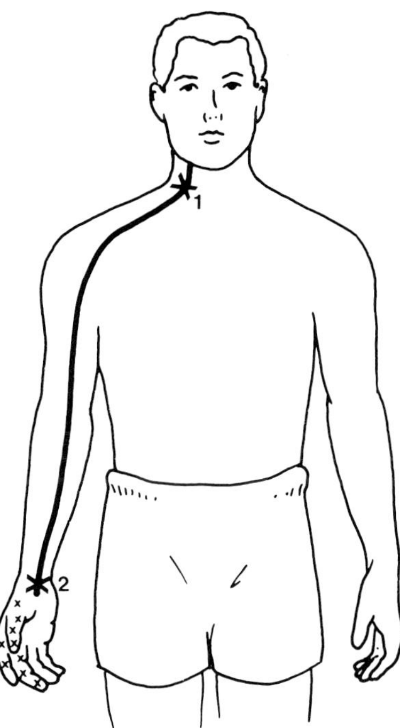

Figure 3.7.   The double crush. The most common double crush combination is C6 root compression in the neck at C5-C6 (*X1*) and carpal tunnel compression of the same fibers at the wrist (*X2*).

- With chronic root compression the axons have more time to accommodate to the pressure, and the root lesion is more incomplete than in the acute syndromes.
- With degenerative narrowing of the disc, the length of the cervical spine shortens and the root relationship to cervical bars may change, increasing or decreasing irritation.
- As mentioned in the Chapter 1, rootlet exit not only varies from patient to patient, but from the right to the left side in the same patient.
- Patterns of innervation through the brachial plexus may vary.
- A brachial plexus may be prefixed (have a lot of fiber contribution from C4 and little from C8) or postfixed (no fibers from C4 and many fibers from C8).
- Degenerative changes may not be isolated to one segment, and two or more nerve roots may be compressed.
- Other conditions such as thoracic outlet, ulnar nerve compression at the elbow or wrist, or median nerve compression at the wrist are more likely to be present in this age group and lead to the so-called double crush (Fig. 3.7).

Investigation of the Patient With Radiculopathy

It should be possible to rule out other conditions and arrive at a clinical diagnosis of radiculopathy. The anatomical level of involvement is not always obvious, but this does not alter conservative treatment intervention until surgery becomes a consideration. Extensive testing to determine root level, with EMG and CT/myelography or MRI, is not only unnecessary but expensive, and should only be done if surgery is indicated.

Plain Radiographs.   Plain radiographs are an inexpensive and reasonable step to take in patients with radiculopathy. They will show changes in cervical contour (loss of lordosis) and disc degeneration (Fig. 3.3), but, most important, they will quickly reveal most tumors and infections (Chapter 9). Occasionally a cervical rib will be seen (Fig. 3.8).

Electromyography.   When a patient's diagnosis is less clear, probably the best test is EMG examination of the arm and paraspinal muscles. This assumes the diagnosis centers around neurological problems rather than an intrinsic shoulder problem causing radiating arm pain. EMG will usually help differentiate root, plexus, and peripheral nerve entrapment, and it will also demonstrate intrinsic muscle disorders (Fig. 3.9).

When you are contemplating surgery, the EMG may pinpoint the abnormal muscle activity. More importantly, because of the tremendous variation in innervation in the cervical spine, EMG will not necessarily reveal the anatomical level for surgery. If you are confident there is a root lesion, EMG offers very limited help in localizing the anatomical level.

CT/Myelography.   If you are sure you are dealing with a radiculopathy, but are unsure of the level, then the test of choice is CT/myelography. Picking the correct level for surgery only occurs if the patient has continuing radicular symptoms. In turn, the patient must state that he or she does not wish to live with the discomfort or the limitations it presents to activities of daily living, that is, the indications for surgery must be clear cut. The use of any expensive investigation as a substitute for a good clinical assessment, in the absence of surgical indications, is to be condemned.

There is a movement towards using MRI for level determination, but for reasons listed below, it is not the best choice. The gold standard for preoperative investigation of a chronic cervical radiculopathy still remains water-soluble myelography. The addition of postmyelographic CT gives another dimension to preoperative assessment (Fig. 3.10) (1).

Discography.   No topic turns friends into acquaintances more quickly than mentioning discography among a group of spine surgeons. There is no clear consensus as to the role of discography in localizing levels for surgery in cervical disc disease. Opinions on it range from "useless" to "the test of first choice."

We will take the middle road—discography is sometimes necessary to help localize the level of surgical intervention, but it is not nearly as reliable as a good clinical exam in combination with CT/myelography. If, after clinical assessment and CT/myelography, you are still unsure of the level that is the source of radicular pain, then discography may be useful. In this situation you are probably dealing with a patient who has mechanical neck pain and referred arm discomfort, rather than true radicular irritation or compression. When operating for neck pain rather than radicular pain, the chance of a successful surgical outcome is greatly reduced. There is no series in the literature to show that the outcome of surgery in this group of patients is raised to an acceptable level by discography.

Discography has many inherent problems that makes it an unreliable test:

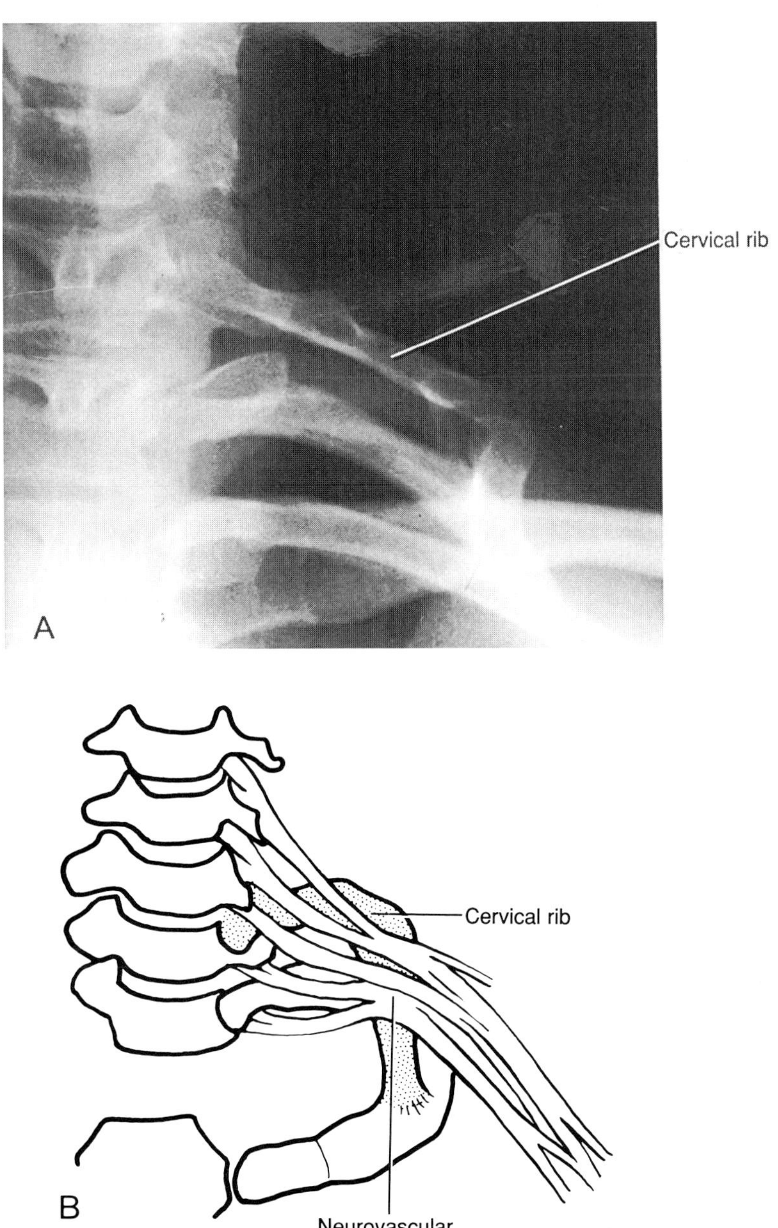

Figure 3.8.   A cervical rib attached to C7 may result in pressure on the neuro (brachial plexus) vascular (axillary artery) bundle.

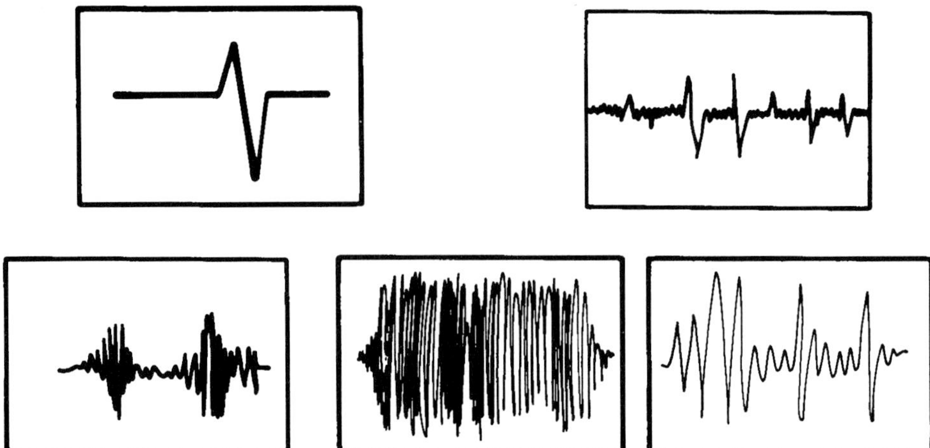

Figure 3.9.   Electromyographic patterns. *Top left*—normal muscle response. *Top right*—spontaneous fibrillation potentials at rest. Normal muscle is electrically silent at rest. *Bottom left*—polyphasic motor unit potentials; an abnormal response seen in neuropathies. *Bottom center*—maximum voluntary contractions are normal. *Bottom right*—maximum voluntary contractions are abnormally reduced in radiculopathy or polyneuropathy.

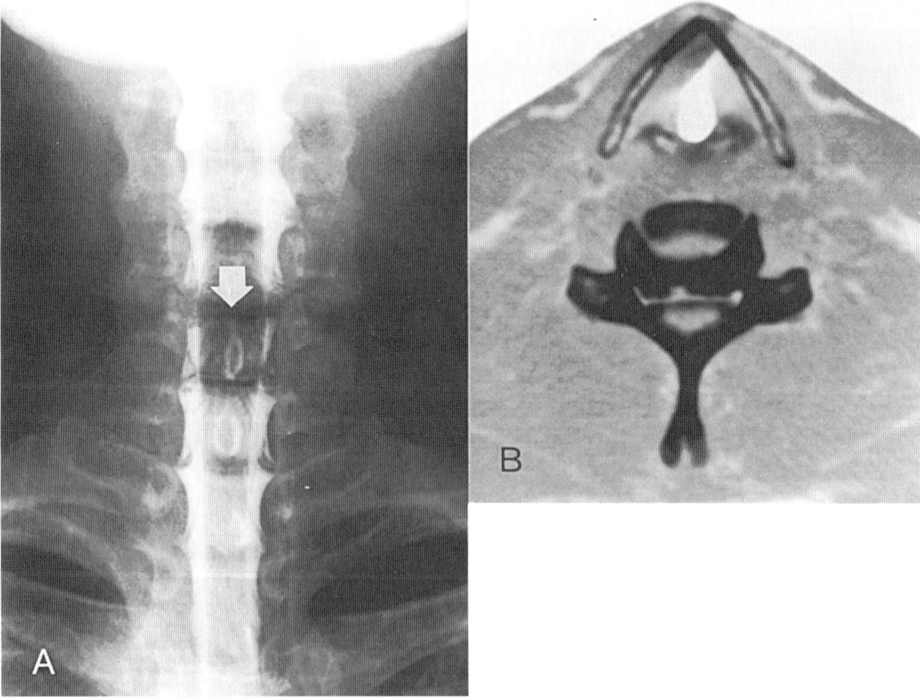

Figure 3.10.   A, myelography showing a localized stenotic lesion at C5-C6. **B,** postmyelographic axial CT showing the narrowing of the thecal sac and space available for the cord at C5-C6. The technique used reverses black/white and is much easier to interpret.

1. It is technically more difficult than lumbar discography even though it is done anteriorly and the distance from the skin to the disc can be reduced to near zero with finger pressure by the investigator. The reasons for the difficulty are:
   a. The disc you are trying to examine is not only narrowed; it often has anterior osteophytes.
   b. The slope of the disc from its anterior margin is upward, and it is necessary to start at a skin level lower than the anterior margin of the disc.
   c. It is relatively easy to perforate the esophagus before entering the disc space and introduce gastrointestinal flora into the disc space, leading to a disc space infection. There have been occasional reports of serious complications when this occurs, including patient death.
2. Any test that depends on patient response for interpretation is immediately suspect. Some patients simply are not reliable witnesses to events, especially when lying on a cold x-ray table in a dark room while some person they have never met is shoving needles into their throat! If you do need discography to help localize a level, make sure:
   a. You are satisfied that you are dealing with radicular involvement.
   b. You have a reliable patient whose disability is not complicated by a motor vehicle accident claim or worker's compensation claim.
   c. You have a radiologist skilled in the technique of discography and the interpretation of patient response.

One of the authors (J.M.) uses discography with all of the above limitations when a patient with obvious radicular pain, but a less obvious anatomical level clinically, has two or more lesions on CT/myelogram. Given a preference to do single-level surgery for radicular pain, discography is sometimes useful to pinpoint the clinically symptomatic level. The discogram cannot be equivocal. The patient has to state clearly on repeated gentle testing, that one level, and one level only, consistently produces pain in the correct arm in the correct distribution of his or her clinical complaint. Anything less, such as inconsistent reproduction of arm pain, reproduction of neck pain only, or reproduction of some arm discomfort at multiple levels immediately reduces the value of discography in surgical decision-making.

Magnetic Resonance Imaging.   In the lumbar spine, MRI is the test of choice to document a surgical lesion. In the cervical spine, the state of the MRI art has not reached the point where MRI is the "test of first choice" (Fig. 3.11).

Nerve Root Infiltration.   In chronic radiculopathies it is often difficult, because of subtle neurological changes, to determine which root is being irritated and/or compressed. In these patients the most useful diagnostic test is nerve root infiltration (9). If injection of local anesthetic into the nerve root emerging from the suspected segment abolishes the pain, the symptomatic level has been irrefutably confirmed.

Nerve root infiltration can be carried out from an anterior approach, a lateral approach, or a posterior approach (Fig. 3.12).

Anterior Approach.   The technique is simple. The sulcus between the anterior border of the sternomastoid and the midline structures is palpated with the tips of the fingers of the left hand; an 18-gauge needle is then inserted into the

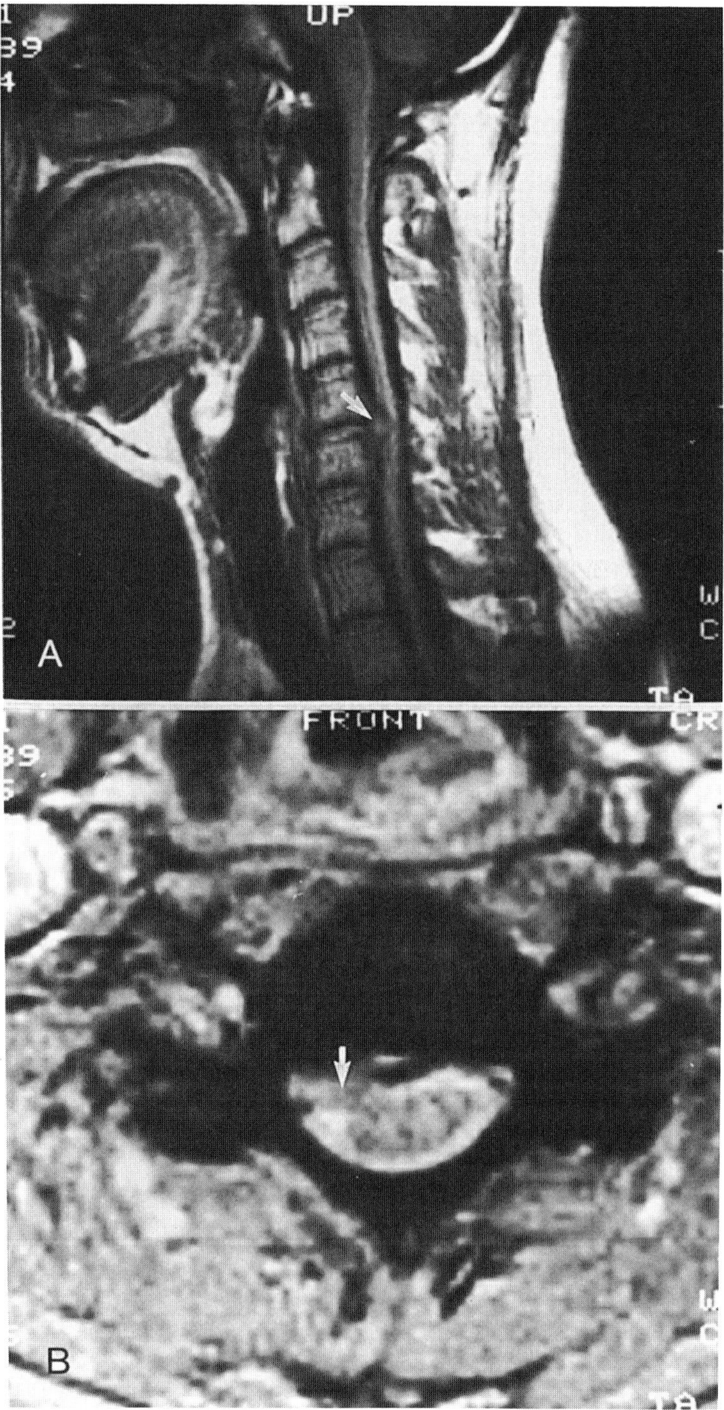

Figure 3.11.   **A**, a sagittal MRI showing an HNP at C5-6 and **B**, an axial at the same level (*arrows*).

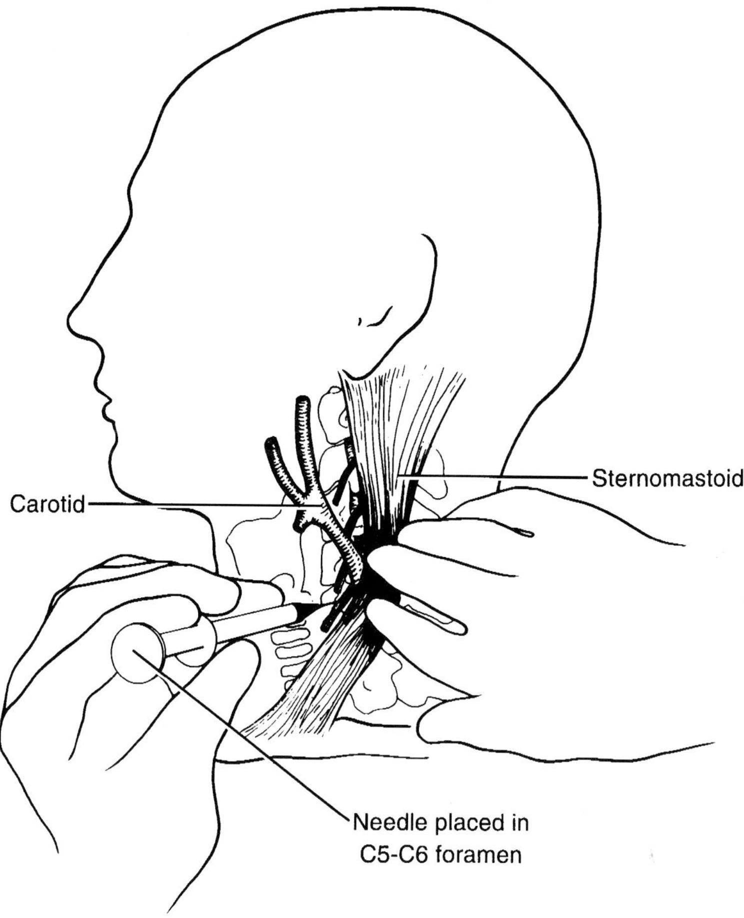

Figure 3.12. Technique of nerve root block, anterior approach. Obviously this is a percutaneous procedure, but in this schematic the important deeper structures have been drawn in. Do you remember Chassaignac's tubercle from Chapter 1? Figure 1.43 shows a nerve root block.

sulcus and directed posteromedially toward the tip of the transverse process immediately lateral to the vertebral artery. When the epidural sleeve is entered, the patient generally experiences a stab of pain radiating down the arm. Frequently, this is similar in character and distribution to the clinically experienced discomfort.

A small quantity of water-soluble contrast is now injected to outline the epidural sheath. If the needle has been correctly placed, the injected dye will assume a tubular configuration outlining the emerging nerve root (Fig. 1.43). Having confirmed the correct position of the needle, 1 ml of 2% lidocaine is now injected. Temporary abolition of symptoms following this injection confirms the site of the lesion.

Lateral Approach. The patient is placed in the supine position with the chin pointing upward. The transverse process is identified with the fingers. The needle is entered .5 cm anterior to the line joining the tip of the mastoid process to the tubercle of Chassaignac and directed to hit the transverse process one level above the suspected root. The needle is then withdrawn and directed downward and medially. This technique avoids the danger of inadvertently inserting the needle into the intervertebral foramen.

Posterior Approach.   The patient is placed on his or her side with the affected extremity uppermost. To inject the C3, C4, C5, and C6 nerve roots, the needle is inserted at a 45° angle—5 cm from the midline—and advanced until it abuts the transverse process. To inject the C7 and C8 nerve roots, the needle is inserted 7 cm from the midline at an angle of approximately 60°. The injection of the C7 and C8 nerve roots by the posterior approach is difficult because of the thickness of the tissues between the site of the puncture and the transverse process.

Three possible complications are associated with cervical nerve root infiltration:

1. It is possible to puncture a major vessel.
2. It is possible to penetrate the dura and injure the cord.
3. It is possible to penetrate the cupola and cause pneumothorax.

To avoid these complications, it is important that the superficial landmarks are strictly observed and identified. Gentle suction may be applied to the needle before injection of contrast material to make certain that neither blood nor cerebrospinal fluid is withdrawn.

Cervical Spondylotic Myelopathy (CSM)

Although it is unusual to have a patient with a chronic radiculopathy slip into a myelopathic state, it is not at all uncommon for a patient with myelopathy to have associated radicular symptoms. Although this section will describe a pure myelopathic clinical picture, be apprised that any of the previously described radicular symptoms and signs may be added to the myelopathic picture.

Myelopathic changes within the cervical spinal cord are due to the combination of:

1. A congenitally small bony spinal canal.
2. Degeneration in the cervical motion segment with
   - annular bulging and osteophytes.
   - facet hypertrophy.
   - ligamentum flavum infolding.
3. An abnormal cervical segment motion (i.e., forward or backward subluxation).
4. Vascular impairment of the substance of the spinal cord (8).

The four etiologic factors cause compression (1, 2, 3) and ischemia (4).

Changes in the upper extremities (mixed UMNL and LMNL) and lower extremities (UMNL) represent the most common cause of spastic paresis in the over-50 age group (5, 6). Men are affected more than women, and once symptomatic there is a better than 50% chance symptoms, signs, and functional impairment will deteriorate to the point of incapacity.

The condition was only clearly delineated in the 1950s by Brain (3, 4), and Clarke and Robinson (5), who pointed out the source of myelopathy as gradual encroachment by degenerative changes (spondylosis) rather than an acute disc herniation.

Clinical Presentation of Myelopathy

There are two patterns of neurological deficit, radicular (LMNL) and myelopathic (UMNL) that may affect both the upper and lower extremities, usually asymmetrically. If you're alert, you will have realized how LMNL in the lower extremities can occur with a lesion in the cervical spinal cord. Lumbar spinal canal stenosis occurs regularly in patients with CSM (it is known as tandem stenosis); it produces a concomitant LMNL in the lower extremities and confuses the neurological presentation of CSM. Patients with tandem stenosis will often have hyperreflexic knee jerks (UMNL), absent ankle jerks (LMNL), and equivocal toes. The examiner focused on lumbar canal stenosis will miss the cervical lesion, and an examiner similarly focused on the neck will miss the tandem lumbar stenosis.

In pure CSM the following findings may occur:

LMNL (radicular involvement in the upper extremity). The spondylotic bar or spur may cause LMNL changes at the level of the lesion. For example a bar and/or osteophyte at C5-C6 may cause biceps pain, biceps weakness, thumb and index paresthesia, and a depressed biceps reflex. Often described, but not always present in a C5 segment myelopathy, is the inverted supinator reflex (decreased or absent supinator reflex and finger flexion on tapping the brachioradialis at the wrist).

UMNL (upper extremity). In the example of a C5-C6 bar, below this level you will have brisk reflexes (e.g., triceps) and spastic weakness in the hands, often described as clumsiness by patients—they can't do up shirt buttons as readily as before, and they are starting to drop things.

Of course, multilevel spondylotic changes, more prominent on one side than the other, can present a very confusing neurological picture. As mentioned earlier, CSM is often but not always accompanied by radicular (LMNL) symptoms and signs.

UMNL (lower extremity). The first disturbance is usually in gait (10). The English expression is, "the patient is going off his or her legs." Patients describe a slowness and stiffness when walking, which progresses to unsteadiness. They describe difficulty with stairs and scuffing of shoes. As with the upper extremities, the symptoms may be more pronounced in one leg. As CSM progresses, the gait becomes broad based (to compensate for the imbalance from posterior column compression) and jerky (spastic from the lateral column compression). Patients quickly learn that flexing the neck relieves symptoms (by opening the spinal canal) and as a result, walk stooped over. The Romberg sign may be positive. Neurological examination of the lower extremities demonstrates increased tone, increased reflexes, upgoing toes, and clonus in varying stages of development (i.e., early and hard to find vs. late and obvious) with or without asymmetry.

Miscellaneous Symptoms and Signs in Myelopathy

Neck Pain and Stiffness. Often, CSM patients have little neck pain (except in the past) and lots of neck stiffness. As the condition developed over the years, the normal range of movement (ROM) was painful, only to be reduced in range by the spondylotic changes that, in turn, stiffen the neck and reduce neck pain, but encroach upon spinal column territory.

Table 3.4.   Assessment Scale Proposed by Japanese Orthopaedic Association

1. Motor dysfunction of the upper extremity
    Score
    0 = Unable to feed oneself
    1 = Unable to handle chopsticks, able to eat with a spoon
    2 = Handles chopsticks with much difficulty
    3 = Handles chopsticks with slight difficulty
    4 = None
2. Motor dysfunction of the lower extremity
    Score
    0 = Unable to work
    1 = Walks on flat floor with walking aid
    2 = Up and/or down stairs with handrail
    3 = Lack of stability and smooth reciprocation
    4 = None
3. Sensory deficit
    A. The upper extremity
        Score
        0 = Severe sensory loss or pain
        1 = Mild sensory loss
        2 = None
    B. The lower extremity, same as A
    C. The trunk, same as A
4. Sphincter dysfunction
    Score
    0 = Unable to void
    1 = Marked difficulty in micturition (retention, strangury)
    2 = Difficulty in micturition (pollakiuria, hesitation)
    3 = None

Bladder and Bowel.   Bladder and bowel symptoms are rare early in the disease. Later, when the lower extremities have reached paresis, the bladder sphincters may also be incontinent.

Lhermitte's Phenomenon.   Flexion or extension of the neck that sends lightening-like sensations down the trunk, arms, and legs is known as Lhermitte's phenomenon. This symptom occasionally occurs in CSM.

Differential Diagnosis in CSM

The aging process and all its potential diagnoses, the mixture of UMNL and LMNL, and the asymmetry of CSM—all combine to make the diagnosis very difficult. For this reason a complete chapter (Chapter 21) has been set aside to discuss the differential diagnoses of all conditions of the neck and shoulder.

Progression of CSM

There is no set pattern to progression of neurological changes and functional impairment (10). It is likely that 50% of symptomatic patients will gradually deteriorate to significant limitation of functional level. Approximately 5% will do so very quickly, even over a period of hours. This is thought to be due to a vascular lesion and ischemia of the cord (2, 11). The rest will deteriorate slowly over months, some with remission and exacerbation, and some steadily. Less than 50% of patients will plateau and not lose ambulatory ability. The Japanese Ortho-

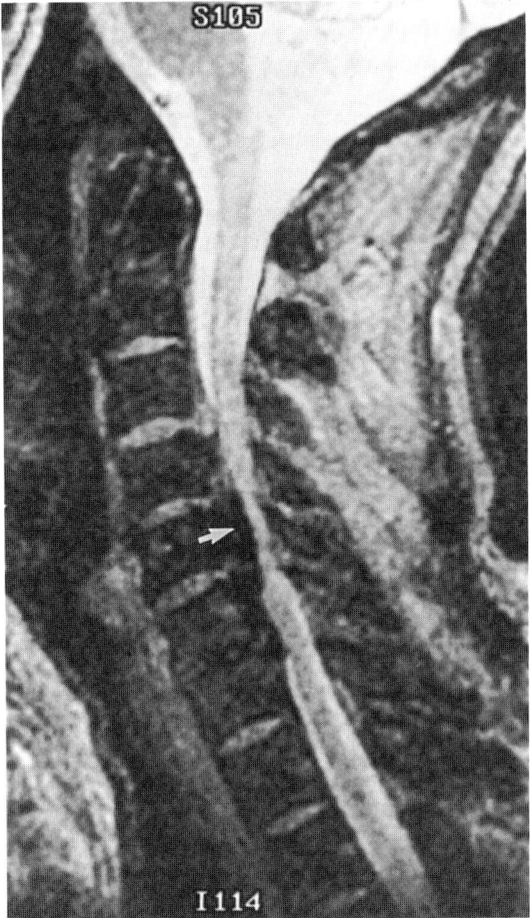

Figure 3.13.   OPLL on axial CT. Note how the calcification extends well down behind the vertebral body (*arrow*).

pedic Association has developed a scale of severity to assess patients with CSM. A patient who scores low is more disabled. The scoring is also useful for postoperative follow-up (Table 3.4).

Ossification of the Posterior Longitudinal Ligament.   Ossification of the posterior longitudinal ligament (OPLL) causing cervical myelopathy is very common in Japan and is assuming a higher profile in other parts of the world (Fig. 2.6).

Ossification of the PLL narrows the spinal canal with resulting cord encroachment. It is usually most pronounced behind C5 but can extend over more than one segment and even skip segments to involve multiple cervical levels.

The best depiction of OPLL is with CT or MRI showing ossification from pedicle to pedicle and behind the vertebral bodies, in contrast to cervical degenerative disc disease, where osteophytes rarely form pedicle to pedicle and are always opposite the disc space (Fig. 3.13).

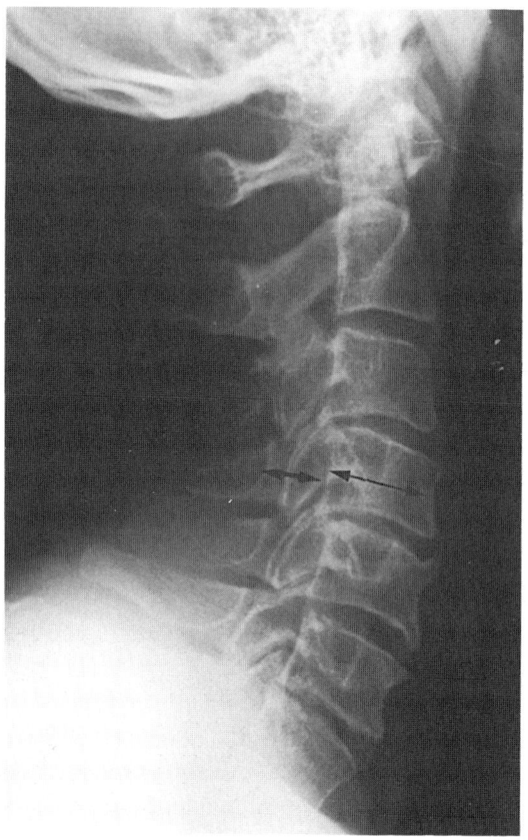

Figure 3.14.   Plain lateral x-rays showing a narrowed spinal canal (*arrows*).

Investigation of the Patient With Myelopathy.   Plain Films.   Obviously, plain radiographs are necessary to build the case for myelopathy (Fig. 3.14).

CT/myelography.   The gold standard for investigation of cervical myelopathy remains CT/myelography (Fig. 3.15). At the time of myelography, CSF must be sent for analysis if there are any differential diagnostic problems.

MRI.   MRI limitations have been outlined in the preceding section on radiculopathy. An MRI of cervical myelopathy is shown in Figure 3.16.

Vertebral Basilar Insufficiency

Osteophytes that project laterally from the uncovertebral joint or anteriorly from the inferior facet can compress and distort the vertebral artery. Because of collateral supply in the vertebral basilar system, a lesion on one side is rarely symptomatic (Fig. 3.17).

Symptomatic patients will complain of vertigo or giddiness, visual symptoms (diplopia), and ataxia with episodes of syncope. All of these symptoms can be exacerbated by neck movements and can sometimes be profoundly aggravated, resulting in death, by therapeutic neck manipulation.

The diagnosis is made by dynamic angiography with the patient positioning the neck in the most symptomatic position during contrast injection. If a discrete

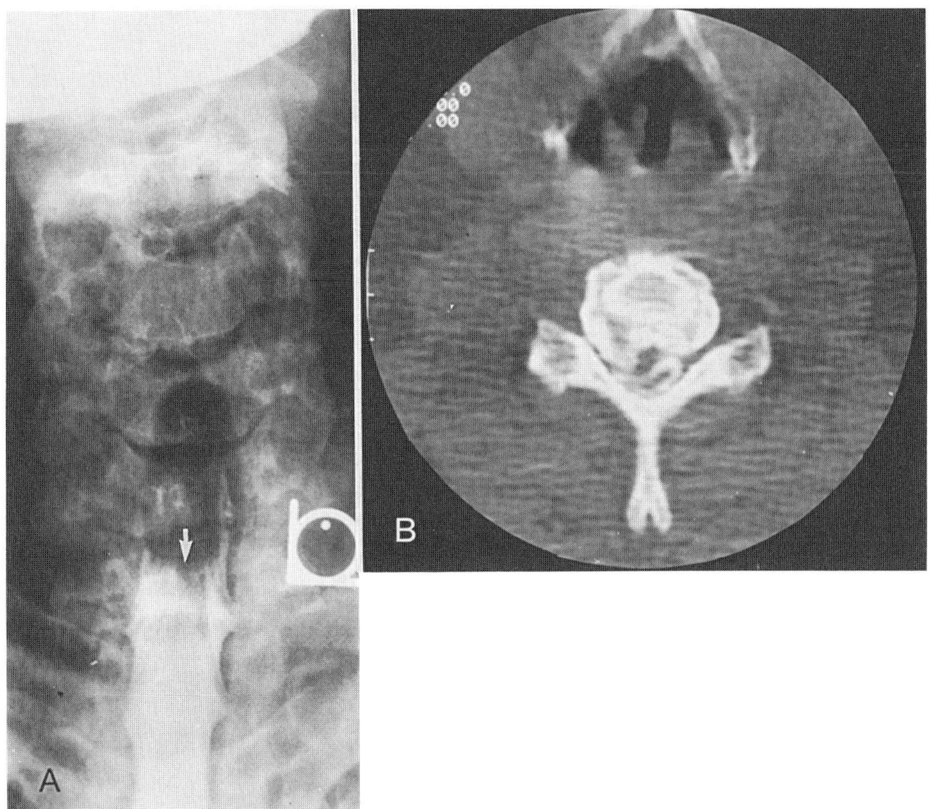

Figure 3.15.   Myelography (**A**) and CT/myelogram (**B**) showing multilevel spondylotic bars interfering with the flow of contrast material (*arrow*).

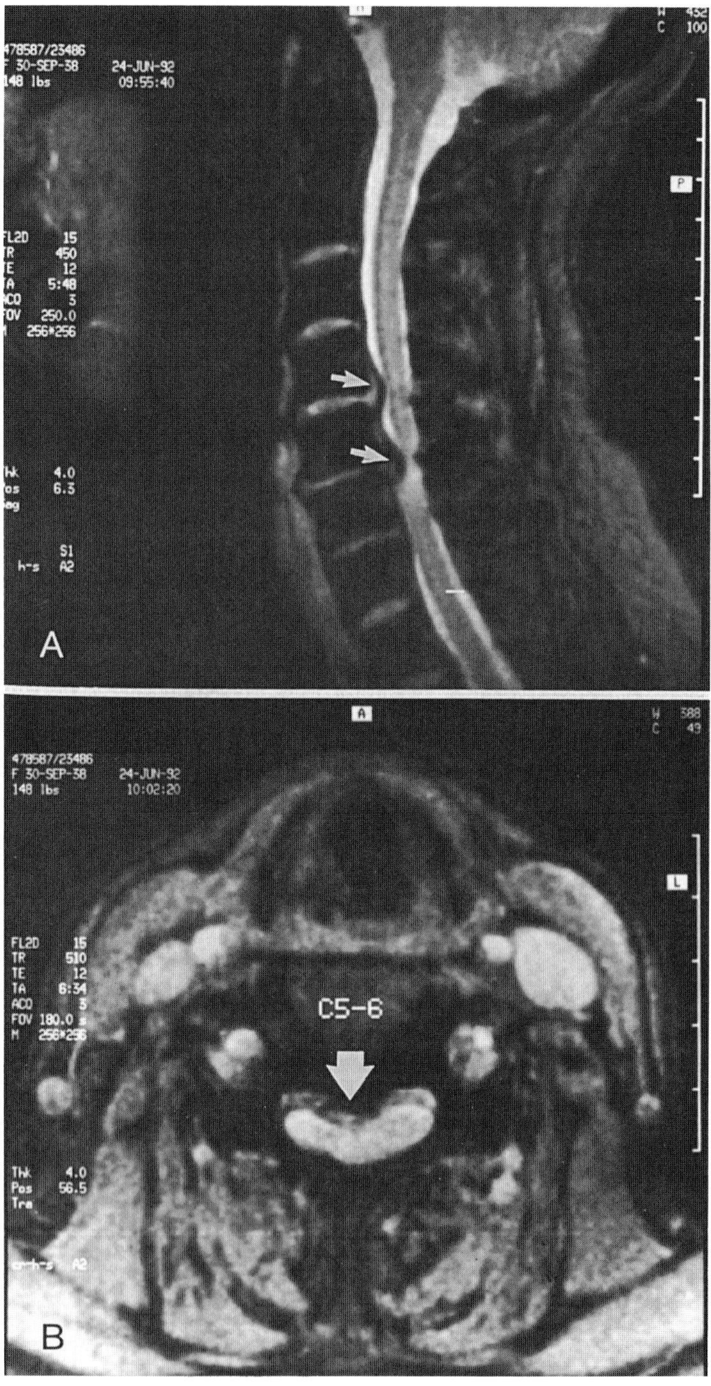

Figure 3.16.   Sagittal (**A**) and axial (**B**) MRI in spondylotic myelopathy (*arrows*).

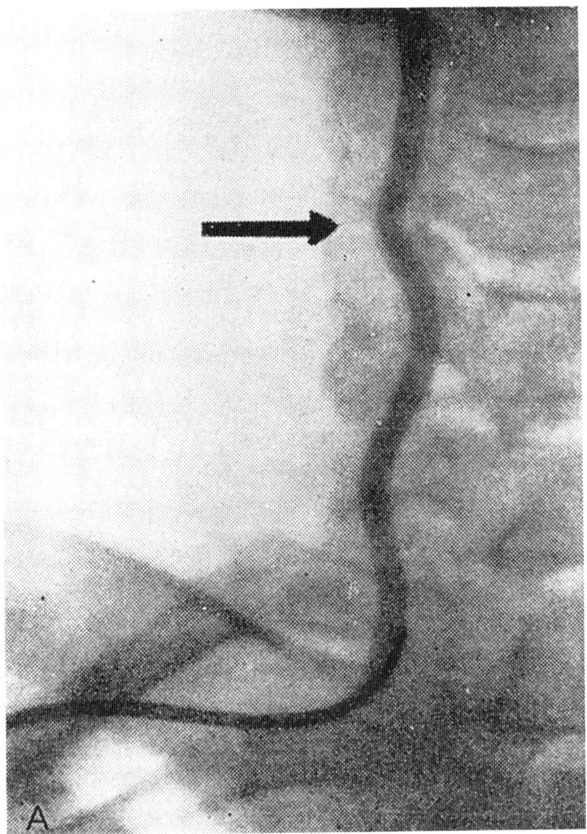

Figure 3.17.   A, vertebral arteriogram showing vertebral artery being deflected by an osteophyte.
B, schematic showing a more severe form of vertebral artery occlusion.

lesion is demonstrated, then an anterior decompression is indicated. Because of
the venous plexus around the vertebral artery, the adhesions that develop, and
the thin friable vertebral artery wall, this can be a very bloody operation.

REFERENCES

1. Bohlman HH: Cervical spondylosis with moderate to severe myelopathy. Spine 2:151–162 (1977).
2. Bohlman HH and Emery SE: The pathophysiology of cervical spondylosis and myelopathy. Spine 13:843–846 (1988).
3. Brain R: Cervical spondylosis. Ann Intern Med 41:439–441 (1954).
4. Brain RW, Northfield D, and Wilkinson M: The neurological manifestations of cervical spondylosis. Brain 75:187–225 (1952).
5. Clarke E and Robinson PK: Cervical myelopathy: a complication of cervical spondylosis. Brain 79:483–510 (1956).
6. Crandal PH and Butzdorf U: Cervical spondylotic myelopathy. J Neurosurg 25:51–66 (1966).
7. Dillan W, Booth R, Cuckler J, Balderston R, Simeone F, and Rothman R: Cervical radiculopathy: a review. Spine 11:988–991 (1986).
8. Gooding MR, Wilson CB, and Hoff JT: Experimental cervical myelopathy: effects of ischemia and compression of the canine cervical spinal cord. J Neurosurg 43:9–17 (1975).
9. Kikuchi S, Macnab I, and Moreau P: Localization of level of symptomatic cervical disc degeneration. J Bone Joint Surg 63B:272–277 (1981).

10. LaRocca H: Cervical spondylotic myelopathy: natural history. Spine 13:854–855 (1988).
11. Ono K, Ota H, Tadak K, and Yamamoto T: Cervical myelopathy secondary to multiple spondylotic protrusions—a clinicopathologic study. Spine 2:109–125 (1977).

4

Treatment of Cervical Disc Disease

"Physical pain is not a simple affair of an impulse, traveling at a fixed rate, along a nerve. It is the resultant of a conflict between a stimulus and the whole individual."
—René Leriche

INTRODUCTION

The symptoms of cervicobrachial pain derived from disc degeneration are usually insidious in onset. A careful, detailed history commonly reveals that over a long period of time the patient has been "conscious" of his or her neck. Frequently, the patient will relate recurrent episodes of a "stiff neck" or a "crick" in the neck. More commonly, the patients will attribute the onset of symptoms to a specific incident; for example, "I drove home with the car window open."

Occasionally, the onset is sudden, dramatic, unanticipated, and unrelated to any precipitating activity. The patient may awaken one morning with an extremely painful stiff neck; during the passage of the day, the pain may radiate to the shoulders and interscapular region, rendering the patient painfully immobile. Such episodes generally subside within 10 to 14 days with or without treatment but have an unfortunate tendency to recur. Eventually the patient presents continuing symptoms affecting the axial skeleton and/or its neurological contents. With your knowledge of pathogenesis (Chapter 2) and your clinical exam (Chapter 3), you have established a diagnosis and can prepare for treatment.

The treatment decision in cervical disc disease is based on a clear understanding of four factors:

1. Do you have an accurate diagnosis? Is this a soft tissue syndrome, a discogenic problem, a root encroachment problem, a cord encroachment problem, or a combination of various syndromes?
2. Do you know your anatomical level? Compared to lumbar disc syndromes, determining symptomatic anatomical levels in cervical disc disease is much more difficult for reasons mentioned in Chapter 3.
3. Do you know your patient? Is he or she accurately reporting the disability, or is there some embellishment for medical-legal or compensation purposes?
4. What is the functional limitation? Is this collection of minor symptoms of nuisance value to the patient, or is there cord compression to the point that the patient needs aids for ambulation?

CONSERVATIVE TREATMENT

Choices in conservative treatment can be classified into:

1. Rest

2. Medication
3. Modalities
4. Manipulation, mobilization, and massage
5. Miscellaneous (e.g., transcutaneous electric nerve stimulation (TENS) unit, trigger point injections, and epidural steroids)
6. Exercise
7. Education

Probably the most important treatment decision is to be patient. Don't get too aggressive, because most of the symptoms associated with cervical disc disease are self-limiting and will go away spontaneously whether or not a doctor, physical therapist, or chiropractor is involved. How many spectacular cures have been claimed by these disciplines, when in fact the resolution of symptoms was due to the wonderful ability of the neck to spontaneously stabilize a segment and abolish symptoms!

Rest

There are many forms of rest, including bed rest, external collars, and traction. Even exercise, by rebuilding muscular strength, which in turn reduces stress on joints, can be included as a restful treatment modality.

Bed Rest

Occasionally, the pain is so severe that patients cannot cope with the daily rounds of life, even with the help of analgesics, sedation, and wearing a cervical collar. Under such circumstances, patients should be advised to go to bed. It must be remembered that the strained posterior joints of the cervical spine have to support the weight of the head, which is approximately 15 lb. The only way to take this weight away from the posterior joints is to persuade the patient to lie down in bed. Some patients are most comfortable sitting in bed with the head and shoulders supported by two or three pillows. Others prefer to use the "dog bone" pillow (Fig. 4.1). Still others prefer to wear a cervical collar and have just a baby pillow under the occiput. There is no general rule. During the day, there is no reason patients should not prop themselves up with several pillows and entertain themselves, either by reading or watching television; nothing is more soul-destroying than lying in bed glaring balefully at the ceiling without any promise from the physician about the cessation of their tribulations.

Modification of Activities

It is an unusual situation in which modification of activity can play a significant role in the management of neck pain. In the low back, bending and lifting may aggravate back pain, and it may be possible to eliminate that activity and effect treatment. In the neck, about the only activity that consistently bothers patients is extension, for example, homemakers working in high kitchen cupboards or construction workers doing a lot of overhead work. In today's tough economic times, a suggestion to modify work too often leads to a layoff. For this reason we play down work modification unless the pain is terribly acute and requires bed rest, or the chronic pain is not resolving with other treatment measures and there is a clearly defined work aggravation. Overall, work modification

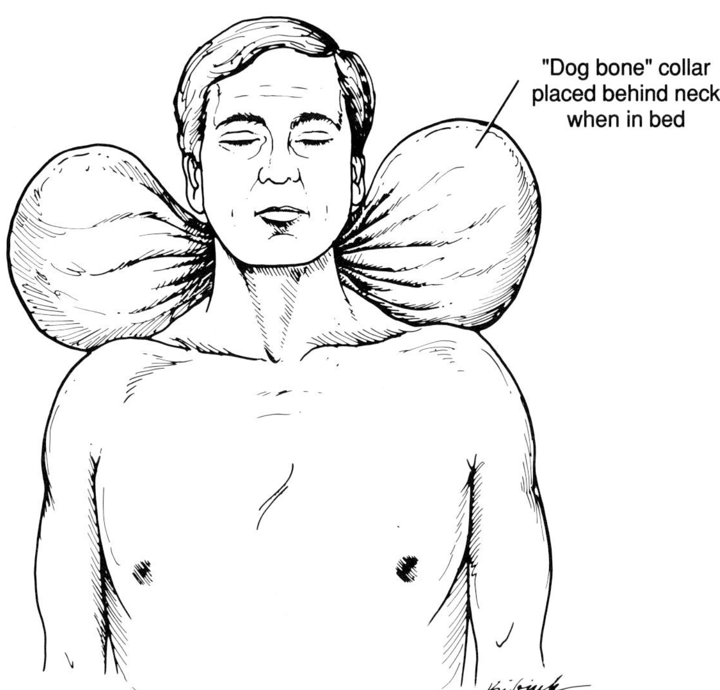

Figure 4.1.   There are many varieties of cervical pillows. This is the so-called dog bone pillow, which the patient can make out of an old feather or down pillow by removing some of the stuffing.

is not a high-priority conservative treatment modality for management of cervical disc disease.

Cervical Collars (Orthoses)

There is a long history of neck bracing extending back to Hippocrates. As the years rolled by, braces were designated by various descriptive terms, such as what they looked like (e.g., four-poster) or where they came from (Philadelphia collar). Recently, Krag (13) has tried to bring some clarity to cervical orthoses, and his modified classification is presented in Table 4.1. Table 4.2 is adapted from Johnson et al. (12) and shows the extent of decreased movement that can be expected when using various collars. The use of more rigid collars is discussed in the chapters on fractures, tumors, and infections.

For degenerative conditions of the spine, cervical and cervical–base of skull: high thoracic collars (Table 4.2, *a* and *c*) are the most frequently used varieties (Figs. 4.2, 4.3, and 4.4). The soft cervical collar, with no base of skull extension or thoracic extension, offers very little immobilization of the neck. It is something for the chin to rest on and reminds the patient that a treatment program is in progress. As such, it is largely a decorative placebo device. For more limitation of neck motion, the Philadelphia collar is the best choice for degenerative cervical conditions. At night, the patient may wear a soft cervical collar—it is impossible to sleep for any length of time in a Philadelphia collar. Better still, prescribe a cervical pillow that holds but doesn't restrict the neck (Fig. 4.1).

Table 4.1.   Classification of Cervical Bracing (modified from Krag) (13)

Classification	Types
a) Cervical	Soft foam in stockinette (Fig. 4.2) Rigid
b) Cervical-base of skull	Mandibular and/or occipital support added to cervical collar (e.g., Queen Anne) (Fig. 4.3)
c) Cervical-base of skull -high thoracic	Shoulder support added to collar b) e.g., 4-poster (Thomas) and Philadelphia (Fig. 4.4)
d) Cervical-base of skull -low thoracic	Chest extension added to collar c) e.g., extended Philadelphia or Somi brace (Fig. 4.5)
e) Cranial-thoracic	Halo (Fig. 4.6)

Table 4.2.   Amount of Movement Decreased by Various Cervical Orthoses (modified from Johnson et al.) (12)

	Flexion/Extension	Lateral Flexion	Rotation
a) Cervical	25%	10%	20%
b) Cervical-base of skull	25%	10%	20%
c) Cervical-base of skull: high thoracic	75%	30%	50%
d) Cervical-base of skull: low thoracic	80%	50%	80%
e) Halo	Decreases all movements close to 100%		

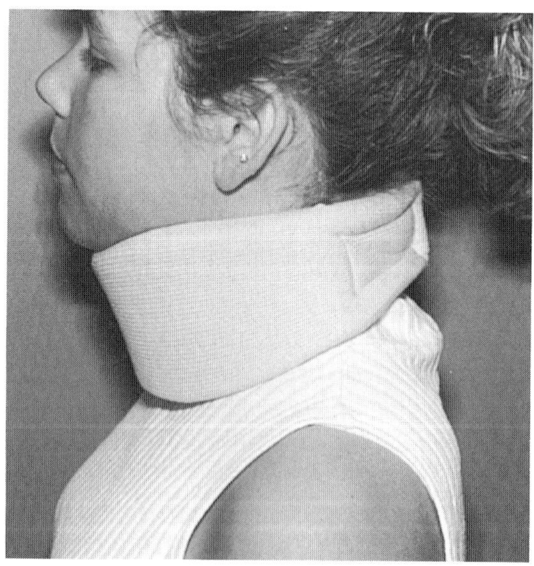

Figure 4.2.   A soft cervical collar.

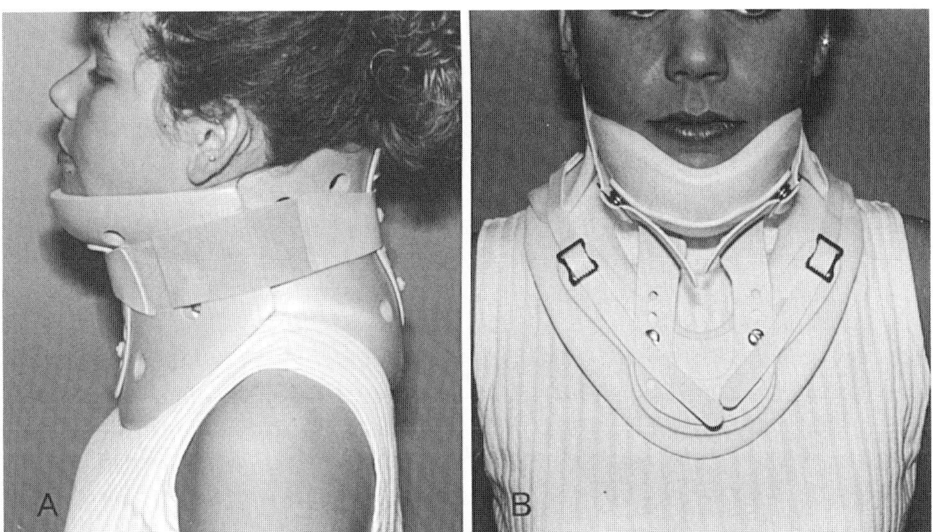

Figure 4.3. **A,** Philadelphia collar (cervical-base of skull: high thoracic). **B,** Malibu collar (cervical-base of skull: high thoracic).

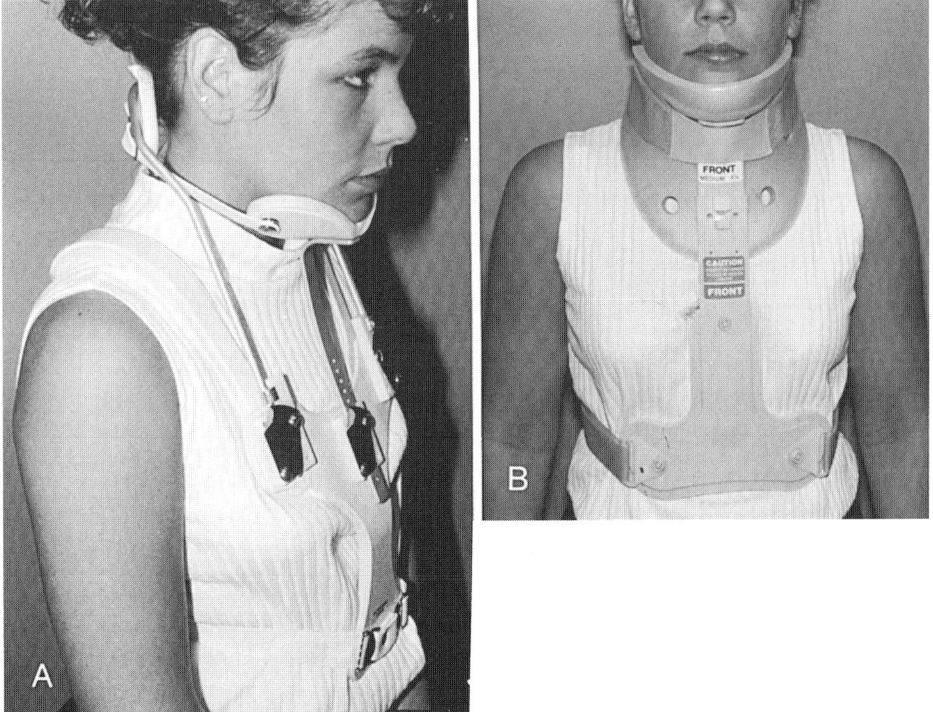

Figure 4.4. **A,** Somi collar (sternal-occipital-mandibular immobilizer) (cervical-base of skull: low thoracic). **B,** an extended Philadelphia collar (cervical-base of skull: low thoracic).

Traction

Traction, or stretching of the neck, is thought to passively lengthen muscles and ligaments, resulting in a decrease in intradiscal pressure. To test its value, do some stretching in the office. Have the patient lie down on the examining table and place your hands around the angle of the jaw. Longitudinal traction should be applied by holding the neck in slight flexion. The traction should be applied gently and maintained for one or two minutes. If the patient admits to some relief of discomfort on application of manual traction, then a course of traction is a logical form of treatment.

If traction is to be considered, a good place to start is under the supervision of a physical therapist. The physiotherapist should be requested to attempt to relax some of the spasm of the paracervical muscles with one of the modalities of heat prior to the application of traction. Traction should be applied with the patient reclining; the angle of traction should have the neck pulled in slight flexion. Because the mandibular portion of a head halter is shorter than the occipital sling, there is a built-in tendency to pull the neck into extension. The traction cord must be pulled forward so that the major force is exerted on the occiput. Excessive pull on the anterior portion of the sling may produce discomfort in the temporomandibular joint, and this must be avoided. Occasionally, the patient has to wear a bite plate while traction is applied. The precise angle of flexion is extremely important and varies from patient to patient. The angle of traction should be altered until the patient feels relief. To begin with, the effect of minimal traction (10 lb) should be assessed. If the patient is comfortable during the application of such traction, the weight can be increased to 12–20 lb, provided this produces a greater degree of relief from discomfort.

Traction should not be continued unless the patient experiences relief of pain while traction is actually being applied. Once the patient has been shown how to apply traction in a manner that relieves pain, he/she should continue this form of therapy at home to avoid the time-consuming daily trips to a physiotherapy department.

Although many home traction kits are available, probably the simplest and best is the gibbet-like device that hangs over a door frame. The traction is applied with the patient sitting in a chair facing the door (Fig. 4.5). By moving the chair, the patient can alter the angle of traction applied. A doorstop should be put under the open door. The patient must be given detailed instructions on the use of cervical traction, and the traction should be applied for 15 minutes, three times a day, with 12 to 20 lb.

Remember, traction is only of value if the patient experiences significant relief from discomfort during the application and for some time afterwards. Once the patient notices little change in symptoms while the traction is being applied, or if the patient notices that pain is aggravated after a period of traction, treatment should be discontinued. However, because of the unfortunate propensity of symptoms to recur, the patient should keep the apparatus against the evil day when the pain may return.

Although the mode of action of traction is not understood, the fact remains that traction appears to shorten the duration of arm symptoms in particular.

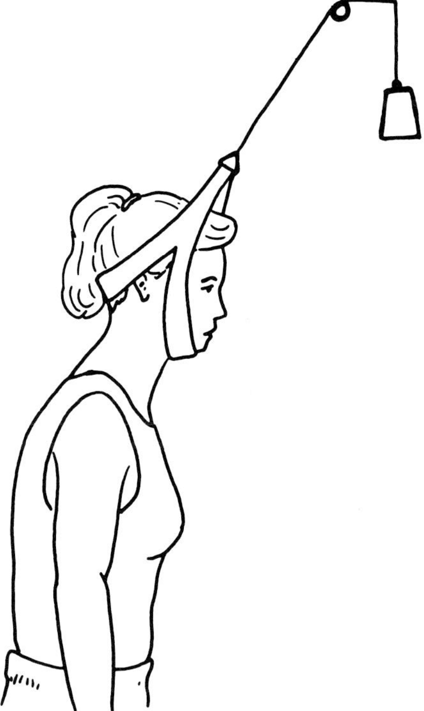

Figure 4.5. Cervical "home" traction.

Because of the intermittent decrease in discomfort, traction also cuts down on the need for analgesics.

Medication

Analgesics

Analgesics are usually the first line medications for pain (9). The choices are simple—use nonnarcotics (acetaminophen [Tylenol]) or narcotic medication in increasing potency (Table 4.3) for more severe pain. There are obvious problems with the introduction of pain medication in a potentially chronic neck problem; the use of narcotics and the symptom of neck pain may become chronic together (23). For this reason nonsteroidal anti-inflammatory drugs have become a very popular method of dealing with musculoskeletal pain.

NSAIDs (Nonsteroidal anti-inflammatory drugs)

Because of their analgesic, anti-inflammatory and antipyretic actions, NSAIDs have become a popular group of drugs (3, 22). They are thought to act at the (peripheral) site of injury, rather than centrally, by blocking prostaglandin synthesis; prostaglandins supposedly sensitize free nerve endings to nociceptor impulses. The equation is simple: inflammation leads to increased prostaglandin synthesis and thus pain: anti-inflammatories decrease the prostaglandin synthesis of inflammation and thus decrease pain. At low doses NSAIDs are analgesic and at higher sustained doses they are anti-inflammatory.

Table 4.3.   Analgesic Medications

1. Nonnarcotic-ASA, NSAIDs
2. Narcotic Analgesics
   a) Moderate pain (agonists)
        Codeine
        hydrocodone (Vicodin)
        oxycodone (Percodan, Percocet, Tylox)
        propoxyphene (Darvon)
   b) Moderate to severe pain (agonists)
        meperidine (Demerol)
        Morphine
        hydromorphone (Dilaudid)
        levorphanol (Levo-Dromoran)
   c) Moderate pain (mixed agonists/antagonists)
        pentazocine (Talwin)

Table 4.4.   Commonly Used NSAIDs

Class	Chemical Name	Trade Name
Salicylates	Aspirin	Numerous
	Enteric Coated ASA	Ecotrin
Salicylate Substitutes	Diflunisal	Dolobid
	Salsalate	Disalcid
Propionic Acid Derivatives	Ibuprofen	Motrin
	Naproxen	Naprosyn
	Ketoprofen	Orudis
	Flurbiprofen	Ansaid
	Ketorolac Tromethamine	Toradol
Indoles (Acetic Acids)	Sulindac	Clinoril
	Indomethacin	Indocin
	Tolmetin	Tolectin
Oxicam	Piroxicam	Feldene
Pyrazalones	Phenylbutazone	Butazolidin

Metabolism of NSAIDs occurs in the liver but side effects are largely confined to the gastrointestinal tract and the kidneys. Indomethacin and phenylbutazone have the added toxicity of bone marrow suppression. The older patient is especially prone to these side effects from those NSAIDs with a long half life (Dolobid, Naprosyn, Clinoril, Feldene, and Butazolidin). Doses of these drugs have to be lower in the geriatric population; anyone with GI upset—young or old—has to receive gastric protection (e.g., H2-receptor antagonists like Tagamet) or come off the NSAID. Because they lead to water retention, hypertensive patients need careful monitoring of blood pressure. NSAIDs also inhibit platelet aggregation, and most surgeons ask patients to stop anti-inflammatory drugs for 10 days prior to surgery. Table 4.4 lists the commonly used anti-inflammatory drugs.

Gastrointestinal complications are the most common side effects of NSAIDs and deserve special mention (2). The chance of a patient on NSAIDs developing an ulcer (gastric or duodenal) range from 2%–20%; approximately 20%–40% of patients admitted to hospitals with acute upper GI bleeding have been on NSAIDs. To prevent these complications Babb recommends:

1. Prescribe the lowest possible dose, and avoid combinations with other NSAIDs and corticosteroids.
2. If patients especially at risk for NSAID gastropathy (the elderly, the chronically ill, and those with a history of peptic ulcer disease) have to be given an NSAID, prophylactic ulcer therapy should be considered.
3. The prevention of NSAID ulcers remains controversial. Misoprostol (Cytotec) helps to prevent gastric ulcers, but its use in duodenal ulcer prophylaxis is unclear. H2-receptor antagonists, such as ranitidine (Zantac), help prevent duodenal ulcers but not gastric ulcers.

Corticosteroids

Corticosteroids are mentioned mainly to caution against their use. On occasion, an acute radicular pain is so severe that a very aggressive short-term therapy program lasting three to seven days may be instituted. A Medrol dose pack is a convenient way to prescribe. Frequent use of this treatment modality in your practice, or prolonged use in an individual, is simply not good medical judgement.

Muscle Relaxants

The next most-used group of drugs for cervical conditions is the muscle relaxants—and nobody can explain why. They all work on the central nervous system with hopeful transfer of the action to the peripheral site of muscle spasm (6). No scientific proof exists to support this transfer phenomenon. The common muscle relaxants are cyclobenzaprine (Flexeril), orphenadrine citrate (Norflex), chlorzoxazone (Parafon Forte), methocarbamol (Robaxin), carisoprodol (Soma), and diazepam (Valium). To make them even more attractive, drug manufacturers have parceled them together with analgesics: Norflex + acetylsalicylic acid (ASA) + caffeine (Norgesic), methocarbamol + ASA (Robaxisal), and carisoprodol + codeine (Soma Compound). When the side effects of depression and a "spaced-out" feeling are combined with the potential for habituation—and in light of their cost and the lack of scientific support for their usefulness—one has to wonder why so many muscle relaxants are prescribed.

Antidepressants

Patients who suffer from chronic pain are thought to become depressed because of, or in addition to, depletion of serotonin in the brain. Antidepressants supposedly increase serotonin production in the CNS, which in turn inhibits pain (20, 25). Other antidepressant effects are to increase activity in the endogenous opiate system and to decrease anxiety and muscle tension. Commonly used antidepressants are imipramine (Tofranil), amitriptyline (Elavil) and doxepin (Sinequan).

Antidepressants have a high incidence of side effects including frequent cross-drug reactions with antihypertensive and glaucoma medication. Unless you are prepared to closely monitor the patient for side effects, don't use these drugs.

Modalities

How often have you written a prescription for physical therapy and wondered: "What will happen to the patient in that department in the basement?" One of the common things a physical therapist does is change the temperature of the affected body part (14).

Ice

Ice packs decrease circulation to the area of contact which reduces swelling, spasm, and therefore pain.

Heat

Heat may be superficial (hot packs or infra red) or deep (ultrasound or short-wave diathermy). The heat increases blood flow to the damaged or inflamed tissue, clearing away noxious metabolites and bringing oxygen to the area. Heat also increases the stretch ability of collagen tissue.

Manipulation, Mobilization, and Massage

The laying on of hands! This act alone has a significant placebo effect on patients. Controversy surrounds these modalities, yet the practitioners of these manual efforts continue to make patients better (7, 8, 11, 19, 24). Massage is designed to break down scar tissue and stretch local muscles. It is a very soothing therapy.

Manipulation is practiced largely by the chiropractic community, while mobilization is a tool of the physical therapist (21). The latter feel it is safer and gentler to mobilize a painful joint by passively coaxing a joint (or joints as in the case of the neck) to its normal physiological range of movement. Chiropractors, on the other hand, propose that sudden, assisted, passive joint motion—just beyond the normal range of movement—is more effective in stretching muscles, reducing subluxated joints, and increasing joint movement.

Miscellaneous

Transcutaneous Electric Nerve Stimulation. Live better electrically! TENS units theoretically close gates in the CNS (Fig. 4.6). By transcutaneously sending an electric impulse into the peripheral nerve, the large (fast conducting) myelinated A-alpha nerve fibers are stimulated such that the smaller (slower conducting) unmyelinated C-fibers are blocked at the gate from transmitting their nociceptor impulses. It is sort of like the big guy beating up on the little guy so that he is not heard from! Whether this concept works is under serious scrutiny (4, 5, 26).

Acupuncture. Again controversy abounds! The theory makes sense: acupuncture is a counterirritant and a stimulator of endorphin release. It is also thought to close gates and modulate the transfer of painful stimuli to higher CNS centers (16). In North America, it is hard to find scientific evidence to support its efficacy.

Injections. Injections of local anesthetics and/or steroids may be given to painful muscles (trigger point injections) (15), painful joints (facet joint injections) (17), or the epidural space. There is little scientific evidence to support their use. Rather, claims of effectiveness are founded in placebo effect, an excellent doctor-patient relationship where everything works, or a functional patient taken in by the power of suggestion. These particular treatment modalities cry out for randomized clinical trials to test their efficacy.

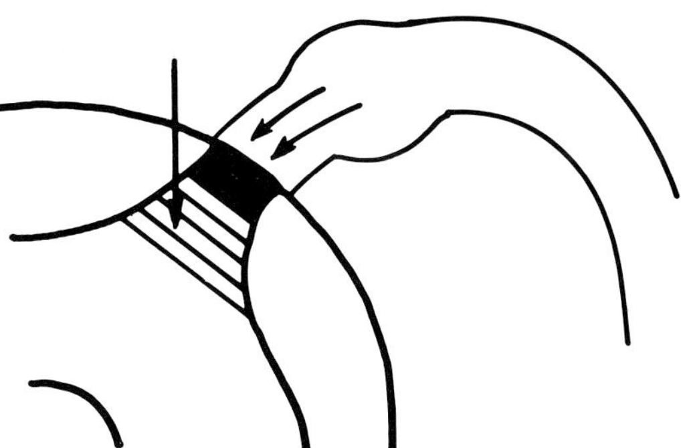

Figure 4.6.   The gate control theory of pain: sensory fibers (*double arrows*) arrive in lamina of dorsal horn. Higher centers (*single arrow*) influence whether or not "gate" opens for transmission of pain impulses. Peripheral nerve stimulation (TENS) is thought to close the gate from below.

Exercise.   All of the various modalities discussed in the preceding section are attempts to help the patient cope with the pain. Exercises, by strengthening muscles and mobilizing joints, have the potential to speed up the body's natural healing powers (10). They should be started as the pain subsides. They represent active efforts on the part of the patient and may be resistive or aerobic in nature. Resisted exercises are isometric (producing an increase in muscle tension without a change in muscle fiber length), isotonic (decreasing fiber length with no change in tension) or isokinetic (moving muscles and joints at a resisted but controlled rate of speed). For neck disorders, active and passive range-of-movement exercises are followed by isometric strengthening exercises (see Appendix for neck exercise programs).

Education.   Education for neck pain takes many forms. Relaxation techniques and biofeedback are attempts to teach patients how to control pain (18). There are a lot of back schools around but no schools for chronic neck pain (1). It is left to the supervising therapist or doctor to assure the patient that, with time, all will be better, and that it is unlikely any crippling side effects will be forthcoming. Using a model of a neck, it is often possible to give a patient some understanding of the anatomy and biomechanics of the area. This little bit of medical knowledge, with reassurance, helps the patient cope with the problem. Next to the passage of time, this step is the most useful of all modalities previously discussed.

Duration of Treatment

Most cervical degenerative conditions, except for CSM, are self-limiting. There is no rush to the operating room. It is recommended that a minimum of six weeks of conservative treatment be tried before considering investigation that may lead to surgical intervention. Before taking this step, emphasize to the patient that there is hurt, not harm, in living with neck and/or arm symptoms, and only when symptoms interfere significantly with activities of daily living should investigation and surgery be considered.

Specific Conservative Treatment

The three most common modes of presentation are: acute neck pain without neurological involvement, recurrent or chronic neck pain without neurological involvement, and cervical disc degeneration with neurological involvement (radicular and/or myelopathic).

Acute Incapacitating Pain Without Root Compression.   Some patients, with or without a provocative incident, develop an acute onset of pain of incapacitating severity. Any attempt to move the neck is associated with an exacerbation of pain radiating along the trapezii and posteriorly to the rhomboids. Commonly the patients place their hands around the back of the neck to obtain some relief.

The patient is usually reluctant to move his or her neck and moves the body as a whole to look from side to side. On examination, all supporting muscles of the neck are prominent and taut. Active movement is limited in all ranges and passive movement in any direction evokes pain. The trapezii, the sternomastoids, the interscapular muscles, and, occasionally, the posterior cervical muscles are tender on palpation.

Even if a patient does not complain of pain or paresthesia in his or her arms, a neurological examination should be conducted and x-rays of the neck should be taken to exclude malignancy or infection. If there is no evidence of nerve root involvement and if serious bone pathology has been excluded by radiological examination, the patient is probably suffering from an acute posterior joint strain. How do you treat it? First, know the prognosis—this patient will get better quickly. Try a collar and pain medication. Modalities such as heat or ice (depending on patient preference) are usually helpful. Within a few days to a week these patients are better with little else being needed.

Recurrent or Persisting Pain.   The common clinical picture is of a grumbling discomfort, radiating from the neck to the shoulders. The pain may radiate to the occiput, the interscapular region, or the chest. Any one of these discomforts may be the major or indeed the only complaint. Patients may complain of a dull, constant, aching pain over the trapezii and the rhomboids; they may be plagued with a persistent nagging pain in one or both arms, sometimes associated with paresthesia in the fingers, even in the absence of root irritation; or their major problem may be a neck pain associated with occipital or suboccipital headaches.

Recurrent pain in the chest over the pectorals, aggravated by activity, may be the patient's major worry—a worry that he/she is suffering from angina. This lesion, commonly caused by segmental instability at the C6 segment, has been referred to as a "cervical coronary." Although the patient may complain of one site of pain, careful questioning frequently uncovers pain radiating to other regions. The patient may admit to intermittent vertigo of brief duration, for example, when standing up from a sitting position. Intermittent blurring of vision and a sensation of dysphagia, particularly when tired, are also common but minor symptoms.

These symptoms are rarely volunteered by the patient; the physician must specifically inquire about them.

Cervical Disc Degeneration.   The chronic debilitating pain of cervical disc degeneration may be punctuated with episodes of acute incapacitating pain: "My neck froze—the pain was so intense I could not move my head. I also had this sudden stabbing pain between my shoulder blades, and I had difficulty even breathing." These episodes may only last a few hours or may persist more than a week. In addition to the burden painful necks impose on everyday living, they cause difficulty in sleeping. Sometimes, the only way patients can sleep is to sit up in a chair with their heads supported by pillows.

During an acute exacerbation of pain, the trapezii may be in "spasm" and are prominent on examination. During these acute exacerbations, all movements of the neck are limited by pain.

Faced with the common clinical picture, namely a grumbling discomfort of nuisance value, it is important to ask yourself, "Why has this patient sought medical advice?" Many patients have friends or relatives with rheumatoid arthritis. The development of pain in the neck or arm without provocative incident may be a frightening experience. The pain may be perfectly tolerable. Many patients do not require, nor are they asking for, specific treatment. They just require a diagnosis. They need to know the cause of this worrisome complaint. With reassurance that they do not have arthritis or cancer, many are perfectly content to carry on with normal activities, scarcely hampered by the discomfort they feel from time to time.

In establishing a routine of management, the clinician must carefully evaluate the purpose of every modality of treatment prescribed. Under the current concept of the pathogenesis of symptoms, it is presumed that, as a result of the instability associated with disc degeneration, abnormal movements are permitted at the involved segments, rendering the posterior joint vulnerable to stress. A strain of the posterior joints in the cervical spine tends to be aggravated and perpetuated by carrying the weight of the head, by muscle splinting, and by extension movements of the neck.

It is, of course, impossible to reverse degenerative changes or induce stability in the damaged segment. All that can be done is to modify the traumatic synovitis in the posterior joints and minimize harmful splinting by prescribing nonsteroidal anti-inflammatory drugs, resting the damaged joints, dulling the patient's discomfort with analgesics, and finally, modifying activities of daily living to shorten duration of the attack and minimize chances of recurrence. In attempting to achieve these goals, the following guidelines may be of value.

Rest.   Obviously, apply the principles of rest discussed previously. This will include use of a cervical collar, bed rest, and activity modification.

Not every patient finds comfort from a cervical collar. Before ordering a special collar, the patient must acknowledge some relief of symptoms while wearing a soft cervical collar. Patients with cervical disc degeneration have a long row to hoe. Although periods of remission increase, the pain may persist intermittently for many months, occasionally for years. Although cervical collars are an effective method of treating an acute episode of pain, they are cumbersome and irksome to the patient. When a prolonged period of disability is anticipated, a more comfortable, well-contoured collar should be prescribed. Strict instructions should be given to the supplier that the collar stand higher at the back than at the front when fitted; the main purpose of the collar is to limit extension of the neck.

During a period of exacerbated pain, most patients prefer to wear the collar all day long. When discomfort has subsided, and during remissions, patients only need to wear the collar when they engage in provocative activities, such as long car drives, golf, gardening, etc. Following such activities, it may be necessary to use a soft collar in bed at night.

Even the prescription of a collar carries a certain inherent danger. Although there is no evidence that wearing a cervical collar weakens the neck muscles, patients may come to believe that the collar is an essential component in the cure of their complaints. With this belief, they tend to wear the collar as a talisman to guard against the possibility of any recurrence of pain. It is essential that the patient be informed that the collar has no influence on the progress of symptomatic disc changes and functions solely as a means of external splinting that is to be replaced, as soon as possible, by the "internal splint" of stronger muscle support.

Physiotherapy.   An exercise program can be initiated, the function of which is to increase the tone of the paracervical muscles and, later, to attempt to restore normal joint mobility. It is best to teach isotonic contractions first, that is, contraction of the muscles without movement of the neck. Initially, this should be taught in a physical therapy unit. The therapist holds the patient's head between his or her hands and starts a slow lateral movement of the neck. The force applied by the therapist is resisted by an equal force applied by the patient. No movement takes place. Each contraction is followed by a rest period and is repeated at different degrees of lateral flexion and rotation.

The patient can continue isotonic exercises at home using barbells. The bar is held at shoulder level with the head in the neutral position. Without moving the head or neck, the bar is pushed up over the head, held for a moment, and then lowered behind the neck. During this action the neck does not move at all but the muscles contract. The cycle is repeated 10 times (Fig. 4.7). Barbells can be cheaply constructed by the patient. Plastic milk bottles filled with sand can be strapped to the ends of a broom handle. This homemade apparatus can be used as described above. Once the symptoms have abated, the patient can start a program of assisted active exercise to restore normal mobility. Many patients will require postural reeducation to overcome the tendency to stand and sit with an exaggerated cervicodorsal angulation.

Medication.   Medication will not reverse the degenerative changes that have occurred. The so-called muscle relaxants have little or no value apart from a tranquilizing effect. Anti-inflammatory drugs may speed the resolution of the posterior joint synovitis associated with acute exacerbation of pain. Any of the newer group of anti-inflammatory drugs may be given to the patient, but it must be remembered that they all have the danger of producing toxic gastritis or kidney failure especially in the older age group.

Modification of Daily Activities.   Among the major factors perpetuating pain arising from cervical disc degeneration are the activities of daily living that require holding the neck in extension. This will not always be apparent to the patient, and it is important that the patient be given instructions, preferably written, on how these extension strains may be avoided.

In the highly concerned patient, there is a constant danger of overtreatment:

Doctor: Is your pain more severe after activities such as making beds or vacuum cleaning?
Patient: I never do those things.

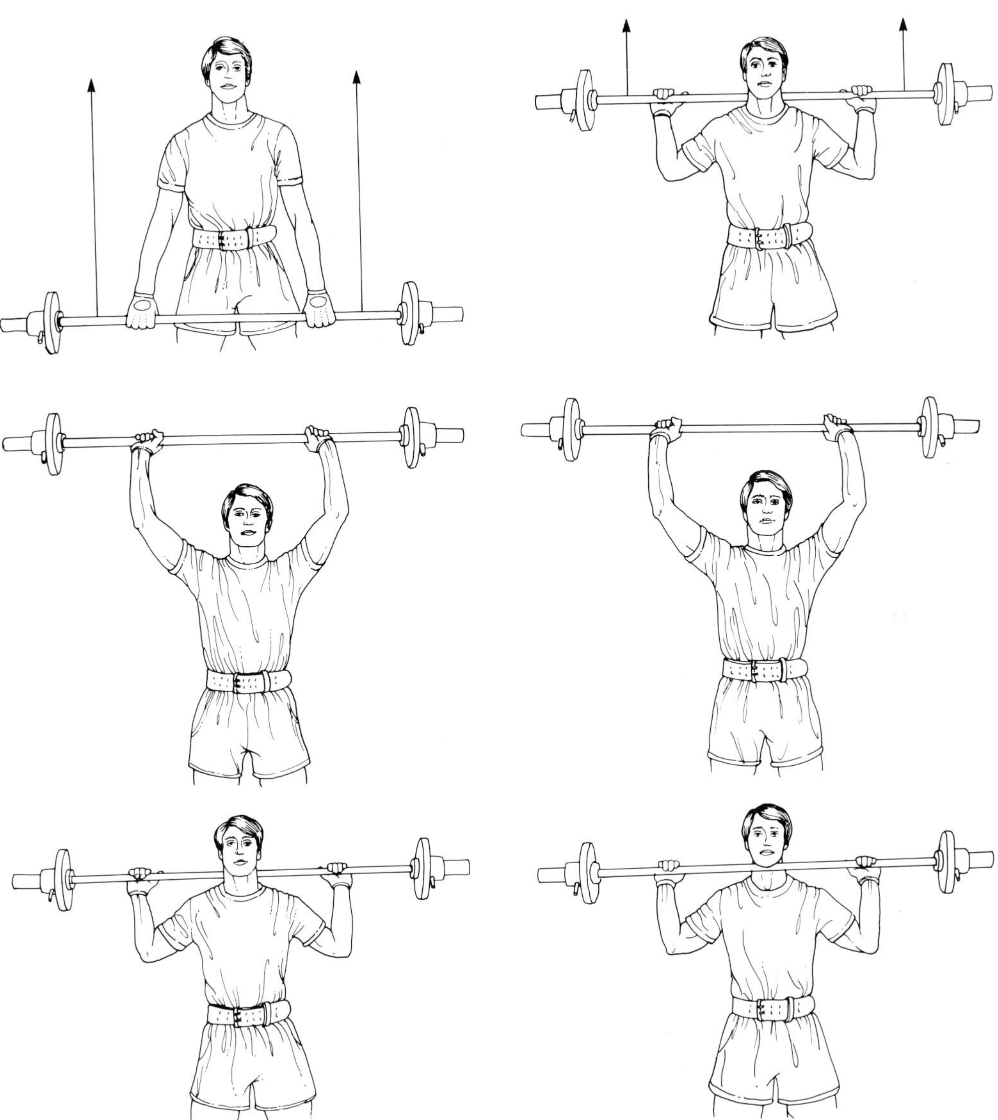

Figure 4.7.   Barbell exercises.

Doctor: Why not?
Patient: My doctor said I shouldn't.
Doctor: When did you go back to work?
Patient: I haven't gone back to work yet.
Doctor: Why not?
Patient: My doctor said I wasn't able to work.

When instructing patients to modify activities in order to minimize discomfort, it is of vital importance to distinguish for them the difference between hurting and harming. Patients must be told that although many things they do may give rise to pain, a flare-up of pain does not signify that they have damaged their necks or slowed their progress. It must be emphasized that suggested modifications of daily activities are merely guidelines for reducing pain. They are not orders to follow a new way of life. Patients must understand it is permissible to engage in all activities within the limits set by the their personal tolerance of discomfort. Limitation of activity is a personal decision.

As mentioned previously, under stressful situations such as anger, frustration, or fear, patients commonly adopt the fight-or-flight position with the neck muscles isometrically contracted and the chin thrust forward. Maintaining this posture, even in the absence of disc degeneration, may cause ischemic muscle pain, experienced not only locally in the neck but commonly referred to the occiput.

Recurrent occipital headaches are a common manifestation of sustained tension states. Indeed, the expression, "tension rheumatism," coined by the late Dr. Wallace Graham (personal communication) to describe persistent or recurrent discomfort over the geographical area of the trapezius, is an apt description of this clinical syndrome—probably more accurate than a mythical pathological diagnosis of "fibromyalgia."

If patients develop symptomatic degenerative disc disease and then emotionally induce tightening of the cervical muscles, they will increase the amount of pain. The intensification of pain hampers patients' abilities to carry out normal activities and thereby increases the stress under which they normally live.

These patients badly need an explanation of the mechanism that produces their pain—in particular, the role played by associated emotionally induced muscle tension. No form of medication will change these patients' fragile emotional makeup. By reducing the patient's drive, some tranquilizing drugs may only induce more frustration; by lowering the patient's affect, other drugs will decrease the patient's tolerance of pain during drug-induced depression.

Physicians must take time to talk to their patients and be careful of the expressions they use. "Neurotic" is not a diagnosis acceptable to any patient. On the other hand, patients may accept that the pressures placed upon them have brought them to the "verge of a nervous breakdown," especially if it seems to imply that they are working too hard. They may accept the fact that they are "tense" if the expression is expanded to describe them as "intensive, hard-driving individuals." In this sphere of medical practice, euphemisms are not only acceptable, they are essential.

Voluntary muscular relaxation is frequently taught as an antenatal routine, and in this manifestation of cervical disc degeneration, patients will derive far greater benefit from instruction in voluntary muscular relaxation than from medications designed to achieve the same objective.

The chronicity of symptoms is the most frustrating aspect of the disease; even more devastating is the patient's erroneous belief that he or she will be miraculously relieved of the burden of pain by some new pill or new modality of treatment at a physiotherapy department. Physicians must be honest. They must let the patient know that the symptoms may continue intermittently for more than a year. Yet, in making this gloomy prognosis, they should encourage the patient to engage in normal activities within his or her ability to tolerate inevitable discomfort, with full knowledge that, with time and patience, the body has a natural ability to stabilize the painful segment and reduce symptoms.

Manipulation.   Manipulation is most effective in the management of these patients. In the hands of a skilled practitioner of the art, discomfort can be reduced dramatically. Prolonged manipulation is not advisable; rather, an exercise program should be initiated, and it should gradually take over as manipulation decreases discomfort.

Multisegmental Degenerative Disc Disease.   On occasion, patients suffering from multifocal, multisegmental, degenerative disc disease fail to obtain any relief of symptoms from the usual methods of conservative treatment and are not suitable for any operative intervention. These patients are an unhappy group. They are disabled by pain that arises from degenerative changes at multiple levels. They derive little benefit from conservative routines. They cannot hope to expect any cure from surgical stabilization.

Fortunately, despite the apparent hopelessness of the pathetic picture they present, many obtain dramatic relief of symptoms from rigid fixation of the neck afforded by halo vest immobilization over a period of three or four months. Fortunately these are rare occasions, but the patient with multilevel disease that has not responded to conservative care should at least be considered for external splinting.

Cervicolumbar Syndrome.   Some patients have the misfortune of combining symptomatic lumbar disc degeneration and cervical disc degeneration. The common picture is initially of pain in the lower back. When the lower back is painful, patients tend to stoop forward and assume a flexed position to avoid stresses placed on hyperextended posterior intervertebral joints in the lumbar spine.

However, because it is natural for patients to allow their eyes to remain parallel to the horizon, the neck will then be held hyperextended. This position will cause pain in the neck. In order to get relief from the ensuing cervicobrachial pain, patients have to flex their necks. They now have to hyperextend the lumbar spine to allow their eyes to remain parallel to the horizon.

This is almost a Catch-22 situation. On occasion, the patient will present the unbelievable picture of "total body pain"—pain in the occiput, pain in the neck, pain in one or both arms, interscapular pain, lumbar pain, and pain radiating down one or both legs. It is highly tempting, of course, to regard this type of presentation as largely functional in origin. The physician, nevertheless, should be aware of the possibility of a physiogenic basis for this unusual and distressing symptom complex.

Cervical Disc Degeneration With Neurologic Impairment.   Neurological involvement may be isolated radicular, isolated myelopathic, or combinations of the two. Our clinical experience is that 90% of patients with neurological involvement will have radicular involvement alone, with most of the rest presenting a combined radicular/myelopathic picture, and very few presenting as a pure CSM.

The symptoms produced by cervical disc degeneration associated with root involvement may have an acute onset, or they may be insidious. Pain in the arm is the major symptom and is commonly associated with paresthesia in the hand or fingers. Subjective weakness of muscle groups may develop, but this weakness is often slow in onset and gradual in development. As mentioned previously, the neurological deficits resulting from compression of any one cervical root vary from patient to patient, and do not adhere to a rigid sclerotome or dermatome distribution described in standard texts of neuroanatomy.

Root compression in the vast majority of cases is produced by osteophytic excrescences on the neurocentral joints (Fig. 4.8), and the resulting syndrome is chronic radicular pain. Discal ruptures protrude into the spinal canal medial to the neurocentral prominence and may therefore not only give rise to root compression but also to cord compression. Acute radicular syndrome has been described in the previous chapter.

Treatment of Acute Radicular Syndrome

Traction.   It is in this group of patients that traction has the most benefit. It is especially important that traction be applied so as not to aggravate the arm pain. This usually means a neutral or slightly flexed neck position (Fig. 4.5). After learning the traction technique in a physical therapy department, home traction can be used.

Collar.   Rest is the cornerstone of reducing the compressive and irritative effects of a soft disc pressing on a nerve root. For the first few days of onset of acute radicular pain, the patient rarely obtains relief in bed, but rather sits in a high-back chair with pillows propped in various positions. A soft or semirigid collar is useful to splint the neck. Its function at this stage is to reduce the movement that aggravates the compressive and irritative effects of the disc rupture.

Medication.   Initially, strong analgesic, muscle relaxant, and/or sleeping medications are useful. Most physicians also prescribe anti-inflammatories, so the patient is taking a lot of medication to "cool off" the severe pain.

As the severity of the pain declines, use of medication can be reduced accordingly. The relaxant and sedative medications can be dropped, and the nature and/or dose of analgesics can be reduced. The last medication to be reduced and discontinued is the anti-inflammatory.

Exercise.   As the acute arm pain settles, the medication regime is reduced, the collar is weaned, and an exercise program is started. Both isometric and range-of-movement exercises are useful, and institution is gradual. With increasing comfort and increasing compliance with exercise, the collar, traction, and medication can be reduced.

Manipulation.   Manipulation of a patient with neurological consequences to cervical disc disease is not indicated. The potential for increase in neurological consequences is too great (19).

Prognosis.   It is unusual for a soft cervical disc causing acute arm pain to persist. Almost all patients respond to conservative care, with few requiring surgical intervention.

Treatment of Chronic Radicular Syndrome

In contrast to the soft cervical disc causing acute arm pain, the bone spur causing a chronic radicular pain is more resistant to conservative care.

All the conservative care proposals made in the section on acute radicular pain need to be tried, with confidence that some patients will improve. Recovery will rarely be in a straight line, more commonly resembling a bouncing ball, with exacerbations and remissions.

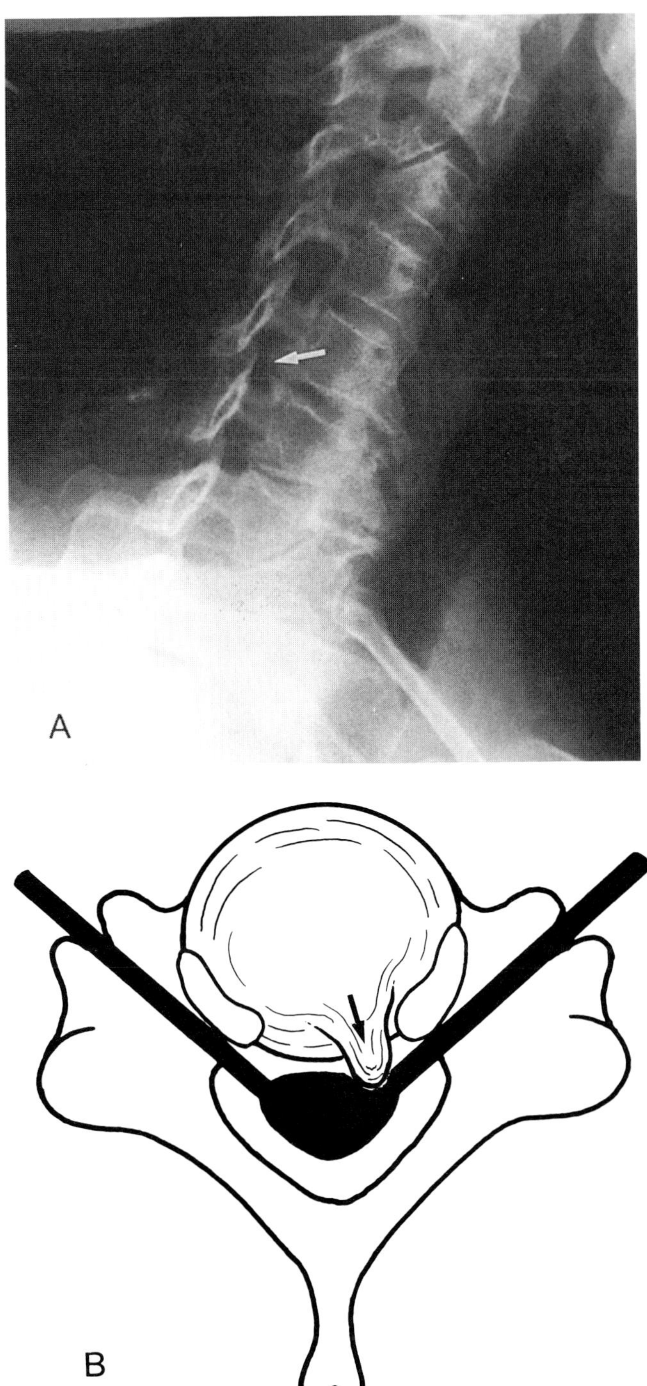

Figure 4.8.   A, neurocentral osteophyte (*arrow*) closing down the foramen. **B,** disc rupture medial to the uncovertebral joint (*arrow*). Note how it may compress the root and the cord.

Table 4.5.   Clinical Aspects of Cervical Spondylotic Myelopathy (CSM)[a]

	Symptom	Sign

Lower Extremities	• Gait deterioration
	  Weak, stiff,
	    unsteady (very
	    little pain)
		• Spastic gait
		  Shuffling
		• Spastic lower extremities
		  Hyperactive reflexes, Babinski, Clonus,
		    mild diffuse weakness, no sensory
		    loss (rare posterior column loss)

Upper Extremities	• Myelopathic hand
	    (UMNL)
	  Clumsy finger use
	  Diffuse paraesthesia
	  Diffuse weakness
		• Myelopathic hand (UMNL)
		  Inability to open and close fist rapidly
		  Nondermatomal hypalgesia
		• LMNL at level of spondylotic bar
		  Weakness appropriate to anatomical
		    level
		  Sensory loss appropriate to anatomical
		    level
		• UMNL below level of spondylotic bar
		  Inverted radial reflex (C5-C6)
		  Spastic upper extremities
		  Hyperactive reflexes, Hoffman reflex

Miscellaneous	Lhermitte's	
Sphincter	Bladder and bowel symptoms and signs occur late in CSM	

[a]Remember:
1. Any one or more of these findings may or may not be present.
2. There may be a painful radicular component at the level(s) of the spondylotic bar(s).

As long as there is not worsening of neurological status, conservative care can
go on as long as the patient wishes. However, if the patient presents a significant
neurological deficit, or the neurological deficit increases during treatment, surgery is indicated. The most common indication for surgery in this group of patients is persistent arm pain, unresponsive to conservative care and interfering
with functional activities to a degree the patient will not accept.

Cervical Spondylotic Myelopathy (CSM).   A chronic myelopathy caused by
a posterior cervical osteophytic bar may develop insidiously. The patients are
generally older than 50 and the most common symptom is difficulty in walking,
often described as a heaviness in the legs, or the patient complains that, "I can't
get my legs to do what I want them to do." Many give a history of frequent
stumbling. Most of the patients also complain of arm pain associated on occasion
with subjective weakness (Table 4.5).

The combination of upper and lower motor neuron lesions make for confusion
in diagnosis with a cervical myelopathy mimicking a cervical cord neoplasm, sub-
acute combined degeneration, syringomyelia, or disseminated sclerosis. It is important that the diagnosis be established, because when left untreated, the lesion
is relentlessly progressive. It is advisable to include a CT scan or an MRI in
routine assessment.

It is almost impossible to prescribe a universally accepted treatment to this
patient. Most would agree that if the patient has moderate functional impairment, surgery is indicated without trial of conservative treatment. Further, if
the patient is on conservative treatment, and functional capacity is decreasing
and/or the neurological deficit increases, surgery is indicated.

This leaves only the mildly impaired and neurologically stable patient as a conservative treatment candidate. At the onset, let us set aside the use of traction in this patient population. In addition, with cord encroachment there is no margin for error in manipulation. Although manipulation can be used in a majority of patients with no consequences, the occurrence of a paralyzing disc rupture during manipulation is reported in the literature (19). Those using manipulation in this patient population are exposing the patient and themselves to dire consequences.

Postural Training. On the theory that neck flexion unbuckles the ligamentum flavum and increases the space available for the spinal canal, patients should receive postural training. Probably the most important is keeping the neck out of extension for all activities. Neck flexion is obviously a better position but limits a number of activities.

Immobilization. A number of CSM patients with mild functional impairment will report relief of symptoms with a custom-fitted cervical collar that will be worn long term.

Exercise. To limit the term of collar use, patients should be started on an isometric neck strengthening program. Range-of-movement exercises are not indicated for fear of worsening the neurological lesion.

Medication. Because of the older age group in which CSM occurs, and the chronicity of the lesion, addicting analgesic medication, mood altering relaxants and sedatives, and ulcerogenic anti-inflammatories have to be carefully controlled and monitored.

SURGICAL INTERVENTION

Absolute indications for surgery in degenerative disease of the cervical spine largely center around neurological involvement.

They are:

1. Severe neurological radicular deficit on presentation. The exception to this is the soft cervical disc, symptomatic less than six weeks with no prior significant conservative care. Most of these patients will get better without surgery.
2. Increasing neurological deficit in the face of conservative care.
3. A neurological deficit and pain that persist in spite of conservative care.

A relative indication for surgical intervention is:

4. Persisting arm pain, without neurological signs (but usually with neurological symptoms) that persists in spite of conservative treatment and additionally is painful enough to interfere too much with the patient's pattern of living.

Soft Tissue Syndromes

There is no indication for surgery in this situation—especially if the patient has an attached litigation or compensation claim.

Cervical Disc Degeneration Without Root Involvement

Neck pain from degenerative disc disease rarely constitutes an indication for surgery. The condition is self-limiting, and with appropriate conservative treatment symptoms can usually be brought into the range of a patient's functional demand. In addition, cervical degenerative disc disease is multifocal. Picking the

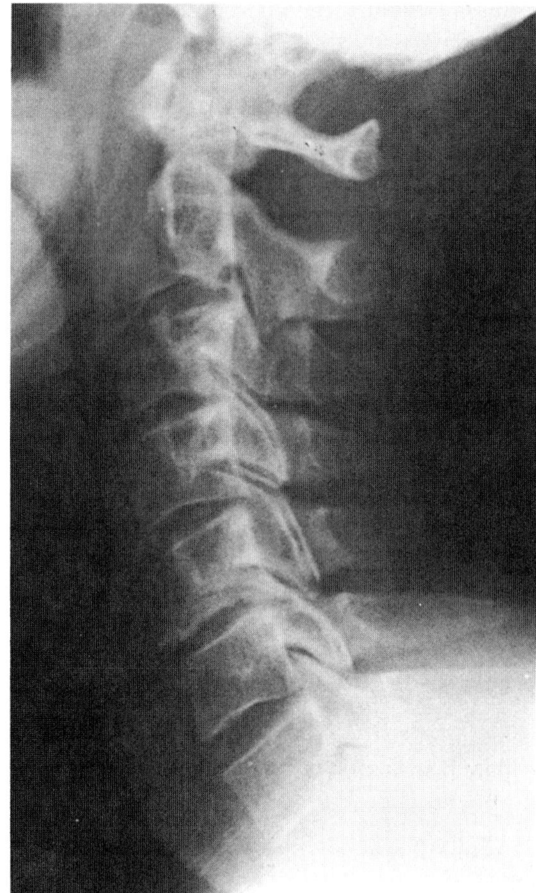

Figure 4.9.   Single level degenerative disc disease (DDD), C5-C6.

correct level is impossible with CT/myelography and/or MRI. Surgeons then reach for discography, a test with many pitfalls surrounding its interpretation.

About the only patient with neck pain who should be considered for anterior fusion of the offending segment is:

- A patient with single level disease on plain x-ray and either discography or T2-weighted MRI (Fig. 4.9).
- This patient must have failed extensive conservative treatment.
- This patient should not have any secondary gain factors deflecting the disability towards a surgical decision.

The surgery needed in this rare situation is an anterior discectomy and fusion.

Cervical Disc Disease With Radicular Pain
Acute Radicular Pain

Acute radicular (arm) pain is almost always caused by a soft disc herniation. It is very unusual for a soft disc herniation not to respond to conservative care, making the indication for surgical intervention rare in this patient population. Even in the presence of a neurological deficit, such as a depressed biceps reflex and weak elbow flexion in a C6 root deficit, conservative care (especially traction) will often be successful, including a return of neurological function.

The indications for surgery in acute radicular pain are:

1. A major neurological deficit such as cord compression.
2. A major root deficit such as an absent triceps reflex and a significant weakness in elbow extension (C7). Partial root lesions, as mentioned above, will likely respond to appropriate conservative care.
3. Persistent radicular pain in spite of good conservative care.
4. Recurrent radicular pain after successful conservative care.

Obviously, in each of these situations, there must be some correlation between the distribution of the patient's arm pain, neurological symptoms, and neurological signs, and the appearance of a lesion on investigation. In the young patient with normal plain x-rays, verification of the lesion may be made on MRI. If the MRI is at all equivocal, then a CT/myelogram becomes mandatory, and if this does not reveal a root or cord compression deficit, you do not have an indication for surgery. In this situation, it is necessary to start from the beginning with a history, a physical examination, and other tests such as a chest x-ray with apical views, EMG, etc. (see Chapter 21 on Differential Diagnosis).

Surgical Approaches

Chemonucleolysis.   A few European and Asian investigators have successfully used chymopapain in soft cervical discs. Although the classic indication for chemonucleolysis in the lumbar spine is a contained soft disc herniation, it is the manufacturer's recommendation that chymopapain not be used at cord levels, i.e., the cervical spine.

Anterior Cervical Discectomy With/Without Fusion.   The majority of orthopaedic surgeons, and a reasonable number of neurosurgeons, would recommend, when indicated, an anterior discectomy for a soft cervical disc rupture. Only if the disc herniation is lateral would some neurosurgeons recommend a posterior approach. If there is any central component to the disc rupture, an anterior approach is mandatory, because manipulation of the spinal cord from behind to retrieve central fragments has a high risk of quadriplegia.

Anterior Discectomy Approach.   It is much easier and safer to use the anterior approach for lesions anterior to the spinal cord, for example, a cervical disc rupture. This approach cannot be used if there is an enlarged thyroid gland. Examine the thyroid before starting this approach.

Surgical Anatomy

The approach is through the anterior triangle of the neck (Fig. 4.10). The skin incisions for various levels are shown in Figure 4.11. Most right-handed surgeons use the right-sided approach. Some surgeons prefer the left-sided approach to avoid stretching the recurrent laryngeal nerve. For the right-handed surgeon this approach presents too many obstacles (Table 4.6). It is much easier, technically, for the right-handed surgeon to operate from the right, elevate the longus colli very carefully, and place the retractor blades under the longus colli—rather

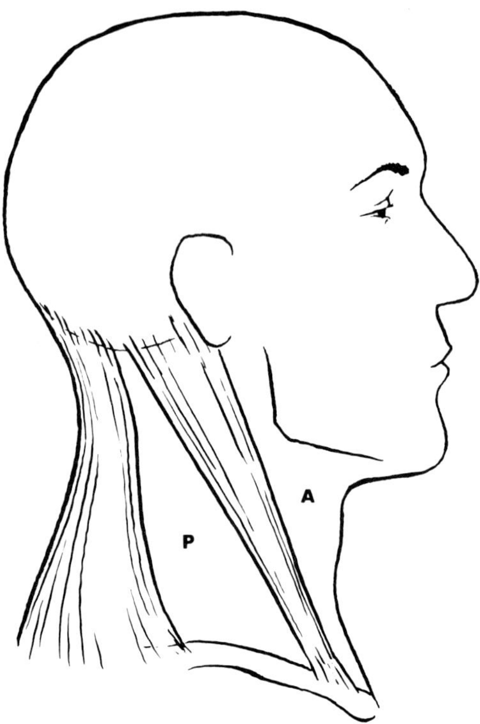

Figure 4.10.   The anterior (*A*) and posterior (*P*) triangles of the neck, divided by the sternomastoid muscle.

than the esophagus—to prevent excessive traction on the recurrent laryngeal nerve (Fig. 4.12).

An approach medial to the sternomastoid muscle and carotid sheath, and lateral to the strap muscles (Fig. 4.13), takes you to the front of the vertebral column C3-T1. In a bullnecked individual with a stiff neck, the approach is more difficult, but this is a patient who seldom has a soft disc herniation. It is more likely that this patient has chronic neurological syndromes as discussed in the next section. At the higher levels, C2-C3 and C3-C4 neurological structures—such as the hypoglossal nerve and the superior laryngeal nerve—must be avoided. At all levels care must be taken not to stretch or damage the fragile venous system.

The plane between the strap muscles medially and the sternomastoid muscles laterally is developed by keying on the anteromedial border of the sternomastoid muscle and the deeper carotid artery. At all times these two structures must be identified and kept lateral to the dissection. On the way in, the omohyoid muscle will be encountered and can be retracted inferiorly, superiorly, or it can be transected. Almost all of this dissection is done bluntly with a finger or the tips of the closed Metzenbaum scissors.

Neurovascular structures that may cross the interfascial plane between the carotid sheath and the tracheoesophageal groove are:

- Any of the thyroid arteries or veins.
- The superior laryngeal nerve.

Table 4.6.   Problems With a Left-sided Approach for a Right-handed Surgeon

1. The mandible is in the way.
2. The thoracic duct is easily damaged, especially if it has a high (anomalous) insertion into the judular vein.
3. The recurrent laryngeal nerve may be aberrant, crossing the surgical field left or right (1–200).
4. The left carotid artery is usually the dominant carotid and damage, or dislodging of an atheromatous plaque, has the potential for more complications than if similar problems occurred on the right.

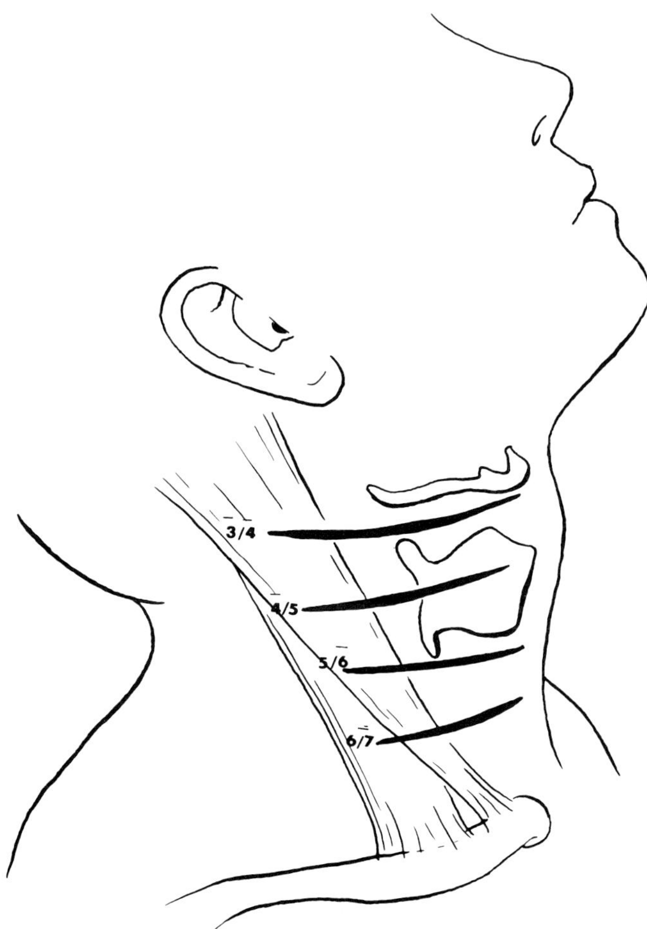

Figure 4.11.   Skin incision levels for C3-C4, C4-C5, C5-C6, C6-C7 approaches. The C5-C6 incision is at the level of the cricoid cartilage and C6-C7 is below the cricoid cartilage.

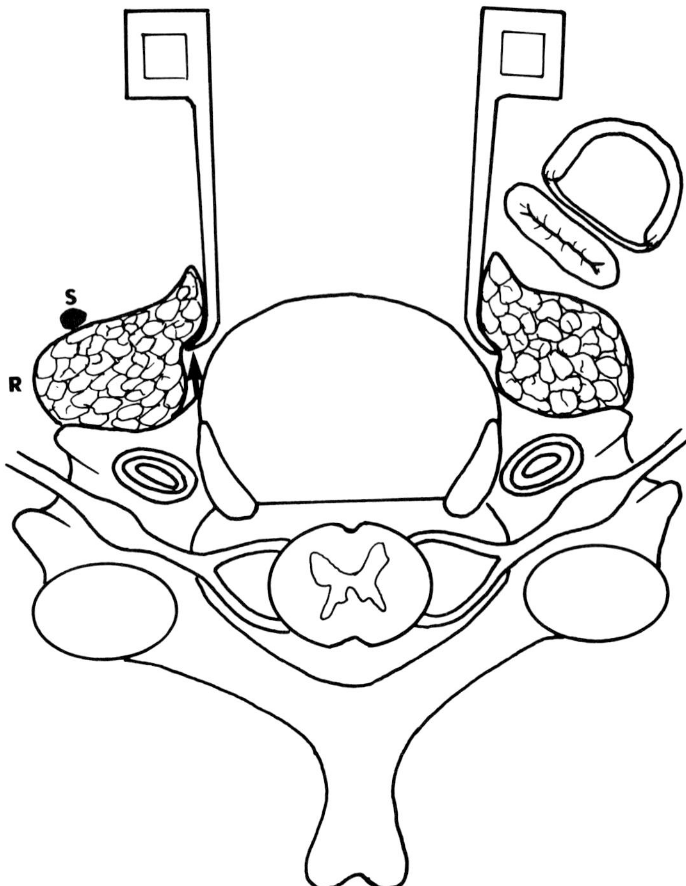

Figure 4.12.   This schematic is drawn as you would look at a CT scan. You are at the patient's feet looking towards the head. The right side is labeled, and the trachea, esophagus, and recurrent laryngeal nerve are retracted to the left. The force of the retraction is applied to the carefully elevated medial edge of the longus colli (*arrow*). Note the sympathetic plexus and how retracting across the front of the longus colli can damage both the recurrent laryngeal nerve and sympathetic plexus (sharp teeth on the retractor blade may even puncture the esophagus). (*R* = right, *S* = sympathetic trunk.)

- The nonrecurrent (aberrant) laryngeal nerve (Fig. 4.14).

Once the plane of the prevertebral fascia is reached it is necessary to do two things:

1. Identify your level with x-ray (using a needle marker as in Fig. 4.15).
2. Clear the longus colli, bilaterally, off the anterolateral aspects of the vertebrae and disc space. Dissecting the longus colli too far laterally can damage the vertebral artery and/or the sympathetic chain (Fig. 4.12).

Disc Excision

The disc is excised with a combination of sharp anterior dissection and blunt pituitary and curette posterior dissection (Fig. 4.16). This is aided by an interspace or vertebra spreader and a microscope.

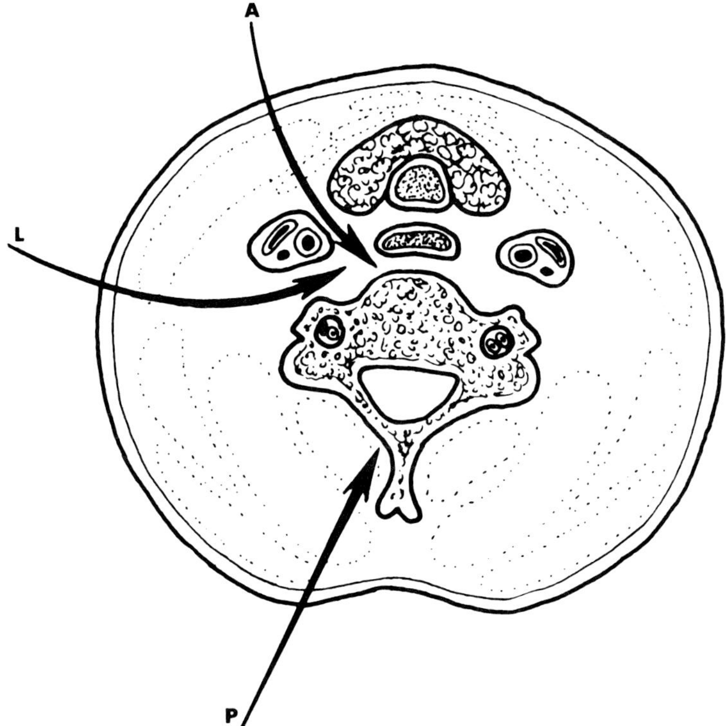

Figure 4.13.   The three approaches to the cervical spine: (*1*) Anterior (*A*), (*2*) Lateral (*L*), (*3*) Posterior (*P*). The anterior approach takes you medial to the sternomastoid and carotid sheath; lateral to the trachea, esophagus, and strap muscles.

If a fragment of discal material has perforated the annular/posterior longitudinal ligamentous complex, it can be retrieved under direct vision with the aid of the microscope. This usually requires wider opening of the rent in the posterior longitudinal ligament. If the fragment of extruded discal material has travelled away from the disc space, as determined by preoperative investigation (fragments usually migrate caudally rather than cranially), the fragment must be retrieved.

Foraminal Exploration

On occasion, fragments of discal material will migrate towards the foramen, necessitating a foraminotomy and removal of discal material. Obviously, the foraminotomy must not extend lateral to the lateral border of the uncovertebral joint for fear of damaging the vertebral artery.

In exploring the foramen note:

1. The nerve root takes a sharp angle anteriorly as it exits, making a hook in the axilla of the root especially dangerous.
2. Root anomalies such as double roots are quite common.
3. Laterally, the annular/posterior longitudinal complex is of variable thickness and provides no reliable landmark into the epidural space.

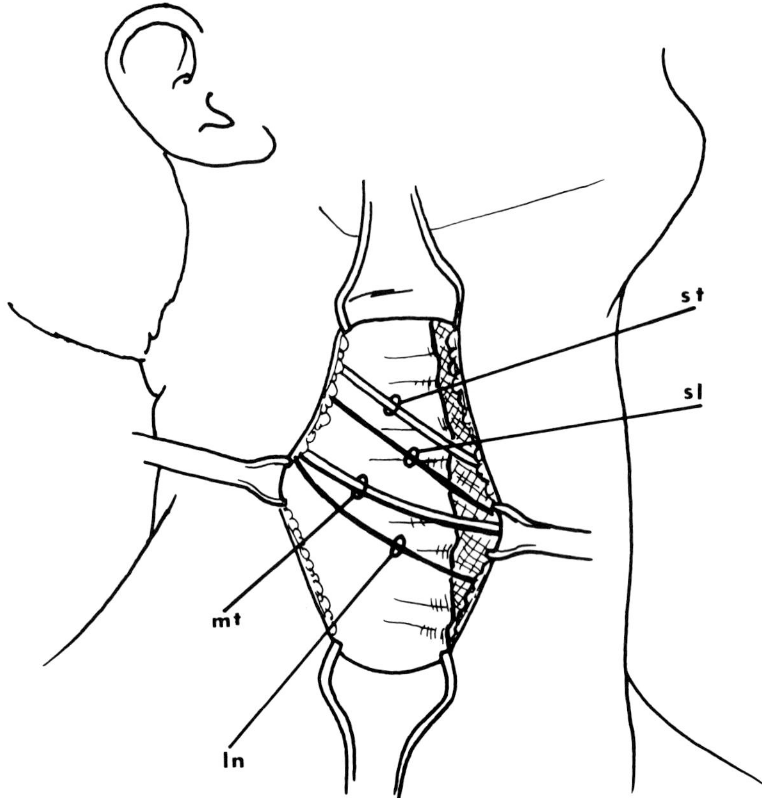

Figure 4.14.   A few surprises may be waiting for you when you use the anterior approach: (*1*) the nonrecurrent laryngeal nerve (*ln*), and (*2*) the middle thyroid vein (*mt*). At the higher levels (C3-C4), you have to deal with the superior laryngeal nerve (*sl*) and the superior thyroid artery (*st*).

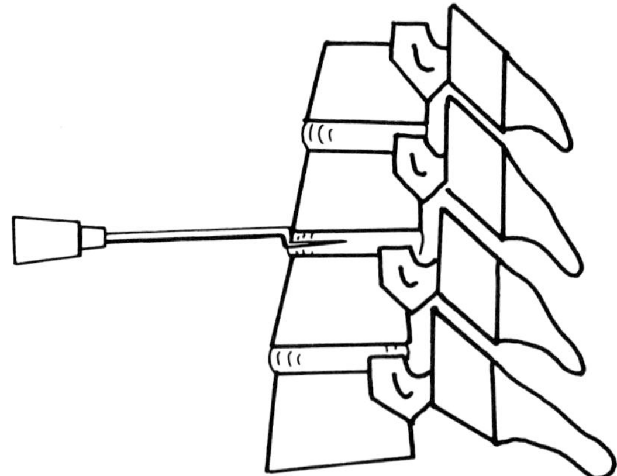

Figure 4.15.   Identify your level. Use a bent needle to mark the disc space for a lateral x-ray.

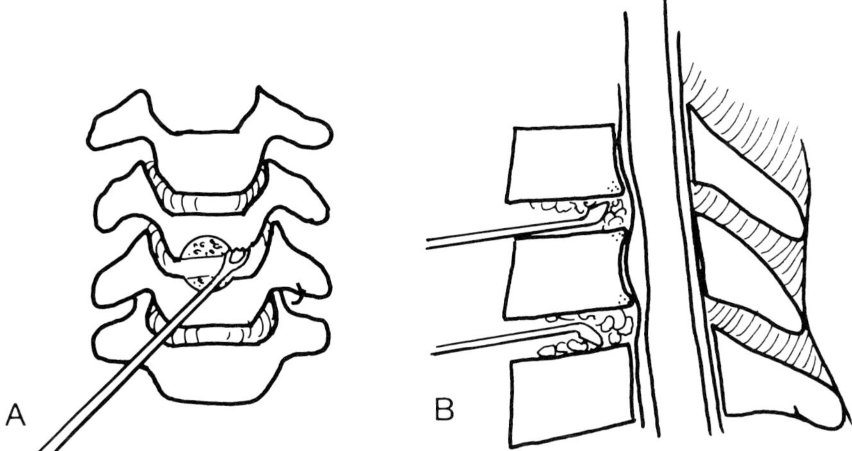

Figure 4.16.   **A,** AP showing use of the curette to remove posterior osteophytes. **B,** lateral showing the Smith-Robinson technique using curettes at two levels (did you notice the Cloward drill hole in Fig. 4.16*A*?).

If a fragment of disc has migrated laterally, the prudent approach is to open the annular ligamentous complex medially to laterally, starting with the rent in the annulus or at the midline.

To Fuse or Not to Fuse

Considerable controversy surrounds the necessity for fusion, and what type of fusion should be done with an anterior discectomy. The choices, advantages, and disadvantages are:

Anterior Cervical Discectomy Without Fusion

Advantages include the speed of operation and the lack of need for a separate incision on the patient's pelvis for donor bone. To avoid the iliac crest incision, some prefer allograft bone, which the authors do not recommend because of a higher pseudarthrosis rate and the remote possibility of disease transmission. The disadvantages of omitting the fusion include increased neck pain immediately after surgery and a higher incidence of long-term neck pain, especially in patients with degenerative disc disease and preoperative neck pain.

Anterior Cervical Discectomy With Fusion

The authors prefer this method, using autogenous bone. It takes longer, but the results are better (Fig. 4.17).

Posterior Approach to Soft Disc Herniation

Indications.   The authors see very little indication for this approach, but others would recommend it for the lateral or foraminal soft disc herniation.

Preparation.   Considerable controversy surrounds the use of the sitting or prone position for posterior approaches to the cervical spine. The advantage of the sitting position is decreased bleeding and thus less impairment of visualization of neurological structures. Disadvantages of the sitting, compared to the

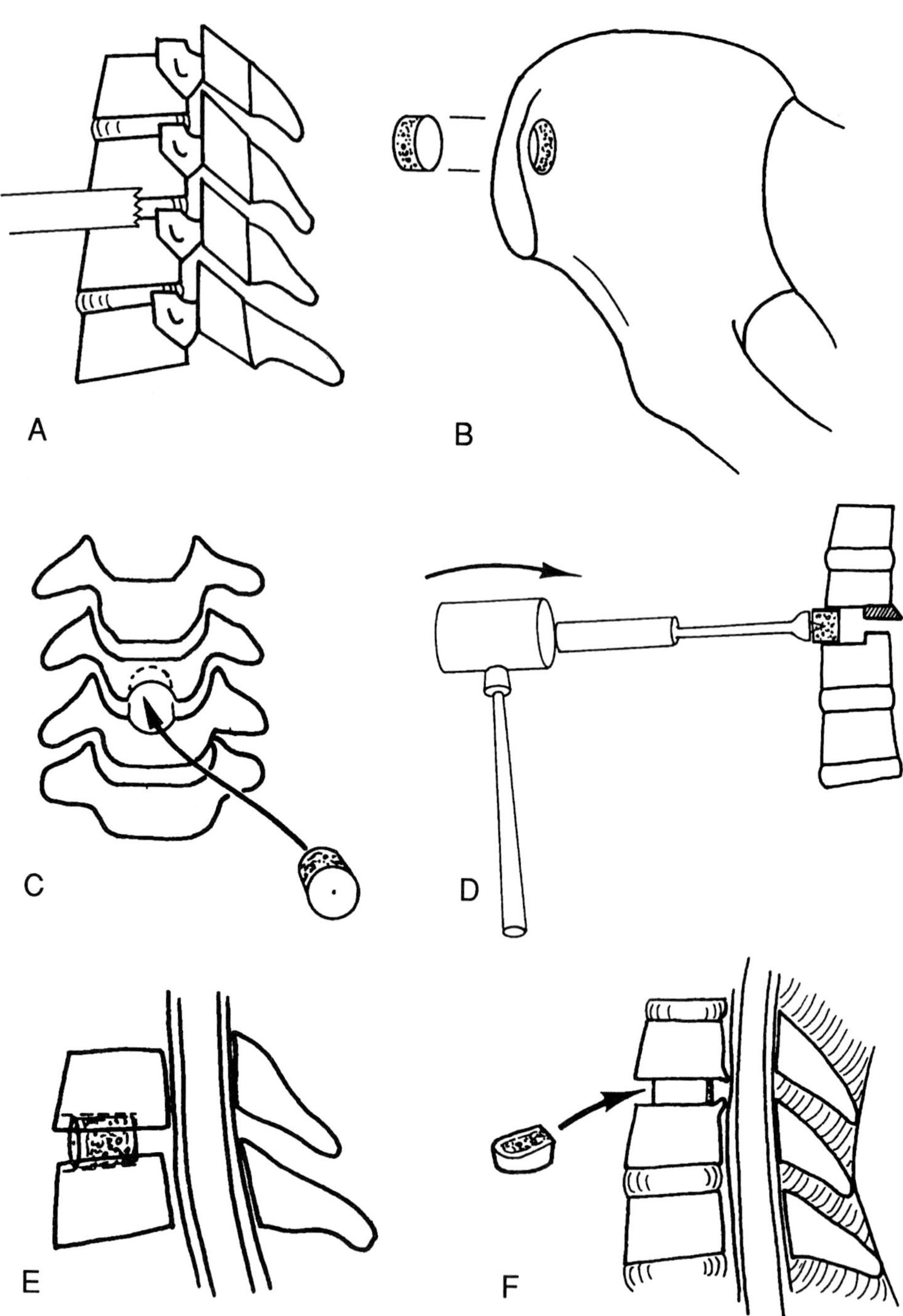

Figure 4.17.   **A,** drilling the vertebrae adjacent to the disc space with a Cloward or Crock drill. **B,** remove a corresponding plug of autogenous bone from the pelvis. This plug is usually 2 mm larger than the hole drilled in the vertebral bodies. **C,** insert the bone plug between the vertebral bodies. **D,** the bone plug being inserted. It is hard to obtain a plug of bone too long for the predrilled hole, but it is easy to insert it too deeply and cause cord damage! **E,** the Cloward bone plug in place. **F,** the Smith-Robinson bone plug in place. Note the remaining posterior osteophytes, usually left alone by those using the Smith-Robinson technique.

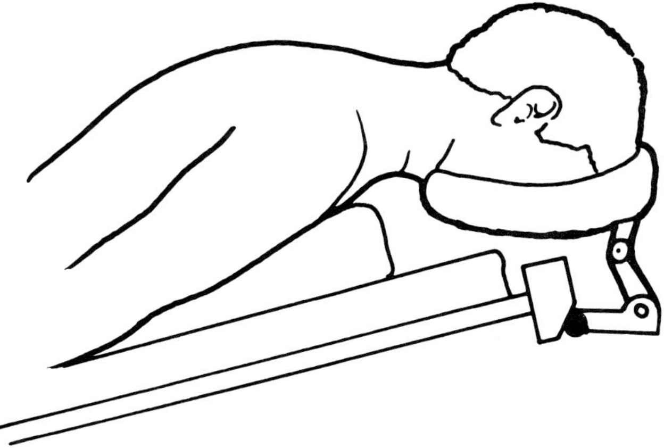

Figure 4.18.   The prone position for a posterior approach. Most neurosurgeons prefer the sitting position for this approach.

prone, position are the cumbersome efforts needed by the operating room staff to get the patient into position and the possibility of air embolism. For routine posterior approaches, we recommend the prone position.

In preparing for the prone position, it is necessary to be sure there has been no past excessive bleeding during surgery and that there are no coexistent bleeding disorders. The patient should be off all platelet inhibiting drugs such as NSAIDs.

Positioning of the patient on the OR table should allow for decreased pressure on the abdomen, careful preparation of the head to prevent pressure on the eyes, and free access to the endotracheal tube (Fig. 4.18).

Incision and Exposure (Single Level).   The spinous process landmarks are used to roughly identify your level:

1. C2 and C7 are the most prominent spinous processes.
2. C6 is shorter than C7 and sometimes bifid.
3. C5 is usually bifid.

A marking needle and image intensifier is then used to mark the bottom (inferior) edge of the disc space (Fig. 4.19). After suitable prepping and draping, a short 3 cm incision is made, straddling the marking line. After exposing the ligamentum nuchae, an elliptical incision is made in the fascia (Fig. 4.20) and the muscle is elevated subperiosteally off the interspinous and interlaminar intervals. After positioning a suitable retractor (Fig. 4.21), the microscope is positioned for the laminotomy.

Laminotomy.   The extent of the laminotomy/facetectomy is shown in Figure 4.22. If osteophytes are present, they are removed from the anteromedial aspect of the inferior facet and adjacent superior facet. The lateral extent of the ligamentum flavum is removed to identify the nerve root. After exposure of the nerve root, the superior and medial boundaries of the pedicle below are identified. Following the medial border of the pedicle anteriorly will keep you away from the cord and take you to the disc space just above the superior edge of the

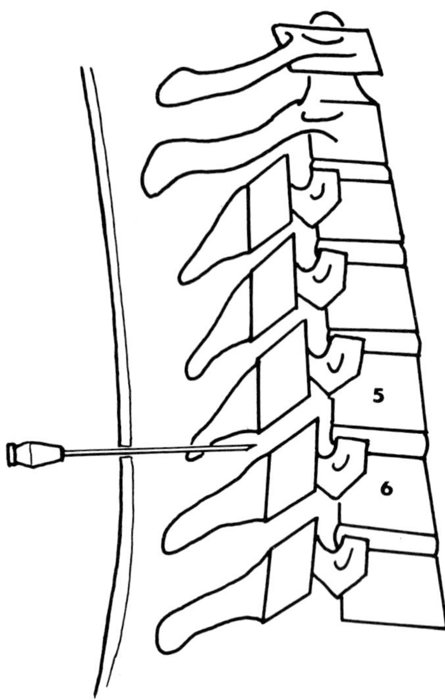

Figure 4.19. A needle in position marking the inferior edge of the disc space at the level to be exposed.

pedicle. There the soft disc herniation will be found anterior and inferior to the nerve root. It will be more readily seen by retracting the nerve root cranially.

Following the nerve root into the foramen usually requires bipolar coagulation of venous bleeders and the gentle blunt dissection of adhesions.

Excising the Disc.   The disc will be found in the axilla of the nerve root and can be gently removed with pituitary forceps. As the nerve root is retracted cranially, the absence of muscle-paralyzing agents by anesthesia will allow for muscle reaction or evoked response if the root is being excessively manipulated. No attempt should be made to evacuate intradiscal material.

Closure.   No interposition fat or gelfoam is used and, after removing the retractor, it is a simple matter to close the fascia and skin.

Cervical Disc Disease With Radicular Pain

Chronic Radicular Pain

Chronic radicular pain has many characteristics that distinguish it from acute radicular pain:

1. By definition, it has been present longer than acute syndromes.
2. It is usually less severe pain in a radicular distribution.
3. It waxes and wanes over time but eventually becomes persistent. This is unlike painful shoulder conditions where shoulder movement produces sharp immobilizing pain followed by lingering aching discomfort.
4. It often has neurological symptoms (paresthesia).

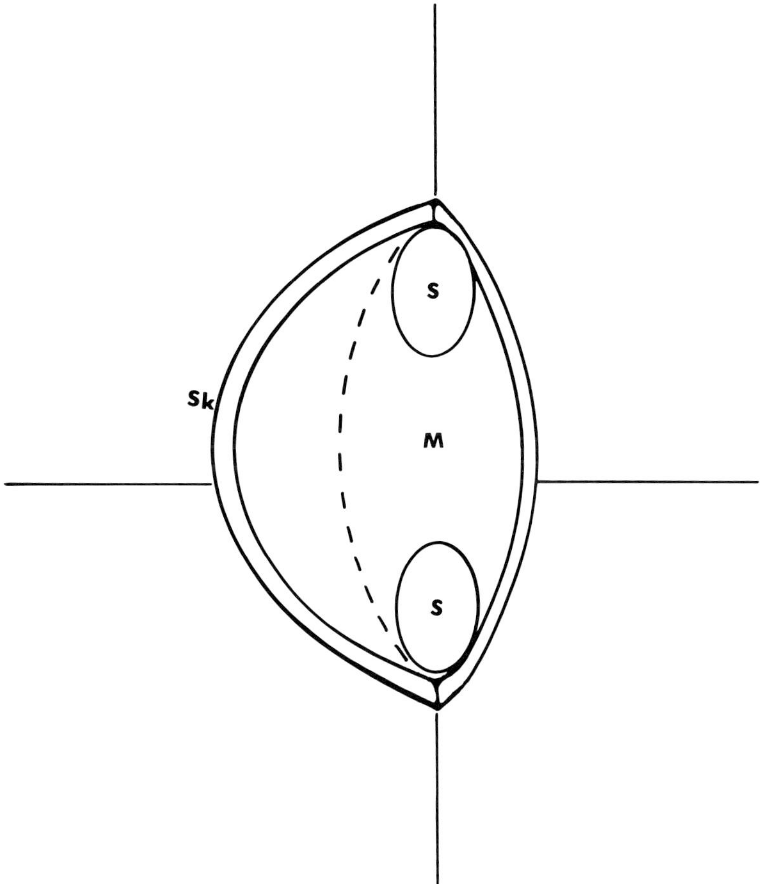

Figure 4.20.   The partial elliptical incision in the fascia (*broken line*). Spinous process (*s*), midline (*m*), and skin edge (*sk*).

5. It rarely has significant neurological findings compared to acute radicular pain. This is because neurological tissues that are very slowly compressed have more time to adapt and resist the pressure.
6. The pathology is due to osteophytic encroachment on the neural foramen (Fig. 4.23), rather than a soft disc herniation, making it impossible for the compression to spontaneously disappear. Once the symptoms of chronic radicular pain become persistent, conservative treatment will make little difference and the patients are forced to make a decision between:
   a. No surgery, and coping mechanisms such as mild analgesic medication and intermittent traction and collar use, or
   b. Surgical decompression.

Surgery for Chronic Radicular Pain

Anterior Approach

Discectomy.   A discectomy is necessary to get to the back of the disc space where the osteophytes are located. It is similar in approach to acute radicular pain.

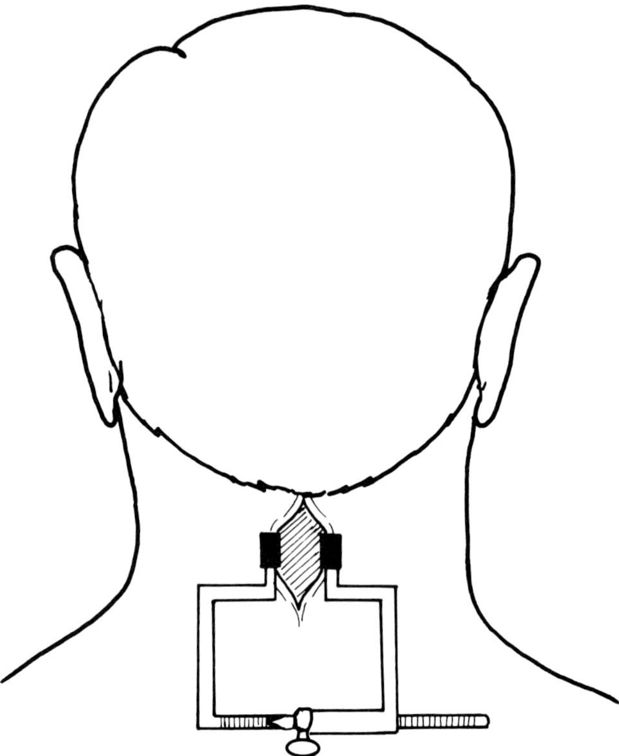

Figure 4.21.   The frame retractor is in position to expose the interlaminar interval.

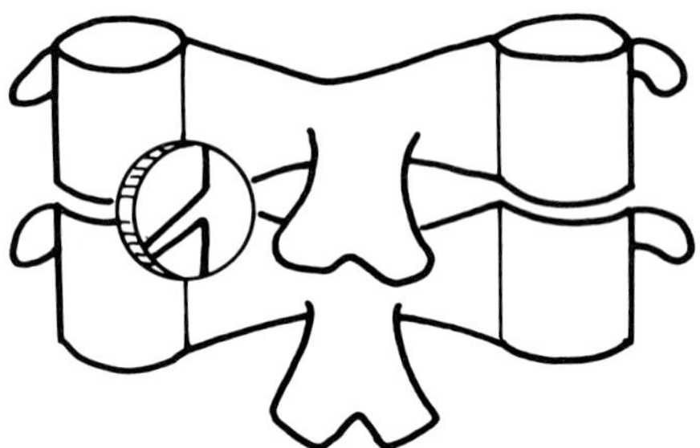

Figure 4.22.   The extent of the keyhole laminectomy centered just medial to the medial border of the facet joint. The edge of the cord (dura) and nerve root are shown.

Osteophytic Removal.   Only the uncovertebral osteophytes can be removed from an anterior approach. If it is necessary to remove osteophytes from the facet joint that encroach upon the neural canal, a posterior approach is necessary. Removal of the anterior osteophytes is greatly assisted by the microscope.

Fusion.   Since these patients usually have neck ache in association with their chronic arm pain, it is even more important to do a fusion at the time of discectomy (Fig. 4.17).

Posterior Approach

This is an approach more frequently used in the neurosurgical community for:

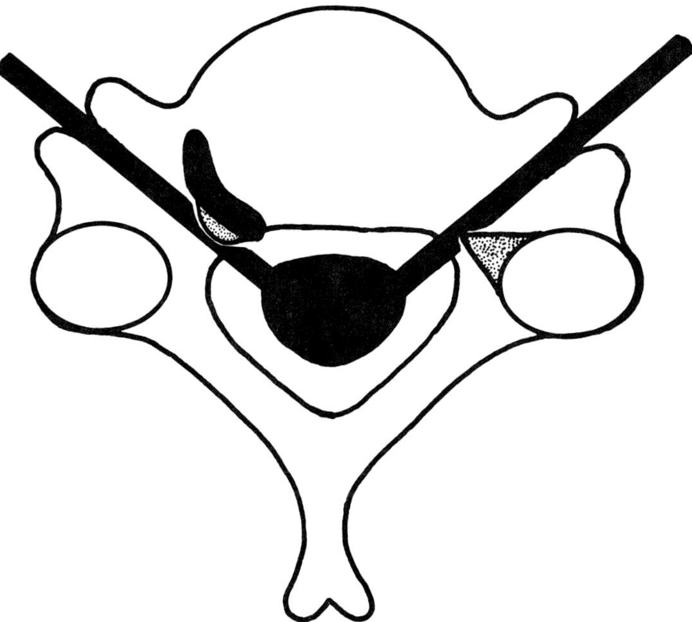

Figure 4.23.   The two forms of osteophytic encroachment. On the left, the more usual form of an uncovertebral osteophyte. On the right, a facet joint osteophyte (*stippled areas*).

1. Lateral or foraminal disc herniations with root compression.
2. Facet joint osteophytes (Fig. 4.24) encroaching upon nerve root territory, causing radicular pain.
3. The patient who has had anterior cervical surgery with adequate decompression and fusion persists with arm pain, and another level has been ruled out as the source of symptoms.

Before considering a posterior foraminal decompression you must be absolutely sure the correct anatomic segment has been approached and that there is a facet osteophyte encroaching on the nerve root. It is far more likely that failed anterior surgery was due to an incorrect diagnosis or the wrong level operated upon. The technique is no different than that described in the section on soft disc herniations except that this is a much easier decompression since it all occurs posterior to the nerve root.

Surgery for Cervical Myelopathy

Although it is uncommon for operative intervention to reverse the myelopathic deficit completely, the patient's function can be improved and the relentless progression of the lesion can be stemmed to some extent by enlarging the spinal canal (Table 4.7). This is the main reason surgeons are so aggressive with surgery in myelopathic patients. Neurological changes, however, are produced by a combination of factors. The spinal canal is narrowed anteriorly by a projecting bar at the back of the vertebral body and is further narrowed posteriorly by the buckled ligamentum flavum. The cord is placed in further jeopardy

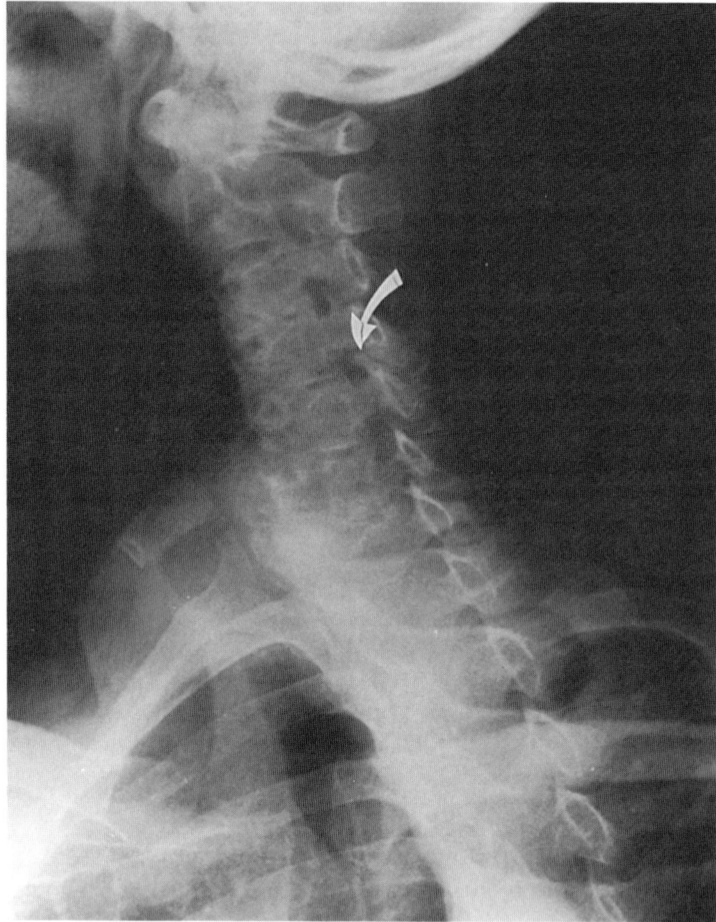

Figure 4.24.   A facet joint osteophyte (*arrow*) encroaching on the foramen.

by abnormal mobility of the involved segments. In addition to this, cervical cord ischemia results from spasm of the lateral spinal arteries and their branches to the pia anastomosis. If the lesion is not corrected, a chronic asphyxia of the Schwann and neuronal cells results and continues beyond the point at which functional recovery is possible.

Operative arrest of the process demands the following: removal of the posterior vertebral body bony spurs, or removal of the lamina and ligamentum flavum, and decompression of the nerve roots. Results are improved with a segmental fusion to overcome the harmful instability.

The choices and controversies in surgery for CSM center around anterior vs. posterior approaches. Those who support the anterior approach feel that since most of the pathology is anterior (posterior vertebral body osteophytes) it is better to operate from the front. The controversy then centers around how many levels to do and by what method (individual disc excision and grafting [Fig. 4.17] or corpectomy and a strut graft [Fig. 4.25]).

Table 4.7.   Factors Affecting Outcome in Surgery for CSM

Better outcomes from surgery occur if:

1. The patient is young.
2. The history of CSM is short (but not of an acute [vascular] onset or sudden deterioration).
3. The spinal canal is not seriously reduced in size from birth.
4. The neurological deficit consists of:
   a. Spasticity more than weakness.
   b. No muscle atrophy.
   c. Unilateral more than bilateral symptoms.
   d. No bladder or bowel symptoms.
   e. No cord atrophy on MRI.
5. Symptoms are benfitted by wearing a collar.
6. There are few significant concurrent medical problems such as diabetes, cardiac disease, pulmonary disease, or CNS dementia or debility.

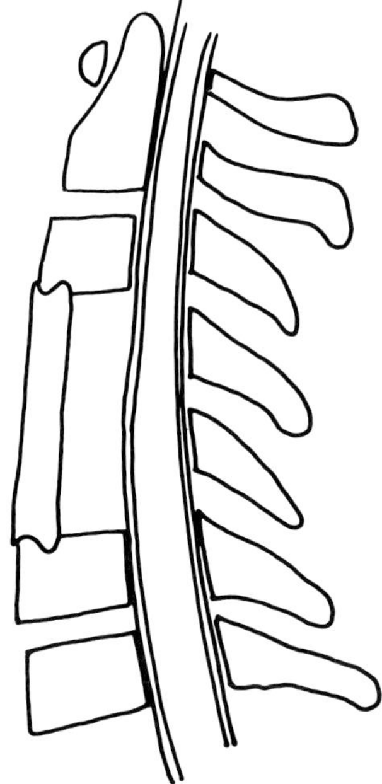

Figure 4.25.   An example of removal of vertebral bodies 4 and 5 and a fibular strut graft.

Anterior Approach

The authors use individual anterior discectomies and Smith-Robinson fusion for single- and double-level procedures; for three or more levels, the authors use a corpectomy and autogenous fibular strut graft. Obviously, in a corpectomy, the posterior osteophytes are removed. It should be just as obvious for individual discectomies and fusions that the posterior osteophytes should also be removed. This is greatly facilitated by the microscope. To leave the posterior osteophytes on the theory that, once a fusion has been achieved, they will melt away is simply not holding up to scrutiny.

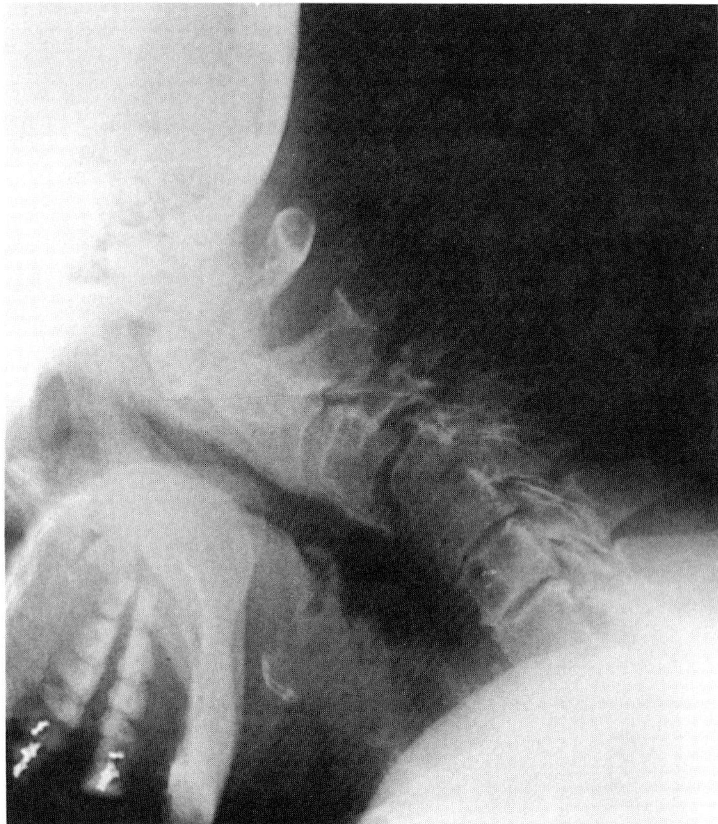

Figure 4.26. A swan neck deformity.

The Posterior Approach

The posterior approach tends to be used for multilevel (three or more segments) stenosis, severe stenosis (a canal less than 13 mm), and OPLL (ossification of the posterior longitudinal ligament). The posterior approach is contraindicated if a swan neck deformity is present preoperatively (Fig. 4.26).

The choices posteriorly are a wide laminectomy (Fig. 4.27) or a laminoplasty (Fig. 4.28). The advantages of laminoplasty include less risk of a postoperative swan neck deformity and more remaining bone with which to effect a fusion, if that is part of the game plan.

Postoperative Care

If a fusion has been part of the operation, patients usually wear a Philadelphia collar for six weeks to facilitate bone graft incorporation. An anterior discectomy without a fusion causes a lot of postoperative pain requiring brace support of the neck. A posterior decompressive operation, unless it is multisegmental, is so benign that no collar support is needed.

Six weeks post surgery, if x-rays show all bone grafts are still in place, start weaning the patient from the brace and begin a gentle exercise program.

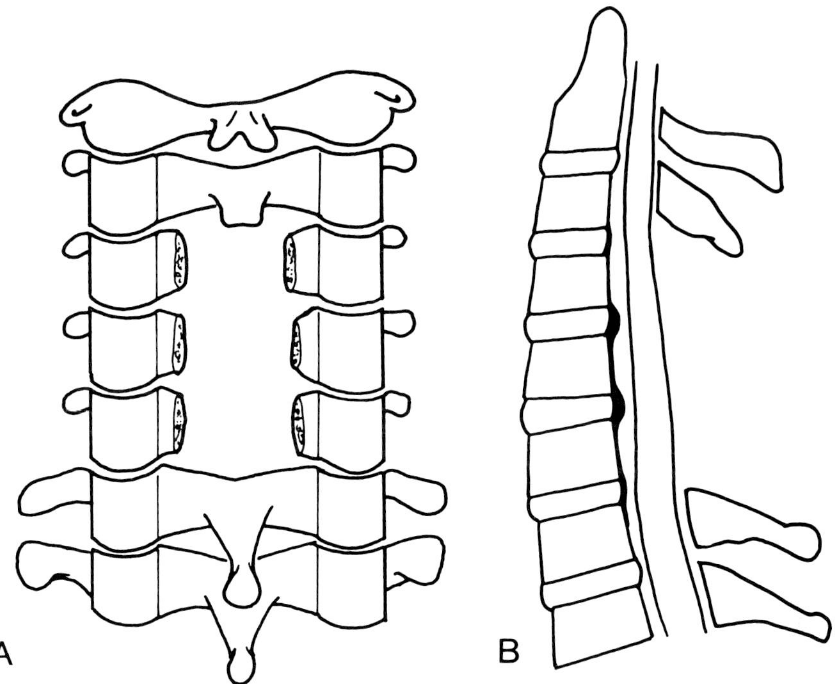

Figure 4.27. **A,** posterior view of a three-level laminectomy (C3, C4, C5). **B,** a lateral view of the same level laminectomy.

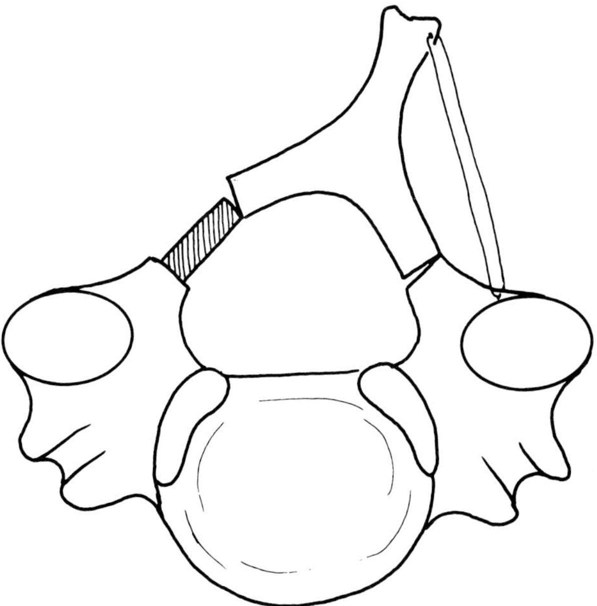

Figure 4.28. A laminoplasty—opening the lamina on one side and blocking the opening with bone graft (*striped area*).

Complications of Anterior and Posterior Spine Surgery

Obviously, any surgical procedure may be followed by general complications of atelectasis, pneumonia, urinary tract infections, and/or phlebitis.

More to the point are the specific complications relative to spine surgery. Far and away, the most common reason for a poor outcome is failure of diagnosis. The patient selection was poor (you operated on a malingerer!), the diagnosis was missed (the patient had a frozen shoulder), or the wrong level was operated upon (your clinical exam and/or your investigation let you down).

Injury to neurological structures may occur with either the anterior or posterior approach. Since the main neurological structure is the spinal cord, injury can be devastating.

Any surgery can be followed by an infection, and the usual perioperative precautions need to be taken.

Complications Specific to the Anterior Approach.   Structures that may be injured on the way in include the carotid artery and jugular vein laterally, and the trachea, esophagus, and recurrent laryngeal nerve medially. More deeply, the sympathetic plexus on the anterolateral surface of the longus colli may be injured. All these complications may be prevented by blunt finger dissection to get to the front of the cervical spine and careful but aggressive elevation of the longus colli so that sharp retractor blades can be placed deeply. Retraction is then on the longus colli and not on all these important structures.

A complication to be avoided at all costs is damage to the vertebral artery (Fig. 4.29). Anomalies of the vertebral artery and variations in dominant supply (right vs. left) take a high toll on the base of the brain when this complication occurs.

Low anterior exposures may result in a pneumothorax or mediastinitis. Injury to the thoracic duct on the left side has already been mentioned.

Almost all anterior approaches are followed by a few days of dysphagia. This should lessen in five to seven days. Be wary of a sudden increase in dysphagia a few days postoperatively—your bone graft has extruded. Serious dysphagia and/or shortness of breath from a hematoma is rare and prevented by draining the wound for 24 hours postoperatively after careful hemostasis on closure. If a hematoma with shortness of breath occurs in the first few days, deal with it on an emergency basis by reopening the wound and evacuating the hematoma.

Complications Specific to the Posterior Approach.   Complications of the posterior approach are less common than those of the anterior approach. Constant dialogue occurs between those who perform the posterior approach with the patient in the sitting position and those who prefer the patient in the prone position. The sitting position lessens bleeding but exposes patients to the possibility of a rush of air entering a vein, traversing the heart, and causing infarction of the brain. This is a rare complication, the fear of which has become the driving force behind the increase in posterior surgery with the patient in the prone position.

Dural tears, especially in the laminoplasty techniques with power tools, are more frequent with the posterior approach, but still very rare.

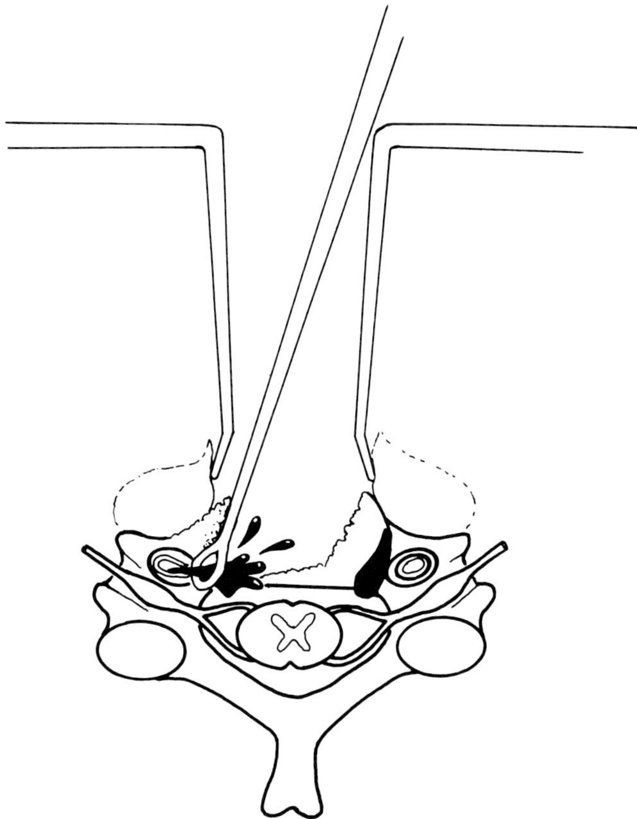

Figure 4.29.   Damage to the vertebral artery can occur lateral to the neurocentral osteophyte.

CONCLUSION

The challenge of treating the diseased cervical spine center around a careful diagnosis, long term conservative treatment efforts and, when indicated, precise surgical techniques to prevent devastating complications.

REFERENCES

1. Andersson GBJ: Back schools. In: The Lumbar Spine and Back Pain, 3rd ed., pp 315–320. Ed: Jayson MIV. Churchill Livingstone, Edinburgh (1987).
2. Babb RR: Editorial: Be cautious in the use of NSAIDs. Orthop Review 21:687–688 (1992).
3. Brooks PM and Day RO: Nonsteroidal anti-inflammatory drugs—differences and similarities. N Engl J Med 324:1716–1725 (1991).
4. Deyo RA: Conservative therapy for low back pain: distinguishing useful from useless therapy. JAMA 250:1057–1062 (1983).
5. Deyo RA, Walsh NE, Martin DC, Schoenfeld LS, and Ramamurthy S: A controlled trial of transcutaneous electrical nerve stimulation (TENS) and exercise for chronic low back pain. N Engl J Med 322:1627–1634 (1990).
6. Elenbaas JK: Centrally acting oral skeletal muscle relaxants. Am J Hosp Pharm 37:1313–1323 (1980).
7. Friedman LW and Galton L: Freedom from Backaches. Simon & Schuster, New York (1973).
8. Godfrey CM, Morgan PP, and Schatzker J: A randomized trial of manipulation for low-back pain in a medical setting. Spine 9:301–304 (1984).

9. Inturrisi CE: Narcotic drugs. Med Clin North Am 66:1061–1071 (1982).

10. Jackson CP and Brown MD: Analysis of current approaches and a practical guide to prescription of exercise. Clin Orthop 179:46–54 (1983).

11. Jayson MIV, Sims-Williams H, Young S, Baddeley H, and Collins E: Mobilization and manipulation for low back pain. Spine 6:409–416 (1981).

12. Johnson RM, Hart DL, Simmons EF, Ramsky GR, and Southwick WO: Cervical orthoses: a study comparing their effectiveness in restricting cervical motion in normal subjects. J Bone Joint Surg 59A:332–339 (1977).

13. Krag MH: Biomechanics of the cervical spine. In: The Adult Spine: Principles and Practice, pp 929–965. Ed: Frymoyer JW. Raven Press, New York (1991).

14. Landon BR: Heat or cold for the relief of low back pain? Phys Ther 47:1126–1130 (1967).

15. McCray RE and Patton NJ: Pain relief at trigger points: a comparison of moist heat and short-wave diathermy. J Orthop Sport Phys Ther 5:175–181 (1984).

16. Melzack R: Acupuncture and related forms of folk medicine. In: Textbook of Pain, pp 691–700. Eds: Wall PD and Melzack R. Churchill Livingstone, Edinburgh (1984).

17. Murphy TM, Raj PP, and Stanton-Hicks M: Techniques of nerve blocks—spinal nerves. In: Practical Management of Pain, pp 597–636. Ed: Raj PP. Year Book Medical Publishers, Chicago (1986).

18. Nouwen A: EMG biofeedback used to reduce standing levels of paraspinal muscle tension in chronic low back pain. Pain 17:353–360 (1983).

19. Paris SV: Spinal manipulative therapy. Clin Orthop 179:55–61 (1983).

20. Pheasant H, Bursk A, Goldfarb J, Azen SP, Weiss JN, and Borelli LL: Amitriptyline and chronic low-back pain: a randomized double-blind crossover study. Spine 8:552–557 (1983).

21. Sikorski JM: A rationalized approach to physiotherapy for low-back pain. Spine 10:571–579 (1985).

22. Simon LS and Mills JS: Drug therapy: nonsteroidal anti-inflammatory drugs. N Engl J Med 302:1179–1186 (1980).

23. Stimmel B: Pain, analgesia, and addiction: an approach to the pharmacologic management of pain. Clin J Pain 1:14–19 (1985).

24. Swezey RL: The modern thrust of manipulation and traction therapy. Semin Arthritis Rheum 12:322–331 (1983).

25. Ward NG: Tricyclic antidepressants for chronic low back pain: mechanisms of action and predictors of response. Spine 11:661–665 (1986).

26. Woolf CJ: Transcutaneous and implanted nerve stimulation. In: Textbook of Pain, pp 679–690. Eds: Wall PD and Melzack R. Churchill Livingstone, Edinburgh (1986).

5

Psychogenic Neck Pain

"It is as important to know as much about the man who has the pain as it is to know about the pain the man has."
—Numerous Great Physicians and Surgeons

That medicine should concern itself with the whole person is often stated but frequently ignored. The hallmark of a good clinician is the ability not only to diagnose disease but also to assess the "whole patient." No test of the art of medicine is more demanding than the identification of the patient with a nonorganic or emotional component to a neck problem.

To start, recognize the disability equation:

$$\text{Disability} = A + B + C$$

where A = the physical component (disease); B = the patient's emotional reaction; C = the situation the patient is in at the time of disability (i.e., compensation claim, motor vehicle accident).

Each patient with neck pain may have a component of each of these entities entwined in his or her disability. For example, a patient presenting a collection of symptoms, with no physical findings evident on examination, should lead one to think of the other aspects of the equation and look for emotional disability or situational reactions.

A classification of nonorganic spinal pain (2) is outlined in Table 5.1. The term nonorganic has been chosen over other terms such as nonphysical, functional, emotional, and psychogenic.

Before even considering this section, recognize that nonorganic syndromes do not occur in a void. There is always a clinical setting that supports the presence of a nonorganic component to the patient's disability, that is, if you make the diagnosis of psychosomatic pain, there must be a patient in anxiety or a tension-producing situation in the patient's life. If you make the diagnosis of psychogenic

Table 5.1. Nonorganic Spinal Pain

1. Psychosomatic spinal pain
   a. Tension syndrome (fibrositis)
2. Psychogenic spinal pain
   a. Psychogenic spinal pain
   b. Psychogenic modification of organic spinal pain
3. Situational spinal pain
   a. Litigation reaction
   b. Exaggeration reaction

pain syndrome, you will find a premorbid personality or emotional state that fostered the reaction. If you make the diagnosis of situational spinal pain, a situation such as a motor vehicle accident—and a lawyer or a compensation claim— will exist. Nonorganic reactions do not occur in a void.

The following definitions are used:

1. Psychosomatic spinal pain is defined as symptomatic physical change in tissues of the spine, which has anxiety as its cause. The expression of anxiety is mediated as a prolonged and exaggerated state that eventually leads to structural change (spasm) in the muscles of the neck or low back.

2a. Psychogenic spinal pain is defined as the conversion or somatization of anxiety into pain referred to the neck or back, unaccompanied by physical change in the tissues of these regions. The pain is variously known in the literature as conversion hysteria, psychogenic regional pain, traumatic or accident neurosis, and hypochondriasis.

   The emotional upset brings pains to the neck just as it may bring tears to the eyes. The reason for the conversion is found in complex psychodynamic mechanisms beyond the scope of this book. The reaction represents a sincere unconscious emotional illness that offers the patient the primary gain of solving inner conflicts, fears, and anxieties. Inherent in the conversion reaction is the concept of suggestion and hypnosis, the importance of which will become apparent later in this chapter.

2b. Psychogenic modification of spinal pain is a sincere emotional reaction that modifies the appreciation of organic pain. Usually, the organic pain by itself would not be disabling, but with the psychogenic modification a significant disability ensues. No associated physical change occurs as a result of anxiety, and a conversion reaction may coexist.

   An example is the patient burdened with situational pressures—mortgage payments, car payments, etc. This patient, because of his or her minor physical illness, feels unable to sustain the effort necessary to meet these demands. A resulting depression may occur, and the symptoms of fatigue, loss of appetite, insomnia, impotence, constipation, etc., so dominate the patient's history that the underlying physical condition is missed. Other examples are patients with passive-dependent personalities, drug or alcoholic dependence, or psychosis. In the face of a minor physical problem, these patients use their illness to step out of the pressures of the real world with frequent demands for mood-altering or analgesic medications.

   Some obsessive-compulsive patients cannot adjust to a minor physical problem, and this personality trait leads them to feel they have a significant disability.

3. Situational spinal pain is a reaction whereby a patient, through a collection of symptoms, maintains a situation (with potential secondary gain) through overconcern or conscious effort.

3a. The litigation or compensation reaction is defined as overconcern by the patient for present and future health, arising out of a litigious or compensable event that initially affected health. The reaction manifests itself in a patient's complaint of continuing neck or back pain coupled with a concern that, upon formal severance from his or her claim to compensation, deterioration in health may occur. The patient with this reaction is neither physically nor emotionally ill.

This reaction is not to be confused with the ambiguous terms "litigation neurosis" or "compensation neurosis." Like "whiplash," these terms have no medical or legal value and should be dropped from our vocabulary. If a patient has a true neurosis arising out of a litigious or compensable event (accident), then those terms listed under "psychogenic spinal pain (2a or 2b)" should be used for diagnostic purposes (e.g., traumatic neurosis or accident neurosis). If the patient's disability appears to be based more on an awareness of the commercial value of his or her symptoms, the reaction should not be legitimized by the use of the term neurosis in conjunction with the words litigation or compensation (hence the classification: litigation reaction).

3b. Exaggeration reactions are attempts by the patient to appear ill or magnify an existent illness. "Malingering" is a term frequently applied to this reaction and is defined as the conscious alteration of health for gain.

As will be described below, it is possible for the physician to detect efforts to magnify, but it is not proper to assign motives, like the desire for gain, to the patient. The lawyer involved is in a reversed role. He or she may raise doubts about the plaintiff's motives (such as desire for gain) but may not be in a position to clinically detect efforts to magnify or exaggerate. The choice of the word "malingering" implies proficiency in two professions, an uncommon occurrence. For this reason, the terms "malingering" and "conscious effort" are best not used by the physician when discussing nonorganic spinal pain.

Alteration of health in order to deceive, evade responsibility, or derive gain does occur. Those who would deny this deny the existence of human nature. The patient who tries to alter or reproduce symptoms or signs of a spinal problem may do so in a number of ways:

1. Pretension. No physical illness exists and the patient willfully fabricates symptoms and signs. Occurring infrequently in the military during wartime, it is a rare civilian event.
2. Exaggeration. Symptoms and signs of a spinal disability are magnified to represent more than they really are.
3. Perseveration. Symptoms and signs that were once present have ceased to exist but continue to be described or demonstrated by the patient.
4. Allegation. Genuine disability is present, but the patient fraudulently ascribes these to some cause associated with gain, knowing that, in fact, his or her condition is of different origin.

Civilian nonorganic situational spinal pain is usually the exaggeration or perseveration type. Pretension and allegation are uncommon forms of gainful alteration of health in civilian practice. Like the patient with the litigation reaction, these patients are neither emotionally ill nor physically ill. However, they differ from the litigation reaction in that they are attempting to demonstrate physical illness through the effort of exaggeration or perseveration. The reason for this effort is usually, but not always, found in secondary financial gain.

CLINICAL DESCRIPTION

Before describing each of these entities, it is important to emphasize:

1. This is a simplistic classification that is useful only to the family practitioner or the spinal surgeon. It does not allow for the more complex assessments done by psychologists and psychiatrists, but it does allow for a foundation on which to build clinical recognition of these entities so that the patient can be referred to others more skilled in the field.
2. One cannot rigidly define nonorganic disability, because there are gray areas. However, there is a tendency for a nonorganic disability to fall largely into one category.
3. It is most important to determine whether the setting exists for one of these nonorganic disabilities.
   a. A patient who has had previous emotional problems is prone to have an emotional component to a disability. Symptoms such as fatigue, sleeplessness, agitation, gastrointestinal upset, and excessive sweating should signal that an emotional component is likely present.
   b. A patient who is in a secondary gain situation such as a motor vehicle accident claim has the potential for these nonorganic reactions. It is important to establish if the incident is a claim type of accident and whether insurance and legal factors are involved. Conversely, if there is no secondary gain detected on history, it is unusual to arrive at a secondary gain diagnosis such as litigation reaction or magnification-exaggeration reaction.
4. A vague and confusing history, a baffling physical examination, and an elusive diagnosis signal a possible nonorganic diagnosis. Reflect on this before taking the expensive step of hospital admission and sophisticated, expensive testing having the potential for a false-positive result.
5. A patient who quickly establishes an abnormal doctor-patient relationship has a potential nonorganic component to his or her disability. These abnormal doctor-patient relationships include patients who are hostile or effusively complimentary, those who have had many other doctors caring for them before your assessment, some who fail to respond to standard (physical) conservative treatment measures, and patients who are critical of other doctors.

Psychosomatic Neck Pain

The psychosomatic phenomenon of muscle spasm arising out of tension usually affects the neck more commonly than the low back. It should be known as the "orthopaedic ulcer," but more often is given the label of fibrositis. Patients with this problem are overtly strained and tense, as evidenced by facial expression. They are fidgety and restless, and may sit on the edge of the chair while they wring their hands. Some of these patients will place their hands on their neck or back during the history, and literally wring the area while describing the pain. They have a general feeling of restlessness and a specific feeling of tightness in the neck, with associated sensations of cracking and a constant feeling of the need to stretch out the neck and shoulder muscles. The pain is not specifically mechanical but does tend to accumulate with the day's activity, especially when that activity is carried out in the tension-producing environment like the workplace.

The pain typically responds to chiropractic or physiotherapeutic intervention, but relief is usually temporary, a fact that makes the patient tend to seek prolonged care.

Physical examination reveals a good range of movement in the back, with a complaint of pain only if movement is done too quickly or carried to extremes. The significant physical finding is the presence of firm, tender muscles or "trigger points" when the affected part is examined in a position of rest. The patient may be able to demonstrate the "cracking" to the touch or auditory perception of the examiner.

No evidence of nerve root involvement exists in the extremities. Skin tenderness, the significance of which is explained below, is not an unusual finding.

Psychogenic Neck Pain

The patient with psychogenic spinal pain is emotionally ill. These patients often have a history of past illness replete with emotional problems. It follows that history of the present illness contains a preponderance of emotional symptoms, and the description of pain will not be typical of any organic condition. The patient is convinced that he or she is ill, and this conviction results in frequent demands for consultation with numerous doctors. Considerable financial hardship and aggravation will occur in some cases where these consultations take the patient great distances to and from major clinics or spas throughout the world. Throughout their constant demand for care, these patients notice times when their symptoms do improve. This is due to the institution of some new form of treatment that affects the patient through suggestion or hypnosis, a fact that makes placebo trial of little value in evaluation of these problems.

It follows that, because these patients are emotionally ill, no causative organic problem will be found on physical examination. The conversion reaction is associated with a distorted appreciation of body image such that a topographical unit (the neck and arm), indifferent to matters of innervation or anatomical relationship, will contain physical findings of skin tenderness and dulled sensory appreciation (3) (Fig. 5.1). The somatization infrequently reaches the stage of weakness, with wasting and depression of all reflexes in the contiguous part, e.g., the arm.

However, the important observation on physical examination of this patient is the paucity of physical findings, which separates him or her from the magnifier and exaggerator, who has, by definition, many "physical" findings.

Psychogenic Modification of Organic Pain

Of all of the nonorganic causes of spinal pain, the patient who psychogenically modifies organic pain presents the most difficult diagnostic and therapeutic challenge. Sometimes, but not always, the organic problem by itself would not be disabling. Thus, the historical and physical component of the disability related to the organicity is not significant. Those findings indicative of a physical illness will be appropriate and serve as a quantitative guide to the extent of physical illness. However, the situational pressures or the personality of the patient modify the disability to a significant degree. In addition, the psychogenic reaction interferes with response to treatment and leads to persistence of the disability. In a surgical practice, this failure to respond to conservative treatment is the classic indication for operative intervention. If the surgeon fails to recognize that the failure

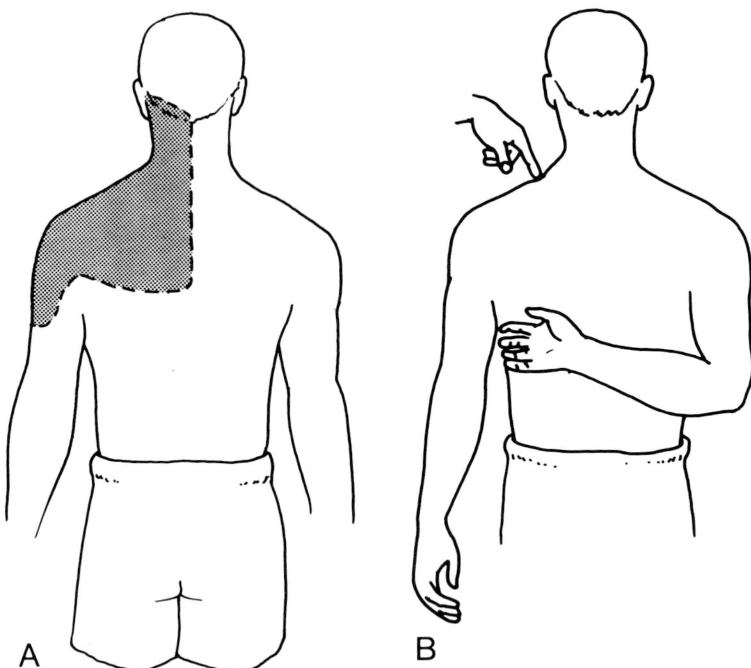

Figure 5.1.   **A,** the shaded area represents a nondermatomal (nonanatomical) area of tenderness, where just lightly touching or pinching the skin will produce pain. The area usually has decreased sensory appreciation that is nondermatomal. **B,** later in the exam, while testing internal rotation of the opposite shoulder, use the same pressure to retouch the shaded area, at which time no pain will be produced. This is a form of distraction testing.

to respond to physical treatment measures is due in this instance to a psychogenic disability, he or she will gradually build a practice containing a number of spinal surgery failures.

Psychogenic modifications are commonly seen in the patient with an inadequate personality. By definition, this patient's personality may limit advancement up the social, educational, and occupational ladder, and confine him or her to the unskilled worker classification. Some of these patients can be found in the Workers' Compensation population, which may be one of the reasons for poorer results of treatment sometimes obtained in this kind of patient.

These patients are seen with a minor physical problem (e.g., neck strain) yet they have total disability. All attempts at treatment fail to return the patient to the workforce. Frequent office visits reinforce the disability for the patient. If the doctor fails to recognize this maladaptive reaction and reinforcement, he or she may initiate treatment that will not help the patient in any way.

Other psychogenic modifications come about through drug addiction and alcohol dependence. Occasionally, psychotic behavior will convert a minor physical problem into a prolonged disability.

Physical examination will reveal the nature and extent of the physical impairment. Usually the physical impairment by itself would not be significantly disabling. The loss of movement in the neck is minor and the neurological changes are of questionable significance. In the face of repeated assessments and a continuing statement of disability, the patient's minor physical problem may become magnified in the mind of the clinician who does not assess personality and life-situation factors.

Situational Spinal Pain

Litigation Reactions

This patient is neither physically nor emotionally ill. Thus, few emotional symptoms will be present on historical examination. The patient is in the process of litigation or under the care of the Workers' Compensation Board. These patients often state that they do not care about the litigation or compensation issue, yet they also state that they are afraid to settle or return to work for fear that further illness will develop. Their continuing complaints are rather vague and would not normally be incapacitating. If they are on treatment, they are not improving. Physically, there may be an increased awareness of the body part as manifested by skin tenderness in the affected area, but no organic illness is detectable, and there is no attempt to exaggerate or magnify a disability.

Magnification-Exaggeration Reaction

Some or most of the following historical characteristics will be obtained from this patient. The most obvious historical point is the secondary gain situation that usually involves the fault of someone else and/or payment of financial compensation. Other secondary gain situations can occur. The initiating event is usually a trivial or minor incident. There may be a latent period of hours or days between the incident and the onset of symptoms, during which time the patient speaks to friends and relatives, and learns of the commercial value of the injury.

The patient describes the pain with some degree of indifference as evidenced by a smile or a laugh when describing his severe disability. He or she is vague in describing and localizing the pain, giving the examiner the impression of someone struggling to remember a dream. Specificity and elaboration require memory for repetition, a quality not present to a significant degree in this type of patient. The individual wishes you to believe this pain is unique and severe. This attempt to have you believe in the pain is often accompanied by a salesman-like attitude, with many examples of the disability spontaneously listed. Inability to engage in sex is usually at the top of the list.

In spite of the trivial initiating event, the disability may have been present for a long time. Three types of treatment patterns occur:

1. The patient follows a "straight line" course of treatment; he or she does not respond to the standard physical treatment or to the suggestion and hypnosis of treatment—that is, he or she does not improve or gets worse.
2. The patient is not on treatment because he or she is "allergic" to all medications prescribed, "suffocates" in neck or back braces, or becomes ill from the "heat" in a physiotherapy department.
3. The patient is not on treatment because he or she has not sought treatment.

Certain behavioral patterns become apparent after seeing a number of these patients. Some never appear for appointments in spite of weeks of notification. Others appear late for the appointment and do not apologize, or they state indifferently that the traffic was heavy. There may be an attempt to manipulate your feelings with a compliment about your reputation or your office. There may be an effort to play one doctor against another by making false statements about another doctor. Finally, hostility may appear during the assessment. A patient who is truly ill will not be aware or afraid of exposure and will not be hostile unless provoked. A patient exaggerating a disability is suspicious. He or she may start out hostile, but the usual pattern is one of developing hostility as discrepancies in the history and physical examination are exposed. Examiners are advised, for obvious reasons, not to precipitate this final behavioral pattern.

The patient who is magnifying or exaggerating a disability can be exposed only through an adequate physical examination. Those physicians who do not physically examine patients will not recognize this reaction, which may explain the reluctance of the psychiatric community to accept this clinical entity.

The physical findings of magnification or exaggerated reaction are classified into those that demonstrate acting behavior, those that indicate anticipatory behavior, and those that fail to support the patient's claim to illness.

Acting Behavior.   Exaggerating a disability requires acting by the patient. This acting may be general in nature, such as the Academy Award performances of some patients, who moan and groan through the examination, walk around the examining room with their eyes closed, and either reach for objects to support themselves or reach for their painful areas. The incongruity of this acting behavior may be evident when the patient mounts the examining table with considerable ease and/or dresses within minutes of the examination and smiles and waves goodbye as he or she leaves the office.

Specific examples of acting behavior are the rigid neck, a condition that disappears on the examining table (Fig. 5.2), the reduction of shoulder movement (Fig. 5.3), tender skin, and the paralyzed insensitive upper extremity. That these findings are a result of acting can be demonstrated through the use of distraction testing (Table 5.2). Using nonpainful, nonemotional, and nonsurprising examination techniques, it is possible not only to change the acting behavior but also to demonstrate normal physical function. The authors' opinion is that proper distraction testing that dismisses a physical finding as acting, and demonstrates normal physical function, is a method of proving magnification-exaggeration behavior. The best distraction test is simple observation of the patient as he or she gets undressed and moves about the examining room.

Varying degrees of acting behavior occur in different patients. In general, the more sophisticated the patient, the more sophisticated the acting behavior—and the more sophisticated the examiner must be.

Anticipatory Behavior.   The second group of physical findings in this reaction represents anticipation on the part of the patient to the test situations. This anticipatory behavior leads to an appropriate response by the patient in an attempt to indicate illness. These tests are illustrated in Figure 5.4.

Contradictory Clinical Evidence.   Statements by the patient to the effect that he or she is unable to work may not be supported by clinical observation. Some patients will say they are unable to drive yet will have driven by themselves a great distance to get to the examination. Some patients will say that they require frequent medication, yet will arrive from great distances without their medication. The patient who claims to wear a neck collar continuously

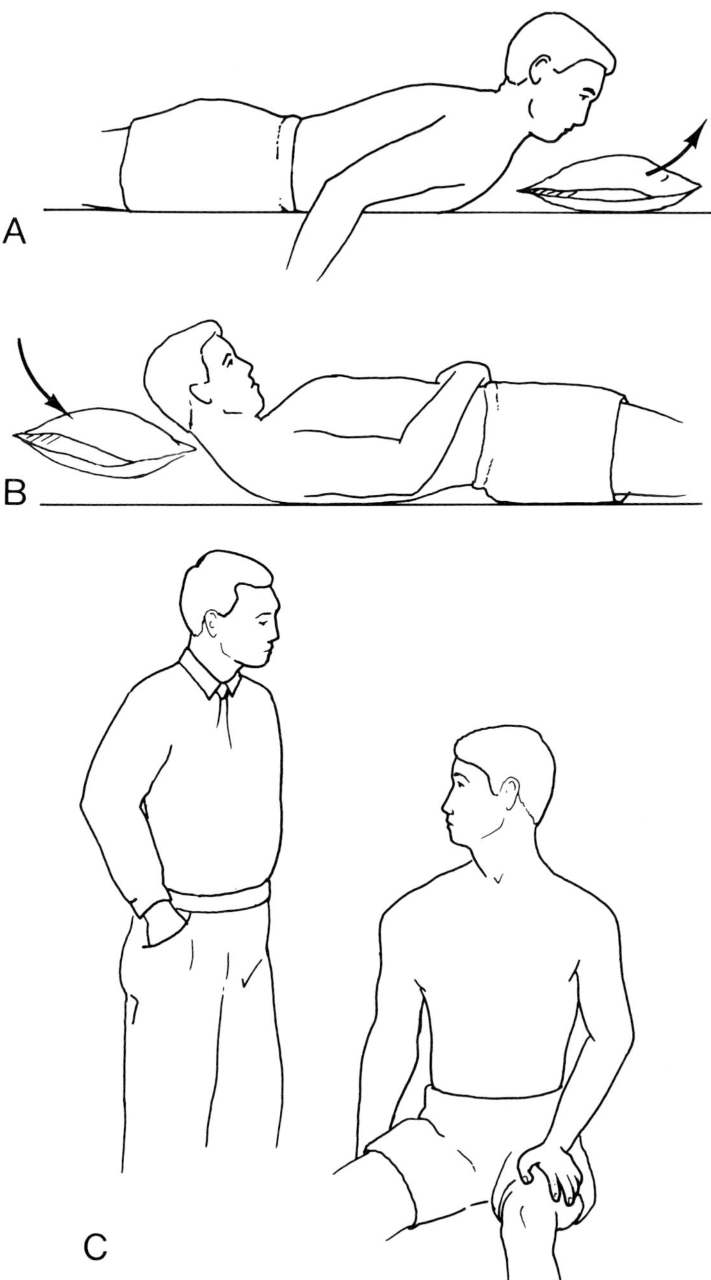

Figure 5.2.   The pillow test for the patient who "acts" out a rigid neck. Early in the exam (usually with the patient sitting), note the "rigid" neck. Later in the exam, with the patient prone (**A**), take the pillow away. Later still, with the patient supine (**B**), offer the pillow back. Each time note the range of movement. There are many variations of this test. A further example of distraction testing for the patient who "acts" out a stiff neck is (**C**). Stand behind the patient and engage him or her in casual conversation, and note the range of rotation.

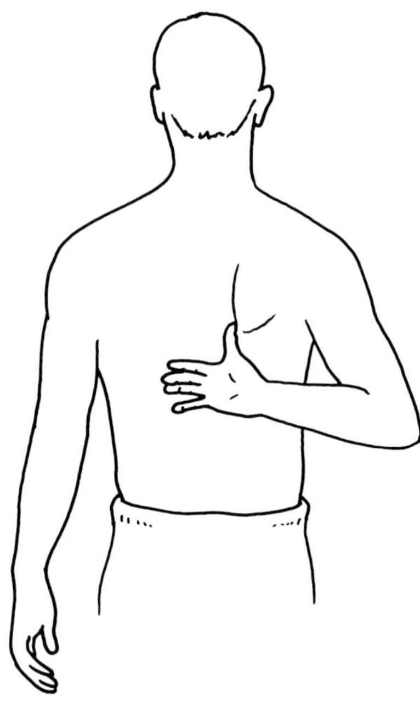

Figure 5.3. The magnifying patient, by definition, often magnifies everything, including loss of internal rotation of the shoulder joint. Later in the exam, ask the patient to point to where his or her scapular pain is located, and you will see a good range of internal rotation.

Table 5.2.   Demonstration of Acting Behavior

	Condition	Response
Step 1:	Physical finding (acting behavior)	Reduction in shoulder movement
Step 2:	Distraction test (e.g., pillow test) Nonpainful Nonemotional Nonsurprising	Normal neck movement
Observation:	Result	Normal physical function

should show signs of this wear on the body and on the appliance. If a patient carries the collar to the examination, ask him or her to put it on. It may turn out to be a friend's brace that was borrowed for the doctor visit, and it either does not fit or the patient does not know how to put it on! Patients with calluses on their hands and knees contradict their story of a prolonged inability to work. Other evidence of work may be in the form of paint stains or a particular distribution to their sunburn. Patients with nicotine stains on a grossly paralyzed limb should start to demonstrate similar stains on the opposite hand. Finally, those patients who attempt to demonstrate a prolonged and profound weakness in an extremity will not have associated wasting of that extremity.

It is important to stress that one swallow does not make a summer! Just because there is one contradictory finding, it does not mean the patient should be classified as a magnifier-exaggerator or litigant reactor. It is important to stress

Table 5.3.   Symptoms and Signs Suggesting a Nonorganic Component to Disability

Symptoms

1. Pain is multifocal in distribution and nonmechanical (present at rest).
2. Entire extremity is painful, numb, and/or weak.
3. Extremity gives way (as a result the patient drops things).
4. Treatment response:
   a. No response.
   b. "Allergic" to treatment.
   c. Not on treatment.
5. Multiple crises, multiple hospital admissions/investigations, multiple doctors.

Signs

1. Tenderness is superficial (skin) or nonanatomic (e.g., over acromion).
2. Simulated movement tests are positive.
3. Distraction tests are positive.
4. Whole arm is weak or numb.
5. "Academy Award" performance.

that a collection of symptoms and signs should be present with the appropriate clinical setting to make the diagnosis of magnification-exaggeration behavior. Waddell et al. (2) have documented the significant symptoms and signs that, when existing together, suggest a nonorganic component to the disability. These symptoms and signs have been scientifically documented as valid and reproducible. As a screening mechanism, they are an excellent substitute for pain drawings and psychological testing (Table 5.3).

It is one thing to have a fancy classification; it is another to make it work. When interviewing the patient, try to place him or her in one of the following categories:

Normal, Everyday Patient With Neck Pain

Fortunately, this group is by far the largest group of patients. It seems, without great socioeconomic research, that people tend to associate with kindred spirits. Turkeys prefer to flock with turkeys, and eagles like to soar with eagles. Similarly, the hypochondriacal patient tends to associate with other anxious, tension-ridden people. If, as a practitioner, you are oversympathetic and solicitous to patients with emotional components to their disability, then soon their friends start appearing as your patients, and soon the bulk of your patient load ceases to be the normal, everyday patient with neck pain!

Stoic

This patient is usually in your office because his wife sent him. When asked why he is there, he may state that there is a little pain in his arm, but "not to worry, I can work and play." Do not be misled. This patient may have no more than 5° of neck movement, no biceps reflex, and no elbow flexion power, that is, he has a significant physical problem due to the ruptured disc at C5-C6. But he does not have time in his busy life for illness. We use the male designation for this example because most (but not all) of these patients are men. They are not always from "management"—many come from the labor sector of the economy

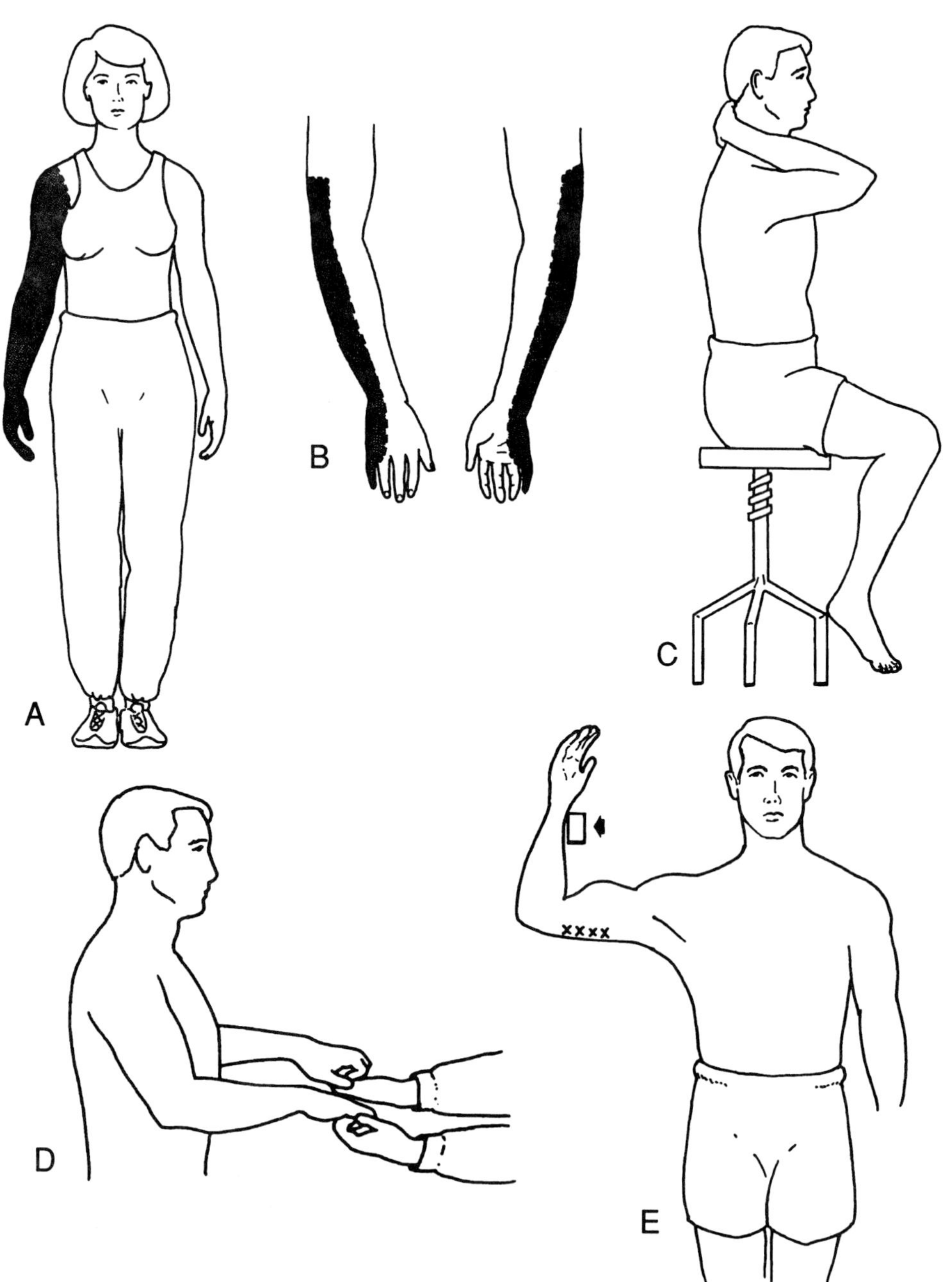

Figure 5.4.

and have yet to succumb to the financial inducements to illness behavior inherent in various Workers' Compensation systems.

Racehorse Syndrome

The racehorse syndrome applies to the group of tense, hard driving, hyper-reactive patients. Under stressful situations, they tend to hyperextend their necks and assume the fight position because of their chronic muscle spasm. Throughout their lives, they have responded to tense situations in this manner without pain. However, once they develop disc degeneration, segmental instability and muscle spasm allow the related posterior joints to be pushed beyond their permitted physiological range when this posture is adopted, and pain results. The pain they experience interferes with their ability to get on with a normal way of life, and the frustration they feel increases tension in the sacrospinalis, thereby aggravating and perpetuating discomfort. In the treatment of these patients, the significance of this postural change must be explained. In addition to routine conservative treatment of discogenic neck pain, they should be taught voluntary muscle relaxation, and they need mild sedation to take the edge off their normal tensions and anxieties. (Classification: This patient has a variety of psychosomatic pain, aggravating the organic condition of degenerative disc disease.)

Razor's Edge Syndrome

The razor's edge syndrome refers to patients who precariously tread their way through life on the razor's edge of emotional stability. These patients with hysterical personalities—like people in show business—play their lives in "high-C."

Before the recent changes in sartorial habits, they could be spotted easily. The women loved outlandish hairstyles and heavy eye makeup. They decorated themselves with large earrings and rows of necklaces. Multiple bracelets and bangles adorned their wrists, and they wore huge garish rings on their fingers. The men grew beards, and both men and women wore dark glasses, even indoors. In today's world, dress and hairstyle can no longer be regarded as having diagnostic significance, but the dramatization of symptoms is characteristic.

Superlatives are thrown around with gay abandon. The pain is "agonizing . . . I was paralyzed with pain . . . It was as though someone was tearing the muscles

---

Figure 5.4.   Examples of anticipatory behavior. **A,** often the whole arm will be numb irrespective of dermatomal innervation. **B,** sometimes only the ulnar side of the forearm will be numb. Test this at various times in supination and in pronation, and note that the extension of the numbness from the forearm into the arm changes from lateral (*left*) in pronation, to medial arm (*right*) in supination. **C,** the simulated movement test. Sit the patient on a rotating stool, ask him or her to close the eyes, and rotate the stool (without rotating the neck). The magnifier will complain of neck pain and may even reach for the neck. **D,** the simultaneous hand strength test. Test each hand grip separately. If the symptomatic arm is weak and the normal arm strong, test bilateral grip strength simultaneously. The mind is not fast enough (without training) to transmit a weak message to one arm and a strong message to the other. With this test, the magnifier will show both weak (usual) or both strong (unusual). **E,** agonist/antagonist testing. The example is testing biceps/brachialis strength (*block and arrow*). In true weakness the triceps (*xxxx*) will relax, but in acting-out weakness, the magnifier will contract the triceps during biceps strength testing (which can be palpated).

out of my shoulder . . . It's like boiling water being poured on my neck . . . I haven't had a wink of sleep in two months."

Examination reveals diverse corporal contortions, such as twitching, turning, writhing, and rolling about, and the examiner's discovery of tender points is invariably acknowledged by wails, moans, groans, sharp intakes of breath, or uncontrolled and alarming shouts.

No drug will give these patients a chemical vacation from their exhausting reaction to life. If the underlying cause of their symptoms can be recognized through their emotional smoke screen, it should be treated along routine lines. When the cause of the pain has been overcome, they will return to a way of life that is normal for them.

Hysterical reactions are common in childhood. When a child grazes his knee, he walks with a stiff leg. There is no need to do this; it is a hysterical response to injury—an exaggerated response for the purposes of gain, namely, attention and sympathy. In a child, this is understood and tolerated with a smile. In an adult, the same response generally irritates the physician; indeed, it may irritate him or her to such a degree that examination and treatment tend to be superficial. At times it is difficult to remember that these patients cannot control or modify their reactions—it is in their genes. The physician is treating a patient, not a neck, and regardless of the bizarre description of the symptoms, and the histrionics on examination, he or she must accept the possibility of a physical disorder and investigate its probability, if indicated. (Classification: This patient is a psychogenic modifier with, more often than not, a minor physical problem.)

Worried-Sick Syndrome

Only a fool would be totally unconcerned about the development of inexplicable symptoms. Most patients are concerned not only about the cause of their symptoms, but also about their significance. Many have seen relatives in the terminal phases of malignancy whose last symptom was spine pain. Many associate pain in the neck with "arthritis," and this fear may be heightened when the patient has previously been told that "x-rays of the neck showed arthritic changes." To most patients, arthritis denotes a dreaded and relentlessly progressive disease leading to confinement in a wheelchair. These fears are common, although not commonly expressed. Above all, the physician must reassure the patient and disabuse him or her of unfounded anxiety. The patient with disc degeneration must never be told he or she has "arthritis of the spine."

Anxiety may be a form of intelligent concern, but in those born to worry, an almost pathological unfounded concern about symptoms may be more disabling than the pain itself. These patients confuse the words "hurting" and "harming." Every time they do something that increases pain, they are terrified they have done themselves irreparable damage. They treat their necks like Dresden china, fearful of doing anything that may aggravate the lesion and prolong their disability. Their problem may be compounded by the physician's advice. In the routine management of discogenic back pain, they may be told to avoid certain activities, such as bending, lifting, playing tennis, or bowling. This is good advice, but they must also be told that these modifications of activity are suggested to decrease discomfort, not to prevent damage. Otherwise, patients may gradually cut themselves off from all activities, and eventually they merely vegetate.

"This neck pain is completely ruining my life—I can't bowl, I can't ski, I can't play golf, I can't do anything," the patient may say. "Do you get a lot of pain when you do these things?" asks the physician. "I don't know—I haven't done anything for two years," replies the patient. "Why haven't you tried to play a game of golf again?" "My doctor told me I shouldn't."

After weeks or months of inactivity, it will be extremely difficult to get these patients back to the business of normal living. Every increase in activity may be associated with a new twinge of pain that may frighten them back to the security of their beds. Their problems are compounded by apprehension and misapprehension, and the physician must deal firmly with both. (Classification: These patients have a variety of situational spinal pain. Although worried about their symptoms, they have not gone through the complex psychodynamic mechanisms resulting in somatization. Rather, these patients simply need encouragement to deal in a more positive way with their symptoms and recognize the significant difference between hurt and harm.)

Last Straw Factor

The havoc wrought by neck pain may destroy the patient's emotional stability as, for example, in the case of a male patient who speaks little English, has no special skills, and works as a laborer in a small town supporting a wife and five children. Because of a recession in the area, an insecure job situation keeps him constantly concerned about his ability to make payments on his debts. The neck pain resulting from an accident stops him from working for a few days. A recurrence without provocative trauma makes both the employer and the patient doubtful about the patient's ability to hold down a job. A third attack finds him unemployed. Inability to find new employment increases his debts, and his family's furniture is repossessed by the finance company. To this patient, neck ache is the major disaster of his life, and his symptoms and signs may well be exaggerated beyond recognition.

This patient cannot be helped solely by measures directed at his neck. His whole problem has to be alleviated, and the help of every available social service has to be enlisted. (Classification: this patient is not uncommon and exhibits a psychogenic modification of organic spinal pain.)

Camouflaged Emotional Breakdown

Depressive states are common between the ages of 45 and 55. These patients, commonly very active when young, find that their psychic energy decreases as they move into life's second gear, and they are increasingly unable to cope with the demands made on them. Despite the term "depression," they do not present a picture of melancholia. They demonstrate concealed or overt hostility. They are more easily provoked to anger and tears. They are increasingly critical of faults they perceive in others. They are constantly tired, and sleep does not refresh them. They do not sleep well and frequently awaken early in the morning. They cannot make decisions. They do not want to go out, and they hate staying in. They lose their sense of fun. They claim that this unsociable state is the result of their wretched spine. Remember, a persistent neck ache seldom makes people miserable, but miserable people frequently have neck ache and complain loudly about it.

The neck pain from which they suffer becomes a scapegoat to explain their inability to cope with life. "I was always a very active woman. I was president of the local PTA. I was one of the campaign organizers for the last election. I always went with my husband on his trips, but, with this neck ache, I am useless." Such patients have an almost delusional belief in the organicity of their symptoms. They believe, and would like you to believe, that they would still be a leader in the community had it not been for the neck ache. Characteristically, when giving the history they will constantly refer to the restrictions placed on their life in nonphysical terms.

The curtailment of their activities is not solely due to neck ache. In better emotional health, they could cope with their discomfort, mollifying and minimizing their pain with mild analgesics and a slight modification of their daily rounds. Simple therapeutic measures directed at the organic basis of their complaints will not permit them to return to normal activities. Failure of conservative treatment may lead to desperation surgery, nearly always with poor results and an aggravated deterioration in the patient's emotional health. Treatment must be directed at the patient as a whole, and psychiatric guidance must be sought early. (Classification: This is simply another variety of psychogenic modification.)

"What If I Settle" Syndrome

These patients bring a vague set of symptoms and little in the way of physical findings to the doctor-patient encounter. They are simply drifting in a sea of minor symptoms. The wind in their sails is sometimes provided by an unscrupulous lawyer hoping for prolonged symptoms, more investigation, and a large green poultice in the end. If an unscrupulous doctor joins the cause, the situation may never end for the patient. These unsuspecting and usually sincere patients have become a pawn of the professionals involved in their claim and their care. Giving them a simple explanation will often bring matters to a satisfactory conclusion. (Classification: Obviously, this patient is in a litigation or compensation reaction.)

"Head to Toe" Syndrome

Although these patients rarely complain outright of pain from the tops of their heads to the tips of their toes, it becomes apparent during their history that there is no part of the body that doesn't hurt. They may represent psychogenic pain or, if secondary gain is involved, they may be magnifying their disability. As soon as we recognize that pain is present from head to toe, our tendency is to fall back on our medical training, which taught us to give the patient the benefit of the doubt. This may be accompanied by a rather perfunctory examination, missing the historical and physical features of magnification behavior. The charade goes on in an attempt to pump up damages, which an unscrupulous lawyer may use to make a substantial claim.

Rather, in this setting, the doctor should attempt to separate these patients into those who have emotional disability and are in need of counseling, and those whose disability will disappear only when contentious issues are removed from consideration (i.e., settlement of a lawsuit).

It is apparent that these everyday clinical occurrences can be classified into psychosomatic, psychogenic, or situational spinal pains with or without some organic component. Once classified, treatment by the appropriate explanation and/or therapy can be instituted.

But wait! Is there any further help in assessing these patients?

ASSESSMENT OF NONORGANIC SPINAL PAIN

There are additional methods of assessing these conditions, including the pain drawing (1), psychometric testing, and the pentothal pain study (3). Although the orthopaedic literature is full of descriptions of these assessment methods, it is probably best if these assessment methods are conducted and interpreted by those skilled in the field. Orthopaedic surgeons, by and large, are not skilled in these fields, and it is somewhat dangerous for them to be using these tests. These tests can be used to suggest the presence of a nonorganic component in the disability, resulting in referral of the patient to someone more skilled in its assessment. We do not use any of these ancillary assessment methods, but rather rely on the history and physical examination findings described in the preceding sections. A brief description of these three assessment methods is offered.

Pentothal Pain Study

The introduction of the thiopental sodium pain assessment by Walters (3) has been of value in assessing the significance of emotional states in the production of the disability presented by the patient. The basis of this test lies is that the patient, in a state of light anesthesia, although unconscious, is still capable of demonstrating primitive reactions to pain. The patient is anesthetized with thiopental in a slow induction fashion, and then is allowed to rouse until the corneal reflex returns. At this stage of anesthesia, the patient will withdraw from a pinprick and will grimace when a painful stimulus is applied, such as squeezing the Achilles tendon. With the patient maintained at this level of anesthesia, maneuvers that were previously painful on clinical examination are reevaluated. An example would be a patient who had limited neck movement before induction of the pentothal anesthesia. Theoretically, two extremes can occur. At one extreme, the significant range of movement reduction will persist under the light general anesthesia, a finding that may be taken as irrefutable evidence of significant root tension. If, on the other hand, neck range-of-movement becomes normal on clinical examination at the stage of anesthesia when the patient withdraws from a pinprick, then the clinician may safely conclude that there is no evidence of neck pathology. It is likely that this patient's disability is due to an emotional reaction rather than to an organic source of pain.

If the patient previously had the diffuse, stocking-type of hypoesthesia at this stage of narcosis, he or she will withdraw the limb when it is pricked by a pin. If, however, in addition to the hysterical response there is a sensory loss due to root compression, then the patient will not show any response on pricking the skin over the dermatome of the root involved.

Pentothal pain assessment is used in the patient with a combined nonorganic/organic disability. Its use is best confined to psychiatrists with an interest in chronic pain, whereas the spinal surgeon relies on the symptoms and signs out-

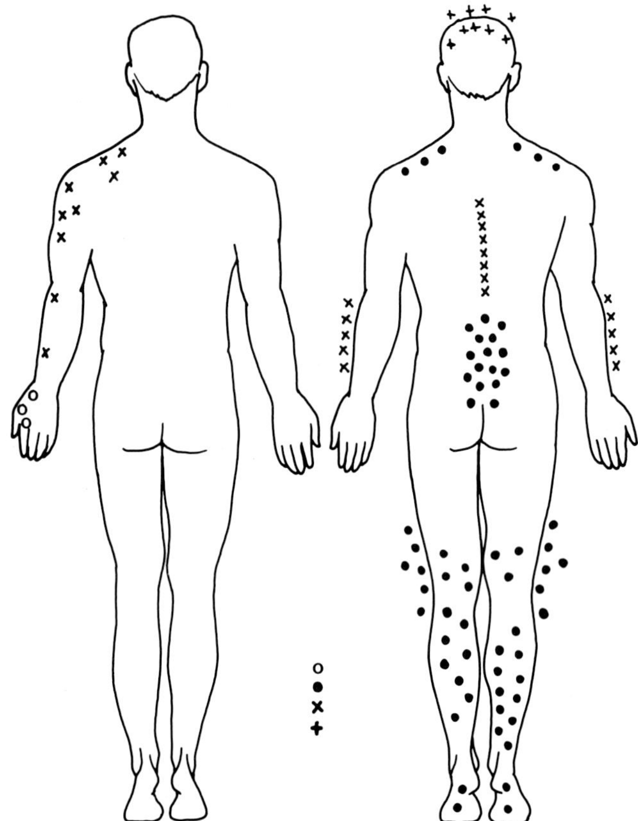

Figure 5.5.   The pain drawing. On the right is the pain drawing for an (organic) radicular syndrome. On the left is the diffuse reaction of a nonorganic reaction. Note that some of the marks are outside the body (the *dots*, *circles* and *xs* are, respectively, sensations of burning, tingling, and pain).

lined in Table 5.3 to detect the potential for a nonorganic component to the disability.

Psychometric Testing

Psychometric testing is a simple rough guide to a patient's emotional health. The use and interpretation of these tests depend greatly on the experience of the user. Wiltse and Rocchio (4) have demonstrated convincingly that patients with a good emotional profile, as shown on the Minnesota Multiphasic Personality Inventory (MMPI) studies, could be expected to obtain better results following chemonucleolysis than those patients in whom a psychological profile was abnormal. There are many psychometric tests, with various strengths and weaknesses. Again, it is suggested that the spinal surgeon refer the patient to someone skilled in the use of these tests when there is evidence of a nonorganic component to the disability.

Pain Drawing

The pain drawing (Fig. 5.5), popularized by Mooney (1), is a simple form of psychometric testing that can be done by patients while in the waiting room.

Patients do not mind doing a pain drawing, as they regard this as cooperating with the physician in keeping an adequate record of their symptoms. They have exactly the reverse reaction to psychometric testing.

The pattern used by the patient to fill out the pain drawing weighs the disability toward an organic or a nonorganic basis. This is probably the safest assessment method for a spine surgical practice. There are, however, pitfalls in its use and interpretation; therefore, it should be used by the orthopaedic surgeon or neurosurgeon in a screening fashion only. An abnormal pain drawing should result in referral of the patient to someone more skilled in the assessment of nonorganic disability.

CONCLUSION

Every human attends the school of survival. Sometimes the lessons lead patients to modify or magnify a physical disability at a conscious or unconscious level. One word of caution—the presence of one of these nonorganic reactions does not preclude an organic condition, such as a herniated nucleus pulposus. The art of medicine is truly tested by a patient with physical neck pain who modifies the disability with a nonorganic reaction, such as tension, hysteria, depression, or other factors.

REFERENCES

1. Ransford AO, Cairns D, and Mooney V: The pain drawing as an aid to the psychological evaluation of patients with low back pain. Spine 1:127–134 (1976).
2. Waddell C, McCulloch JA, Kummel EG et al: Non-organic physical signs in low back pain. Spine 5:117–125 (1980).
3. Walters A: Regional pain alias hysterical pain. Brain 84:1–18 (1961).
4. Wiltse LL and Rocchio PD: Preoperative psychological tests as predictors of success in chemonucleolysis in the treatment of low back syndrome. J Bone Joint Surg 57A:478–483 (1975).

6

Whiplash Injury of the Cervical Spine

"One must not arrogate to oneself the opinion that things that one cannot explain do not exist."
—A. Steindler

INTRODUCTION

If there is one place in this book where the authors part company, it is in the preceding chapter on psychogenic neck pain. The senior author (I.M.), with many years of experience researching the topic and assessing patients, supports the organicity of the lesion. The junior author (J.M.), with 22 years of experience dealing with these patients, is convinced that many of them—with the support of their lawyers—are affected more by the commercial value of the injury. How else do you explain a 1991 study of auto claims in Hawaii by the Insurance Research Council? It reports that medical treatment of a typical neck sprain from whiplash totals $1,300 if handled without a lawyer on a no-fault basis. The cost to treat the same injury if it is part of a tort claim comes to about $8,000. In the beginning, science was reason. What you are about to read is science. Unfortunately, it has run afoul of reason as defined by the judicial system.

Acceleration extension injuries of the neck were first recognized as a clinical entity with the introduction of the catapult-assisted takeoff from aircraft carriers. Many pilots developed persistent neck pain of sufficient severity to warrant medical discharge from the service. Some even lost consciousness on takeoff and crashed. The loss of planes stimulated a more detailed study of the problem. It became apparent that lesions were caused by hyperextension of the neck produced by sudden acceleration. By increasing the height of the back of the seat to support the head, extension strains were prevented and the problems overcome.

Acceleration injuries of the neck were not frequently seen again until the motor vehicle's massive invasion of urban areas in the late 1940s. By the 1950s, rear-end collisions constituted about 20% of all motor vehicle accidents in North America; the incidence is now over 35%.

By law, the striking vehicle was almost invariably at fault, and this fact removed the need to prove liability. The sustained injury rarely presented objective stigmata of an organic lesion. The blameless client, incapacitated by subjective symptoms—the evidence of which could not be proven or disproven—was manna for his or her attorney and pestilence for the defense attorney. For the unscrupulous patient, the injury could mean a paid vacation. Crowe's (2) introduction of the term "whiplash" in 1928 lent an evil connotation to the injury; many patients were more disabled by the diagnosis than by the injury itself.

140

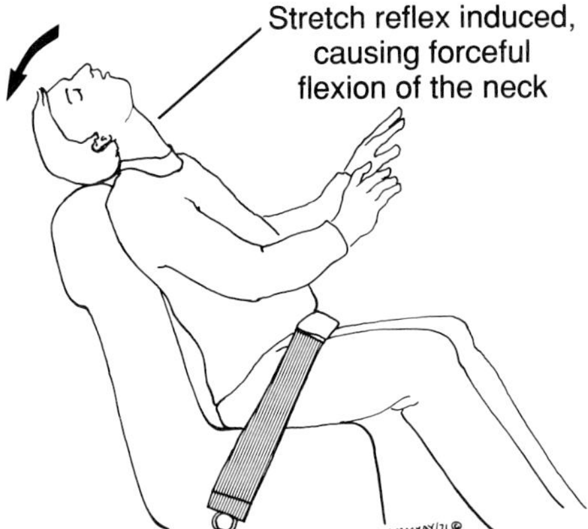

Figure 6.1.   The use of a seat belt (especially the lap portion), unfortunately increases the strain on the neck by preventing the torso from sliding forward on the seat. Extension strains, therefore, are concentrated on the cervical spine.

The emotional overtones associated with the lesion converted it into a cause rather than a clinical syndrome. Lawyers and doctors alike took sides on philosophical rather than scientific grounds. However, anthropomorphic dummies demonstrated that a 15-mph collision could cause the head to accelerate with a force of 10 G. Demonstrating that victims of rear-end collisions are indeed subjected to severe strains of the neck prompted several clinicians to review the problem more objectively.

Mechanism of Injury

When a car is struck from the rear, it suddenly accelerates forward. As it does, the back of the front seat pushes against the torso of the occupant. The back of the seat will bend backward to a degree, varying with the weight of the occupant and the rate of acceleration. If the seat is not equipped with a headrest, there is nothing pushing the head forward as the car accelerates. As a result, during the first few milliseconds following impact, the torso of the occupant is moved forward in relation to the head. When the soft tissues of the neck can no longer stretch, the head falls backward and the neck suffers an extension strain. The force of this extension strain is intensified by the forward recoil of the front seat (Fig. 6.1). There is probably a component of sheer force, before full extension is reached, that has its greatest impact on the disc space and facet joints, especially if they are in the early stages of degeneration.

As the neck is hyperextended and the head rotates, the maxilla rotates away from the mandible and the mouth is flung open, to a degree that may strain the temporomandibular joint.

Backward rotation of the head stretches the anterior cervical muscles; when their tone is overcome, nothing resists the extension movement except the anterior longitudinal ligament and the anterior fibers of the annulus. If the rate of stretch of the muscles is very rapid, there may be insufficient time for muscle fibers to relax, and muscle ruptures may occur.

When the car stops accelerating, the head will rebound forward; this forward movement may be accelerated by contraction of the neck flexor muscles because

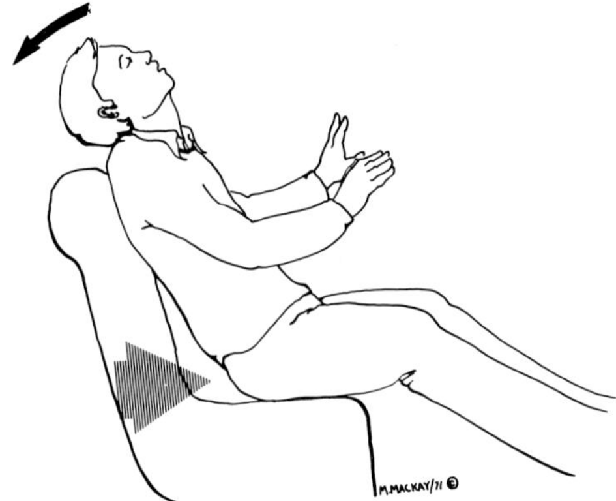

Figure 6.2.   Extension of the neck produces a stretch reflex in the anterior cervical muscles. Contraction of these muscles will bring the head forward.

of the induction of a stretch reflex on the extension phase of the movement (Fig. 6.2). Patients frequently feel as if they are flung forward first and then thrown back, but this is a misconception; if the car now hits the vehicle in front, sudden deceleration will occur. Deceleration will produce forward movement of the occupant's body, resulting in the possibility of the occupant striking the windshield, the steering wheel, or the dashboard.

The force of impact tends to compress the car and, in effect, makes it into a shorter but taller vehicle. A vertical component of the force is therefore also present and tends to push the occupant vertically upward. This may result in the occupant striking his or her head against the top of the car or being thrown over the back of the front seat. This vertical force can be resisted by the shoulder harness.

It is important to recognize this vertical component of the force in construction of the headrest. If the headrest is not level with the top of the occiput, the occupant's head will fall back over the top of the headrest because the occupant is pushed upward by the impact.

To summarize, in rear-end collisions injury may result from the relative acceleration of the head and torso of the occupant, with the degree of injury dependent on the rate of acceleration. Many factors influence the rate of acceleration and must be specifically sought when assessing the severity of injury.

Acceleration will depend on the force applied and the inertia of the vehicle that has been struck. The force is dependent on the weight and speed of the striking vehicle; a streetcar travelling at 3 mph can apply as much force, and initiate the same degree of acceleration, as a compact car travelling at 40 mph. The inertia of the car that has been struck will depend not only on its weight but on factors that might allow it to roll easily: slippery road conditions, whether the brakes were applied, whether the transmission was automatic or standard, etc. A car that is moving slowly will accelerate more rapidly than one that is stationary at the moment of impact; in the latter instance, the inertia of the stationary vehicle will have to be overcome before the car starts moving.

The amount of damage sustained by the car bears little relationship to the force applied to the occupant. To take an extreme example, if a struck car was

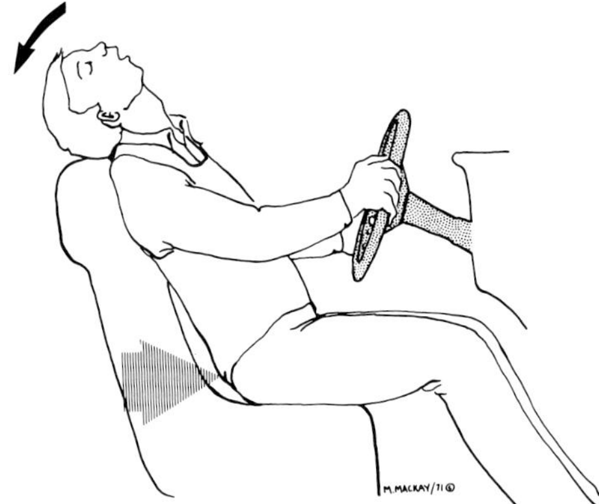

Figure 6.3.   Although the right front passenger is usually more seriously injured than the driver, this is not always the case. On certain occasions, the torso of the driver cannot slide forward on the seat because the driver is holding the steering wheel. The driver, therefore, sustains the more severe extension strain of the cervical spine.

stuck in concrete, the damage sustained by the vehicle might be very great, but the occupant would not be injured because the car could not move forward. In contrast, on glare ice damage to the car could be slight, but the injury sustained by the passenger might be severe because of the rapid acceleration permitted by the ice.

In impacts up to 15 mph, the right front-seat passenger stands in greater danger of injury than the driver. The driver can brace himself or herself to some extent by holding on to the steering wheel. Above 20 mph, the force of acceleration is such that the pelvis of the front-seat passenger slides forward on the seat, causing the torso to recline at an angle. As a result, the extension strain on the neck is correspondingly less. However, the steering wheel prevents the torso of the driver from sliding forward any distance. Therefore, at this speed of impact, the driver may receive a much more serious injury because the forces applied will be concentrated on the neck (Fig. 6.3). Similarly, safety belts tend to aggravate the injury by preventing forward movement of the torso.

During high-speed impacts, the force with which the occupant's body strikes the seat tends to break the back of the front seat (Fig. 6.4). In such instances, as the car accelerates the occupant is lying almost horizontally and a traction rather than an extension strain is applied to the neck. Paradoxically, the occupant is less likely to be severely injured in high-speed collisions. Experimentally, using model cars with monkeys as passengers, the senior author has shown that the injuries received are significantly less when the car is constructed so that the back of the front seat tilts back 30° on rear impact.

Pathology

In an attempt to understand the pathological changes that take place, animals were subjected to an extension strain of the neck produced by sudden acceleration (6). Because of the difficulties of obtaining a standard force, it was decided to use the force of gravity. Anesthetized monkeys were strapped to a steel platform attached to two vertical guide rails and the platform was dropped over a

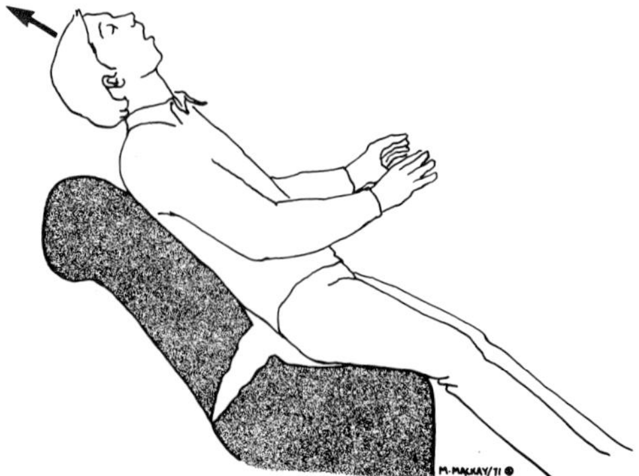

Figure 6.4.   Occasionally, during high-speed impacts, the weight of the passenger breaks the back of the front seat. When this occurs, the passenger lies almost horizontally as the car accelerates. The result is a traction strain rather than an extension strain of the neck.

distance varying from 2 to 40 ft. When the platform struck the bottom of the runway, the animals' heads and necks were suddenly extended over the edge of the platform, producing an acceleration strain as in rear-end collisions. At the conclusion of the experimental drops, a lethal dose of anesthetic was administered. It must be realized, of course, that the experiment using the described apparatus does not accurately reproduce the forces involved in rear-end collisions; the method was used to determine whether recognizable acceleration extension injuries do indeed occur.

By altering the height of the drop, various lesions resulted. Muscle injuries were noted, varying in severity from minor tears of the sternomastoid to more severe tears of the longus colli. Any tear of the longissimus coli, no matter how small, was associated in these experiments with a retropharyngeal hematoma. Hemorrhages were also found in the muscle coats of the esophagus. Damage to the longus colli was occasionally associated with damage to the cervical sympathetic plexus.

One of the most interesting lesions found in the experiments was tearing of the anterior longitudinal ligament and separation of a disc from the associated vertebra (Figs. 6.5 and 6.6). This lesion never occurred without damage to the anterior cervical muscles.

Wickstrom (14) studied the pathological lesions resulting from experimental acceleration extension injuries of the neck in primates. He noted damage to the brain and its coverings, consisting of hemorrhage and edema. He reported sprains of apophyseal joints, subchondral fractures of facets, hemorrhage in muscles, muscle ruptures, hemorrhage about the cord and cervical nerve roots, and hemorrhage under the anterior and posterior longitudinal ligaments. Some animals subsequently showed evidence of concussion with impaired neuromuscular control. Wickstrom stated that the severity of these pathological changes were directly related to the rate of acceleration of the head.

It is always difficult and, at times, dangerous to translate the findings of experimental investigation into the sphere of clinical experience. However, these experiments show that recognizable injuries can be produced. They also suggest that lesions can vary from minor injuries, such as a tear of the muscular fibers, to

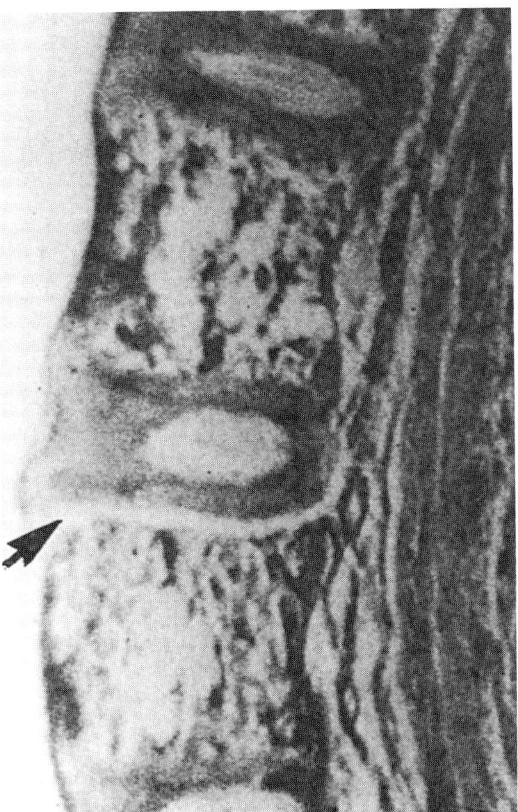

Figure 6.5.   Specimen showing disruption of the anterior longitudinal ligament and separation of the inferior portion of the intervertebral disc from the vertebra below. The detachment of the whole disc is frequently found when performing an anterior cervical fusion for a patient who has suffered an acceleration-extension injury of the neck.

serious lesions, such as separation of the disc or damage to the posterior joints. It is reasonable to assume that the same variation is found clinically, with the majority of patients sustaining minor injuries only; in some patients however, the lesion may be of more serious significance.

Symptom Complex

It is essential to know the pathomechanics of the injury in order to understand the symptoms patients commonly complain about (11). Patients with serious injuries usually experience some pain immediately after the accident, although significant discomfort may be postponed for as long as 24 hours. Later, the pain radiates from the neck to one or both shoulders and down the arms. Patients may not have any pain in the neck and, indeed, the pain may be experienced solely in the shoulders or in the arms. The pain may radiate to the interscapular region, to the chest, or into the suboccipital region. Occipital headaches are common; these may radiate over the vertex or bitemporally, or they may be associated with retro-ocular pain. This pattern of pain radiation is of no value in localizing the site of the lesion. The same pattern of pain can be produced by the

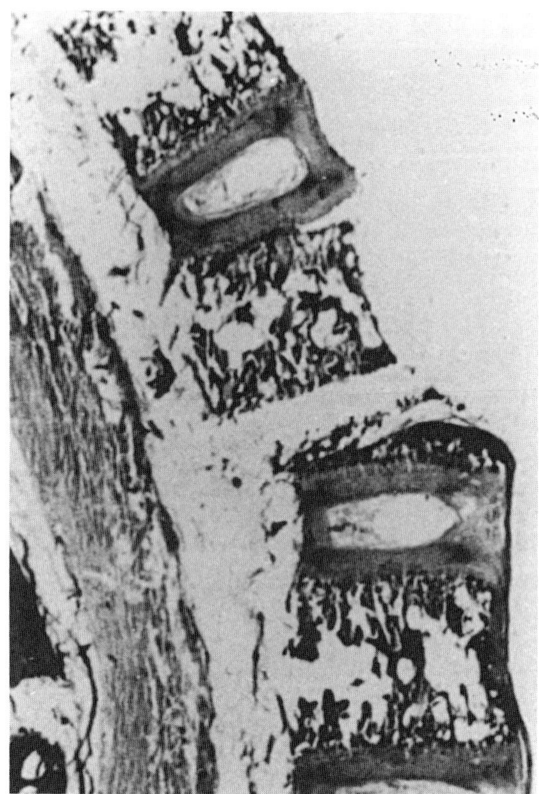

Figure 6.6.   A very severe acceleration-extension injury of the cervical spine showing a horizontal fracture through the vertebral body of C5 and separation of the disc from the superior surface of the vertebra of C6.

experimental injection of hypertonic saline into the supraspinous ligament at any point from C1-C7. Similar pain patterns can be produced on clinical discography at any cervical segment. It is important to emphasize that the presence of persisting suboccipital pain does not necessarily indicate a local lesion at the atlantoaxial region—it may be referred pain, arising from any damaged cervical segment.

Similarly, pain radiating down the arm does not necessarily indicate nerve root pressure. It is frequently another manifestation of referred pain. Disc herniation, with root irritation and impairment of root conduction, rarely results from a whiplash injury of the neck. Rather, patients frequently complain of dull aching in the arm(s) and a subjective numbness in relation to the ulnar border of the hand; indeed, in some instances, there may be a diminished appreciation of feeling a pin prick the ring and little fingers. This is rarely the result of root pressure or even a traumatic ulnar neuritis. Much more commonly, it is caused by scalenus spasm secondary to the painful lesion in the neck.

Severe pain over one rhomboid, associated with spasm and tenderness on pressure, may be caused by a traction lesion of the dorsal scapular nerve as it passes through the scalenus medius. The scalenus medius is placed under tension when the neck is rotated. If the head is turned to one side at the moment of impact, then a traction strain might involve the nerve on the side to which the chin was rotated.

Other symptoms commonly complained of are dysphagia, blurring of vision, tinnitus, dizziness, hoarseness, facial dysesthesia, and temporomandibular joint symptoms.

Dysphagia

When the patient complains of dysphagia shortly after the accident, the cause of dysphagia is either pharyngeal edema or a retropharyngeal hematoma (Fig. 6.7). The latter can be seen on routine lateral x-rays of the spine by observing the forward displacement of the air shadow of the pharynx. The onset of dysphagia is of serious prognostic significance. Dysphagia occurring after the passage of several weeks, however, is usually emotional in origin.

Blurring of Vision

Intermittent blurred vision of short duration is a common symptom. The cause may be damage of the vertebral arteries and their nerve plexus, or the

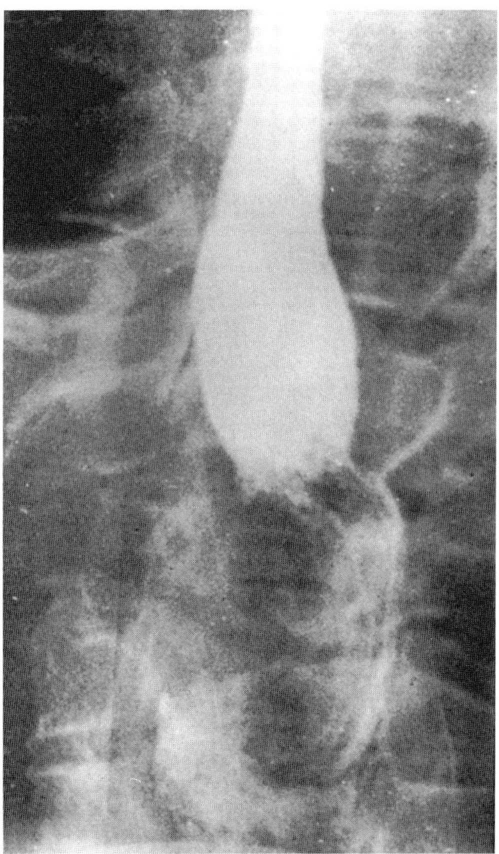

Figure 6.7.   A barium swallow performed in a patient suffering from dysphagia following an acceleration injury of the spine. This x-ray examination reveals obstruction of the esophagus at the level of the thoracic inlet.

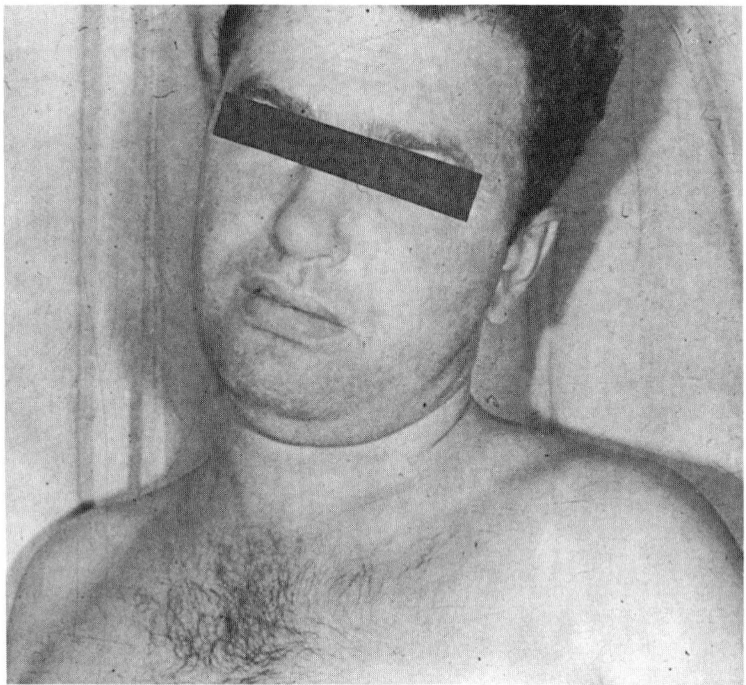

Figure 6.8.   The typical "cock robin" posture frequently adopted by patients with neck pain following an acceleration-extension injury to the neck. This is produced by contraction of rotator muscles passing from the occiput to C1, which may be associated with unilateral spasm of the sternomastoid.

blurring may reflect damage to the cervical sympathetic chain. Blurring of vision by itself is of no prognostic significance, but if it is associated with a Horner's syndrome it indicates extensive soft tissue injury.

Tinnitus

Many patients complain of a buzzing or "popping" sensation in the ears. The pathogenesis of this symptom is not clear (1). The cause may be a temporomandibular injury or temporary occlusion of the vertebral arteries at the time of injury, or the symptoms may reflect direct damage to the inner ear. Although persistent tinnitus is usually associated with some loss of hearing in the upper range, it is very difficult to prove that this is caused by the accident; these patients rarely, if ever, have had any audiometric testing prior to their accident. Usually, tinnitus by itself is of no prognostic significance and is rarely of long duration.

Dizziness

Early severe vertigo caused by vertebral artery spasm or an inner ear disturbance generally indicates a severe extension strain. The veering that many patients complain of can probably be attributed to interference with the neck-righting reflex induced by spasm of the supporting cervical muscles (Fig. 6.8). It can be aggravated experimentally by injecting the sternomastoid with hypertonic saline. This symptom subsides when the neck movements are regained.

Some patients experience severe vertigo on rotation of the head and may indeed lose consciousness. In such instances, the possibility of vertebral artery compression must be investigated.

In most patients, the brunt of the extension force is experienced in the midcervical region. In older patients with pre-existing degenerative changes at the C5-C6 and C6-C7 levels, movement in the midcervical spine is already reduced. In such instances, the major injury occurs in the upper cervical spine, particularly at the atlantoaxial level.

This older group of patients frequently has concomitant atherosclerotic changes involving the vertebral arteries; it is in this group that various types of vertebral artery syndromes may develop. Some patients may go on to present the Wallenberg (13) syndrome (lateral medullary syndrome) caused by thrombosis of the posteroinferior cerebellar artery.

Muscle Rupture

As the head starts to rotate backward, the sternomastoid muscles contract. If the movement rotating the head backward is too great, the muscles, stretched passively and rapidly, do not have a chance to elongate. In such instances, the muscle will rupture with the formation of a hematoma (Fig. 6.7). Hemorrhage and edema of the strap muscles may cause hoarseness and dysphagia, and a similar lesion in the longus colli may make it difficult for the patient to lift his or her head off a pillow.

Lesions of the Upper Cervical Nerve Root

The superficial branches of the cervical plexus (the great auricular nerve, the superficial cervical nerve, and the supraclavicular nerves) pierce the cervical fascia and wind around the posterior border of the sternomastoid to reach the skin. They may be stretched as the neck is extended, particularly if extension is combined with rotation. Traction injuries to these nerves may result in patches of hypoesthesia or dysesthesia in the face, associated with dry skin (Fig. 6.9). There may be tenderness at the point where the nerves emerge through the fascia; percussion at these points may result in paresthesia radiating over the area of skin distribution. This phenomenon may persist for several months after the injury.

Temporomandibular Joint Symptoms

As previously mentioned, as the head rotates backward, the mouth is flung open; this may result in a temporomandibular joint strain. Indeed, the joint may be dislocated. As the joint is flung open, the masticatory muscles are stretched, resulting in a reflexive rapid closing of the mouth. The closing of the mouth may be sufficiently forceful to break the teeth.

Patients with a strain of the temporomandibular joint subsequently complain of pain when chewing and painful limitation of their ability to open their mouths. It is important to note that these symptoms are aggravated by halter traction; indeed, cervical traction may by itself produce a temporomandibular arthropathy in the presence of malocclusion. This syndrome has been referred to as Costen's syndrome (1).

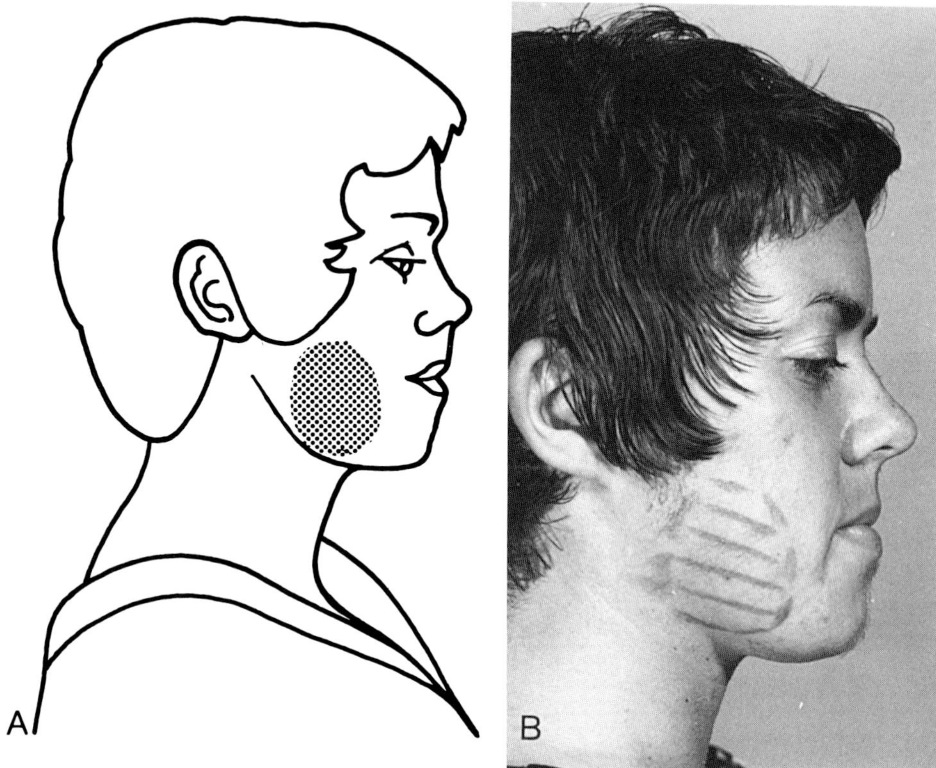

Figure 6.9.   When first seen, patients who have been involved in a rear-end collision frequently have an area of hypoesthesia below the ear.

Significance of Symptoms

Although there is general agreement on the type of symptoms to be expected, widely divergent views are held on their significance. Rigidly held and hotly contested, these diverging viewpoints are usually based on impressions only. In an endeavor to make these impressions more factually significant, the senior author carefully followed the progress of 575 patients (7). Many physicians believe that individuals suffering from the whiplash syndrome comprise a group of hysterical, neurotic—if not dishonest—people. However, certain disturbing features apparent from an analysis of these case histories make it difficult to accept litigation reaction as the sole explanation of this long, drawn-out disability.

Some patients had associated injuries. In addition to injuring their necks, they sprained their ankles or broke their wrists. Normal painless function returned to their ankles and wrists in the expected period of time. These patients did not keep complaining month after month about their painful ankles or their painful wrists, but their necks still hurt. It is difficult to understand why litigation reaction in these instances should be confined to the neck.

When forward flexion of the neck is produced by acceleration or deceleration, the head stops moving when the chin touches the chest. Similarly, in lateral flexion, movement stops in the normal cervical spine when the ear hits the shoulder.

Table 6.1.   Analysis of Whiplash Results Two Years After Settlement of Court Action

Total number of patients available for review	266
Number of patients reviewed	145
Number of patients with symptoms	121
Persistence of symptoms two years after settlement	121 of 266 (45%)

In both these modalities of cervical movement, the range of movement is within physiological limits and, in normal necks even at the extremes of movement, no strain is applied to the intervertebral joints. In extension injuries to the neck, however, nothing blocks movement until the occiput hits the chest wall, and this is far beyond the physiologically permitted limit. In the series of rear-end collisions analyzed, none of the five patients—who at the moment of impact experienced an uncontrolled flexion of the neck—complained of neck pain.

Of 69 patients who were passengers in vehicles involved in side collisions—and, one presumes, experienced lateral flexion movement applied to the neck—only seven suffered neck pain and in only two did significant disability persist for more than two months.

If neck pain following acceleration injuries is purely neurotic in origin, it is difficult to understand why patients frequently become neurotic if their head is thrown backward but rarely become neurotic if it is jolted forward or sideways. This finding suggests that the persistence of pain following forced extension of the neck is related in some way to the fact that the neck can move beyond the physiologically permitted limit. Those who support a high nonorganic component in this injury might discover that patients suffering forward or lateral injuries become either defendants or plaintiffs when litigation occurs—one is no more likely than the other. In contrast, the "rear-endee"—the patient suffering hyperextension injury—is always the plaintiff in tort issues arising out of the accident.

An interesting observation of the significance of litigation reaction emerges from following-up these patients after settlement of court action (Table 6.1). Of 266 patients, all legal problems had been settled two or more years before follow-up. As in any review of this type, it was impossible to recover all these patients for study. Of 145 patients examined personally by the senior author, 121 were continuing to have symptoms. It is obvious in a follow-up such as this—where attendance for review seems pointless, time-consuming, and difficult—that patients most likely to attend are those with continuing symptoms. To avoid bias of this type, we should regard all patients who did not return as having completely recovered.

On this basis, out of 266 patients, 121 continued to have some measure of symptoms. That is, satisfactory conclusion of settlement or court action failed to relieve symptoms in 45% of the group studied.

The group studied is not representative of every whiplash injury. It is a special group. It consists of patients referred for specialist opinion because of severity of symptoms or undue persistence of symptoms; it represents, therefore, the more severe disabilities, whether they be physiogenically or psychogenically induced.

At first sight, the results may appear grossly at variance with Gotten's often quoted review (5). In 1956, Gotten published a survey of 100 cases of whiplash injuries reviewed after settlement of legal action. This review stated that 88% of those injured had "largely recovered" and only 12% were still significantly disabled. Reading these results the other way around, one can say that, out of 100 patients reviewed, many professed some sort of symptoms and, even after the passage of several years, 12%—a significant number—were seriously disabled and 3% were losing time from work.

In other follow-up studies, the results are remarkably constant (3, 8, 9, 12). The majority of patients improve with the passage of time, and they can learn to live with their intermittent residual discomfort. However, about 10%–20% are left with discomfort of sufficient severity to interfere with their ability to do work or to enjoy themselves in leisure hours.

It can be fairly stated, therefore, that careful follow-up reviews strongly support the contention that significant soft tissue damage may result from acceleration-extension injuries and therefore it is not surprising that symptoms may be prolonged in a minority of patients. To identify this group of patients and apply appropriate treatment—and to avoid prolonged treatment of milder injuries and promote early settlement of legal claims—we would suggest the following approach to clinical management.

Clinical Management

Stage 1: Assessing Severity of Injury (Table 6.2)

Sudden death has been reported as a result of acceleration-extension injuries of the neck (13). Serious vascular injuries, including occlusion of the posterior-inferior cerebellar arteries resulting from extension strains, have been reported several times. No one doubts the clinical picture in these findings because of the positive and undeniable physical evidence. However, many clinicians are still reluctant to accept that relatively minor lesions associated with disabling and persistent symptoms may result from this type of injury.

When a patient sustains a simple compression fracture of the cervical spine, even though the injury may involve litigation, an emotional or functional overlay is not common. Similarly, when patients break their wrists or sprain their ankles, even if the lesion is associated with an acceleration-extension injury of the neck, normal painless function usually returns to the ankle and wrist in the expected period of time without any functional overlay. Surely, these observations suggest that broken necks, sprained ankles, and broken wrists are treated adequately; surely, these findings suggest that, by failure to treat a whiplash injury adequately, the physician may be responsible for some of the so-called litigation reactions.

If physicians are to avoid iatrogenic neuroses in their treatment, they must accept the possibility of significant injury and be prepared to investigate its probability.

The first essential is to obtain a careful, painstaking history. Many factors modify the injury received; when assessing the significance of these symptoms, the physician must learn as much as possible about the details of the accident. The rate of acceleration is of vital importance. It is necessary, therefore, to answer the following questions.

What was the type of vehicle in which the patient was sitting and the relative weight of the vehicle that struck the patient's vehicle?

What were the road conditions—slippery or dry?

Table 6.2. Severity of Injury Scale for Whiplash Injury

Factor	Mild Injury	Moderate Injury	Severe Injury
Collision factors (see text)	Minor collision with minimal damage	Moderate collision with moderate damage	Significant impact with extensive damage
Patient position and preparation	Driver prepared by looking in rear-view mirror	Driver or passenger unprepared	Driver or passenger unprepared with neck rotated
Collision effects	Seat intact, hat & glasses still on	Seat back broken	Seat intact, hat & glasses in back seat
Onset of pain	Delayed by 24 to 48 hours	Immediate or delayed by a few hours	Immediate severe pain
Extent of pain	Mild to moderate	Moderate to severe	Severe, to point where patient taken to hospital by ambulance
Associated symptoms	Aside from headache, minimal associated symptoms	A few associated symptoms such as mild dysphagia, blurring of vision	Many associated symptoms, including headache, visual disturbances, dysphagia, tinnitus
Timing of immediate care	Often delayed for days	Emergency care immediately or family doctor care next day	Emergency care
Extent of immediate care	Pain meds, muscle relaxants	Pain meds, muscle relaxants and collar can work	Rigid collar pain meds, muscle relaxants, unable to work
Physical exam on immediate care	Minor reduction in range of movement (ROM)	Moderate reduction in ROM	Significant reduction in ROM, anterior neck swelling, tenderness
X-ray exam on immediate care	No preexisting degenerative changes, normal lordosis	No preexisting degenerative changes, loss of lordosis	Pre-existing degenerative changes & loss of lordosis

Was the patient's vehicle moving at the moment of collision?

How far was the vehicle pushed forward? Did it hit another vehicle in front?

What happened to objects inside the patient's vehicle? Did the glove compartment fly open? Were objects on the front seat thrown into the back seat?

It is necessary to know whether the patient was the driver or the passenger. As mentioned previously, at low-impact speeds the passenger in the right front seat is most vulnerable to injury. The driver, who can often anticipate the accident, may have time to brace himself or herself and firmly hold the steering wheel, thereby decreasing neck movements.

It is also important to know the position of the patient's head at the moment of impact. The physiologically permitted range of extension is much less when the neck is rotated (Figs. 6.10 and 6.11). Normally, at the limit of extension, the occipitomental line is about 20° to 40° above the horizontal when the chin is pointing straight forward. If the neck is rotated to 45°, the degree of extension permitted is only about half this range. Because the permitted physiological range of extension is very short when the neck is slightly rotated, the posterior joints can soon be pushed beyond the physiological range; injury easily results from an extension strain.

Rupture of the anterior longitudinal ligament is much more readily produced experimentally in cadavers when the head is rotated before an extension strain is applied to the neck. If, at the moment of impact, the driver and passenger had their heads turned toward one another while talking, then the presence of right-sided pain in the driver and left-sided pain in the passenger lends "an air of artistic verisimilitude to an otherwise bald and unconvincing narrative" (4).

The movement of the patient is also important. Did the patient's head hit the roof? Did the patient feel his or her head snap back? Did the back of the head go over the top of the headrest? In severe injuries, the neck may be extended to such a degree that the occupant faces the rear of the car. Some information about the severity of the forces involved may be gathered by asking patients what happened to their hats, glasses, false teeth, etc., as a result of the impact. In one patient in the series studied, a plastic Spanish comb she wore was thrown against the rear window and it broke. Conversely, if the patient wore a hat and glasses and neither was dislodged, it is reasonable to assume that the head was not jolted vigorously.

Significant injuries almost invariably cause some pain immediately after the accident. The pain may temporarily subside and then gradually intensify over the next few hours. It is important to inquire specifically about this time period. Patients who have serious emotional upset frequently state that they were unable to sleep on the night of the accident—not because of the pain but because they constantly relived their frightening experience.

If seen shortly after the accident, patients with significant injury will show evidence of damage to soft tissues at the front of the neck, with tenderness on palpation. The physician must be wary of the patient who complains bitterly of pain in the neck and presents marked tenderness over the spinous processes posteriorly without any discomfort on palpating the anterior structures.

At the conclusion of the history, the physician should have a clear impression of the patient and the injury. A clear record of the physical findings must include: permitted range of movement, sites of tenderness, and evidence of nerve root irritation or impairment of root conduction. Remember that apparently bizarre areas of diminished feeling in response to a pinprick on the side of the face or behind the ear may result from stretching the superficial cervical nerves (Fig. 6.9).

Radiological findings must be interpreted with care. Loss of cervical lordosis can be demonstrated in normal subjects just by lowering the chin. The cause of the apparent flattening of the cervical curve, so commonly seen, is usually the position in which the patient holds his or her head when the lateral view is taken. Provided the chin is in the normal position for lateral x-ray, loss of cervical lordosis is of some prognostic significance. Changes in the pattern of movement on

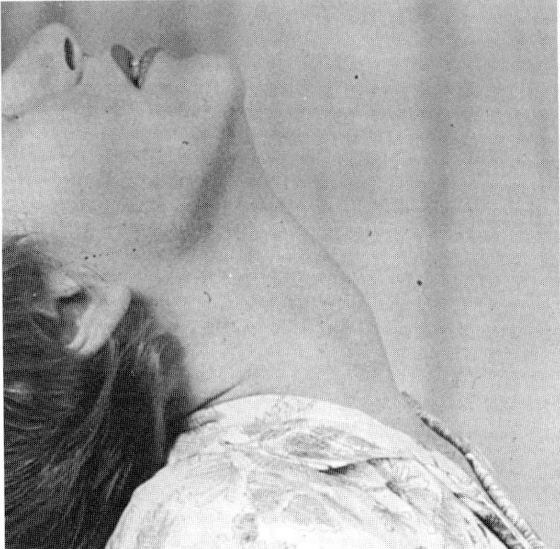

Figure 6.10.   Passive extension of the cervical spine. When the face is pointing straight forward, extension is permissible so that the occipitomental line (a hypothetical line drawn from the tip of the chin to the occiput) is approximately 30° above the horizontal.

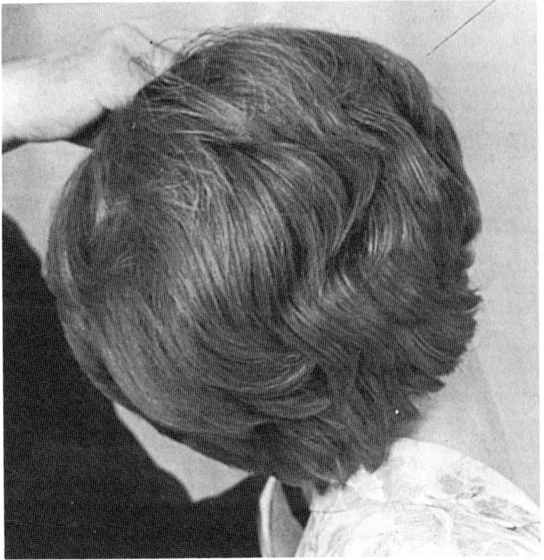

Figure 6.11.   With the head rotated through 45°, it is only possible to extend the cervical spine by 30°. Therefore, if the head is rotated at the moment of impact, the posterior joints sustain a much more serious injury.

flexion and extension do not necessarily indicate damage to the discs or posterior joints, but may merely reflect restricted movements because of pain or fear of pain.

Stage 2: Establish a Prognosis and Target Dates for Treatment Responses

That nonorganic components of disability (see Chapter 5) can coexist with the physical effects of whiplash cannot be denied. The mistake in this injury is two-fold. First, it is possible to miss this nonphysical component in a mild injury and order excessive investigation and treatment, imparting to the patient a severity of illness that doesn't exist. These steps on the part of the treating physician prolong the disability, pad his or her accounts and tax society in a fashion we can no longer accept. The second edge of this sword is to miss the severity of injury and, when the patient fails to respond to treatment, label the patient as neurotic. For these reasons, it is important to have an injury severity scale and attach to it a prognosis well-supported by published studies (Table 6.2). Most patients will fall into the mild or moderate whiplash severity scale.

Stage 3: Establish a Treatment Protocol Based on Injury Severity Scale (10)

Table 6.4 is a summary of the guidelines. If it appears that the patient may have sustained a significant injury as evidenced by the nature of the impact, by marked muscle spasm of the sternomastoid, or by complaints suggesting damage to the anterior tissues of the neck, the neck should be splinted. If the neck needs splinting at all, it needs splinting well. The best way to do this is to apply a molded cervical collar (Fig. 4.3). The only way to rest the neck completely is to remove the weight of the head; the only way this can be achieved is to confine the patient to bed and insist that the patient remain lying down. If, after 12–24 hours of recumbency, the patient is relatively free of symptoms, he or she may get up; otherwise the patient should stay in bed for a week.

Traction can be applied at this stage, but only if manual traction relieves the pain temporarily. The traction must be applied in such a way that a slight flexion pull is applied to the neck. Initially, the patient should have traction applied for one hour and then be freed from traction for the second hour. Thereafter, traction should alternate hourly.

If patients are asked to stay in bed for a week, it is essential that they be given some form of sedation; otherwise, because they feel relatively well, they are unlikely to carry out a form of therapy that seems to them unreasonable. Their only symptom is pain. The need for rest must be explained, otherwise they will not cooperate.

The majority of these patients should be able to return to work at the end of one week. They should be given instructions about how to avoid extension strains to the neck in the activities of daily living.

The patients should not be prescribed unnecessary and expensive medication. As the cost of medication rises, so does the cost of injury. All that is required are mild analgesics to take the edge off discomfort and mild sedation to take the edge off anxiety. The nature and purpose of the drugs must be explained to the patient. It is dishonest, and it is bad medicine, to prescribe tranquilizers and pretend their purpose is to reduce the patient's "neck spasm." If patients are disabled by a psychogenic magnification of symptoms, they must be told of this;

Table 6.3.   Prognosis of Whiplash Based on Injury Severity Scale

	Mild Injury	Moderate Injury	Severe Injury
Duration of symptoms	Symptoms resolved within 2 months	Symptoms may still be present at 2 months but will be largely settled within 2 years	Symptoms will probably persist beyond 2 months and continue for at least 2 years
Probability of continuing symptoms after settlement	None	Likely up to 2 years	High probability
Extent that symptoms will interfere with work or leisure activity	None	Low probability	High probability
Need for long-term care and surgery	None	Very low probability	Probability

they must also be informed that the purpose of the sedative is to treat this aspect of their problem.

Physiotherapy, if ordered, must be along rational lines. If patients do not feel comfortable in a soft collar, try a more rigid type. If they do feel better in a collar and can work more efficiently while wearing it, there is no physiological or psychological reason for withholding it.

If the patient's problems are severe enough to warrant a week of resting in bed, he or she will probably have daily discomfort for six weeks. If, at the end of six weeks, the patient is still conscious of discomfort all day long, intermittent discomfort may be experienced for another six months to one year. Patients must be told the expected duration of symptoms. Nothing is more demoralizing than expecting a cure day-by-day from some new pill or new apparatus at the physiotherapy department. Unless the physician honestly believes that the patient will get better in a week or 10 days, he or she must tell the patient what to expect based on the injury severity scale (Table 6.3). At the same time, the doctor must explain that the lesion in the neck alone, and the discomfort it causes, are not sufficient reasons to withdraw completely from the activities of daily living (Table 6.3).

Chronic Whiplash Symptoms

The patient may not be seen for several months after the injury. At this time, assessing the severity of injury and the cause of continuing disability becomes more difficult. Physicians must ask themselves, "Why is this patient so disabled by the pain?" Many patients are genuinely fearful about perpetuating the damage and permanently crippling themselves. For this reason, they assiduously avoid any activity that provokes discomfort. Their disability is exaggerated by ignorance. Some patients become disconsolate because of the apparent failure of medical therapy. Week after week, they have expected their discomfort to subside as a result of prescribed treatment. Week after week their hopes have been dashed as their symptom continue. The failure of therapy and the continuance of

Table 6.4.   Treatment Guidelines Based on the Injury Severity Scale

Treatment Modality	Mild Injury	Moderate Injury	Severe Injury
Rest in bed	Not indicated	Not indicated	Often indicated
Rest in collar	Often not needed	Usually needed	Always needed
Medication requirements			
• pain	Mild	Mild to moderate analgesia	Moderate analgesia
• anti-inflammatory	Not needed	Often useful	Usually needed
• muscle relaxants/ tranquilizers	Often not needed	Needed in mild form	Needed in moderate form
Mobilization (ROM exercises and manipulation)	Start immediately and decrease medication	As pain subsides, start gentle manipulation and mobilization exercises—will need some medication support	As pain subsides, start gentle manipulation and mobilization exercises—will need lots of medication support
Rehabilitation through exercise strengthening	Can start within a few weeks of injury	As pain further subsides with mobilization, start strengthening exercises	Start as pain decreases with mobilization exercises and anticipate prolonged course
Use of traction	The use of traction in this injury is not well established and should be decided on a case-to-case basis—discontinue early if no response.		

pain often exaggerate the severity of the injury. When told she had not been subjected to a serious neck injury, one patient stated, "If nothing is wrong with me, why is it costing so much to get me better?"

False faith in ineffectual treatment can trigger symptoms of secondary depression. Patients suffering from this disorder are tired all the time; sleep does not refresh them. They are provoked to unreasonable anger and/or to tears more easily than usual, and they become intolerant of faults they perceive in others. They also lose their sense of fun.

It may become apparent that patients' disabilities result from a psychogenic magnification of symptoms derived from the underlying physical disorder. In better emotional health, they would not be significantly troubled, let alone disabled. In this case, the physician must offer an honest opinion of the nature and cause of their continuing disabilities. This situation should be recognized early and a psychiatric opinion should be sought.

In teaching patients to live with minor discomforts, the attitude of the physician is of paramount importance. The physician must accept the possibility of injury and investigate its probability in each patient. The physician must not be perfunctory in treatment, yet must never overtreat the patient. Treatment should not interfere with the patient's daily routine.

Few cases come to surgery. If the patient's pain persists for more than two years and interferes significantly with his or her ability to work or enjoy leisure activities, and if you are satisfied on clinical assessment (Chapter 5) that a significant psychogenic component does not coexist, then the patient requires more detailed investigation to localize the site of the pathological lesion. The investigation will be along the lines suggested in Chapter 3.

If it can be shown that symptoms stem from one or, at most, two adjacent disc units, then these patients will respond well to anterior cervical discectomy and fusion.

In teaching the remainder of patients to accept and live with minor discomfort, physicians must be honest about the treatment that they are giving, about the patient's physical and mental well-being, and about the prognosis. Above all, physicians must take care not to fan the flames of hostility some patients commonly exhibit. This can initiate, aggravate, or perpetuate a financially motivated exaggeration of symptoms.

REFERENCES

1. Costen JB: A syndrome of ear and sinus symptoms dependent on the disturbed function of the temporomandibular joint. Ann Otol Rhinol Laryngol 43:1–15 (1934).
2. Crowe HW: Injuries to the cervical spine. Paper presented at the annual meeting of the Western Orthopaedic Association, San Francisco (1928).
3. Gargan MF and Bannister GC: Long-term prognosis of soft-tissue injuries of the neck. J Bone Joint Surg 72B:901–903 (1990).
4. Gilbert and Sullivan: The Mikado.
5. Gotten N: Survey of 100 cases of whiplash after settlement of litigation. JAMA 162:865–867 (1956).
6. Macnab I: Acceleration injuries of the cervical spine. J Bone Joint Surg 46A:1797–1799 (1964).
7. Macnab I: The "whiplash syndrome." Orthop Clin North Am 2:389–403 (1971).
8. Maimaris C, Barnes MR, and Allen MJ: Whiplash injuries of the neck: a retrospective study. Injury 19:393–396 (1988).
9. Pearce JMS: Whiplash injury: a reappraisal. J Neurol Neurosurg Psych 52:1329–1331 (1989).
10. Pennie BH and Agambar LJ: Whiplash injuries: A trial of early management. J Bone Joint Surg 72B:277–279 (1990).
11. Pennie BH and Agambar LJ: Patterns of injury and recovery in whiplash. Injury 22:57–59 (1991).
12. Theimeyer JS, Duncan GA, and Hollings GC: Whiplash injuries of the cervical spine. Med Monthly 85:171–174 (1958).
13. Wallenberg A: Acute bulbar affection (embolus der art. post. inferior sinistra). Arch Psychiat (Berlin) 27:504 (1895).
14. Wickstrom J, Martinez J, and Rodriguez R: Quoted by Frankel V: Cervical Pain. Pergamon Press, Oxford and New York (1972).

7

Fractures and Dislocations of the Cervical Spine

"I love and honor him, but must not break my back to heal his finger."

—Timon of Athens II

INTRODUCTION

Injuries to the cervical spine involve not only the musculoskeletal system, but may also include neurological system damage. Assessment and treatment depends on the ability to balance aggressive treatment of the neurological injury with judicious preservation of residual stability and painless motion in the spinal skeleton.

Classification of Cervical Spine Injuries
1. Musculoskeletal System
   a. Disco-vertebral column
   b. Soft tissue (see Chapter 6)
2. Neurological System
   a. Cord
   b. Root

Neurological System Injury

Approximately one-third to one-half of cervical spine fractures and/or dislocations will have concomitant neurological injury (14). The damage may be to nerve roots and/or the spinal cord, and is incomplete or complete (Table 7.1).

To plan appropriate treatment, it is essential to clearly classify the extent and level of neurological lesion—only then can you provide meaningful advice to the patient and family.

Table 7.1. Neurological Structures and Injury Extent

		Frankel Grades (12)
No neurological lesion	E	Normal neurological function
Incomplete neurological lesion (distal to injury site)	D C B	Useful motor function Useless motor function Sensory only remains
Complete neurological lesion (distal to injury site)	A	No motor or sensory function

Spinal Shock

The final prognosis in neurological injury cannot be determined until spinal shock has passed. Following a severe injury to the cord, the portion of the cord caudal to the lesion shuts down—it is in a state of shock and no activity, including reflex activity, occurs. That means no cord reflex activity occurs; the bulbocavernosus reflex and anal wink, for example, are absent (Fig. 7.1).

This shock-like state may or may not occur. If present, its duration is variable, lasting from a few hours to a few days. Its end is marked by the return of the bulbocavernosus and anal wink reflexes, at which time a detailed neurological exam can be completed (20). If, after return of these cord reflexes, there is no discernible motor or sensory function below the level of the lesion, the patient is determined to have complete quadriplegia from which no functional recovery will occur. On the other hand, if a patient coming out of spinal shock shows some motor or sensory function, this patient has an incomplete cord lesion with a much more favorable prognosis.

The incomplete Frankel grades (2, 12) of B, C, and D can be further subdivided according to the area of the cord that sustains the most injury (Figs. 7.1 and 7.2):

1. Brown-Sequard Syndrome. In this partial neurological injury, one-half of the spinal cord is damaged. This results in distal motor and posterior column loss on the same side, and sensory loss on the opposite side. Excellent recovery usually follows this lesion.
2. Central Cord Syndrome. This injury damages the central gray matter and the central long tracts of the white matter. Knowing the location of those tracts makes it easy to understand how the upper extremities, especially the hands, are more affected than the lower extremities. This is the most common type of spinal cord injury and is prone to occur in the older patient with spondylotic bars who falls and suffers a hyperextension injury to the neck. A reasonable degree of recovery (except for the hands) is possible after this injury.
3. Anterior Cord Syndrome. This lesion affects the anterior two-thirds of the cord and is the most devastating of the incomplete lesions. Fortunately it is less common than the Brown-Sequard and Central Cord syndromes, and leaves the patient with only posterior cord function (position and vibration sense). There is no significant motor or sensory function distally, and very few patients recover useful function.
4. Root Injury. The nerve root exiting at the level of the vertebral injury may suffer from LMNL and may recover. For example a vertebral lesion at C5-C6 should allow for recovery of the C6 nerve root (Table 7.2).

Summary

The salient features about neurological injury in fractures and/or dislocations of the cervical vertebral column are:

1. Neurological involvement will occur in at least one in three cases (it is very common!).

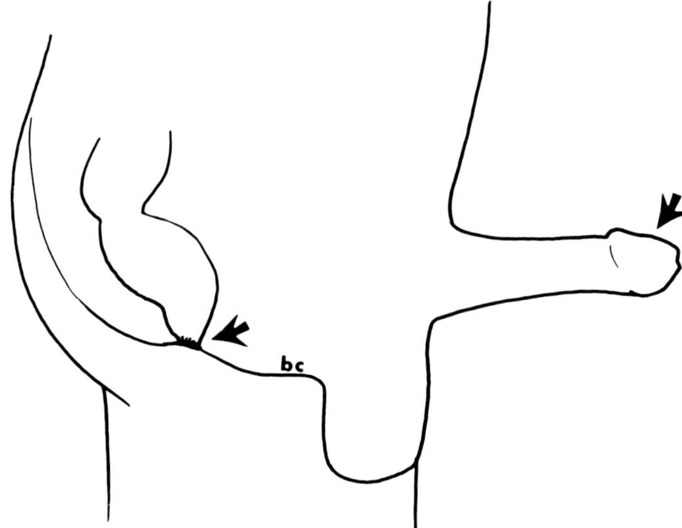

Figure 7.1.   The bulbocavernosus reflex. Normal: squeezing the glans penis will produce (1) a reflex contraction of the bulbocavernosus muscle (*bc*), which you can palpate, or (2) a reflex contraction of the external anal sphincter. In spinal shock these reflexes are absent.

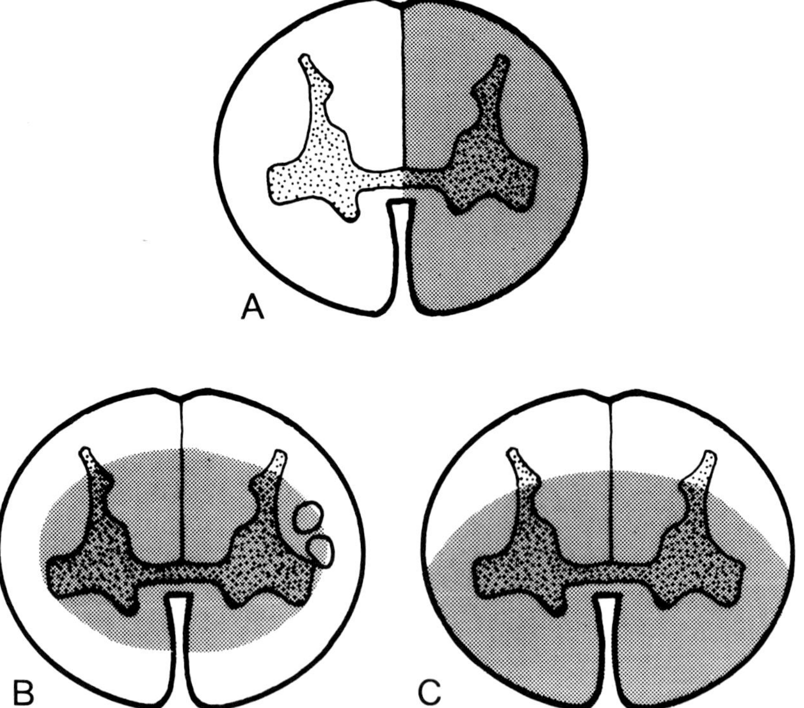

Figure 7.2.   **A,** Brown-Sequard lesion. **B,** central cord lesion. **C,** anterior cord lesion.

Table 7.2.   Law of Spinal Root Recovery in Complete Quadriplegia

Level
C5   Lowest functioning nerve root activates deltoid and biceps
C6   Lowest functioning nerve root activates wrist extensors and elbow flexors
C7   Lowest functioning nerve root activates finger extensors, triceps, and wrist flexor
C8   Lowest functioning nerve root activates finger flexors

2. Detailed initial neurological assessment on presentation in the emergency department is needed to determine whether the patient is intact neurologically, or has a complete or incomplete cord lesion.
3. If the cord lesion appears to be complete below the level of the spine injury, wait for spinal shock to disappear before the final decision about completeness is made.
4. Patients with complete neurological lesions will not experience any useful neurological recovery.
5. If the neurological lesion is incomplete, repeated examinations are necessary on at least an hourly basis to assure that there is no deterioration in function. Any evidence of further loss of neurological function mandates immediate surgical intervention, which usually means stabilization of the spinal vertebral column injury with or without neurological decompression.

Vertebral Column Injury

Throughout this book, the cervical spine has been divided into the upper cervical spine (C1-C2) and the subaxial region (C3-C7). Let's divide fractures the same way:

1. Fractures and dislocations of the C1-C2 region. Common injuries to this region include:
   a. Odontoid fractures.
   b. Fractures of the C1 ring—Jefferson fracture.
   c. Traumatic spondylolisthesis of the axis—Hangman's fracture.
   d. Rotatory subluxation of C1 and C2.
2. Pediatric injuries to the cervical spine
3. Subaxial injuries

Caution!

More often than not, injuries to the cervical spine are missed in emergency. In the unconscious patient, the head-injured patient, the intoxicated patient, and the patient with severe chest and belly traumas, it is easy to overlook the neck (10).

Remember!

For every body bash that appears in the emergency department, obtain at least a lateral x-ray (Fig. 7.3) of the cervical spine that shows C1 to T1 for any patient who is unconscious; for any patient who has a head injury; and for any patient who complains of neck ache.

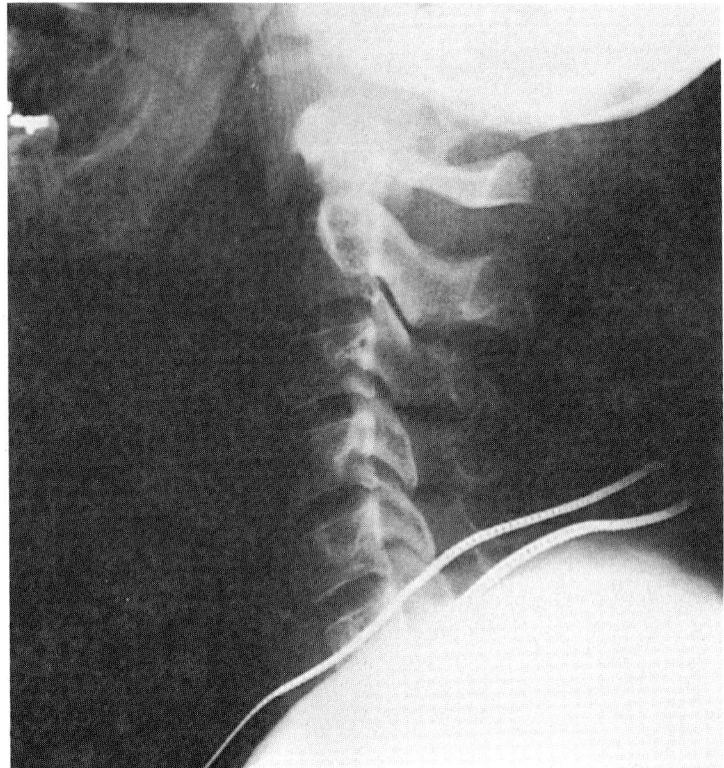

Figure 7.3.   Lateral x-ray of the cervical spine done in emergency (with no time to remove the chain!). Is it acceptable? Read on.

An anterior-posterior x-ray should also be obtained with the lateral because there is potential for missing severe cervical injuries with just a lateral x-ray.

When possible, the routine x-ray series for the cervical spine should include:

- A standard AP and lateral.
- Oblique views.
- Open mouth AP of the odontoid.

If there is any doubt about an injury, or if an injury has been noted on plain x-rays, a CT scan of the area is mandatory. Also remember that fractures of the odontoid occur in the transverse plane and can be missed on routine axial CT scanning, especially with wide spacing of the cuts. For these injuries, sagittal CT reconstructions or polytomography in sagittal plane are needed.

General Clues Pointing to Injury of the Cervical Spine

1. The patient is unconscious.
2. The patient has had a head injury.
3. The patient complains of neck pain.
4. There is an increase in pain and a decrease in range-of-neck movement on examination.
5. There is any neurological injury (root or cord).

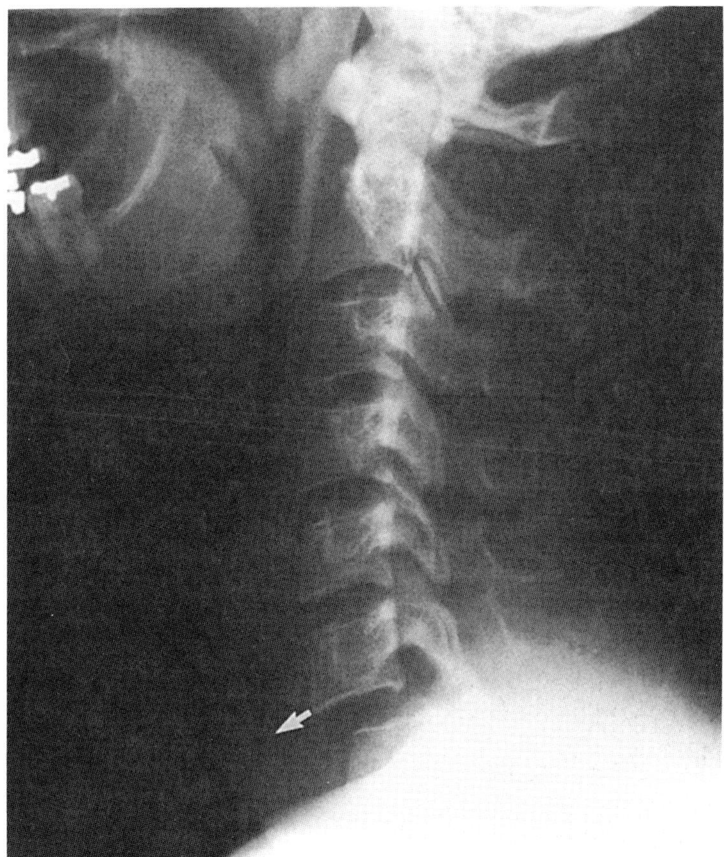

Figure 7.4.   Figure 7.3 wasn't acceptable. This is the same patient with shoulder traction. Also note the soft tissue swelling in front of the dislocation (*arrow*).

6. There is an increase in the soft tissue shadow in front of the cervical spine (Fig. 7.4) on lateral x-ray.

Fractures and Dislocations of the C1-C2 Region

Odontoid (Dens) Fractures

The most frequently used classification of these injuries is that of Anderson and D'Alonzo (3). They divided these fractures into three basic types (Fig. 7.5):

Type 1: Fractures through the tip of the odontoid
Type 2: Fractures through the base of the dens
Type 3: Fractures through the body of the axis that separates the odontoid from C2

Type 1: Fractures Through the Tip of the Odontoid.   This is the rarest of the three types of fractures. There is the potential for confusing this injury with an os odontoideum.

Type 2: Fractures Through the Base of the Dens.   This is the most common odontoid injury. Most occur as the result of motor vehicle accidents, and affect

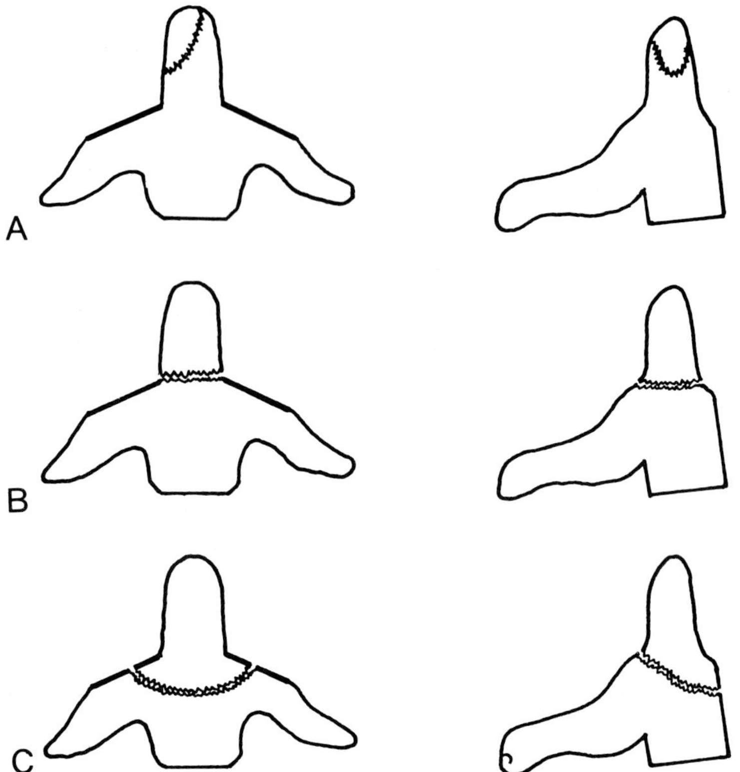

Figure 7.5.   A, Type 1 odontoid fracture. B, Type 2 odontoid fracture. C, Type 3 odontoid fracture.

men more often than women. Neurological injury is uncommon. (If neurological injury occurs in this fracture, it results in instant death.)

The problem with this fracture is the precarious blood supply to the damaged odontoid at the level of the fracture. Displacement of the fracture also interferes with blood supply, making nonunion of this fracture a high possibility.

Once the diagnosis is made, the patient should immediately go into skull tongs or a halo device (8). If there is any displacement of the fractured odontoid (anteriorly or posteriorly), then surgery is indicated. Surgery is either a C1-C2 fusion posteriorly or an anterior screw fixation of the fracture (Fig. 7.6).

Type 3: Fractures Through the Body of the Axis That Separates the Odontoid From C2.   Because there is a good blood supply to this fracture line, union is usual (Fig. 7.7). Treatment should employ halo-vest immobilization until union is complete as documented on flexion-extension films (usually in 12 weeks).

Jefferson Fractures of the C1 Ring

These fractures have always been considered burst fractures (axial load) occurring when a vehicular passenger is thrown against the roof. The mechanism of injury probably includes an element of extension that jams the posterior portion of the C1 ring against the spine of C2. Breaking of the ring allows the lateral masses of C1 to spread on C2 (Fig. 7.7).

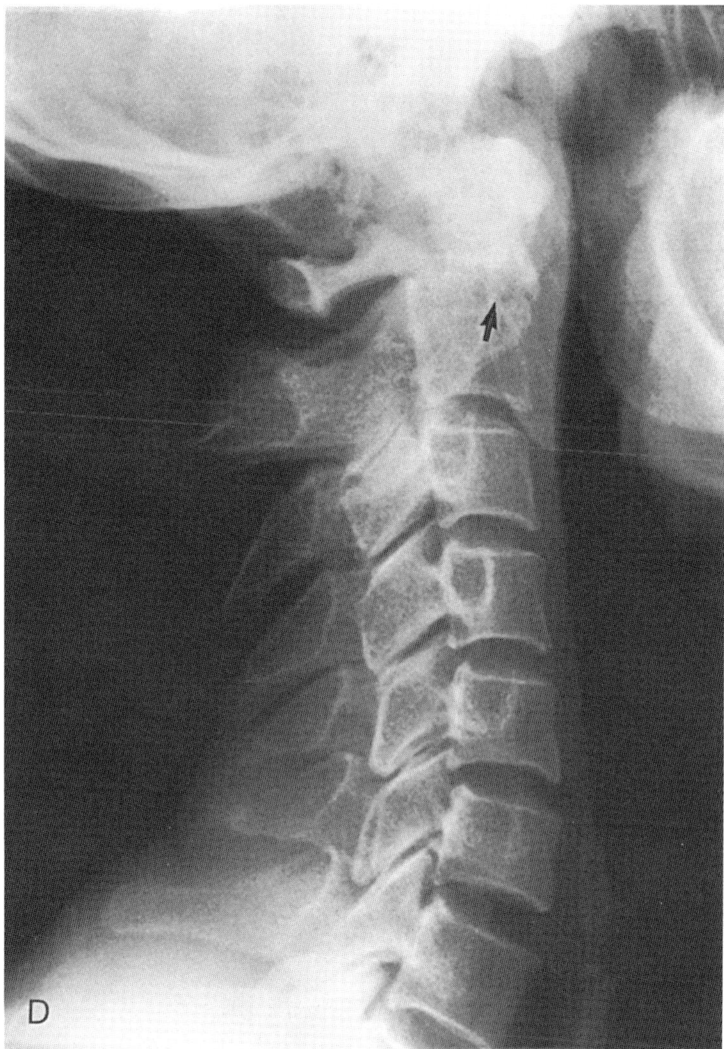

Figure 7.5.   D, Type 3 odontoid fracture (*arrow*).

These are obviously acute fractures, with the patient appearing in the emergency department after a blow to the top of the head, usually in a motor vehicle accident (MVA). The classic symptoms are severe neck pain and inability to rotate the head on the neck. If neurological deficit were to occur, it is a level of the spinal cord incompatible with life; living patients with a Jefferson fracture have no neurological deficit.

Treatment is with skull tongs for a few days to allow all injuries to declare themselves. During this time, a full assessment is completed. A halo vest is then applied for up to eight weeks, followed by a Philadelphia-like collar for another four weeks. It is unusual for these fractures to become nonunion and/or require surgical stabilization.

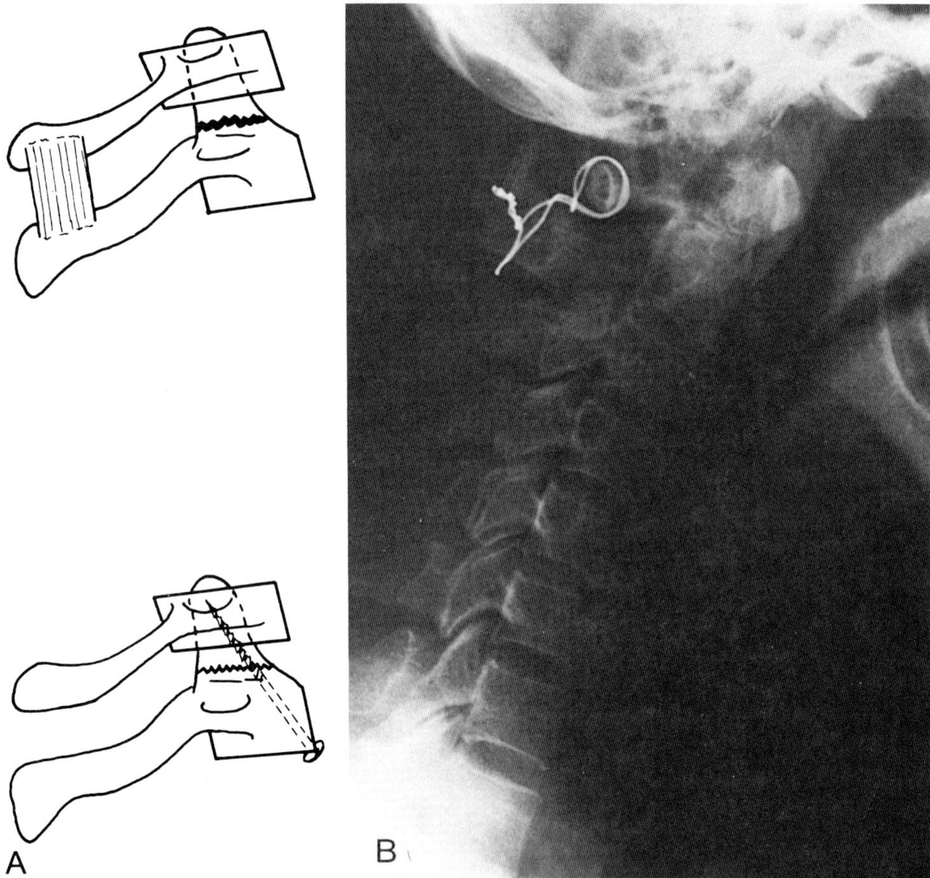

Figure 7.6.   A, posterior C1-C2 fusion (*top*). Anterior screw fixation of an odontoid fracture (*bottom*). **B,** lateral x-ray of a posterior C1-C2 fusion.

Traumatic Spondylolisthesis of C2 (Hangman's Fracture)

Every young resident remembers this fracture, because it is thought to be related to the fracture resulting from execution by hanging. Execution by hanging is designed to end life, yet so few of these patients have neurological deficit! Obviously, the mechanism of injury is different—but just try to get rid of the designation!

Mechanism of Injury

Hyperextension with an axial load is thought to be the mechanism of injury. As a result, the skull and C1 are driven down into the posterior elements of C2, causing the fracture. The axis is the only cervical vertebrae that has a true pars, like the lumbar vertebrae (Fig. 7.8), and the fracture most often crosses the pars separating the superior facet, pedicle, and vertebral body from the remaining posterior elements (inferior facet, lamina, and spinous process). This allows the vertebral body of C2 to subluxate forward on C3 to varying degrees (Fig. 7.9).

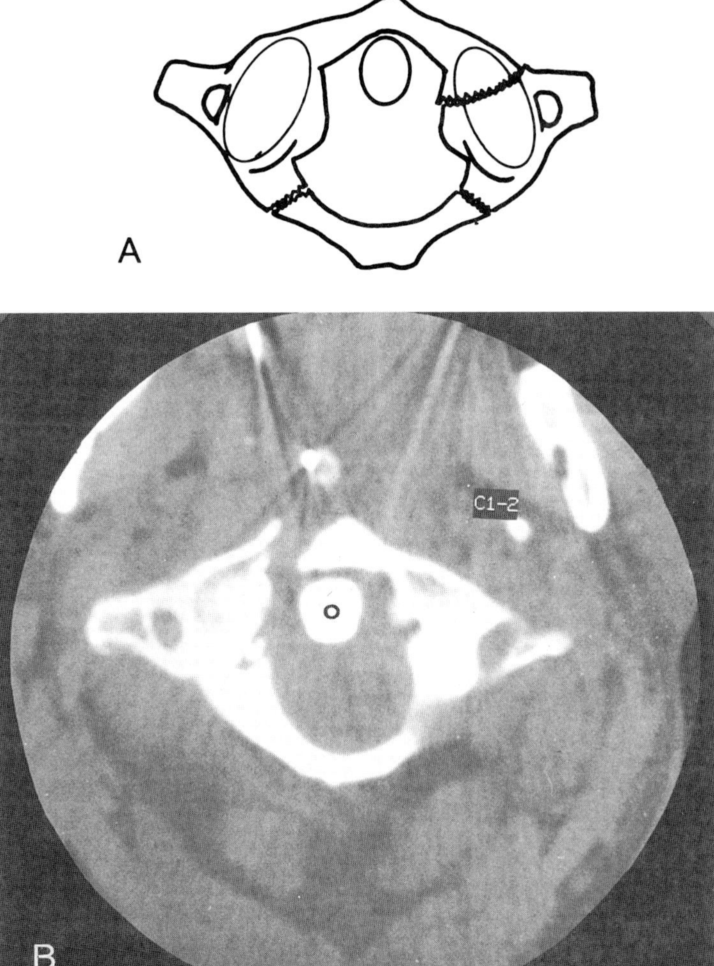

Figure 7.7.   **A**, axial schematic of a Jefferson fracture. **B**, axial CT of a Jefferson fracture (o = odontoid).

This actually enlarges the spinal canal, which accounts for the low incidence of neurological injury. But don't always look for the posterior fractures in the pars—they may be more anterior through the pedicles or more posterior through the lamina.

Classification

As with any cervical fracture, there are different degrees of stability/instability, which has led to the classification of this injury into three types. Based on the definition of instability by White et al. (3.5 mm subluxation and/or 11° angulation), C2 fractures have been classified into three types (25):

1. Minimal displacement of the body of C2 on C3 (less than 3.5 mm)
2. Significant displacement (greater than 3.5 mm)

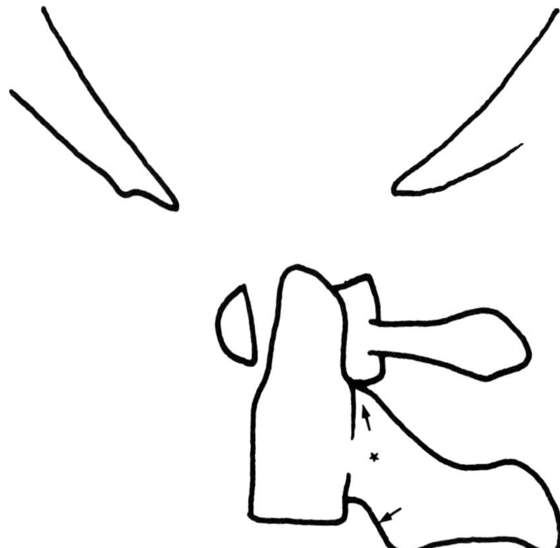

Figure 7.8. The axis (C2) has a true pars interarticularis (*) between a facet joint C1-C2 (*arrow*) and C2-C3 (*arrow*).

3. Significant displacement plus posterior element fractures

Treatment

Since neurological injury is rare, treatment is almost always centered around the fracture (18). Table 7.3 outlines the treatment options. Accurate x-rays, including CT scanning, are necessary to locate where in the posterior elements the fractures have occurred and whether the facet joints are intact. Careful plain x-rays and a CT scan are also needed to rule out other associated spine fractures, the most common being a Jefferson fracture of C1.

Rotary Subluxation of C1-C2

This is a rare lesion compared to fractures of C1-C2. It tends to occur in younger patients as the result of trivial injury. Often it goes undiagnosed for days or weeks until the patient decides that the suboccipital pain and torticollis are persisting too long.

Plain radiographs usually reveal the abnormality (Fig. 7.10). Treatment is by skull-tong traction (Fig. 7.11) and posttraction immobilization in a halo-thoracic orthosis. On rare occasion, the deformity and its pain will persist, requiring a C1-C2 posterior fusion.

Pediatric Injuries of the Spine

Although this is an adult text, we have included some pediatric problems because of the interesting perspective they present.

Injuries to the cervical spine in children differ as follows:

1. Children under 8–10 years of age have a very flexible, short cervical spine with a relatively large head sitting on top. Although young kids tumble and crash into each other on a regular basis, they rarely suffer severe neck injury.

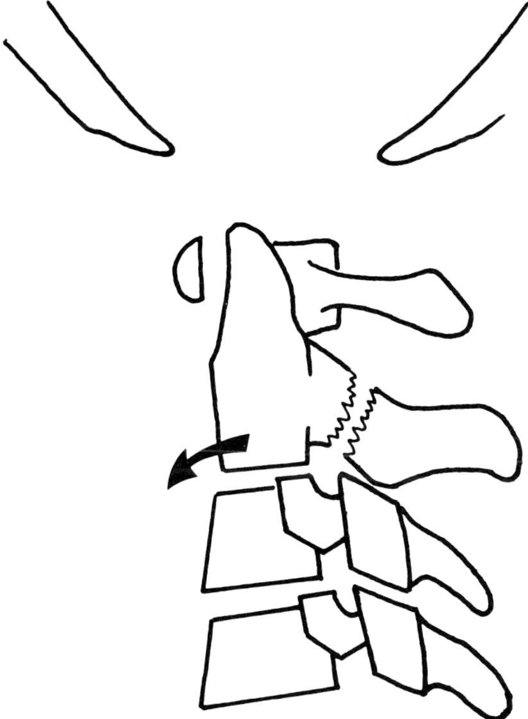

Figure 7.9.   The body of C2 (with C1 and the skull above) subluxates forward on C3, leaving behind some posterior elements of C2 (very much like a lumbar spondylolisthesis).

Table 7.3.   Management of C2 Fractures

	Type 1	Type 2	Type 3
Fracture Location	Pars	More posteriorly	Anywhere in posterior elements
Facet Joint	Not involved	Not involved	Dislocations and/or fractures
Ant. and Post. Longitudinal Lig.	Intact	Usually intact	Both torn
Stable/Unstable	Stable	Unstable	Very unstable
Initial Management	Choice of halo-thoracic or simple Philadelphia collar	Tongs and bedrest—6 weeks, then halo-thoracic—6 weeks	Open reduction posterior facet joints. Tongs and bedrest—6 weeks, then halo-thoracic at least 6 weeks.
Duration	8–12 weeks	12 weeks	12 weeks plus
Chance of Nonunion	Very low	Occurs occasionally	Occurs occasionally
Need for Further Surgery	Not for fracture but for facet degeneration C2–C3	Occasionally	More frequent if not treated aggressively
Type of Late Surgery	Posterior C2–C3 fusion	C2–C3 anterior or C1–C3 posterior fusion	C2–C3 anterior or C1–C3 posterior fusion

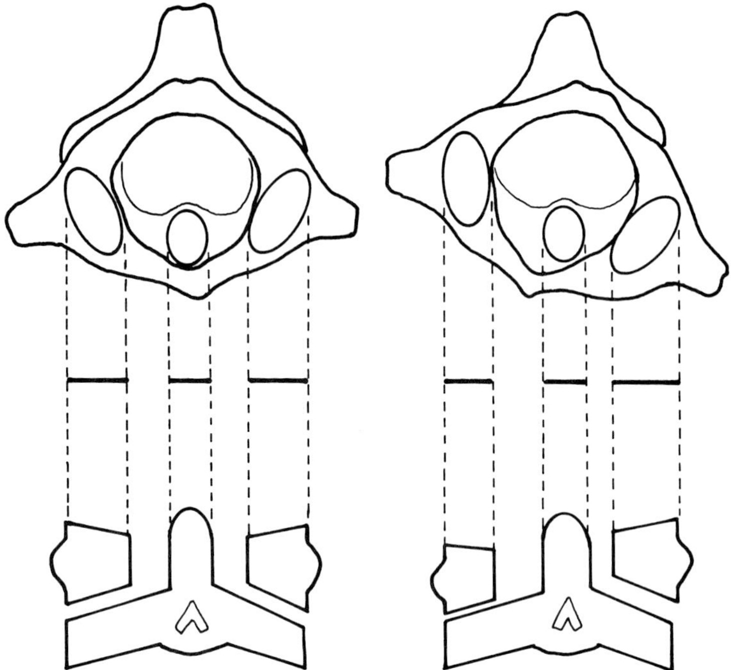

Figure 7.10.   Rotatory subluxation of C1 on C2. *Left*—normal. *Right*—rotatory subluxation. The AP x-ray will show a change in the space between the odontoid and C1 as well as a difference in the lateral masses of C1.

2. Under the age of 8–10 years, injuries of the upper cervical spine (C1-C2) are much more common than subaxial injuries. This is just the reverse of adults. Adolescents over the age of 10–12 years develop an injury pattern very similar to adults.
3. Since the most common injury in young children is at the level of C1-C2, painful torticollis is the usual presentation. Injuries include traumatic ligament disruption and odontoid "epiphyseal" separation.
4. Satisfactory x-rays of the young child's spine are difficult to obtain and interpret because of:
   a. Pain and fear making the child very uncooperative.
   b. A skeleton that is largely cartilaginous.
   c. The high incidence of soft tissue lesions rather than bony lesions.
      Note: Don't be lulled into a false sense of security by apparently normal x-rays. Be especially aware of the child with apparent spinal cord injury who has normal x-rays and has, because of injury, suffered severe soft tissue instability that requires a very diligent search with cine x-rays, with or without myelography and/or MRI to establish the diagnosis.
5. Beware of the pseudosubluxation that occurs at C2-C3 (Fig. 7.12). It is not a significant injury and the x-ray picture will resolve with time and growth.
6. Finally, note some usual occurrences in normal children's x-rays:
   a. The neck is most often straight without the lordotic curve normally seen in adults (Fig. 7.13).

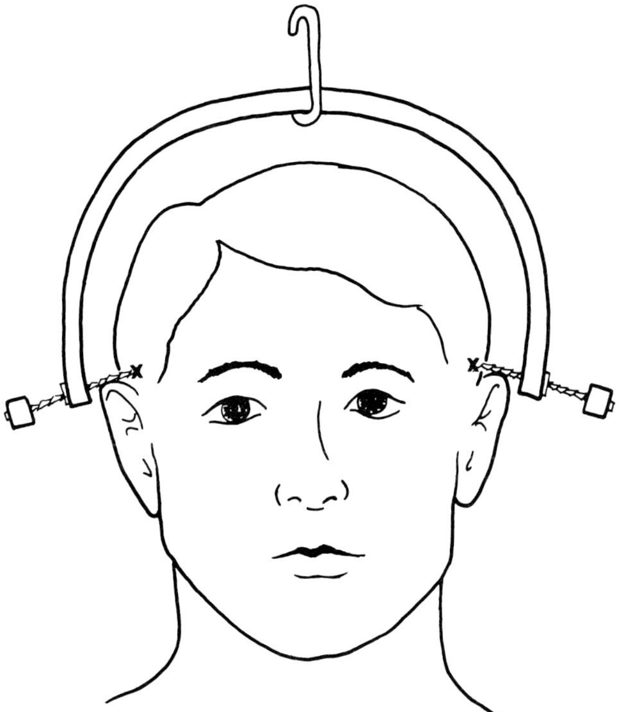

Figure 7.11.   Gardner-Wells skull tongs. These are simple to apply, largely because each tong set comes with easy-to-read instructions!

    b. Crying increases the soft tissue space in front of C2 and is not indicative of a retropharyngeal hematoma from a cervical spine injury.

Subaxial (C3-C7) Fractures and Dislocation in the Adult
Introduction

Neck injury with paralysis is a potential catastrophe. The persisting physical disability and associated morbidity have a long-term negative impact on social, psychological, and financial well-being. Three recent advances are serving to reduce the dimensions of the problem, including:

1. Better emergency medical handling of the injured at the scene of the accident (Fig. 7.14);
2. Development of trauma units to better handle the patient during triage;
3. Better understanding of injuries because of newer imaging modalities (CT and MRI); this in turn has led to better classification of injuries and better treatment (Figs. 7.15 and 7.16) (1, 9, 15, 17, 24).

Associated Injuries

A significant number of cervical-spine-injured (CSI) patients will have associated injuries requiring a multidisciplinary team approach. When assessing the spine implication of the injury, don't lose sight of the whole patient, and always be quick to tap the expertise of your colleagues in other fields.

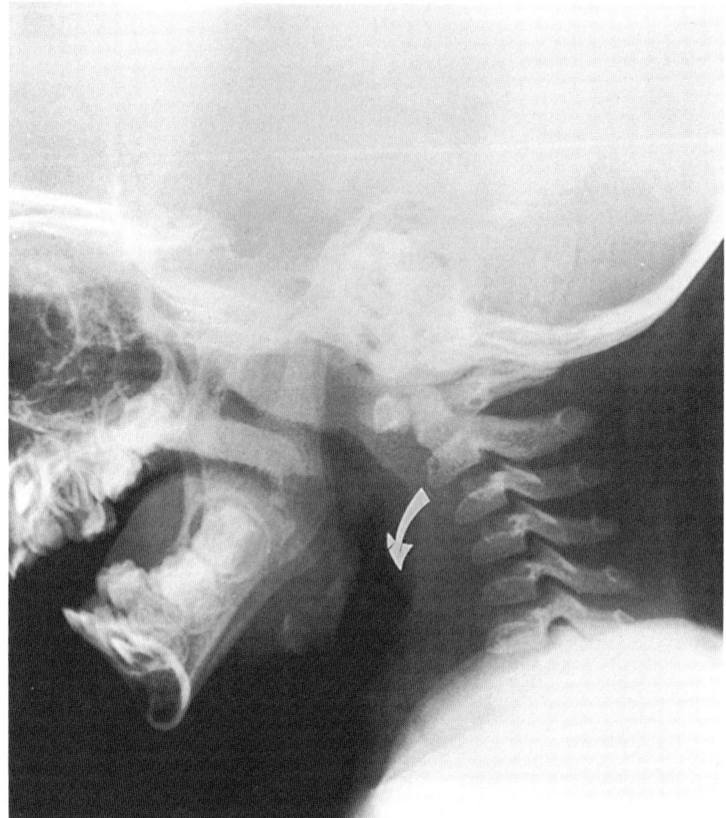

Figure 7.12.   Normal degree of C2 on C3 subluxation in child.

What's Stable? What's Unstable?

The assessment of every cervical spine injury is founded on this question. Instability was defined by White and Panjabi (25) as the inability of the spine to resist physiological loads, which in turn results in neurological injury and/or skeletal deformity. Using this criterion, Table 7.4 outlines instability in cervical spine fractures/dislocations.

Mechanism of Injury

Four groups of individuals have been largely responsible for our understanding of all spine fractures:

1. Holdsworth (15) was the first to separate the thoracolumbar spine into two columns—anterior and posterior (Fig. 7.17).
2. Denis (9) added the middle column, which helped immensely in understanding instability in the thoracolumbar spine (Fig. 7.18).
3. Allen (1) et al. proposed the first working classification of cervical spine fractures.
4. Ducker and McAfee (19) have simplified Allen's classification by proposing we "read the clock" to understand fracture patterns (Fig. 7.19).

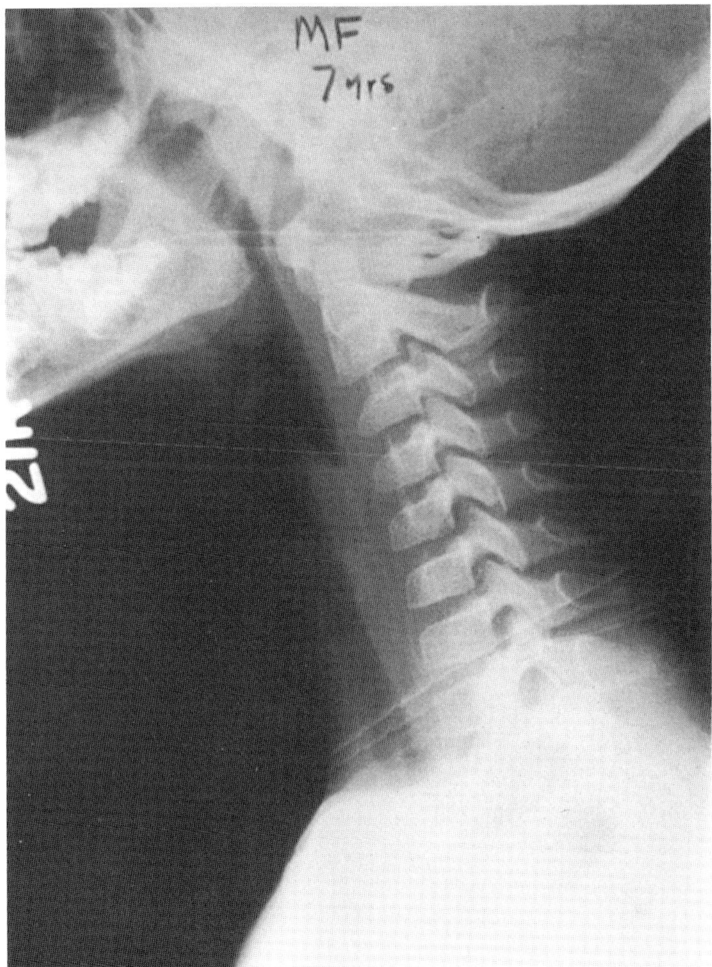

Figure 7.13.   Normal lateral of child's cervical spine showing absence of cervical lordosis normally seen in adults.

Force Directions

Starting at high noon on the Ducker-McAfee clock, there are basically four force directions that injure the neck (Table 7.5). This results in five basic fracture patterns as described by Allen et al. (Fig. 7.19). Unfortunately, assessment and classification of cervical spine injuries is not easy because so many multidirectional forces can occur, more than one injury to the spine can occur (16), and complex single-level injuries perplex even the most astute observer.

Radiological Assessment

Most fracture patterns are apparent on plain x-ray, but it is routine to obtain at least a CT scan, and more often than not, an MRI. The CT scan depicts fine details of the fracture pattern (Fig. 7.15) and reveals other contiguous fractures

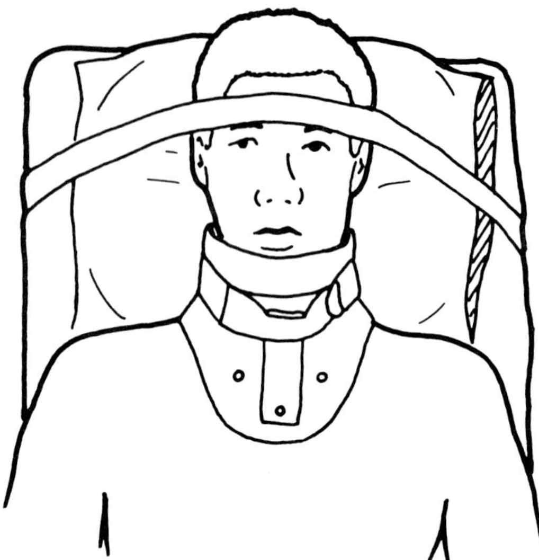

Figure 7.14.   All accident victims should be treated as potential neck injuries and transported in a collar with some form of head immobilization.

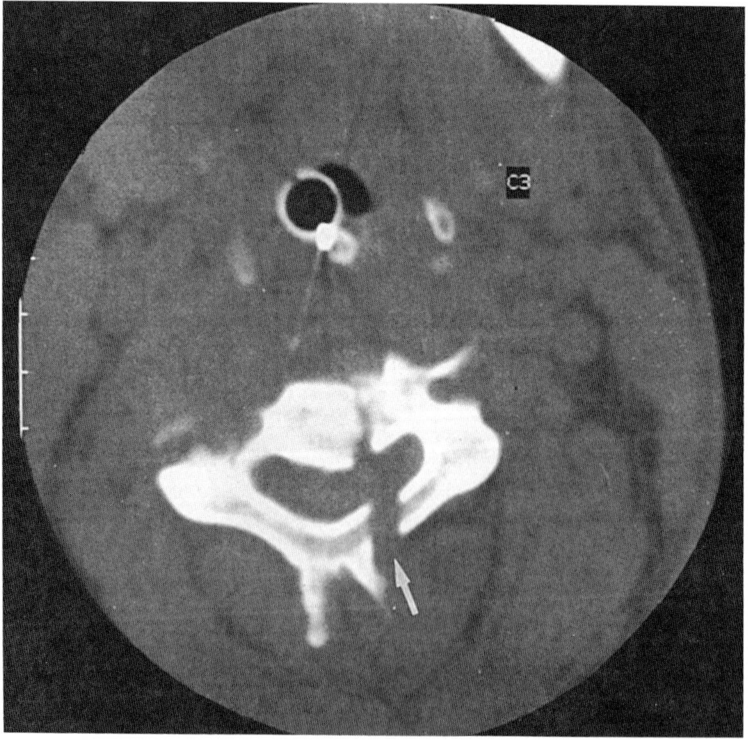

Figure 7.15.   CT scan of the upper end of a burst fracture of C3. Note the laminar fracture (*arrow*).

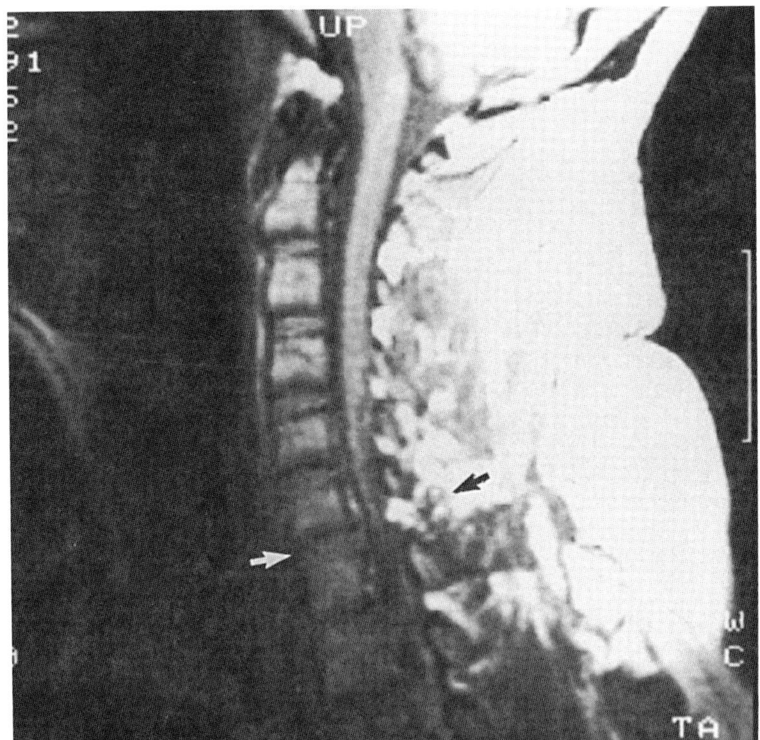

Figure 7.16. MRI showing the extent of soft tissue injury.

Table 7.4. *Instability in Cervical Spine Fracture Dislocation*

System	Mode	Manifestation
Neurological	Clinical	Neurological symptoms at time of injury (Lhermitte's) or neurological deficit on examination*
	X-ray	Mass in canal (bone or disc) seen on MRI or CT/ myelogram
Skeletal	Clinical	Disruption of posterior soft tissue (interspinous/ supraspinous ligaments) on clinical exam
	X-ray (plain)	>3.5 mm forward subluxation of vertebral body >11° angulation of vertebral body on its caudal mate >1 cm separation of vertebral segments on traction test

*Two exceptions:
1. The central cord syndrome that develops in a hyperextension neck injury to a congenitally narrowed canal with degenerative changes.
2. Single-level root lesion in unilateral facet joint subluxation.

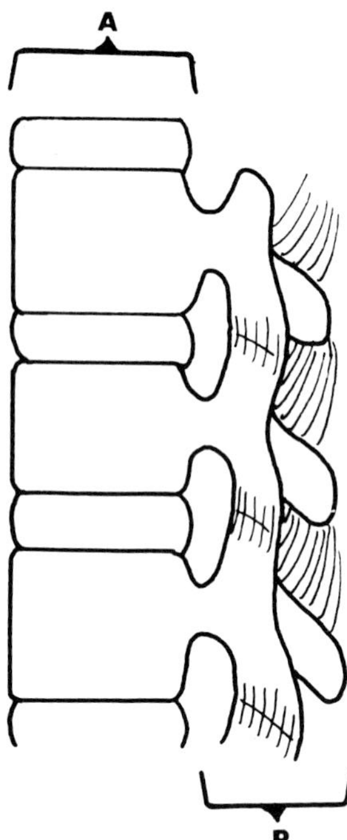

Figure 7.17. Holdsworth separation of the anterior (*A*) column and the posterior (*P*) column. The anterior column included everything back to the posterior longitudinal ligament.

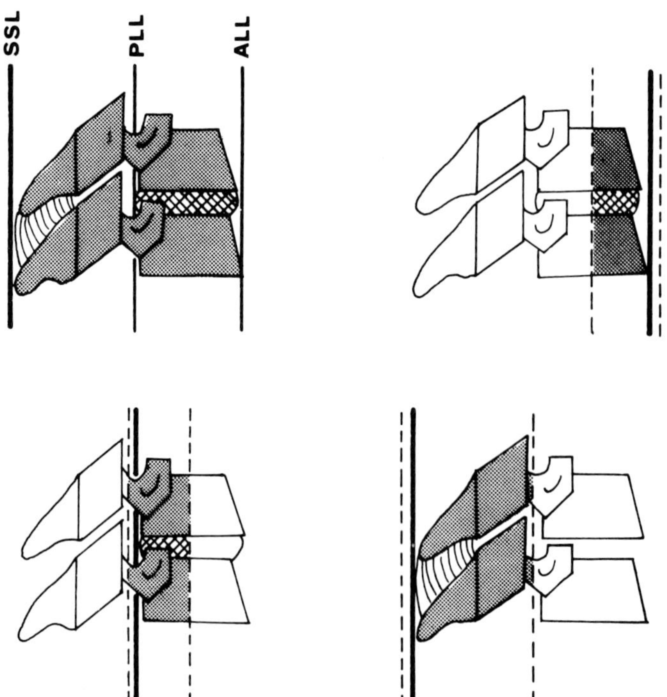

Figure 7.18. Denis "middle column" classification extended to the cervical spine (*SSL* = supraspinous ligament, ligamentum nuchae; *PLL* = posterior longitudinal ligament; *ALL* = anterior longitudinal ligament). *Top right* has the anterior column shaded; on *bottom left*, the middle column is shaded and on *bottom right*, the posterior column is shaded.

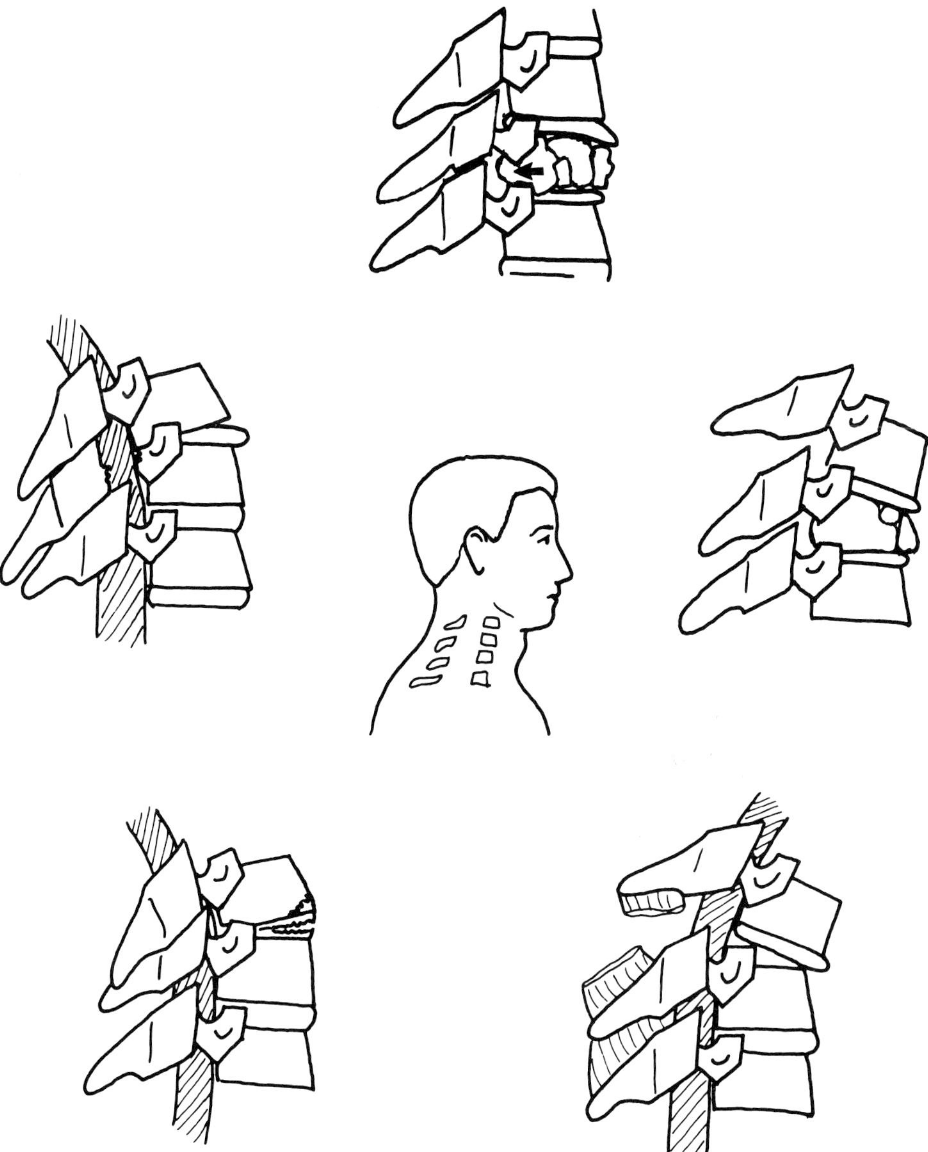

Figure 7.19.   Reading the modified Ducker-McAfee clock.

• 12 noon compression force causing the burst fracture.

• 3 o'clock flexion-compression force causing compression wedge fracture with an anterior tear-drop fragment.

• 5 o'clock flexion-distraction force causing unilateral or bilateral facet dislocation.

• 7 o'clock extension-distraction force causing a tearing of the disc and ALL structure, and a small tear-drop fracture of the anterior inferior vertebral body.

• 9 o'clock extension-compression force causing posterior element fractures as well as disc/ALL injury.

Table 7.5.   Force Directions Injuring the Cervical Spine

1.	Axial up	— Tension, distraction
	Axial down	— Compression
	Axial rotatory	— Rotation
2.	Backward	— Extension
3.	Forward	— Flexion
		— Shear
4.	Sideways	— Lateral flexion

that aid in surgical planning. The MRI shows soft tissue detail in regard to the spinal cord (Fig. 7.16) and disc.

Remember a good general rule in orthopaedics: you must see the joint above and below any fracture. For the cervical spine, this means you must see, on x-ray, the base of the skull (so that you don't miss injuries at C1-C2), and the thoracic spine (so that you don't miss dislocations of C7 on T1) (Fig. 7.4).

Management: General Principles

After assuring that the neck is protected, step aside and let your colleagues stabilize the patient medically. Once this is achieved, you may then focus on the cervical injury and institute a clinical review of the neurological and skeletal status, followed by plain radiographic studies.

If there is obvious instability or a question of instability, the standard is to place Gardner-Wells tongs (Fig. 7.11) and apply traction. Some clinicians prefer the direct application of halo traction (Fig. 7.20) (13) with MRI-compatible halos, which will probably become standard. The use of methyl prednisone within the first eight hours of neurological injury (30 mg/kg of body weight) appears to have some benefit (5), but watch the side effect of stress ulcer.

The next step in management is to clearly decide if the injury is stable or unstable (Table 7.4).

You will then be left with three clinical situations:

1. Stable (neurological and skeletal). This may have been decided on initial assessment when the patient was placed in an intermediate orthosis such as a Philadelphia collar (Fig. 4.3A). Continue this treatment, but be sure you obtain follow-up x-rays, because some of these so-called "stable" injuries go on to late deformity.
2. Skeletally unstable but no neurological injury. In this clinical setting you have to decide if the fracture pattern is such that healing can occur without subsequent neurological damage or skeletal deformity. Keep in mind that predominantly ligamentous injuries (e.g., facet dislocation) do not heal into stability in spite of long-term halo-vest immobilization. If there is potential for instability/deformity problems in this group of patients, operate to stabilize.
3. Unstable skeletally—neurological injury (partial or complete). The first step in handling this patient is a detailed neurological examination that should be repeated at regular intervals. Assess the type, degree, and level of injury (Table 7.1) and whether or not spinal shock is present.

Most of these patients will require some form of surgical intervention. The rules to follow are:

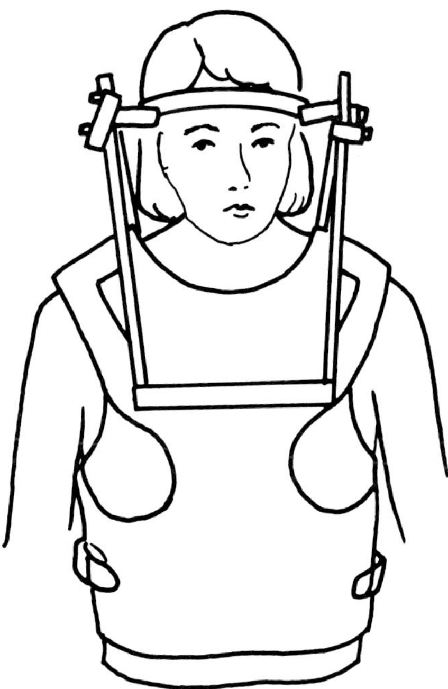

Figure 7.20.   Halo-thoracic orthosis. This is applied by choosing the correct size ring (Fig. 7.21). Using holding devices, place it about 1 cm above the ear and apply 4 pins to hold the halo to the skull. The thoracic orthotic device is then assembled with the vertical rods attached to the halo.

1. Realign the skeleton with external skeletal traction.
2. A partial neurological deficit that is increasing requires immediate x-ray (CT/MRI) investigation and surgery.
3. For incomplete lesions that are improving, it is best to leave things alone for a few days, and then make an elective surgical decision based on skeletal factors.
4. For complete lesions (quadriplegia), surgery is an elective decision and is based on what will get the patient into the rehabilitation stream in the shortest possible time.
5. Bilateral facet dislocations and body displacement (Fig. 7.22) are ligamentous injuries that will not be stable with healing and require posterior stabilization.
6. A unilateral facet dislocation with a unilateral single root involved has the potential, with reduction, to stabilize without surgery. (Remember to do repeat follow-up x-rays at regular intervals.)
7. Although central cord injury is a neurological deficit, it usually occurs in the stable spine of an older patient who started with congenital narrowing and has additional degenerative changes. It is usually not an indication for surgery except when dealing with significant narrowing of the developmental/degenerative condition.
8. Spinal cord monitoring should be part of the surgical procedure (sensory or motor-evoked potentials).

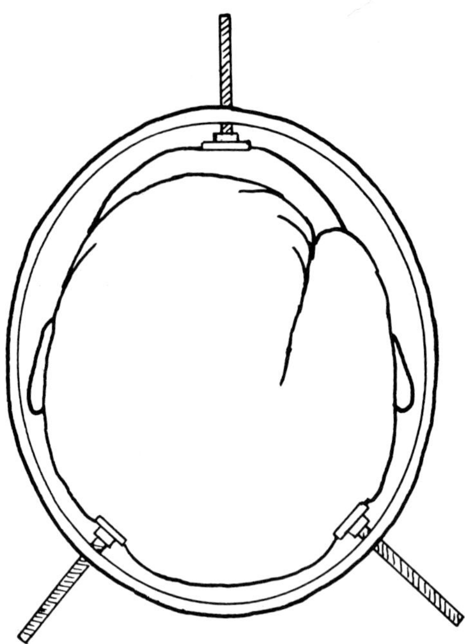

Figure 7.21.   The simplest example of approaching instability from its force vector. This flexion-distraction injury caused bilateral facet dislocation after tearing the posterior soft tissues. After open reduction posteriorly, the soft tissue damage was treated with a posterior fusion and spinous process wiring.

Surgical Approaches

The three basic rules are:

1. Approach the neurological compression from the direction of injury (22). If this is anteriorly, as is usually the case, you must add internal and/or external skeletal stabilization at the same time (Fig. 7.23*A*) (4, 6, 7, 11, 21, 22, 23, 26).
2. Approach skeletal instability from the direction of the greatest damage (force vector) (Fig. 7.22).
3. Be prepared to do both anterior and posterior approaches, especially in multisegmental and/or very unstable injuries (Fig. 7.23*B*) (25).

Common (Subaxial) C-Spine Fractures/Dislocations

The two most common fractures you will see are (1) the flexion-compression injury, and (2) the burst fracture.

Flexion-Compression Injury

This injury is usually the result of an MVA or diving accident. The combination of flexion and compression collapses the anterior aspect of the vertebral body (usually C5) and splits the vertebral body into an anterior tear-drop fragment (Fig. 7.22*A*) and a larger posterior body fragment. The posterior fragment is displaced posteriorly into the spinal canal, which explains the very high incidence of neurological injury in this fracture. Note in Figure 7.24 that the height of the anterior vertebral body is less than posteriorly, and there is a kyphotic

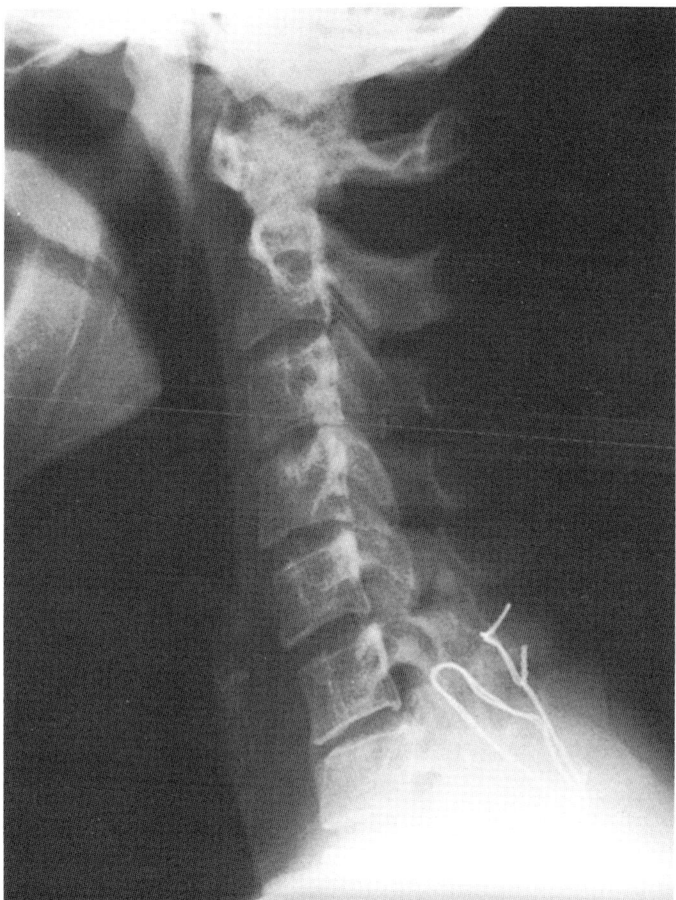

Figure 7.22.   The flexion-compression injury with vertebral body wedging and tear drop anteriorly.

deformity. This helps distinguish this injury from the burst fracture. With the kyphosis comes a widened interspinous interval.

Unfortunately, there is a high incidence of complete neurological injury (quadriplegia) in this fracture. Management is usually surgical, with anterior debridement of the fracture fragments from the spinal canal, bone grafting, internal fixation, and continuing external support.

Burst Fracture

This fracture results from a pure compressive load to the cervical spine and splits the vertebral body into two relatively equal portions. As with the flexion-compression injury, the posterior fragment can be retropulsed into the spinal canal, causing severe neurological damage (Fig. 7.25). Most of these fractures are caused by blows to the top of the head in MVAs and diving accidents. Compressive forces often cause additional posterior element fractures that are only evident on CT scan (Fig. 7.15).

If there is no neurological injury, a burst fracture may be treated nonoperatively in the halo-thoracic orthosis.

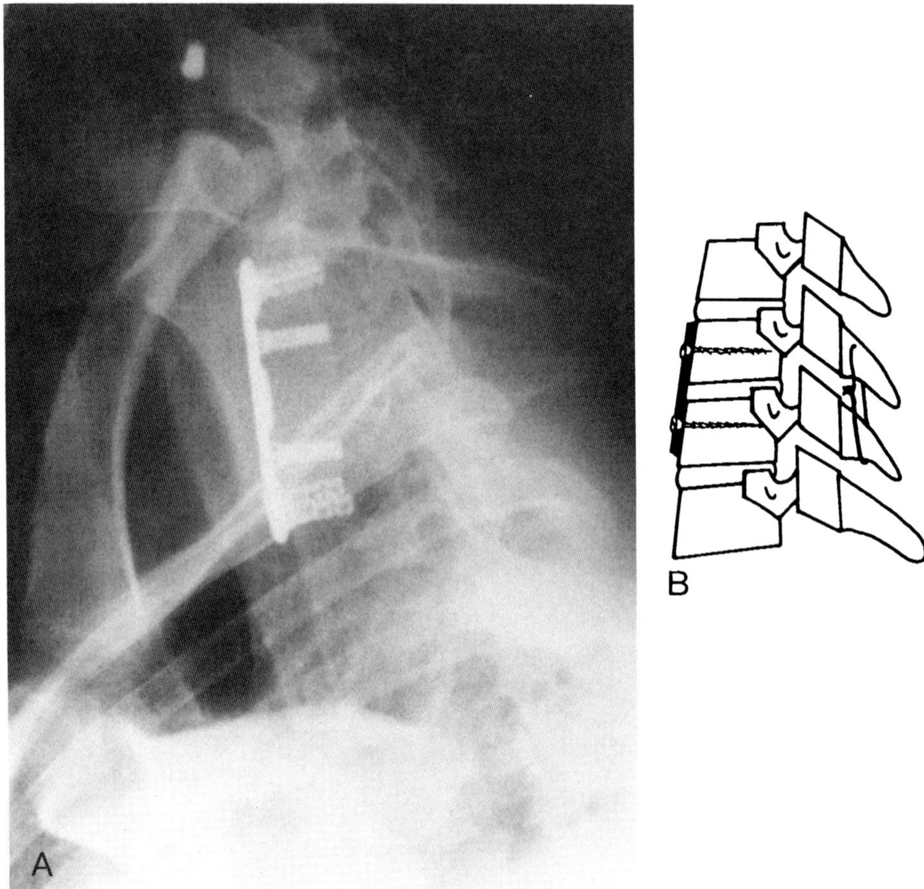

Figure 7.23.   A, anterior plating. **B,** schematic of anterior plate and posterior wiring done for a very unstable injury.

A partial neurological injury, associated with a large fragment of bone in the spinal canal (Fig. 7.26), merits urgent anterior decompression and fusion. A partial cord deficit, with a small fragment of bone in the spinal canal, may initially be treated nonoperatively in a halo, but more than likely will lead to an anterior decompression and fusion.

Complete neurological lesions, with large fragments of bone compromising the canal, are more often than not decompressed, with the slimmest of hope that some neurological function will return. Smaller fragments associated with a complete cord transection are treated nonoperatively in a halo.

The standard of operative care is identical to the flexion-compression injuries, that is, an anterior approach to excise the bone fragment, autogenous bone grafting, internal fixation to hold the bone graft in place, and external halo-thoracic immobilization to hold the neck in alignment.

Less common cervical spine injuries include flexion-distraction, extension-distraction, and extension-compression.

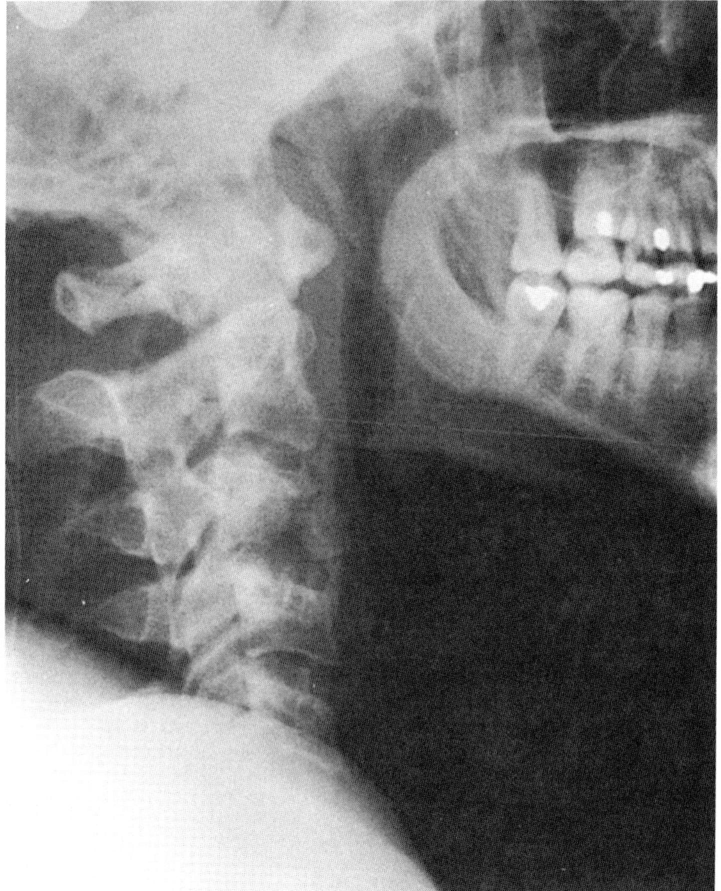

Figure 7.24.   The burst fracture (C3).

Flexion-Distraction Injury

This injury results in varying degrees of tearing of the posterior soft tissues, including the supraspinous/interspinous ligaments, facet capsule, posterior longitudinal ligament, and annulus. The result of this injury is facet subluxation, either unilateral or bilateral (Fig. 7.4). The addition of a rotation component will subluxate one facet joint more than the other; the purer the flexion force and the greater the flexion force, the more likely it is that both facets will dislocate. Bilateral facet dislocation will cause quadriplegia in 50% of victims.

For unilateral or bilateral subluxation or dislocation, immediate closed reduction via halo traction is indicated. If unable to effect a reduction this way, look for the presence of a disc herniation (MRI). The presence of a disc herniation that may be further dragged into the spinal canal requires anterior decompression prior to any posterior approach. Careful neurological assessment is needed during traction reduction.

Unilateral facet subluxation or dislocations must be reduced. Unfortunately, many of these injuries are missed for days, weeks, or longer, making closed re-

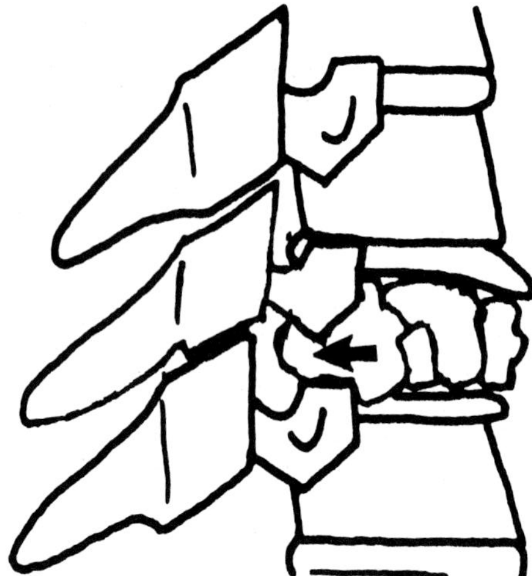

Figure 7.25.   Burst fracture with the posterior vertebral fracture fragment (middle column, *arrow*) in the canal.

duction impossible. Unsuccessful reduction requires an open posterior reduction and internal fixation. Whether a successful closed reduction of a unilateral facet dislocation should be subsequently managed operatively or nonoperatively is not yet settled.

All bilateral facet subluxation or dislocations are unstable and must be fused posteriorly in the reduced (realigned) position (Fig. 7.22).

Extension-Distraction Injury

This is a troublesome injury because the patient often presents neurological damage (central cord syndrome) but no obvious bony injury on conventional x-ray. The injury usually occurs in the older patient as a result of blunt facial trauma (falling down stairs or a dashboard injury).

On lateral x-ray, careful inspection will usually reveal soft tissue swelling anteriorly and a small avulsion fracture from the inferior corner of the involved vertebrae (Fig. 7.19). The small size of the fragment and the usual absence of kyphosis separate this injury from the flexion-compression fracture.

The diagnosis is greatly assisted by MRI, which shows the anterior soft tissue disruption.

After initial stabilization with Gardner-Wells tongs and observation, these patients are best managed with anterior stabilization using bone graft and plates. If there is pre-existing cervical canal stenosis from degenerative disc disease, this will have to be addressed at the time of surgery.

Extension-Compression Injury

This is "the least common of the common" and results in posterior element fractures. The incidence of neurological injury is low, and treatment is usually by way of external immobilization only.

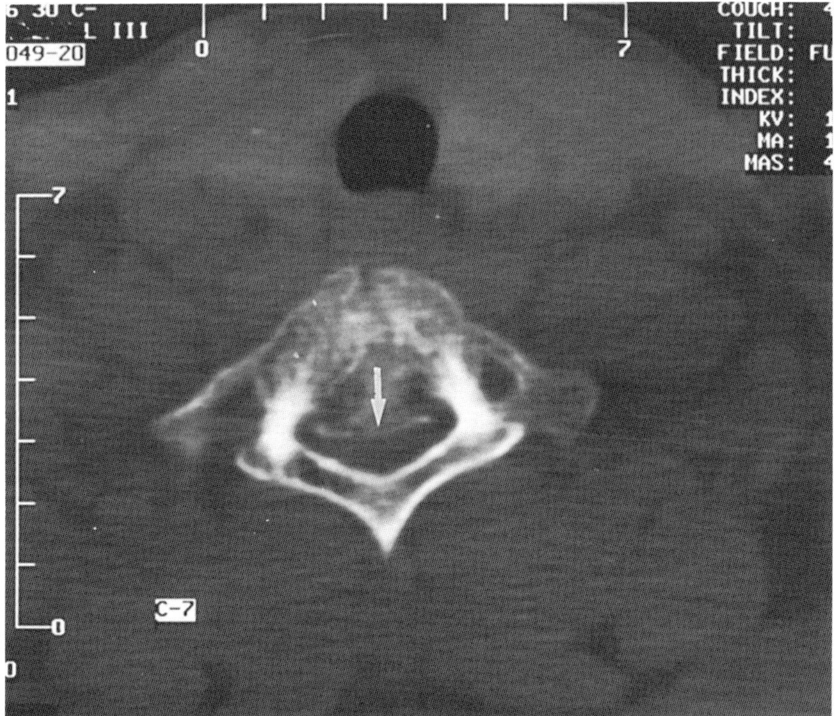

Figure 7.26. A burst fracture C7.

Postoperative Management

Postoperative management of these patients is intense. The most important aspect of immediate postoperative care is maintenance of neurological function and skeletal alignment. Obviously, general bodily functions need careful monitoring. Local wound and pin tract complications need to be prevented; you must be on constant watch for pulmonary, gastrointestinal, bladder, and skin problems.

Once the patient and the injury are stabilized, mobilization and ambulation in the rehabilitation unit are started.

Summary

There is no easy way to understand cervical spine trauma. The generalities discussed above, and the five common fracture patterns, will fall far short of the situations faced by the skilled spine trauma surgeon. Fortunately, experienced trauma surgeons can be found in most centers, and they can bail you out if necessary.

REFERENCES

1. Allen BL Jr, Ferguson RL, Lehmann TR, and O'Brien RP: A mechanistic classification of closed, indirect fractures and dislocations of the lower cervical spine. Spine 7:1–27 (1982).
2. American Spinal Injury Association and American Spinal Injury Association Foundation Guidelines for Facility Categorization and Standards of Care. Spinal Cord Injury, p 7, Chicago (1987).

3. Anderson LD and D'Alonzo RT: Fractures of the odontoid process of the axis. J Bone Joint Surg 56A:1663–1674 (1974).

4. Bohlman HH: Acute fractures and dislocations of the cervical spine: an analysis of three hundred hospitalized patients and review of the literature. J Bone Joint Surg 61A:1119–1142 (1975).

5. Bracken MB, Shepard MJ, Collins WF, et al: A randomized, controlled trial of methylprednisolone or naloxone in the treatment of acute spinal cord injury. N Engl J Med 322:1405–1411 (1990).

6. Caspar W: Anterior cervical fusion and interbody stabilization with the trapezial osteosynthetic plate technique. Tuttlingen: Aesculap-Wissenschaftliche Informationen in Selbstverlag der Aesculap-Werke AG (1984).

7. Caspar W and Harkey HL: Anterior cervical fusion: Caspar osteosynthetic stabilization. In: Microsurgery of the Cervical Spine, pp 109–142. Ed: Young PH. Raven Press, New York (1991).

8. Clark CR and White AA III: Fractures of the dens: a multicenter study. J Bone Joint Surg 67A: 1340–1348 (1985).

9. Denis F: The three-column spine and its significance in the classification of acute thoraco-lumbar spinal injuries. Spine 8:817–831 (1983).

10. Ducker TB: Treatment of spinal cord injuries. N Engl J Med 322:1459–1461 (1990).

11. Dunn EJ: The role of methyl methacrylate in the stabilization and replacement of tumors of the cervical spine. A project of the Cervical Spine Research Society. Spine 2:14–24 (1977).

12. Frankel HL, Hancock GH, Melzak J, Michaelis LS, Unqar GH, Vernon JDS, and Walsh JJ: Postural reduction in closed injuries of the spine. Paraplegia 7:179–192 (1969).

13. Garfin SR, Botte MJ, Centeno RS, and Nickel VL: Osteology of the skull as it affects halo pin placement. Spine 10:696–698 (1985).

14. Harris JH Jr, Edeiken-Monroe B, and Kopaniky DR: A practical classification of acute cervical spine injuries. Orthop Clin North Am 17:15–30 (1986).

15. Holdsworth F: Fractures, dislocations and fracture-dislocations of the spine. Review article. J Bone Joint Surg 52A:1534–1551 (1970).

16. Kewalramani LS and Taylor RG: Multiple non-contiguous injuries to the spine. Acta Orthop Scand 47:52–58 (1976).

17. Kulkarni MV, McArdle CB, Kopanicky DR, Miner M, Cotler HB, Lee KF, and Harris JH: Acute spinal cord injury: MR imaging at 1.5T. Radiology 164:837–843 (1987).

18. Levine AM and Edwards CC: The management of traumatic spondylolisthesis of the axis. J Bone Joint Surg 67A:217–226 (1985).

19. McAfee PC: Cervical spine trauma. In: The Adult Spine: Principles and Practice, pp 1063–1106. Ed: Young PH. Raven Press, New York (1991).

20. Meyer PR Jr (ed): Surgery of Spine Trauma. Churchill Livingstone, New York (1989).

21. Robinson RA and Southwick WO: Indications and techniques for early stabilization of the neck in some fracture dislocations of the cervical spine. South Med J 53:565–579 (1960).

22. Smith GW and Robinson RA: The treatment of certain cervical spine disorders by anterior removal of the intervertebral disc and interbody fusion. J Bone Joint Surg 40A:607–624 (1958).

23. Stauffer ES and Kelly EG: Fracture-dislocation of the cervical spine: instability and recurrent deformity following treatment by anterior interbody fusion. J Bone Joint Surg 59A:45–48 (1977).

24. Weir DC: Roentgenographic signs of cervical injury. Clin Orthop 109:9–17 (1975).

25. White AA III and Panjabi MM: Clinical Biomechanics of the Spine, p 223. JB Lippincott, Philadelphia (1978).

26. Whitehill R: Fractures of the lower cervical spine: subaxial fractures in the adult. Seminars in Spine Surg 3:71–86 (1991).

8

Rheumatoid Neck and Miscellaneous Arthritic Afflictions

"I cannot conceive why we who are composed of over 90 per cent water should suffer from rheumatism with a slight rise in the humidity of the atmosphere."
—John W. Strutt, Baron Rayleigh

INTRODUCTION

The classic noninfective condition universally affecting the spine as we grow older is cervical degenerative disc disease (Chapter 2). More devastating, but fortunately less common, are the effects of rheumatoid arthritis and ankylosing spondylitis on the neck.

Rheumatoid Arthritis (RA)

Rheumatoid arthritis represents the classic diffuse connective tissue disease. It has the potential to seriously disrupt the cervical spine with dire consequences. The etiology of RA is unknown, but it is thought to be a combination of genetic predisposition in the immune system triggered by infectious or chemical agents (7). Other factors—nutritional, metabolic, occupational, and geographic—have been implicated, but it is likely they only modify an autoimmune reaction centered in the synovia. The characteristic of the disease is production of an antibody known as rheumatoid factor (RF), detectable in the serum by the latex agglutination test. Although characteristic for rheumatoid arthritis, its presence in the serum does not secure the diagnosis of RA, nor does its absence rule out the condition (1).

The antibody/antigen-induced inflammatory reaction in the synovia is manifested by exudation of destructive enzymes into the synovial fluid, cellular infiltration by acute and chronic inflammatory cells in the synovial membrane, and subsequent granulation tissue (pannus) formation over the cartilaginous surfaces of joints. In the beginning, the inflammatory synovitis causes joint pain and stiffness. In the end, the cartilage destruction and capsular and ligamentous damage lead to joint subluxations and deformity. The neck is no exception to the disease's progress.

Although the disease afflicts only 1%–3% of the 35–45-year-old population (females more than males by a 3-to-1 ratio), and although the hands and wrists are involved more often than the neck, the disease can be devastating to the cervical spine. Interestingly, RA has limited effects on the lumbar spine.

Effects of rheumatoid arthritis on the neck can be divided into early and late (7).

Early

Rheumatoid arthritis seldom appears as neck ache. The presence of other obvious manifestations of RA, especially in the wrists and hands, makes the recognition of early symptoms of RA in the neck very straightforward.

Early in the disease, the synovitis causes neck ache and stiffness. No significant findings are noted, either in the musculoskeletal confines of the neck or the neurological tissues. Treatment is directed by the rheumatologist and includes use of appropriate analgesic and anti-inflammatory medication, along with intermittent collar support for rest and a strong emphasis on strengthening exercises (4).

Late

Unfortunately, the disease is often relentlessly progressive, especially in the younger patient who has other significant joint involvement and a high RF titer. If it attacks the neck, the erosive synovitis in these patients can affect stability most frequently in the upper cervical spine (C1-C2) or less frequently in the subaxial spine (below C2). The three most common deformities are C1-C2 subluxation, cranial migration of C2, and the subaxial stair-step subluxations.

Upper Cervical Spine

The destructive synovitis of RA can destroy:

1. Soft tissues (ligaments and capsule) of the atlantoaxial joint.
2. Cartilaginous joint surfaces of the atlanto-occipital and the atlantoaxial joints.

The type of deformity that results depends on the pattern of soft tissue and cartilaginous destruction, but can be divided into (3):

a. Anterior atlantoaxial subluxation—most common (10%–40%);
b. Vertical subluxation of the odontoid (5%–25%)—may occur with *a.*;
c. Miscellaneous subluxations such as lateral, posterior, and rotatory—least common.

Anterior Atlantoaxial Subluxation.   Forward instability is defined as a distance of more than 3 mm between the ring of C1 and the anterior aspect of the odontoid on either lateral static or flexion-extension x-rays of the cervical spine (Fig. 8.1).

Surgery to stabilize this subluxation is recommended if the subluxation exceeds 9 mm and/or neurological symptoms of cord compression appear (3). The operation of choice is a C1-C2 posterior fusion (Fig. 8.2). The fusion should be done in situ with only the most mobile subluxations reduced. Because of the subluxation, anesthetic intubation is difficult and usually has to be done nasally. Because of overall disability and attendant medications, such as NSAIDs, steroids, and antimetabolites, the successful fusion rate is low. This low fusion rate is further aggravated by the patient's inability to tolerate postoperative immobilization in halo or cervical collar support. Obviously, this is a frustrating condition for the patient in the late stages of RA and for the surgeon trying to alleviate suffering.

Vertical Subluxation of C2.   More as a result of cartilaginous destruction than ligamentous laxity, the odontoid peg migrates into foramen magnum territory (Fig. 8.3). The cartilaginous destruction affects all of the articulations in the

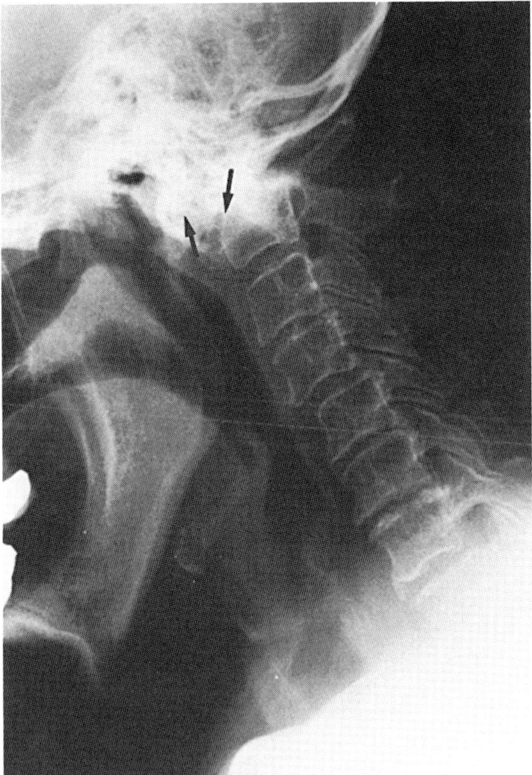

Figure 8.1.   Forward subluxation of C1 on C2 by at least 3 mm. One *arrow* marks the back of C1, the other *arrow* marks the location of an almost nonexistent odontoid (C2).

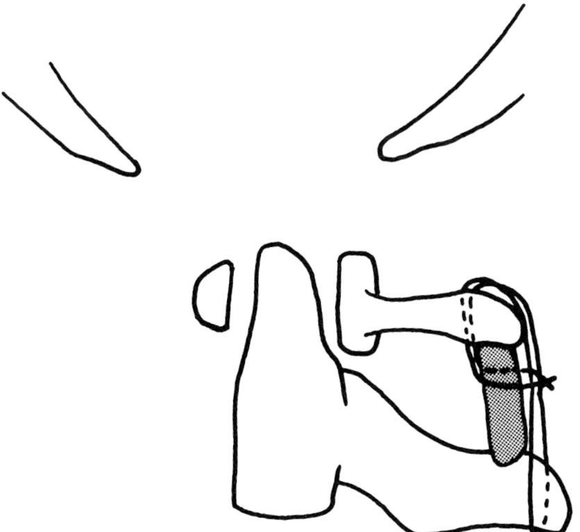

Figure 8.2.   Schematic lateral to show a C1-C2 posterior fusion with wires and bone graft.

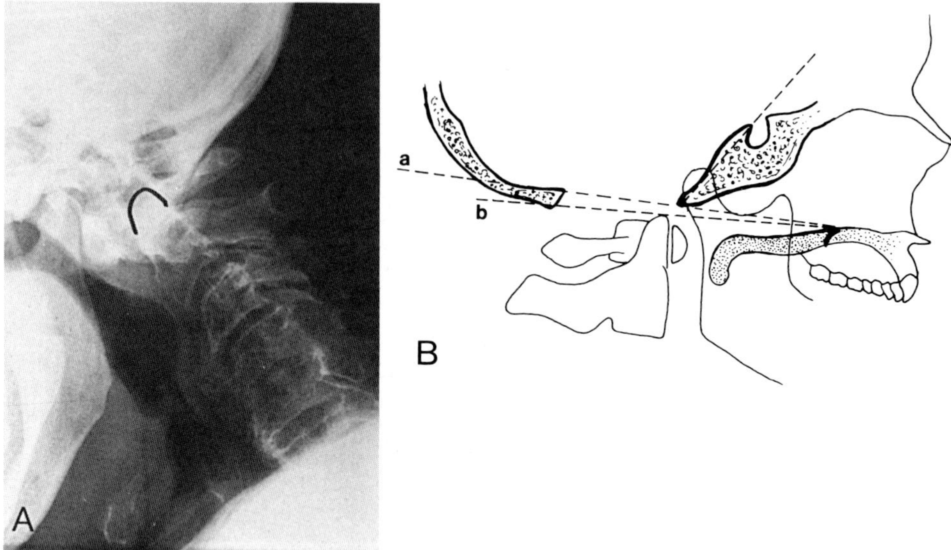

Figure 8.3.   A, vertical subluxation of C2. The dome of the odontoid lies above the foramen magnum. **B,** two lines used to measure upward migration of the odontoid: (*a*) Chamberlain's line, from the posterior margin of the foramen magnum to the posterior margin of the hard palate, and (*b*) McGregor's line, from the posterior margin of the hard palate to the most inferior (caudal) point of the occiput. If the tip of the odontoid is above either of these lines, the odontoid has migrated vertically.

occiput/C1 and C1-C2 junction, allowing for collapse of the area on C2. The skull and C1 sink on C2 and the odontoid, by default, protrudes into the foramen.

Matthews (8) found long tract signs in half the patients with vertical subluxation. Crockard (5) has proposed that these patients undergo transoral excision of the odontoid, followed immediately by posterior occiput-to-C2 wiring and bone graft. Needless to say, the surgery and the postoperative course are difficult, but the morbidity and mortality of untreated myelopathy in conjunction with C1-C2 vertical migration of the odontoid are so great that patients will often choose the surgical option.

Subaxial Subluxations (SAS).   The classic subaxial involvement in the rheumatoid neck is the so-called "stepladder" or "staircase" deformity (Fig. 8.4). Rheumatoid synovitis destroys the facet joints—cartilage and capsule, the joints of Luschka, the disc space (spondylodiscitis), and most importantly, the soft tissue supporting ligaments (especially interspinous). The resulting multilevel instability produces multiple degenerative spondylolisthetic levels and the deformity in Figure 8.4*B*.

Clinically, these patients present a long history of neck pain and stiffness, accompanying all their other RA complaints. Neurological involvement in the form of radicular pain and myelopathy will occur in 20% of these patients (Table 8.1).

Early in the disease, conservative treatment in the form of NSAID, collar support, and neck strengthening exercises will control the symptoms. If neck

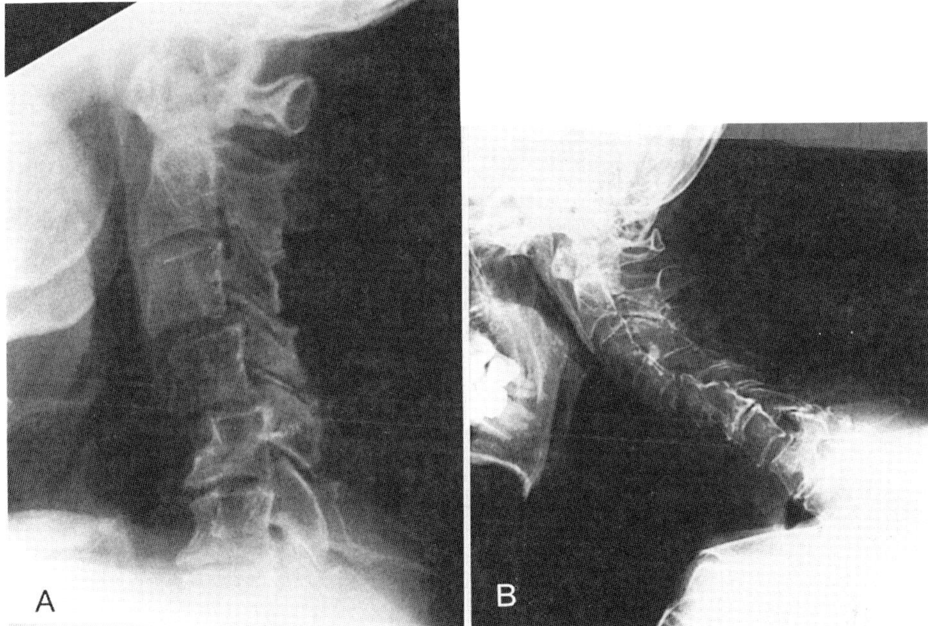

Figure 8.4.   **A,** multiple-level subluxations on a lateral x-ray. The step off from C3-C4 and C4-C5 gives the effect of a stair step. **B,** very late stage of a stair step deformity with one level spontaneously fused.

Table 8.1.   Characteristics of Subaxial Subluxation in RA

1. Occurs in severe RA with articular and nonarticular involvement
2. Usually on significant medical treatment, e.g., steroids, antimetabolites
3. Osteopenic bone (because of criterion 2)
4. Lack of osteophyte formation when compared to DDD (Fig. 8.4)
5. Midcervical involvement (C3–C4 most common) (Fig. 8.5)

pain increases to intolerable levels and/or neurological changes appear, surgery is indicated.

The MRI has revolutionized the assessment of these patients (2). Because of its superior soft tissue depiction, MRI will demonstrate intracanal lesions such as pachymeningitis, arachnoiditis, pannus formation, and extradural nodules, which along with subluxations may compress the cord (Fig. 8.5).

Preoperative halo traction is useful to obtain some degree of reduction. Most spinal surgeons prefer a posterior approach to the rheumatoid SAS (9). Obviously, if myelopathy is part of the problem, a laminectomy and excision of extradural canal pathology are required. All patients require a fusion with some form of internal stabilization (Fig. 8.6). Multilevel involvement and poor graft incorporation have led most surgeons to abandon the anterior approach.

Because of the severity of the associated RA, these patients are difficult surgical management problems with difficult anesthetic intubations, difficult postoperative courses with serious medication requirements, and a high incidence of wound infections and dehiscence. They frequently have fair-to-good, rather than

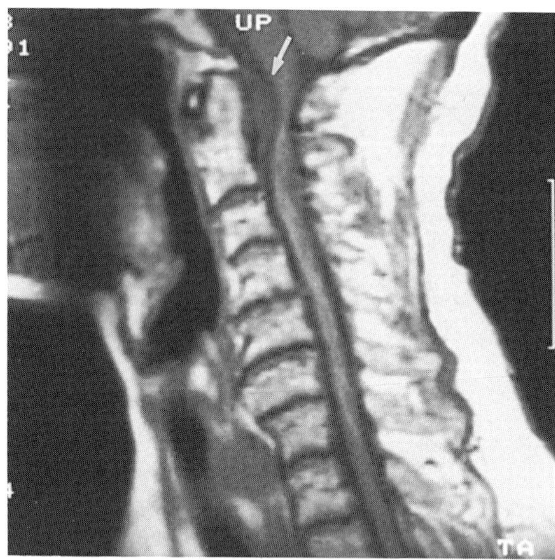

Figure 8.5. Pannus formation behind C2, compressing the cord (*arrow*).

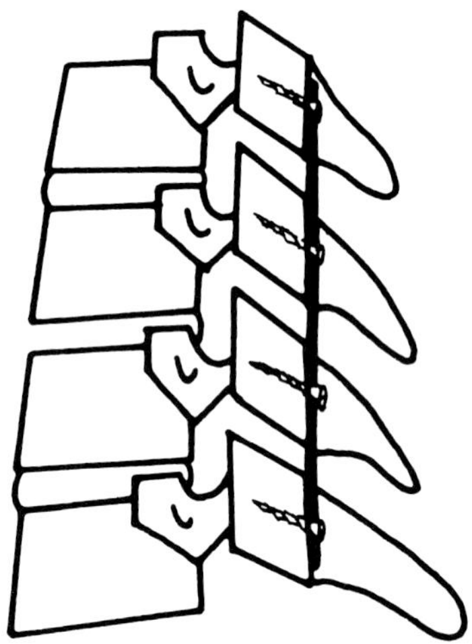

Figure 8.6. A method of posterior plating for RA multilevel stair step deformity. This method of lateral mass screw and plate fixation can be used when a laminectomy decompression has been done.

excellent outcomes and usually have a shortened life span. The management of these problems are not for the faint-of-heart.

Juvenile Rheumatoid Arthritis

It is uncommon for juvenile RA to cause a serious clinical problem in the cervical spine (6). Although facet ankylosis in the higher cervical regions occurs, it is rare that this and other changes in the cervical spine in juvenile RA require surgical intervention.

Table 8.2.   Natural History of Ankylosing Spondylitis[a] (Criteria for Diagnosis)

1. The onset is insidious.
2. There are exacerbations and remissions.
3. Morning stiffness becomes a dominant symptom.
4. Spinal movement limitation and deformity are progressive.
5. If peripheral joints are involved, it happens early.
6. Iritis is early and recurrent.
7. A more severe course has an earlier onset.
8. The course in women is milder than in men.

[a]Adapted from Little H: Editorial: the natural history of ankylosing spondylitis. J Rheum 1988;15:1179–1180.

Ankylosing Spondylitis

The other arthritic condition to be discussed in this chapter is ankylosing spondylitis (Marie-Strumpell's disease). At one time it was regarded as the spinal variant of rheumatoid arthritis; it is now known that they are two distinct diseases.

Epidemiology

With the standardization of criteria for the diagnosis of AS (Table 8.2), better scientific studies of epidemiology have been completed. Initially, it was thought to be a disease predominantly affecting men (male-to female ratio = 10:1), but more recent studies suggest women are affected quite commonly, although with a milder form of the disease. It usually has its insidious onset in 20–35-year-olds and is rare in onset after the age of 40.

The progress of the lesion and its major pathological features are well demonstrated on repeated x-ray examinations. Because the disease does not have a clear clinical presentation, a criteria approach to diagnosis is used (Table 8.2).

Etiology

The cause of AS is unknown except that individuals with the HLA-B27 antigen are predisposed to develop the syndrome. Relatives of people with AS are 20 times more likely to develop the disease and have a much higher incidence of HLA-B27 than the normal population. It is unknown whether the B27 antigen is the primary cause, or whether it acts as a receptor for an infective and/or environmental agent that triggers the disease.

Pathology

AS affects both synovial and fibrous joints with pathological changes in the form of chronic synovitis. The chronic synovitis is followed by cartilage destruction, erosions, sclerosis of underlying bone, and, finally, fibrosis and ankylosis of the affected joints. The sacroiliac joints are involved 100% of the time (Fig. 8.7); the intervertebral discs, symphysis pubis, and manubriosternal joints are frequently involved. Two categories of extra-articular involvement are characteristic:

1. Inflammatory lesions of articular capsule and ligament insertion into bone occur.

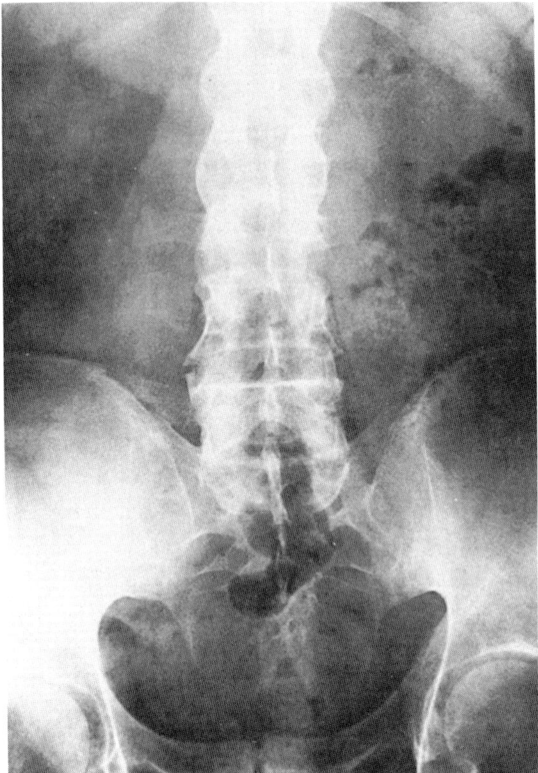

Figure 8.7.   Involvement of the SI joints (late). Also notice the bamboo rod-like spine above.

2. Extraskeletal lesions may occur in the eye (uveitis), aortic root, and pulmonary tree.

Clinical Features

The usual presentation is a young man who reports the insidious onset of grumbling low back pain. Characteristically, there are remissions and exacerbations over the months. The pain may refer to the buttocks and upper thigh and may even be unilateral, leading to ready confusion with the diagnosis of a ruptured disc. But in the absence of neurological symptoms and in the presence of good straight leg raising in AS, the diagnosis of a disc rupture should be immediately suspect. Eventually, the lumbosacral area becomes stiff, especially in the morning, with a hot shower and/or the morning's activity alleviating this complaint. Eventually, the pain and stiffness affect the entire spine, causing clinically detectable range-of-movement loss. The condition spreads to the peripheral skeleton and most often affects the shoulders and hips. Other symptoms are listed in Table 8.3.

Physical Findings

Early in the disease, there is little to find on clinical examination, often leading to delay in diagnosis. Probably the two most commonly mistaken diagnoses are to label the patient "fibrositis" or to mistake unilateral sacroiliac pain for a

Table 8.3.   Less Common Symptoms in AS

1. Constitutional symptoms, such as fatigue and weight loss
2. Chest pains from costosternal involvement
3. Eye symptoms (uveitis)
4. Extra-articular bony tenderness (enthesopathy)

disc rupture. To the careful examiner, there will be detectable loss of lumbar motion in all three planes: flexion, extension, and lateral flexion. This is in contrast to a patient with a herniated nucleus pulposus (HNP), who usually has limited flexion, good backward extension, and limitation of lateral flexion more pronounced on one side than the other (determined by the location of the disc fragment on the nerve root). In AS, there may be pain on direct pressure on the sacroiliac joint, and various tests that stress the sacroiliac joint may increase the pain.

As the disease progresses, there is loss of lumbar lordosis and a decrease in ability to expand the rib cage. Contrary to other reports, these two changes occur early in the natural history of the disease. The loss of chest cage mobility occurs because of involvement of the posterior costovertebral and costotransverse articulations, and the anterior costochondral junctions. The normal chest expansion (measured at the level of the fourth rib) is reduced from over 5 cm to under 2 cm.

The final stage of advancement in the disease is ankylosis of the spine (Fig. 8.8), and if this occurs in a poorly supervised or poorly motivated patient, severe flexion deformities of the spine may occur.

Early in the disease, the enthesopathy may present a tenderness over bony prominences of the ischial tuberosity, greater trochanter, calcaneum, spinous processes, and other bony prominences.

The course of AS is unpredictable. Women tend to have a less severe form of involvement, as do men with later onset. The most severely involved tend to be younger men, but the variability in progression is striking. With proper supervision and an exercise regime, even the most severely affected can maintain long-term, gainful employment.

Aside from severe extraskeletal involvement of the aorta and pulmonary tree (fortunately rare), the most limiting symptoms come from ankylosis of the hips, a spondylodiscitis causing severe back pain, or an atlantoaxial subluxation causing severe neck pain. The ankylosed patient is very susceptible to minor accidents causing fractures of the spine.

Laboratory Tests in AS

Ninety percent of symptomatic patients are positive for the antigen HLA-B27. The incidence of HLA-B27 in the normal Caucasian population is about 8%. Most patients will have some elevation in the sedimentation rate, although it is rarely dramatic.

Radiographic Findings

The diagnosis of AS is made on x-ray. The characteristic involvement of the sacroiliac joints in the presence of the criteria in Table 8.2 confirm the diagnosis.

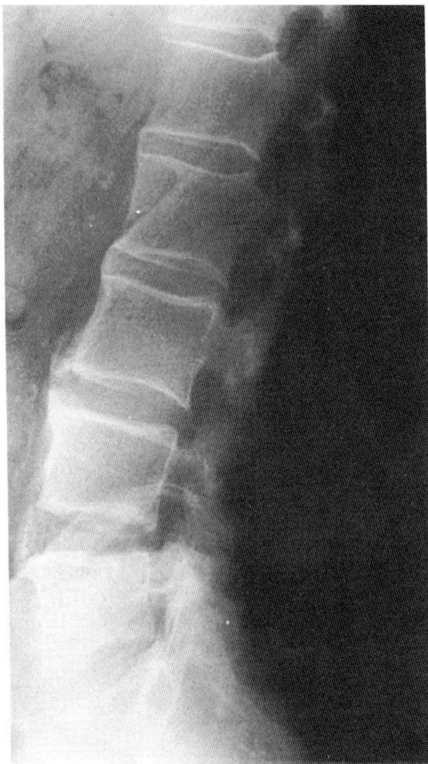

Figure 8.8.   The bamboo spine, with syndesmophytes bridging each segment.

Stages of Changes in the Sacroiliac (SI) Joints.   The x-ray involvement is usually symmetrical in spite of lateralization of symptoms:

Early (Fig. 8.9)
- Blurring of the joint margins
- Erosions and sclerosis of bone

Both of these changes may occur throughout the SI joint but are seen earliest in the lower two-thirds (the synovial portion) of the SI joint. The erosions eventually leave the appearance of widening (pseudowidening) of the SI joints.

Late (Fig. 8.7)
- With progression, calcification and interosseous bridging of the sacroiliac joints occur.

The early radiological changes must be distinguished from osteitis condensans ilii. In this lesion, almost invariably found in multiparous women, there is a wedge-shaped area of sclerosis confined to the iliac side of the joint (Fig. 8.10). It should be noted that there is no evidence that osteitis condensans ilii is ever a source of low back pain.

Development of Syndesmophytes.   Initially, there is inflammation of the annulus fibrosus and the corners of the vertebral bodies. With subsequent erosion of the corners of the vertebral bodies, the anterior aspect of the vertebral body

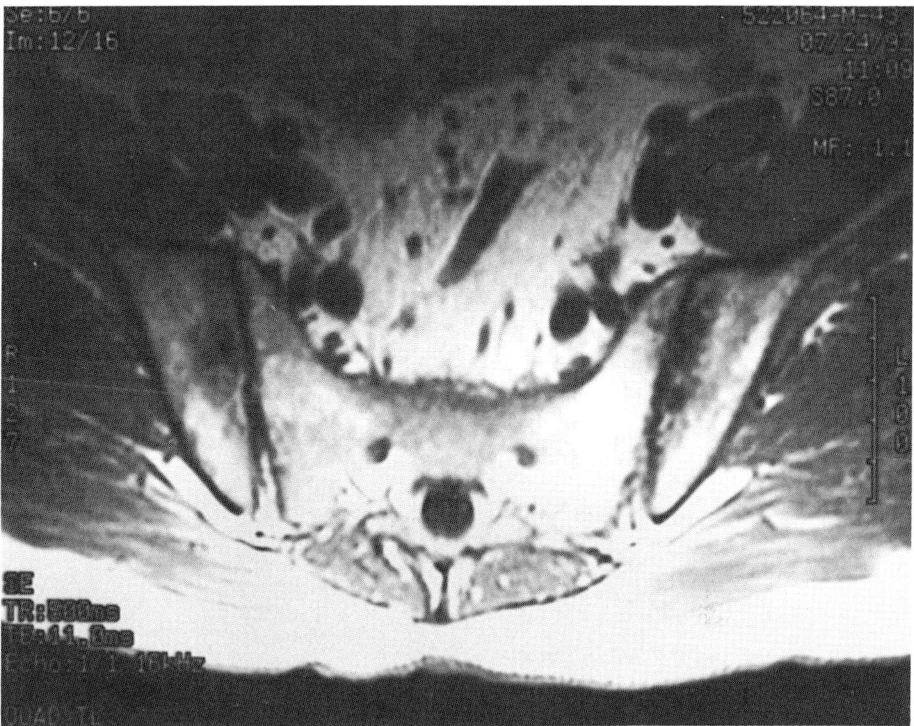

Figure 8.9.   MRI of the SI joints early in the disease. The erosive changes are more obvious on the left.

appears squared (Fig. 8.11). This is soon followed by ossification of the annulus fibrosus, bridging the disc space (syndesmophytes). The ultimate fate is ossification of all ligaments to the spine and complete fusion of the vertebral column (bamboo spine) (Fig. 8.8).

Other Skeletal X-ray Changes.   Characteristic changes may occur in the manubriosternal joint and symphysis pubis (Fig. 8.12). Bony erosions and whiskering at sites of osseous-tendon attachments may be seen on x-ray (Fig. 8.13).

Diagnostic Choices Early in the Disease

The clinician seeing many patients with spinal pain is usually very sensitive to the diagnosis of AS. When AS is suspected clinically, but not supported by plain films of the sacroiliac joints, what x-rays should be done? It has been suggested that the following x-ray studies are useful: special views of the SI joints, bone scans of the SI joints, and CT scans of the SI joints.

The yield of useful information with these tests is so low that, when balanced against the financial cost of routine use, it is probably not worth doing the tests. Provided other disease entities have been ruled out, the most reasonable choice is to treat the patient as a suspected AS and repeat the plain x-rays in a number of months, rather than chase the diagnosis with expensive tests.

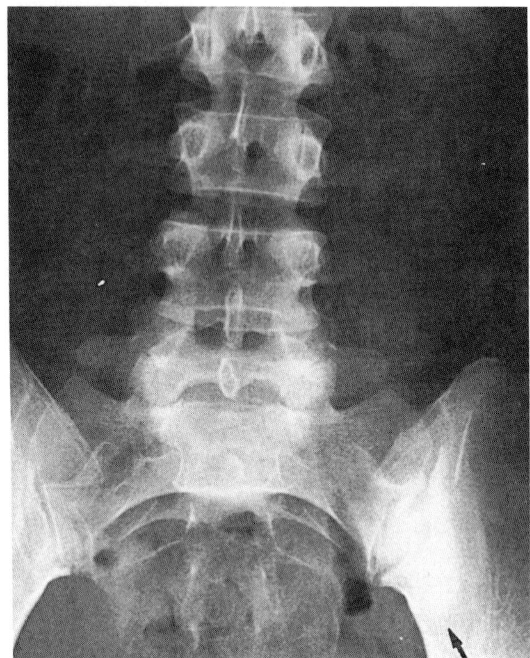

Figure 8.10.   Osteitis condensans ilii (*arrow*).

Treatment of AS

No specific treatment of a curative nature presently exists. The role of the physician is diagnostic awareness of the disease, amelioration of symptoms with carefully controlled use of anti-inflammatory medications, patient education, attention to the possibility of spinal deformities, and management of peripheral joint arthropathies.

It is essential for the patient to understand the natural history of the disease so that he or she sees the need for reasonable rest and a continuing program of postural education and exercises. The exercise program is designed to maintain a straight spine or to attempt to increase lumbar lordosis. Every attempt must be made to maintain the already reduced respiratory excursion.

Occasionally, despite anti-inflammatory medication and excellent continued physical therapy, the spinal deformities progress relentlessly and inexorably to a stage where the patient can only see a few feet ahead when standing (Fig. 8.14). The patient may also have difficulty sitting and eating. In such instances, surgical correction of the deformities must be considered. Operative correction is undertaken at the site of the maximal deformity, taking into full account the serious surgical hazards of respiratory problems and the danger of producing irreversible neurological damage.

Ankylosing Spondylitis Affecting the Cervical Spine

Affliction of the cervical spine occurs late in the disease as the ankylosis and stiffness ascend the spine after starting in the lumbar region (Fig. 8.15). By the

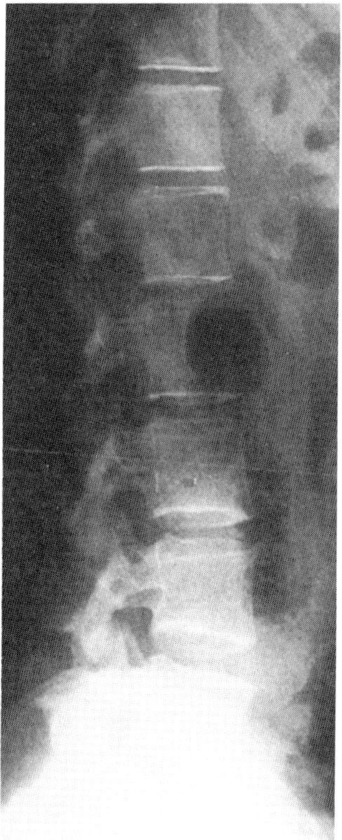

Figure 8.11.   Squaring of the corners of the vertebral bodies, which is most obvious at the thoraco-lumbar junction.

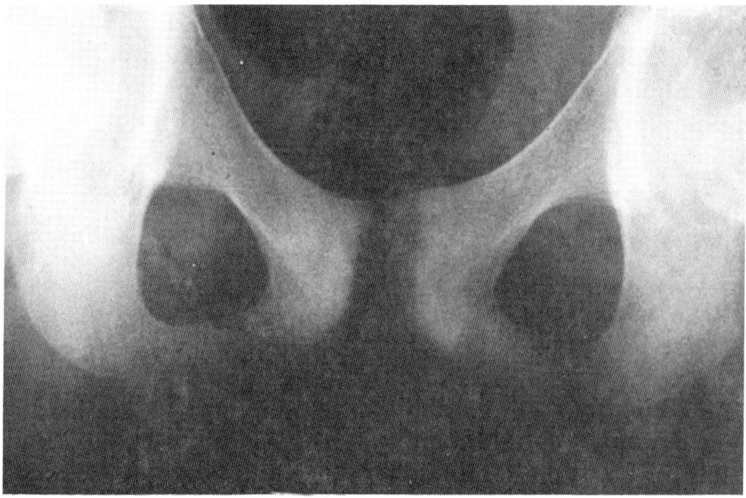

Figure 8.12.   Blurring of the margins of the symphysis pubis.

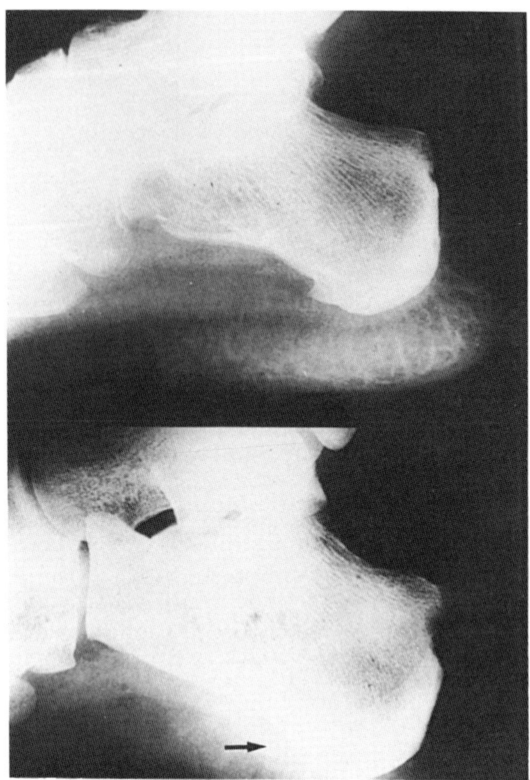

Figure 8.13.   Whiskering at the edges of the os calcis *(top*, early; *bottom*, late).

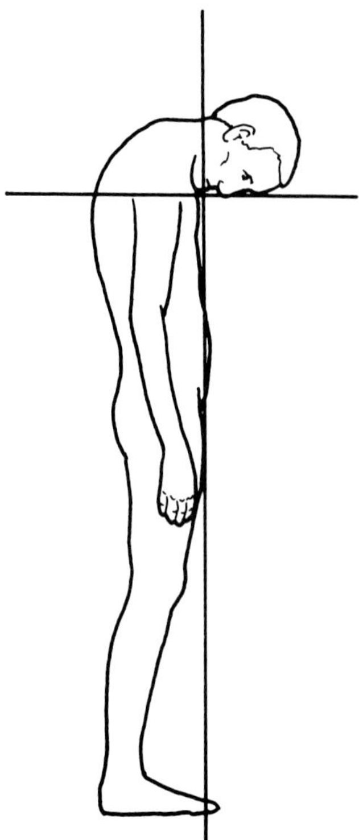

Figure 8.14.   A severe cervical flexion deformity in AS.

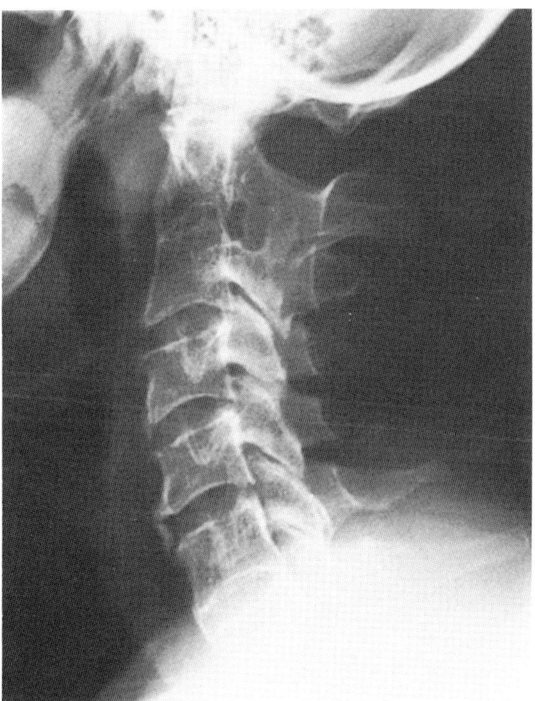

Figure 8.15.   AS ascending the cervical spine. Note the syndesmophyte bridging C5-C6 and early syndesmophytes forming at C4-C5 and C3-C4.

time significant cervical spine involvement occurs, the diagnosis is well established.

Three problems occurring in the cervical spine are (10):

1. Occult fractures
2. C1-C2 subluxation
3. Flexion deformities

Occult Fractures.   As the disease progresses, the neck becomes not only ankylosed but osteopenic. This combination renders the neck very vulnerable to serious injuries, such as falls and MVAs. Often, the result is a fracture. The minor trauma will be a trap for the unsuspecting examiner. Most of these fractures occur at the C6-T2 area, which may not be readily seen on routine emergency-room x-rays (Fig. 8.16). This results in a high incidence of missed diagnoses. Live by the following rule: In spite of apparent minor trauma, the sudden increase in neck pain in ankylosing spondylitis, no matter how trivial the injury, is a fractured cervical spine until proven otherwise. Sometimes polytomograms or CT are necessary to establish the diagnosis. The problem with CT axials is that the cuts may be through the fracture, so CT may miss the axial lesion.

If a fracture occurs, immediate halo vest, without attempts at pre-existing deformity correction, is the treatment of choice. If the fracture is missed at injury, the patient will probably experience increasing flexion deformity and neu-

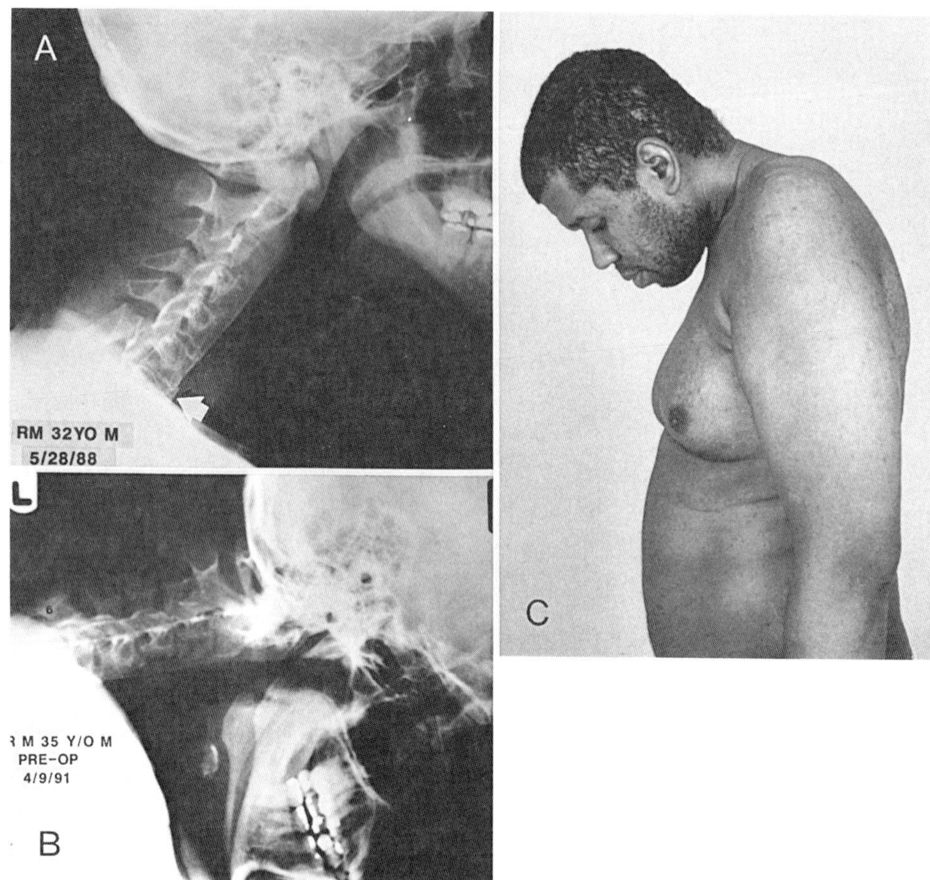

Figure 8.16.   Hidden fracture at the C7-T1 junction in AS with *arrow* showing fracture (**A**). One year after missed fracture, the patient is subluxated at C7-T1 (**B**). The patient's appearance one year later is shown in (**C**) (Courtesy Ed Simmons, Sr., Buffalo NY.).

rological complications, necessitating more significant surgical treatment intervention (10) (Fig. 8.17).

C1-C2 Subluxations.   This cannot be overemphasized: trivial trauma followed by neck pain in a patient with an ankylosed spine is a fracture (or dislocation) until proven otherwise. The top end of the cervical spine is not immune to these injuries—usually they occur in the form of a fractured odontoid or disrupted transverse ligament.

Ankylosis of the spine often spares the C1-C2 junction, but the rigid spine from C3 down leaves the C1-C2 area vulnerable to trauma. If a fracture and/or dislocation occurs at this level in an ankylosed spine, the patient requires urgent halo vest immobilization in the hope that healing may occur and preservation of motion will follow. Unfortunately, there is a high incidence of nonunion in these fractures, necessitating a C1-C2 or occiput-to-C2 fusion that removes the last vestige of movement in the neck of a patient with advanced ankylosing spondylitis.

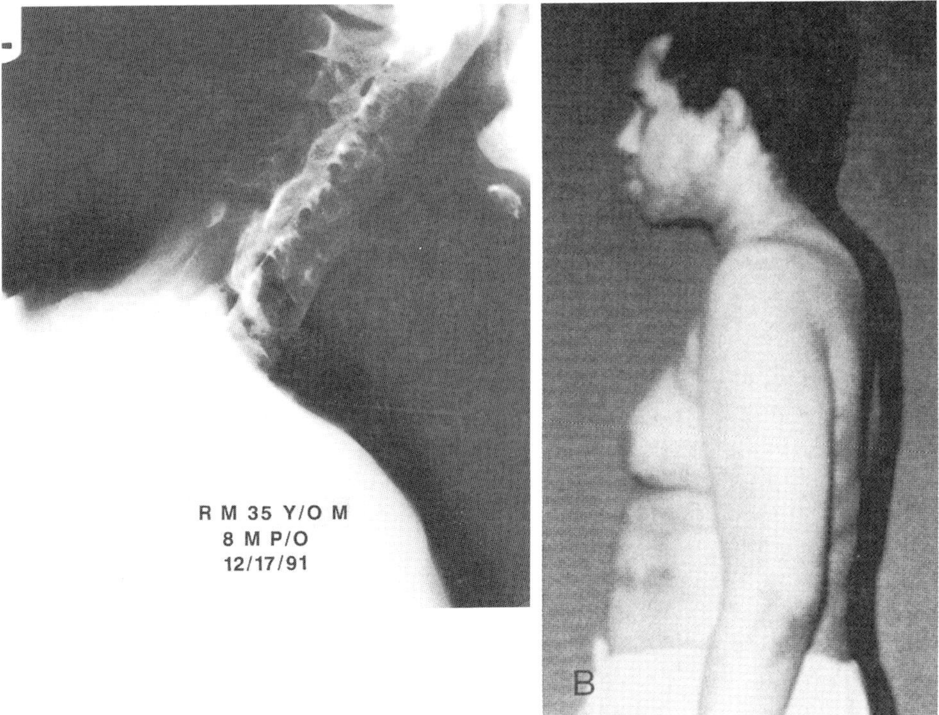

Figure 8.17.   A follow-up to Figure 8.16. Three years later, a posterior closing wedge osteotomy has been done at C7-T1. Note the fusion mass posteriorly from C6-T1. (Courtesy of Ed Simmons, Sr., Buffalo, NY.)

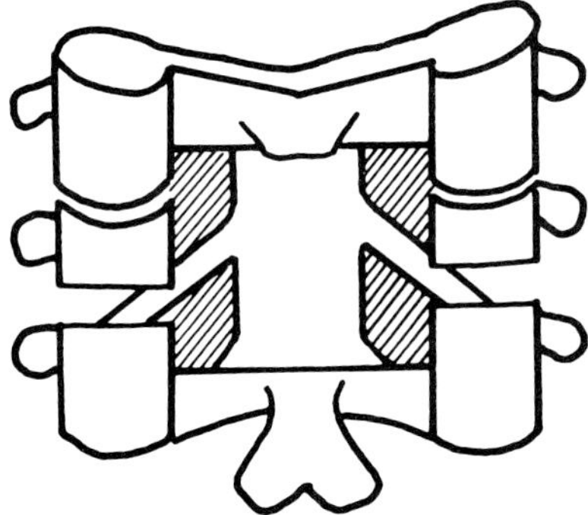

Figure 8.18.   A Simmons closing-wedge osteotomy done at C7-T1. This is almost always below the vertebral artery entrance into the cervical spine. The bone has been removed from the lower portion of C6 and the upper portion of T1. All the lamina and spine of C7 have been removed, and there has been a wide decompression of the C8 nerve root canal.

Flexion Deformities

The final neck problem to discuss is severe flexion deformities that occur in the ankylosed spine (Fig. 8.14). Although most flexion deformities occur in the

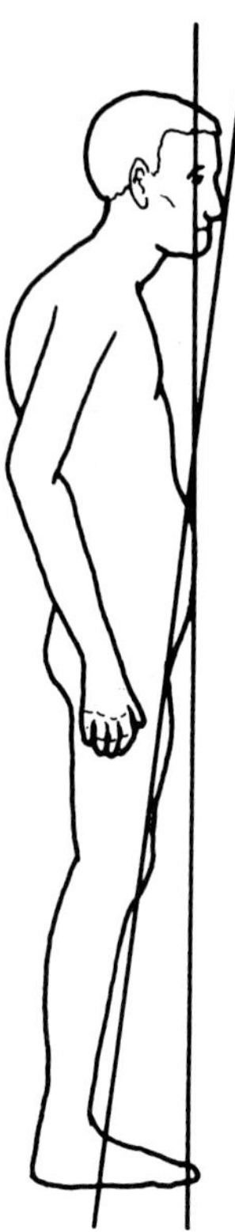

Figure 8.19. The patient drawn in Figure 8.14 has been surgically corrected with the Simmons technique.

hips and lumbar spine, occasionally a patient presents a cervical spine ankylosed in a severely flexed position. If the patient is relatively healthy, motivated to look straight ahead instead of at the ground, and prepared to accept the rigors of postoperative care, Simmons (10) has described a C7-T1 posterior closing-wedge osteotomy under local anesthesia that will correct some of the deformity (Figs. 8.17, 8.18, and 8.19).

Summary

Rheumatoid arthritis and ankylosing spondylitis fortunately are rare, but when afflictions of the cervical spine occur, one or the other is the probable cause. These are relentlessly progressive diseases that, in most patients, eventually affect the cervical spine. In the final phase of the natural history of the disease, the potential for severe debility is great.

REFERENCES

1. Bennet PH and Burch TA: New York symposium on population studies in the rheumatic diseases: new diagnostic criteria. Bull Rheum Dis 17:453–458 (1967).
2. Breedveld FC, Algra PR, Vielvoye CJ, and Cats A: Magnetic resonance imaging in the evaluation of patients with rheumatoid arthritis and subluxations of the cervical spine. Arthritis Rheum 30:624–629 (1987).

3. Clark CR, Goetz DD, and Menzes AH: Arthrodesis of the cervical spine in rheumatoid arthritis. J Bone Joint Surg 71A:381–392 (1989).

4. Conlon PW, Isdale IC, and Rose BS: Rheumatoid arthritis of the cervical spine: an analysis of 333 cases. Ann Rheum Dis 25:120–126 (1966).

5. Crockard HA, Pozo JL, Ransford AO, Kendall BE, and Essigman WK: Transoral decompression and posterior fusion for rheumatoid atlanto-axial subluxation. J Bone Joint Surg 68B:350–356 (1986).

6. Fried JA, Athreya B, Gregg JR, Das M, and Doughty R: The cervical spine in juvenile rheumatoid arthritis. Clin Orthop 179:102–106 (1983).

7. Lipson SJ: Rheumatoid arthritis in the cervical spine. Clin Orthop 239:121–127 (1989).

8. Matthews JA: Atlanto-axial subluxation in rheumatoid arthritis. Ann Rheum Dis 28:260–266 (1969).

9. Santavirta S, Konttinen YT, Sandelin J, and Slatis P: Operations for the unstable cervical spine in rheumatoid arthritis (sixteen cases of subaxial subluxation). Acta Orthop Scand 61:106–110 (1990).

10. Simmons EH: The surgical correction of flexion deformity of the cervical spine in ankylosing spondylitis. In: The Cervical Spine, The Cervical Spine Research Society, pp 573–598. JB Lippincott, Philadelphia (1989).

9

Tumors and Infections of the Cervical Spine

"As it takes two to make a quarrel, so it takes two to make a disease, the microbe and its host."
—Charles V. Chapin

INTRODUCTION

Tumors of the cervical spine region are rare. They can be broadly classified into four groups (in the order in which they occur):

1. Metastatic disease
2. Benign tumors of bone
3. Primary malignant tumors of bone
4. Cervical cord tumors

Metastatic Disease

The spine is the most common sight for secondary (metastatic) tumor deposits, but they are more likely to occur in the thoracic and lumbar regions. Although only 10% of spinal metastases occur in the cervical spine, they still represent the most common tumor in the region. Primary sources are breast, lung, and prostate, and occasionally thyroid and nasopharynx because of their close proximity (11).

Stages of Involvement

Patients exhibit various stages (2, 26) of metastatic involvement, from early to advanced disease:

Stage 1—asymptomatic bone lesion detected on plain x-ray or, more likely, on bone scan.

Stage 2—symptomatic, where the usual symptom is pain that increases over time. It is most troublesome at night and is not particularly aggravated by activity. Even at this stage, the plain x-ray may be normal because 30%–50% of trabecular bone has to be destroyed before plain x-ray changes appear (Fig. 9.1) (14).

Stage 3—vertebral segment instability; occurring because the tumor has destroyed enough bone to allow for collapse (usually producing a kyphos deformity (Fig. 9.2).

Stage 4—neurological compression from tumor ingrowth into nerve root territory and/or spinal cord from the vertebral body. The neurological involvement may be complete or incomplete, root or cord. Stage 4 in isolation is not nearly as common as Stage 5 (Fig. 9.3).

208

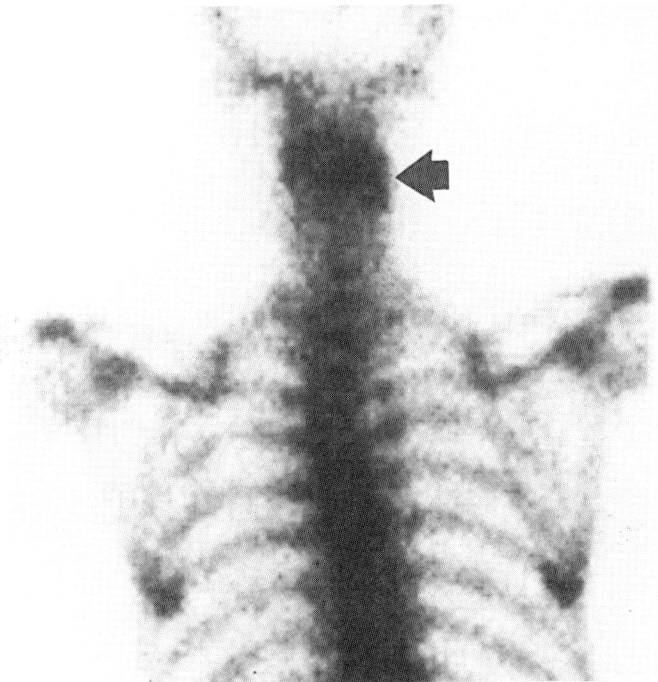

Figure 9.1.   Bone scan (^{99m}Tc) showing multiple hot spots due to metastatic deposits from breast carcinoma.

Stage 5—a combination of instability (vertebral segment collapse) and neurological involvement.

Diagnosis

Most often, the primary tumor location is known and the appearance of a cervical metastatic deposit is merely advancement of the disease process. Occasions will arise when the patient's initial complaint is neck pain; only until the completion of appropriate investigation is the diagnosis of metastatic malignancy made (13).

Steps in Diagnosis.   Plain x-rays are always the first step, but remember, 30%–50% of the trabecular bone has to be lysed before plain x-ray changes are apparent (Fig. 9.4).

Bone scanning with technetium-99 is the most sensitive test (Fig. 9.1) (10, 14, 16). Although it is sometimes difficult to distinguish tumor from infection, fractures, and severe osteoarthritis, the bone scan is the most sensitive investigation to pinpoint lytic or blastic tumors that have osteoblastic activity. The rapid destruction of bone (e.g., multiple myeloma) or osteoblastic activity suppression by chemotherapy will negate the value of the bone scan.

Nonspecific blood tests such as the sedimentation rate and alkaline phosphatase are often elevated. Blood chemistry may also point to the primary source (e.g., an elevated acid phosphatase in prostatic carcinoma).

Magnetic Resonance Imaging (MRI) has replaced CT and CT/myelography as a screening investigation because of the superior depiction of soft tissue involve-

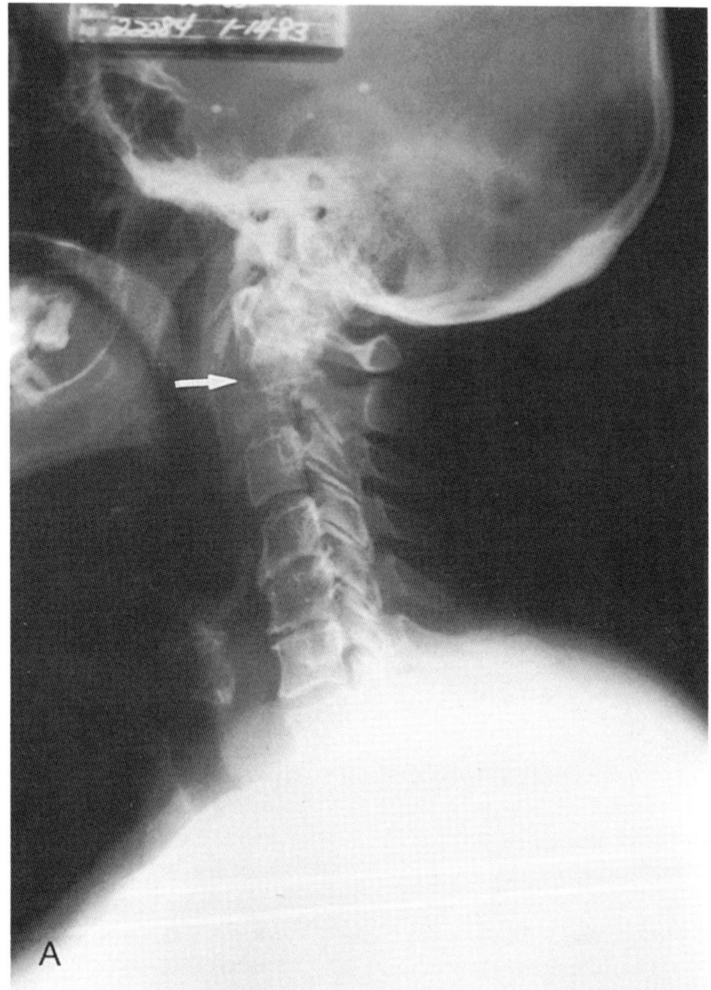

Figure 9.2.   **A,** metastatic carcinoma (C2) with pathological fracture of odontoid (*arrow*) and an extension deformity. Lower in the (subaxial) cervical spine, a pathological fracture will result in a flexion deformity or kyphos (courtesy of Dr. Mark Leeson, Akron General Medical Center).

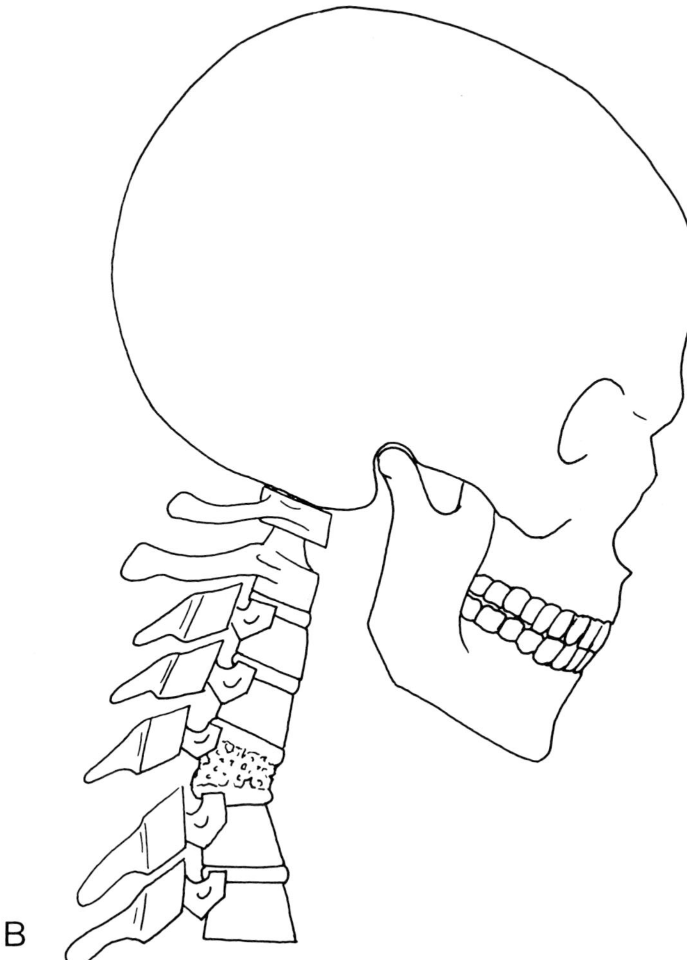

Figure 9.2.   B, schematic of tumor in C5 with the usual kyphotic deformity that results from vertebral body collapse and maintenance of posterior element height.

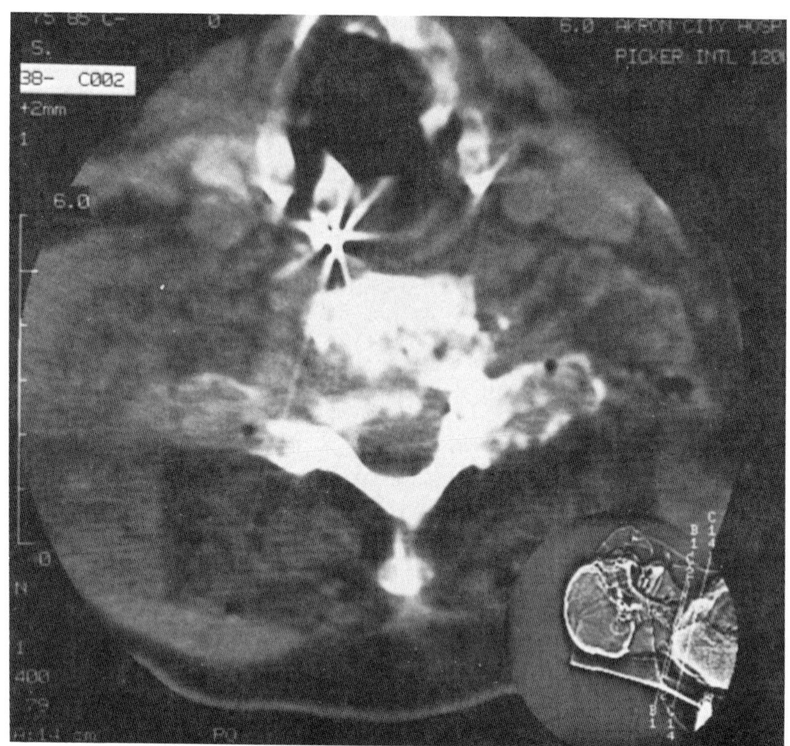

Figure 9.3. Metastatic tumor on CT that is invading spinal canal, especially on right side.

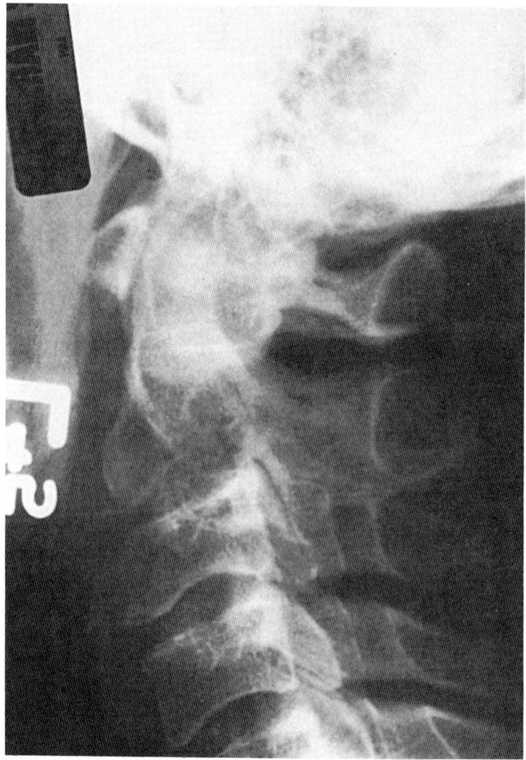

Figure 9.4. Lateral cervical spine x-ray in a patient with a metastatic lesion. Do you see the tumor location? Read on.

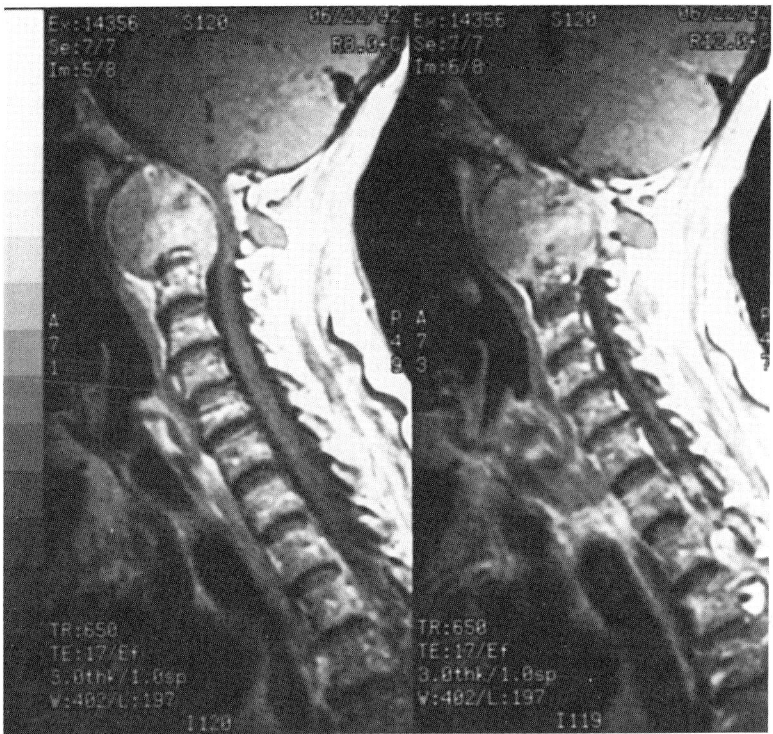

Figure 9.5.   Sagittal T1-weighted MRI showing extensive metastatic lesion replacing C1-C2 level, with soft tissue detail superior to CT (courtesy of Dr. Jim Weinstein, University of Iowa).

ment on sagittal and axial cuts (20) (Fig. 9.5). The use of contrast enhancement with gadolinium does not seem to be routinely useful (32). With a body coil survey, it is possible to localize single or multiple metastatic sites (Fig. 9.6), which may not be seen on myelography. Some patients with neurological involvement become worse after myelography (15), suggesting that the advent of MRI has displaced myelography in studying the extent of neurological involvement. One of the major weaknesses of MRI is the lack of bony detail, making plain CT a valuable surgical planning tool (Fig. 9.7).

Treatment

Treatment of cervical secondary tumors should follow certain principles:

1. Management, because of the complexity of the disease, requires multidisciplinary input from the oncologists, the radiation therapist, and the spine surgeon (3, 30, 33).
2. A tissue diagnosis must be at hand; if it is not obvious from the primary tumor diagnosis, a percutaneous or open biopsy is necessary.
3. Treat the patient first, the disease second. If the patient is medically unstable, with an anticipated short life span, it makes no sense to propose a major surgical procedure. Surgery is only indicated in Stages 3 to 5 in a patient who has a life expectancy of at least three months, is well enough to withstand surgery, and has tissue nutrition that will allow for successful wound healing

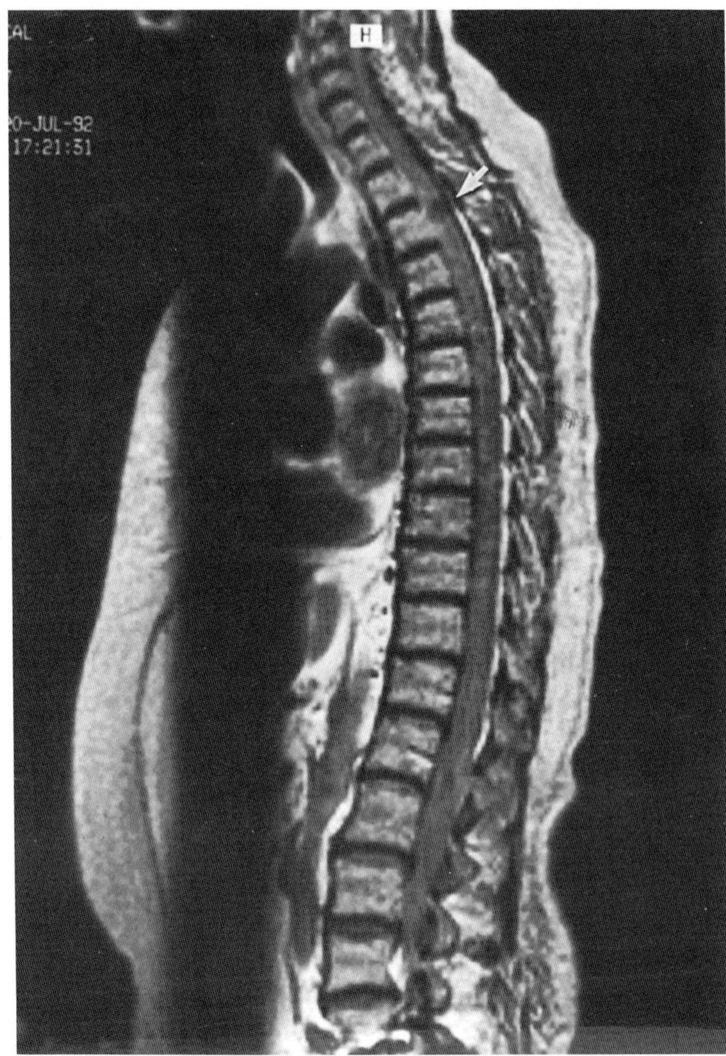

Figure 9.6.   A body coil MRI searching for the cause of a lower cervical or upper thoracic neurological lesion. A meningioma (*arrow*) was located in the C7-T1 region.

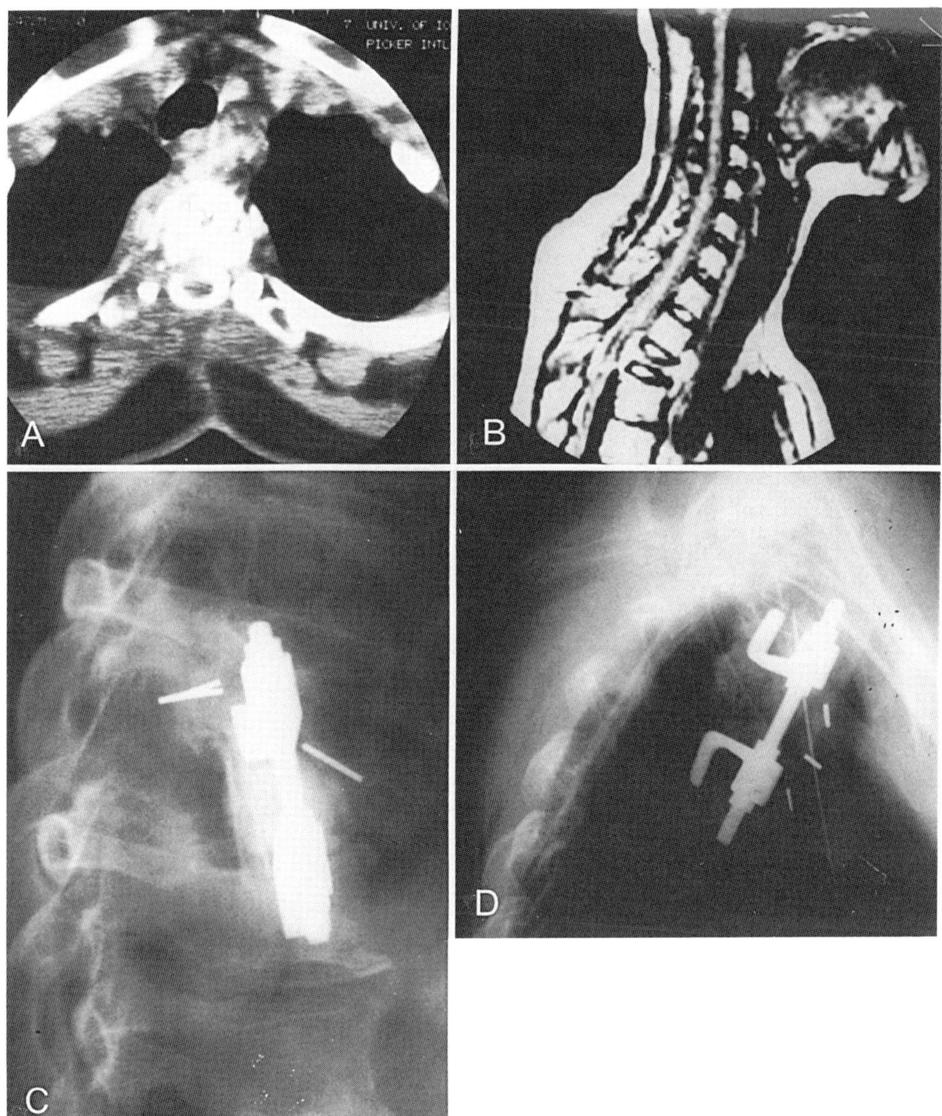

Figure 9.7.   CT (**A**) and MRI (**B**) in a young woman with breast carcinoma metastatic lesion. The combination allowed for a carefully planned anterior surgical procedure (**C**, **D**) (courtesy of Dr. Jim Weinstein, University of Iowa).

(Fig. 9.8). Patients with Stage 1 or 2 lesions are best treated by chemotherapy and/or radiation, depending on the nature of the primary tumor.

4. Patients with hormone-dependent tumors (e.g., breast, prostate, and thyroid) have a better prognosis than patients with poorly differentiated histology, or lung and nasopharynx as primary sites. Multiple metastatic deposits are usually a contraindication to aggressive surgical treatment.

5. In treating the disease second, neurological status is the main determinant. Patients with rapid onset of total paralysis will not do well. Patients with slower onset of paresis (more than 7–10 days), which by definition is incomplete, are likely to experience neurological recovery with radiation and/or surgical decompression (3). In the past, neurological compression from tumor was often treated by laminectomy, that is, make the spinal canal bigger to accommodate the cord and the tumor mass. All too often, the laminectomy failed to arrest neurological deterioration and, worse, it made the diseased vertebral column even more unstable. Laminectomy is mentioned only to condemn it as a surgical method of dealing with metastatic epidural neural compression. Surgery is the primary procedure for neurological lesions that appear to be progressing quickly and for radioinsensitive tumors. Today's standard of surgical intervention for cord compression is to approach the mass from the direction of neurological compromise. Since most secondary deposits occur in the anterior spinal elements (the vertebral body and pedicles), most surgical approaches to decompress the cervical cord should be from the front. The use of steroids (dexamethasone is the choice) preoperatively and postoperatively is useful to reduce inflammation and edema of the cord.

6. Radiation plays a key role in the management of radiosensitive tumors. It is used prior to surgery for slowly progressive neurological lesions or for patients with paralysis who need pain control. For patients with a secondary deposit only—and no neurological involvement—radiation without surgery is the treatment of choice.

7. In treating neurological compromise, the team is most often confronted with associated spinal instability that obviously alters a surgical game plan. Still, the neurological compression must be dealt with, followed by surgical stabilization of the skeleton (Fig. 9.9) (3).

Benign Tumors of Bone

Next to metastatic lesions, benign lesions are the most common tumor to be seen in the adult cervical spine (7, 9). Even in the face of this statement, the authors can count on two hands the number of benign lesions of the cervical spine seen in their combined 50 years of practice. For children, almost all primary tumors of the cervical spine will be benign. Finally, almost every tumor located in the posterior elements will be benign (33).

As a general statement, benign tumors are usually nothing to worry about. The neck is an exception for two reasons:

1. The tumor may grow to compress neurological structures.
2. The tumor may be in a location that makes excision difficult (e.g., wrapped around the vertebral artery).

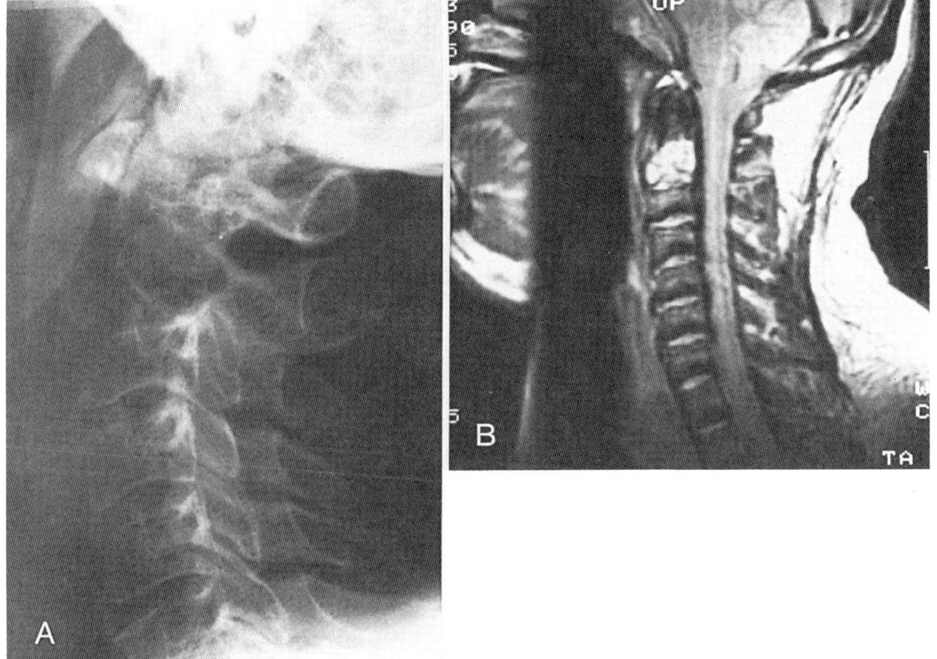

Figure 9.8. **A,** now do you recognize the location of the metastatic deposit from Figure 9.4? **B,** sagittal gradient echo MRI showing the patient is in Stage 3 cervical spine involvement from a renal cell carcinoma. He did well with anterior surgical intervention.

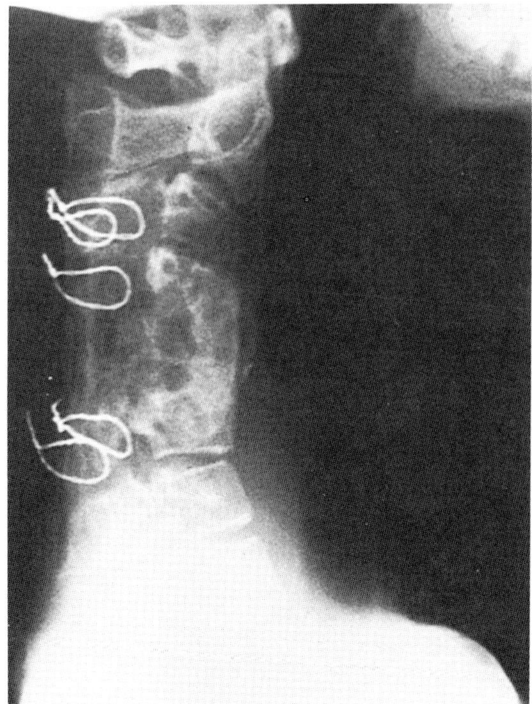

Figure 9.9. Cervical spine lateral x-ray showing an anterior bone graft inserted after excision of C5. A posterior decompression bone grafting and wiring was the first stage of the tumor decompression and excision.

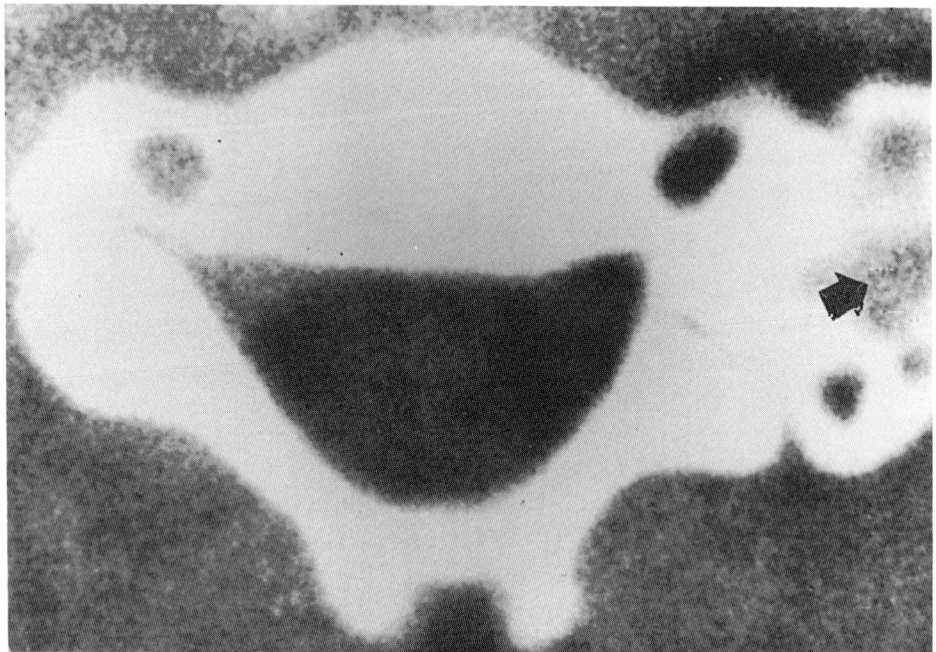

Figure 9.10.   Osteoid osteoma with *arrow* pointing to nidus.

Plain x-rays usually reveal the lesion but CT scanning is usually needed to establish a surgical game plan.

Specific Benign Tumors

Osteoid Osteoma.   This is the classic benign tumor seen in the posterior elements under the age of 30 years (Fig. 9.10). It produces nighttime pain that is relieved by aspirin. On x-ray the tumor appears as a radiolucent nidus with surrounding sclerosis. Treatment is directed at excising the central nidus if technically feasible.

Osteoblastoma.   This is the most common benign tumor in the cervical spine, affecting children and teenagers, and usually located in the posterior elements. The pain is not relieved by aspirin. Plain x-rays usually reveal the lesion (Fig. 9.11*A*). Treatment is directed at excision, and because of the size of the lesion, concomitant bone grafting is usually necessary.

Osteochondroma (Exostosis).   If this tumor is located in the spine, it usually appears in the neck. It is a bony prominence tumor with a cartilage cap that has the potential to cause neurological pressure (Fig. 9.11*B*). If the tumor becomes symptomatic, excise it—otherwise leave it alone.

Hemangioma.   This is a perfectly benign tumor that should be left alone (Fig. 9.12). It is no threat to the patient's well-being and surgical misadventure will lead to a bloody mess.

Aneurysmal Bone Cyst (ABC).   Although nonaggressive, this tumor can land the patient and the surgeon in a tough spot because of its propensity to grow into tough corners in the cervical spine. Fortunately, it is more common in

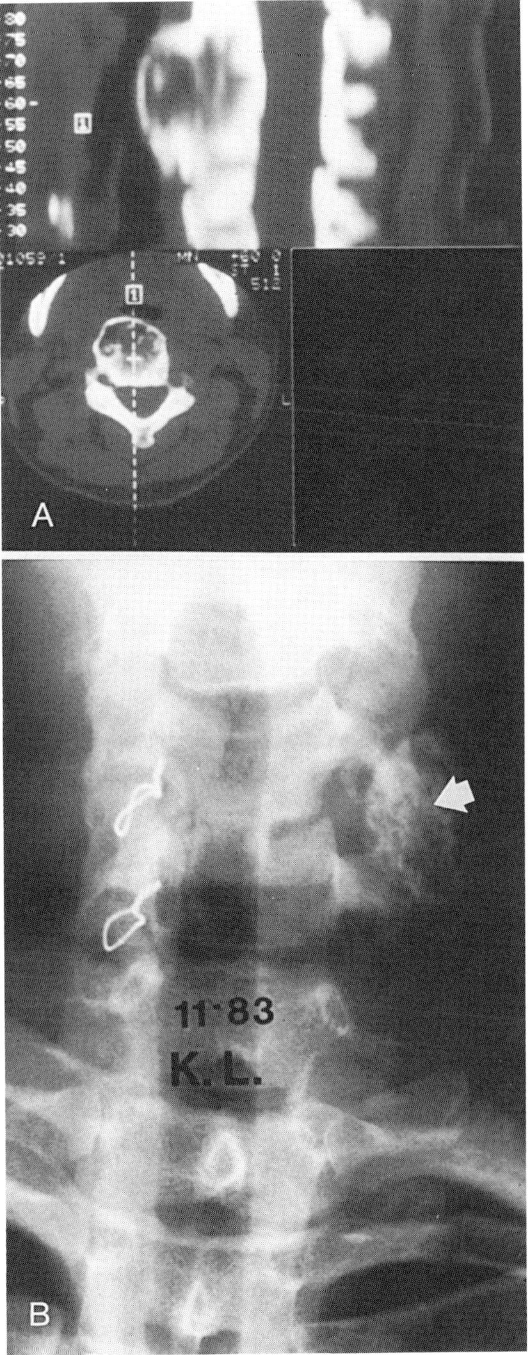

Figure 9.11.   **A,** osteoblastoma C5 on sagittal CT. **B,** osteochondroma (*arrow*). Previous surgery on the opposite side has been done to remove another osteochondroma.

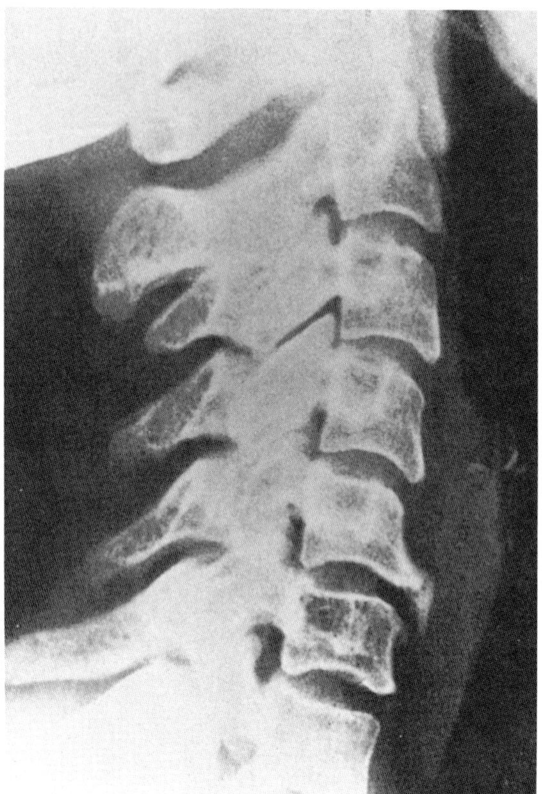

Figure 9.12. Hemangioma in C6.

the lumbar spine. It is an expansive osteolytic lesion that can affect contiguous vertebrae (Fig. 9.13). Treatment is usually by curettage and bone graft.

Giant Cell Tumor. Although giant cell tumor is a relatively common benign tumor of long bones (most common on either side of the knee joint), it is relatively rare in the spine. When it does occur in the spine, it is most common in the sacrum and more prevalent in the female patient. It tends to occur in patients who are older than patients with osteoid osteoma or osteoblastoma. It is rare in the neck (Fig. 9.14).

The clinical presentation is no different from the other benign lesions and includes pain with occasional neurological compromise.

Although the lesion is not commonly malignant, it is certainly more malevolent than benign. From the moment the lytic, expansive lesion with little cortical reaction is seen on plain x-ray, the chase is on to separate it from malignant lesions, with laboratory tests and pathology examination. All laboratory tests will be normal and pathological examination will reveal multiple giant cells. They can be confused with aneurysmal bone cysts, Brown tumor of hyperparathyroidism, and osteoblastoma—as well as osteogenic sarcoma. They can be graded histologically—those lesions that are benign versus those lesions that are more aggressive and malignant. Some would say that grading is not significant because, regardless of grade, if the tumor is not totally excised at initial surgery, it will

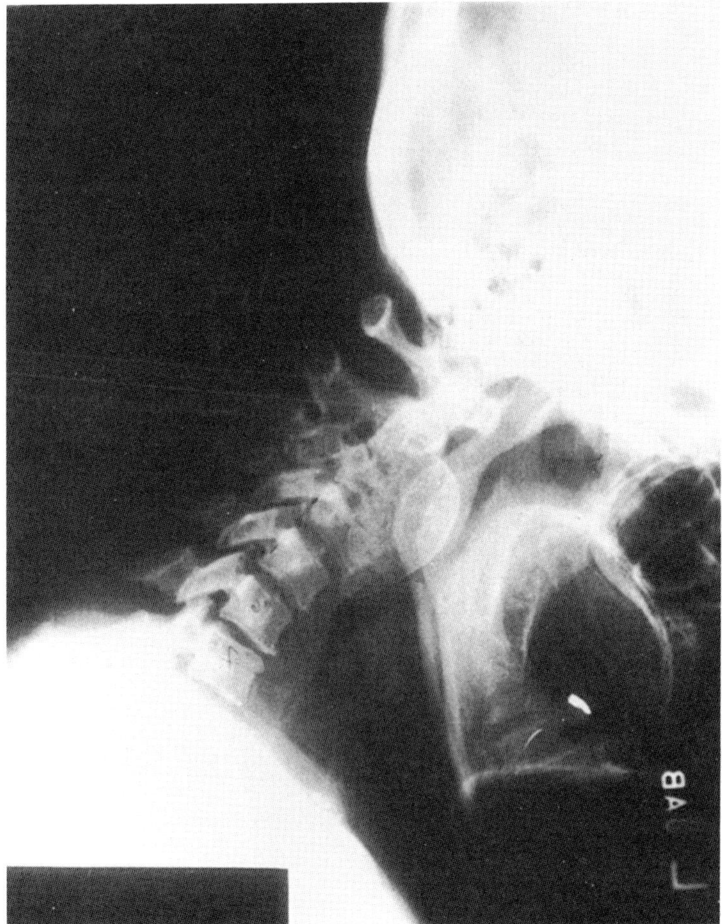

Figure 9.13.   A large ABC extending from C2-C4.

recur and be more aggressive the next time around. Unfortunately, some of the lesions in the cervical spine cannot be totally excised because of size and location. Radiation in these patients has the possibility of increasing the chances of malignant transformation.

Of all benign tumors of the spine, giant cell is the most difficult to treat, and if it is not treated aggressively, it will quickly change its behavior to a more aggressive and, eventually, malignant lesion.

Eosinophilic Granuloma.   This is a proliferative disorder of histiocytes. Vertebral involvement presents early as a lytic lesion and, subsequently, as a variable degree of compression of a vertebral body without evidence of adjacent soft tissue mass. In the extreme form, the vertebra is flattened to a thin disc, the so-called vertebra plana (Fig. 9.15). This spontaneous collapse of the vertebral body in children was first described by Calvé (4). It was thought to be a manifestation of osteochondritis juvenilis and is still referred to as "Calvé's disease." The disease may be part of the complex of histiocytosis X disorders, which include the more sinister forms of multiple histiocytic deposits in Hand-Schüller-Chris-

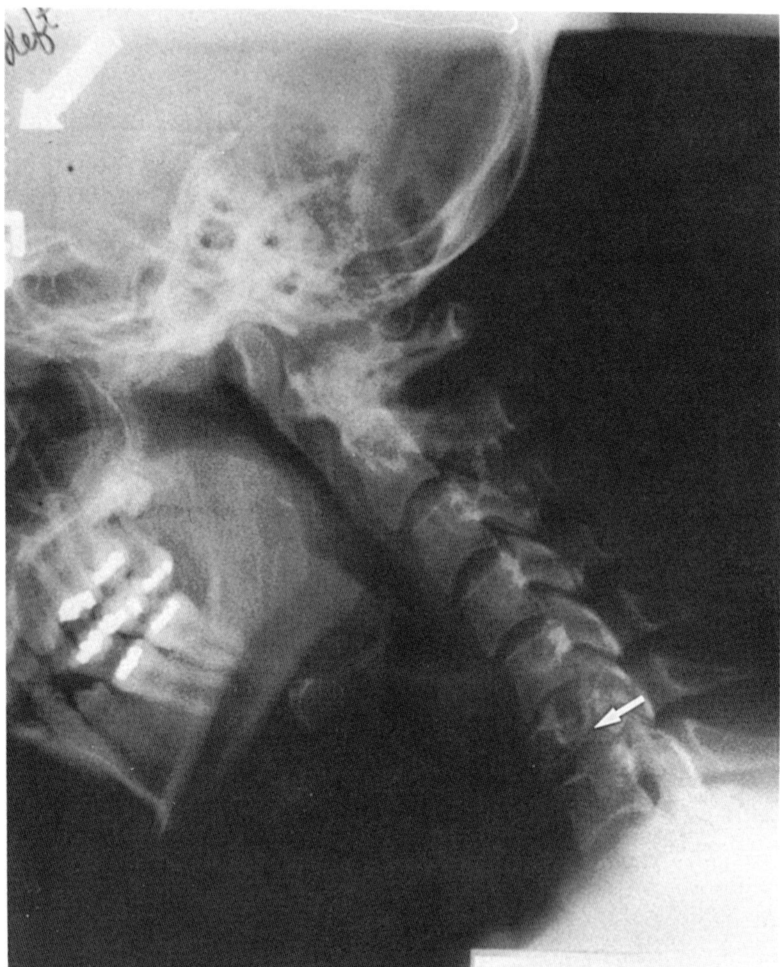

Figure 9.14. Giant cell tumor of C6 (*arrow*) with contiguous involvement of C7.

tian and Letterer-Siwe diseases. As long as the disease remains monostotic, it is the benign form of eosinophilic granuloma. The lesion usually requires a biopsy to distinguish it from Ewing's sarcoma. When biopsied, the eosinophils may be mistaken for neutrophils and the diagnosis of osteomyelitis may be made; likewise, the phagocytic histiocytes may be erroneously confused with Hodgkin's disease.

The prognosis for the solitary lesion is excellent, with no treatment necessary. A word of caution: any secondary deposit may cause wedging of a vertebral body, and this possibility must be carefully considered before making the diagnosis of Calvé's disease.

Primary Malignant Tumors of Bone

Primary malignant tumors of the cervical spine are rare. They largely affect the over-40 population, their incidence increasing with age. The tumors almost invariably involve the body, and occur as neck ache. Neurological manifestations

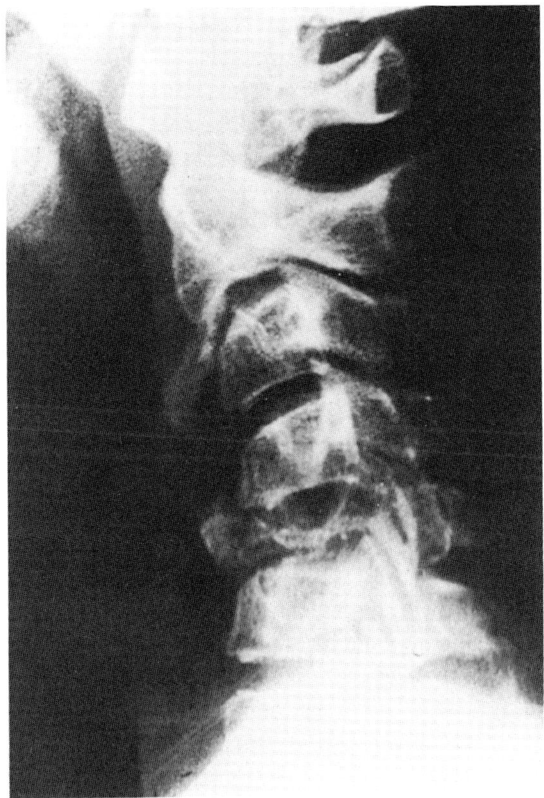

Figure 9.15.   Eosinophilic granuloma of C5, which is a flattened vertebrae (vertebra plana).

may arise, not only because the lesion is expansive but also from vertebral collapse and direct extradural extension. Early in the natural history of the disease, the lesion may not be demonstrated on x-ray. Remember again that 30% of the osseous mass of a bone must be destroyed before a lesion is radiologically evident. In autopsy specimens, only 15% of grossly affected vertebrae demonstrated recognizable lesions when the excised spines were x-rayed. When routine x-rays fail to demonstrate any abnormality, a bone scan can be of value in defining the presence of the lesion and the extent of spinal involvement. CT and MR imaging are more sensitive and detect these lesions before plain x-ray changes become evident.

Chordoma

This is a slowly developing, locally invasive and destructive tumor originating from remnants of notochordal tissue, with a distinct predilection for the midline position at either end of the spinal column.

It is uncommon before the age of 30 and is found mostly in men. Interestingly enough, although the tumor is locally aggressive with a 10% incidence of metastases, the symptoms are frequently of long duration. They are most common in the low back and present as persistent pain. Characteristically, as with all tumors of the spinal column, the pain is not relieved by recumbency. As the tumor encroaches on the cervical foramina and cord, neuropathies and long tract symptoms appear. Neurological involvement is usually later in the natural history of the tumor.

X-rays reveal a large lytic lesion of the neck with a large soft tissue mass almost indistinguishable from the x-ray appearance of a giant cell tumor. However, a chordoma is much more commonly seen in men, whereas giant cell tumors occur with greater frequency in women. A chordoma is not seen until well beyond the third decade, whereas giant cell tumors are more frequently encountered before the age of 30. A giant cell tumor usually progresses more rapidly than a chordoma, and unlike a chordoma, may be situated away from the midline.

Therapeutically, both lesions present problems. Total excision is the goal of any surgery, which is often an impossibility in the cervical spine. In addition, chordomas are very resistant to chemotherapy and radiation.

Myeloma

This is the most common primary malignant tumor of the spine. It is a malignant tumor of plasma cells that produce immunoglobulins and antibodies. The disseminated form of myeloma is uncommon before the age of 50 and is more often seen in men. Clinically, neck ache, weakness, weight loss, and other constitutional symptoms occur in nearly every patient with the generalized disease. The onset of pain may be sudden and is usually produced by the occurrence of a pathological fracture. The tumor is more common in the thoracic and lumbar spine but does occur in the cervical spine.

The sedimentation rate is consistently elevated and is usually greater than 50. Laboratory investigations may reveal hypercalcemia, hyperuricemia, and an elevation in the alkaline phosphatase. Characteristically, the disease is associated with abnormal proteins, best demonstrated on serum protein electrophoresis (Fig. 9.16). Bence Jones proteinuria may be demonstrated in about 50% of the cases. Generally, when the globulins are normal, the albumin is normal. The albumin decreases when the globulins are elevated, reflecting damage to the renal tubules.

On x-ray the solitary lesions are purely lytic and do not show any attempt at regeneration of bone, a fact that renders bone scans negative in a high percentage of cases (Fig. 9.17). The disseminated form frequently shows nothing more than a diffuse osteopenia with or without vertebral body crush. Bone marrow and lesion biopsy will reveal many plasma cells.

Treatment of solitary plasmacytoma lesions is predicated on preservation of spinal stability and cord function. In the absence of gross spinal instability, management with radiation and chemotherapy is probably the best mode of treatment. Spinal instability may require excision of the lesion and bypass grafting.

Cord impairment makes decompression mandatory. Depending on the number of segments affected and the type of encroachment on the cord, decompression may have to be performed either anteriorly or posteriorly, or both. Because the neurological encroachment is coming from an anterior direction, the anterior approach to decompression, if feasible, is preferred. This may seem excessive surgery for a malignant lesion, but it should be remembered that solitary lesions have a 5-year survival rate of about 60%.

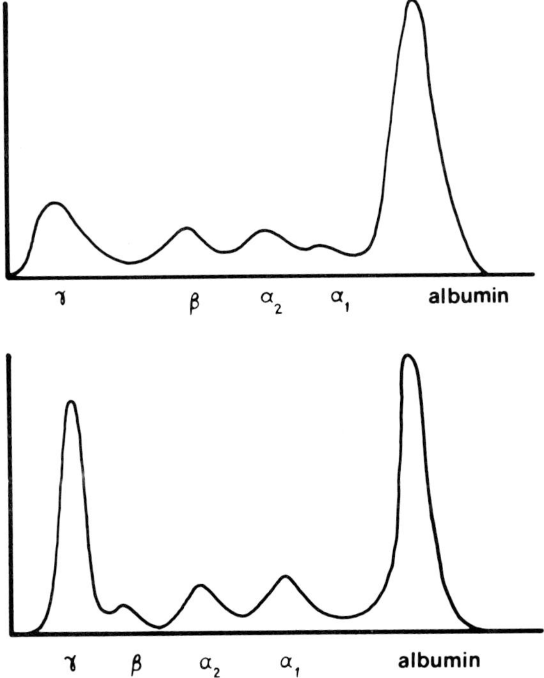

Figure 9.16. *Top*, normal serum protein electrophoresis (SPEP). *Bottom*, SPEP in multiple myeloma showing spike in gamma region.

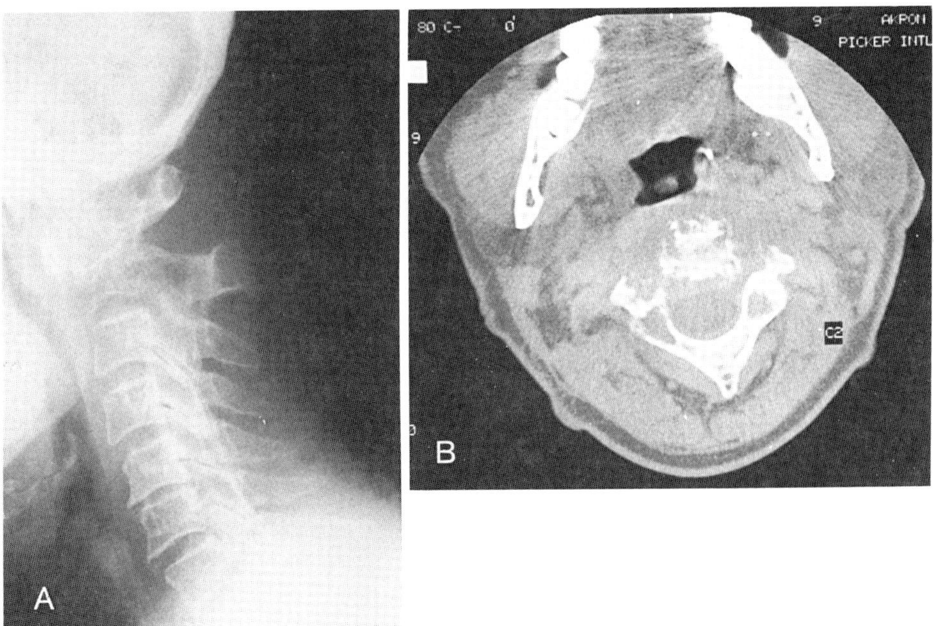

Figure 9.17. Plain x-ray (**A**) and CT scan (**B**) of multiple myeloma in the vertebral body and posterior elements of C2.

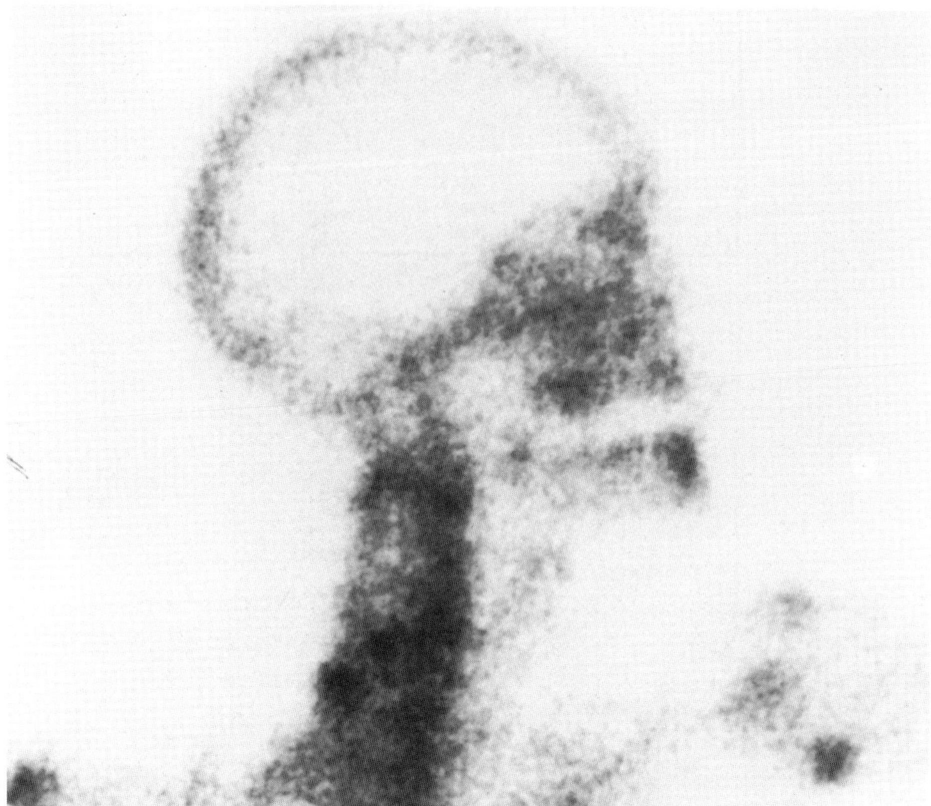

Figure 9.18.   Bone scan showing a scant increase in uptake in C2 in same patient as Figure 9.17.

Cervical Cord Tumors

Spinal cord tumors are traditionally classified as extradural, intradural-extramedullary, and intradural-intramedullary (inside the spinal cord). They are all extremely rare.

Extradural

The extradural tumors are the metastatic and primary bone tumors discussed in previous sections (12).

Intradural-Extramedullary

The two most common tumors in this classification are benign meningiomas and schwannomas (Fig. 9.19) (29). They usually present as slowly progressive radicular pain. Late in the process, a Brown-Sequard cord lesion may occur. The diagnosis is made on MRI and treatment is surgical excision.

An arteriovenous malformation of the cervical cord is predominantly an extramedullary lesion that also exhibits radicular or cord symptoms and signs. A characteristic of this lesion is aggravation with exercise that increases the blood flow through the malformation, or a stealing of blood away from the lesion. Exercise-induced quadriparesis is the hallmark of an arteriovenous (A-V) malforma-

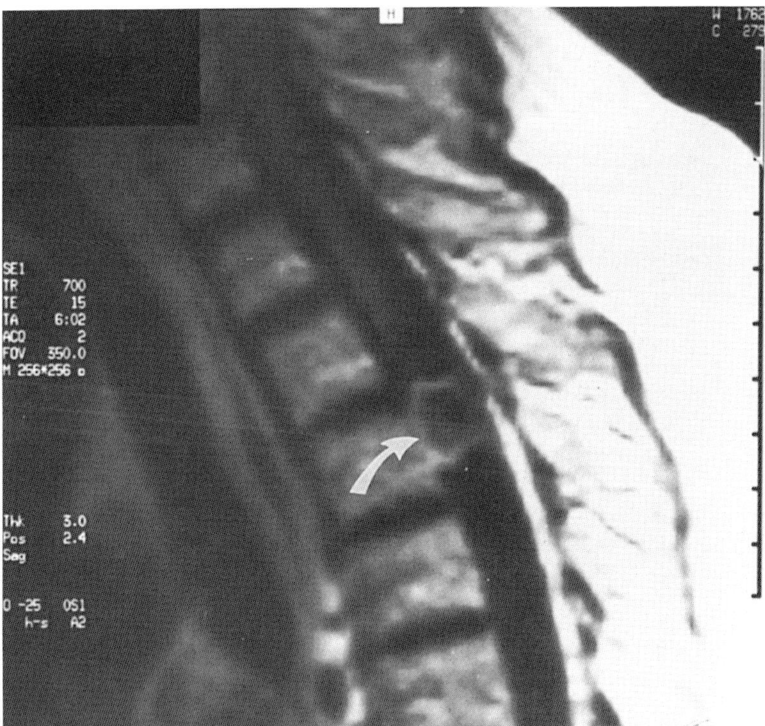

Figure 9.19.   Sagittal T1 spin echo with gadolinium highlighting a meningioma C7-T1 (see Fig. 9.6 for the body coil image).

tion. The diagnosis is confirmed on MRI. For surgical planning, angiography is necessary to define the extent of the malformation and its feeding vessels. Tedious microsurgical removal of the malformation with bipolar coagulation is the method of treatment.

Intradural-Intramedullary

Most intramedullary tumors are either benign astrocytomas or ependymomas (6). There are a number of other miscellaneous intramedullary tumors, gliomatous in nature, which are too infrequent to list.

The presentation is usually characteristic (in retrospect), with vague pain at the level of the lesion, usually without radicular distribution. The sensory and motor loss is significant at the level of the lesion and out of proportion to the minimal pain. Long tract findings, such as a spastic gait, are late to develop and usually follow upper extremity LMNL. Bladder and bowel symptoms are the last symptoms to appear.

The MRI scan is essential for diagnosis, allowing differentiation of syringomyelic cysts from solid tumors (Fig. 9.20).

Treatment is surgical excision using tedious microsurgical techniques to preserve as much neurological function as possible. This is often possible with the well-circumscribed ependymoma, but rarely possible in the more diffuse astrocytoma.

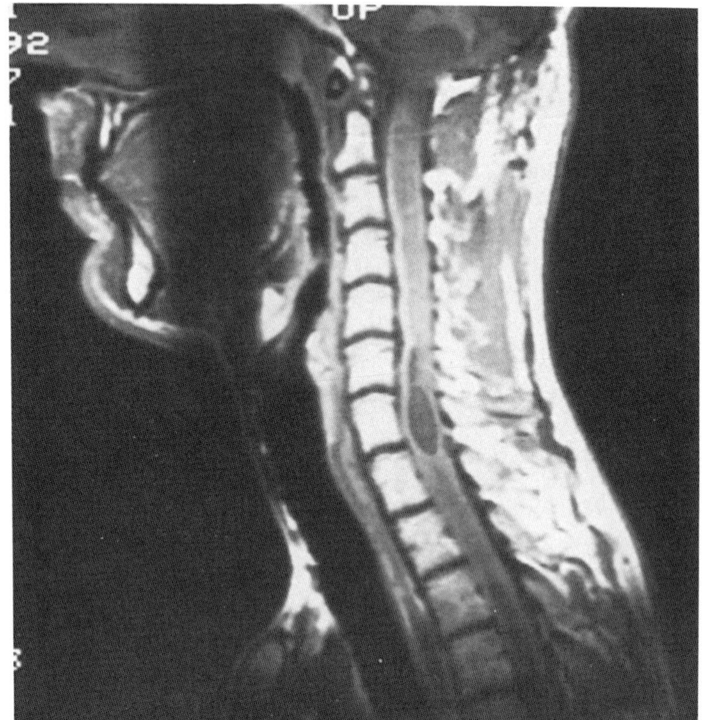

Figure 9.20.   Sagittal T1 spin echo image shows a fluid-filled cyst opposite C7.

Table 9.1.   Classification of Spinal Infections

Host Response	Anatomic Localization	Cause	Age
1. Pyogenic	1. Osteomyelitis/ Discitis	1. Hematogenous	1. Child
2. Granulomatous	2. Discitis of children	2. Invasion (surgery needle puncture)	2. Immunocompetent adult
	3. Epidural abscess	3. Direct spread	3. Immunocompetent adult

Infections of the Cervical Spine

As with tumors, infective lesions of the spine are more likely to involve the thoracic and lumbar spine segments. Even so, you will see these occasional cervical spine infections (Table 9.1):

1. Pyogenic osteomyelitis/discitis
2. Epidural abscess
3. Discitis of childhood
4. Tuberculous spondylitis

Pyogenic Osteomyelitis/Discitis

The most common cause of osteomyelitis/discitis in the cervical spine is iatrogenic—surgical intervention or diagnostic testing such as discography. The tendency is increased by long cases (more than three hours), extensive dissections, and the use of allograft bone and/or instrumentation. The postoperative cervical spine patient, who a few days after surgery stops progressing, stops eating, complains of increased neck pain, spikes a temperature, and has a high white blood cell (WBC) count is an obvious infection.

The next most common setting for osteomyelitis/discitis is spontaneous hematogenous infection in the immunoincompetent patient. These patients may complain of local neck pain, but they are already sick from their debilitation, and they cannot mount a normal resistance to infection signalled by high fever and a high WBC. Their diagnosis is not obvious at all. Their sedimentation rate is usually very high, but it is not until bone scanning or MRI that the true diagnosis is recognized.

The third setting for osteomyelitis/discitis is the so-called classic pattern of severe pain, nuchal rigidity, fever, high WBC, and high ESR. It is a rare event in the cervical spine, especially in the immunocompetent adult.

Pathogenesis. Hematogenous spread in the immunocompetent or immunoincompetent patient is via small arterioles that deposit the bacteria in the metaphysis of the vertebral body. From there, bone is destroyed, a pyogenic abscess is formed, and the disc is quickly invaded (Fig. 9.21).

The chief infecting organism is staph aureus, even in the immunocompromised patient. Occasionally, an IV drug abuser will spring a gram negative surprise such as pseudomonas. In the thoracic and lumbar spine, gall bladder manipulation or genitourinary manipulation can also be followed by a gram negative osteomyelitis/discitis, a rare event in the cervical spine.

Clinical Presentation. Local neck pain, moderate to severe, that does not improve with resting the neck is the classic presentation. In acute cervical disc herniations, the same failure of pain relief with rest occurs, but the pain in this patient is predominantly arm pain. Neck pain that increases in severity over a short time, and is not improved with local cervical collar rest or bed rest, should immediately lead you to consider a spinal infection (or tumor).

Often the pain will radiate into both shoulders, and occasionally radicular pain will occur if the inflammatory reaction or abscess affects a nerve root. Spread into the epidural space can occur late in the disease and produce myelopathic symptoms or paralysis (see section on epidural abscess below). In the neck, swelling may lead to dysphagia (rare) and/or shortness of breath (rarer still).

Diagnosis.   If you have an awareness for the occasional osteomyelitis/discitis that occurs, the diagnosis will be quickly apparent. Fever, elevated WBC, and ESR will point the way. The location of the pain will indicate a bone scintigraphy and MRI. Plain x-rays often do not show changes before four weeks from the onset of infection and can be misleading.

Bone Scanning for Spinal Infections. The chief advantage of bone scintigraphy is its ability to show increased osteoblastic activity and vascularity of infection days or weeks before plain x-ray changes occur (18, 28). Various compounds are available:

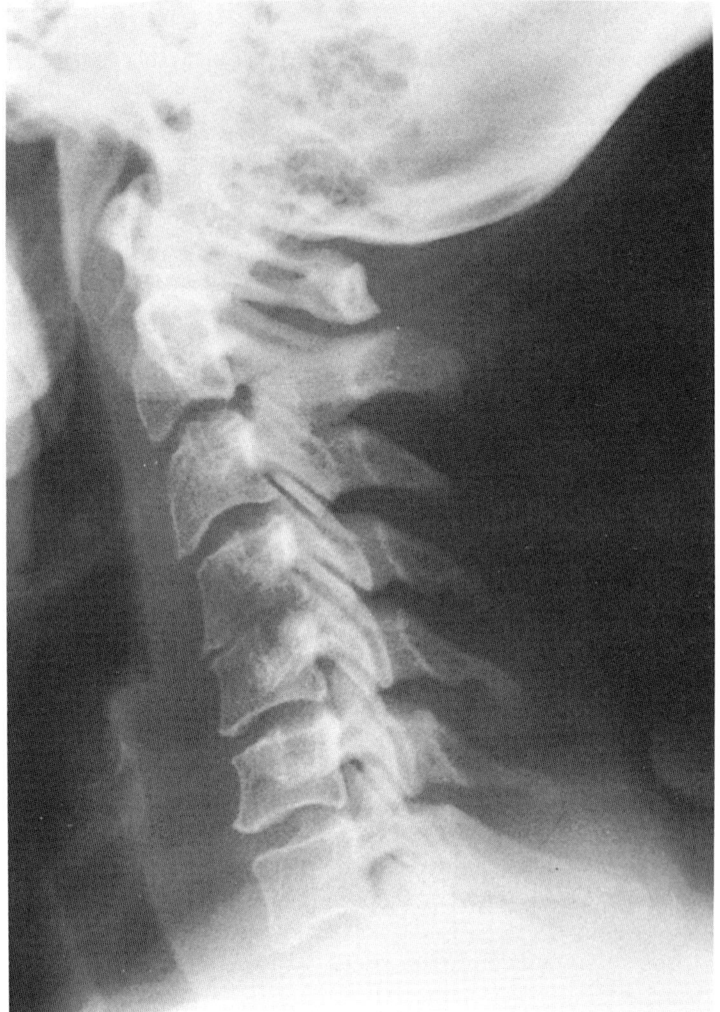

Figure 9.21.   Vertebral body osteomyelitis affecting adjacent vertebral bodies with invasion of disc space and collapse of that space. This is the classic picture of spinal osteomyelitis/discitis.

- Technetium-99m-Labeled Phosphorus (31)
- Gallium-67 Citrate
- Indium-III-Labeled Leukocytes (21, 23)

Technetium-99m-Labeled Phosphorus (^{99m}Tc). ^{99m}Tc is currently the most frequently used radionuclide in nuclear medicine (18). It is so because it is readily available, it is cheap, and it has an ideal biological behavior pattern. This includes easy incorporation into bone, timing of incorporation that suits hospital procedures, and a low radiation dose to the patient.

So that it will target the bone cell, ^{99m}Tc has to be linked to phosphorus before intravenous (IV) injection. Linkage to other compounds will change its specificity to other parts of the body (e.g., linked to macroaggregated albumin, it is

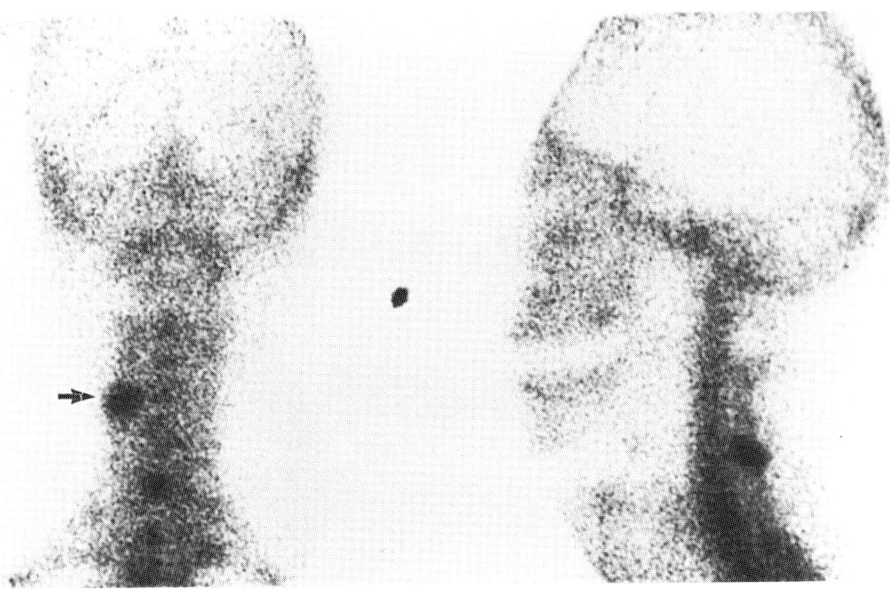

Figure 9.22.   A "hot spot" of activity in an arthritic facet joint (*arrow*).

deposited in the capillary beds of the lung for lung scanning). The fact that ^{99m}Tc in phosphorus quickly incorporates into bone (within 15 minutes of IV injection) points to its mechanism of action. The exchange occurs at the interface of bone and extracellular fluid, where active osteoblastic-directed mineralization is taking place. The ^{99m}Tc-labeled phosphorus incorporates into bone by becoming one or more of the inorganic components of hydroxyapatite. From there it emits gamma rays that are detectable by a gamma camera. The faster the bone turnover (the faster the mineralization of osteoid), the greater the ^{99m}Tc deposited and the more gamma radiation emitted by the site. This is the basis of the "hot spot" (Fig. 9.22). Immediately after injection, the vascularity of the area of interest may provide useful information, in particular in long bone or limb problems.

Technique. ^{99m}Tc is shipped in a parent form of molybdenum-99, which in its container spins off ^{99m}Tc. The container, depending on volume of usage, will deliver useful product for a few weeks. The phosphorus-labeled compound is injected intravenously, and three phases of scans are completed (18):

Phase 1. The perfusion scan is done immediately after IV injection to show whether the area of interest has a vascular supply. This scan is also known as the nuclear angiogram. It is of little use in spinal scanning but is often mentioned in the literature.

Phase 2. The blood pool scan is done a few minutes after the Phase 1 scan and will show the internal vascular status of the lesion. Higher counts signify a vascular lesion; lower counts, a less vascular lesion. It is also of limited use in spinal scanning.

Phase 3. The delayed bone image scan is done three hours after injection, at which time bone incorporation of the tracer isotope is maximum and back-

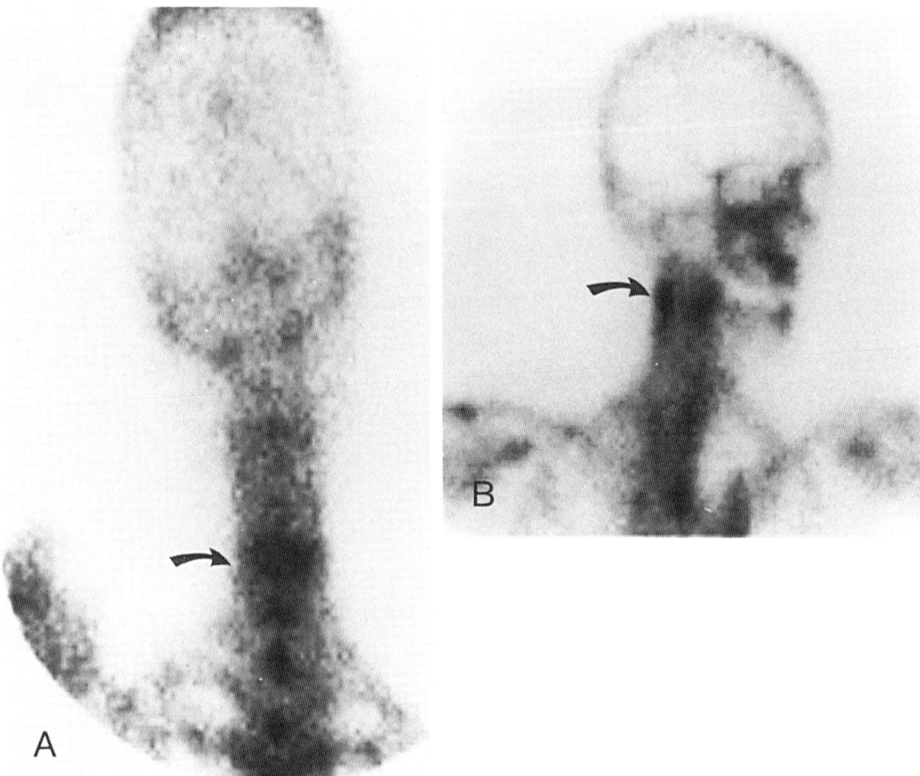

Figure 9.23. **A,** increased tracer uptake in a disc space (C5-C6) after a discogram. The patient had an early disc space infection. **B,** hot spots in metastatic carcinoma of the spine.

ground tracer has been excreted by the kidneys. The half-life of ^{99m}Tc is six hours; by this time, the gamma count becomes too low to be a useful measure.

Technetium-99-labeled phosphorus is deposited where bone turnover is greatest. These sites are normally located in growing bones at the epiphysis, metaphysial regions of long bones, and the sacroiliac joints (this limits the usefulness of bone scanning in ankylosing spondylitis). Abnormal (faster) bone turnover occurs in tumors, infections, and fractures, as well as bone-soft tissue junctions where increased metabolic activity is occurring. Sites with decreased bone activity, such as osteonecrosis or highly destructive tumors (multiple myeloma), will show no activity change (normal bone scan) or a "cold spot" (decreased tracer activity compared with surrounding normal bone). Examples of scans are show in Figures 9.23 and 9.24.

Dose. The usual dose of ^{99m}Tc is 10–20 millicuries. Radiation doses to various tissues of the body are well within acceptable levels (18). The greatest exposure (500–1000 millirads) occurs in the bladder and is best handled by good patient hydration before and after the scan. The height of kidney excretion and bladder exposure occurs three hours after injection, when at least one-third of the amount of tracer injected has been cleared by the kidneys. With this timing,

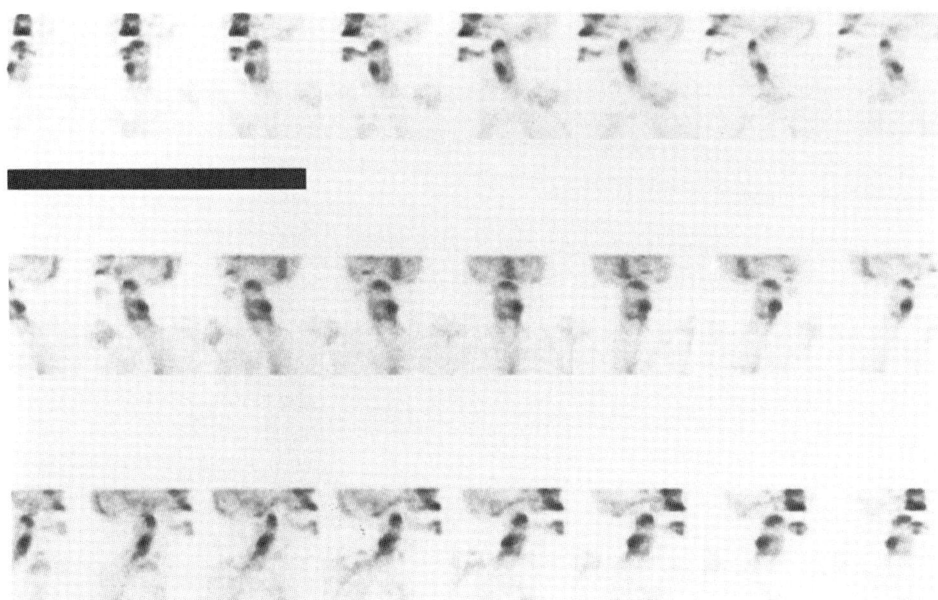

Figure 9.24.   SPECT of neck. This was done to establish age of an odontoid fracture—"fresh" from the examination of the scan.

30%–40% of the tracer is bound in bone, 10%–15% is bound in other tissue, and 5% is in blood.

Gallium Scanning.   Technetium-99-labeled phosphorus identifies areas of increased bone turnover and is nonspecific for infection. This led to the search for compounds that would specifically bind to sites of infection, the most popular (until recently) being gallium-67 citrate. This tracer is taken up by bacteria, leukocytes, and lymphocytes, and thus will localize infections and tumors containing high concentrations of these white blood cells.

Limitations of Gallium-67 Citrate.   Gallium is slowly excreted through the kidneys and bowel such that the optimal time of scanning—that time when concentration in the area of interest is potentially highest and background contamination by blood and soft tissue content is lowest—is 48 hours. This has the potential for contaminating other scanning efforts, such as ^{99m}Tc, for taxing the scheduling efforts of a large hospital department, and for testing patient compliance.

More recently, a number of reports on the limited accuracy of gallium scanning, especially in low-grade infections, have appeared in the literature (23).

The value of gallium scanning appears to be enhanced by doing ^{99m}Tc/gallium-67 scanning sequentially and comparing the uptake of the two scans. A hot ^{99m}Tc bone scan with increased ^{67}Ga activity is suggestive of a bone infection. The trend today is away from gallium scanning for spinal infections when indium-III-labeled leukocytes are available.

Indium-III-Labeled Leukocytes.   Because of the limited accuracy of ^{67}Ga scanning, further research has led to the proposal that indium-III-la-

Table 9.2.   Advantages of MRI for Spinal Sepsis

1. Body coil will show full extent of lesion(s) throughout spine.
2. Surface coil can then be used to home in on area of interest.
3. Images at 90° to each other are available, i.e., sagittal and axial.
4. Marrow changes (extent and nature) are obvious.
5. Disc changes are obvious.
6. Soft tissue extension into the spinal canal and paravertebral soft tissues are well demonstrated.
7. Gadolinium enhancement is available to further document the lesion.
8. Needle penetration of the infected spine (e.g., myelogram) is avoided.

beled leukocytes have a greater specificity for musculoskeletal (and other) infective foci.

Technique.   After harvesting the patient's own blood, the WBC are separated by centrifuge and chemical means, and labeled with the radioactive tracer indium-III. These labeled leukocytes are resuspended in the patient's plasma and injected to seek out foci of infection. Twenty-four hours later, gamma activity is measured with a gamma radiation detection camera.

The higher sensitivity and specificity for indium scanning appear to be well established in the literature. Other advantages of indium scanning include a maintenance of this accuracy in the presence of low-grade chronic infection and in patients on antibiotics and steroids. That scanning can be done 24 hours after injection facilitates hospital scheduling, although the front-end load of harvesting and labeling the leukocytes offsets this benefit.

A number of studies show the value of labeled leukocytes for diagnosis of peripheral skeletal changes, but be aware of the potential for false-negative scans in the axial skeleton.

When interpreted in light of clinical findings (fever) and laboratory findings—WBC count and erythrocyte sedimentation rate (ESR)—indium-III scans are more accurate for the detection of musculoskeletal infections than gallium-67 scanning (21). ^{99m}Tc/indium-III scanning is probably the scintigraphy method of choice for investigating a patient suspected of having increased bone turnover from tumor or infection. In the absence of the clinical suspicion of infection, ^{99m}Tc scanning alone is sufficient.

Conclusions.   Newer techniques are in the research stage and include ^{99m}Tc labeling of leukocytes and labeled antigranulocyte antibodies. In addition, SPECT (single photon-emitted computerized tomography) (Fig. 9.24) is pinpointing the exact location of increased tracer activity in the axial skeleton.

MRI in Osteomyelitis/Discitis.   MRI is now the standard for investigation of spinal sepsis. The advantages are listed in Table 9.2 and are so numerous as to sweep away other approaches (24, 25).

The basis of MRI in infection is the appearance of increased water content of inflammation (Fig. 9.25). On T1-weighted images, water will have a low signal intensity relative to fat, and vice versa on T2. Also observe the pattern of marrow infiltration and the intact cortices (not usually the case in tuberculosis and tumor). Gadolinium enhancement will also light up the infection on T1 spine echo images.

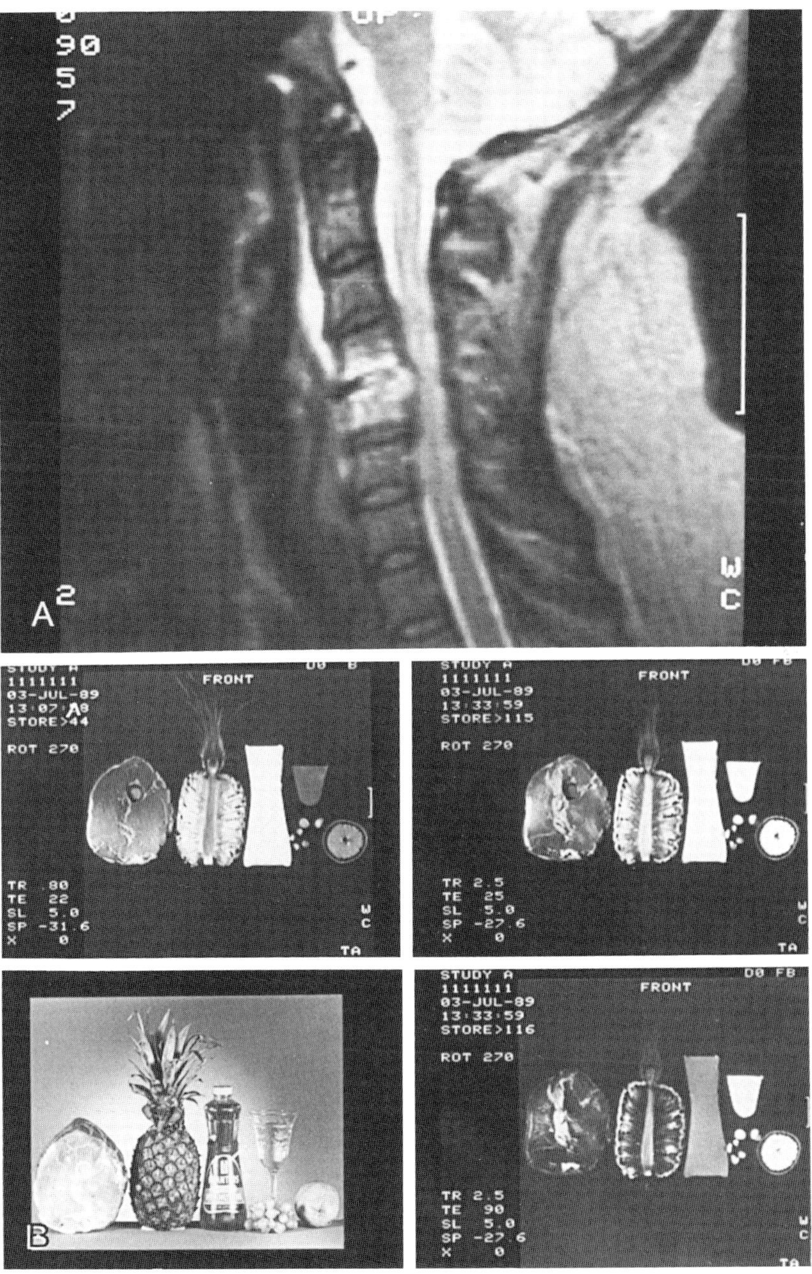

Figure 9.25. **A**, sagittal T2 spin echo image of C4-C5 osteomyelitis/discitis. Note bright signal of edema. **B**, ham, pineapple, peanut oil, water, grapes, and an orange! What are they doing in this text? They show what happens to oil and water when you switch from T1 protocol (*top left*) to T2 protocol (*bottom right*). Water (inflammation) gives off a higher (brighter/whiter) signal. Oil does the reverse—it goes from bright to darker. Look at muscle (ham) and bone (ham) and fiber (pineapple), and practice reading T1-weighted and T2-weighted scans. (Exercise courtesy of Dr. Ed Bury, Akron City Hospital.)

*Table 9.3. Indications for Surgical Intervention in Osteomyelitis/Discitis**

Timing From Onset of Symptoms	Type of Complication (Necessitating Surgery)
Early (hours to 1 or 2 days)	Neurological encroachment
Intermediate (1st week)	Abscess formation
Late (beyond 1st week)	Failed conservative care, instability

*Any of these complications can occur at any time in the disease development.

Although MRI has become the diagnostic gold standard, preoperative planning should almost always include CT to more accurately depict the extent of bony involvement.

Management of Osteomyelitis/Discitis.   First obtain a bacteriological diagnosis. This is done with blood cultures, cultures of a remote source, and most often a biopsy of the spine. The biopsy may be closed (percutaneous) and CT-guided or it can be an open biopsy that immediately becomes part of the definitive operative procedure.

The most common scenario is recognition of the potential diagnosis of a spinal infection, making a quick diagnosis with plain x-rays, bone scanning and MRI, establishing a baseline with a WBC and ESR, and then obtaining a tissue diagnosis—all within 24 hours of hospital admission. Appropriate antibiotics are instituted and the patient's fever, WBC, and ESR are monitored along with the status of local tissues on imaging studies. Indications for surgical intervention are listed in Table 9.3. Neurological compromise at any time is an indication for urgent intervention but tends to occur early in pyogenic osteomyelitis/discitis.

Surgical Approach to Osteomyelitis/Discitis.   If the disease process is caught early with no complications, the antibiotic coverage (IV to start) and a simple cervical brace will suffice. If some bone destruction has occurred, the potential for collapse and a cervical kyphosis dictates use of a halo-thoracic jacket. If complications occur (Table 9.3), and surgery becomes necessary, the approach is from the direction of trouble, that is, anteriorly. We mention cervical laminectomy for osteomyelitis/discitis only to condemn it. At the time of surgery, a decision must be made about bone grafting for fusion and some fixation. It is prudent to fuse with autogenous bone and use a halo frame for external immobilization, rather than an internal fixation device.

Antibiotic Coverage.   A successful outcome in spinal sepsis is far more dependent on successful long-term antibiotic therapy than on any short-term surgical intervention. Antibiotic coverage should continue until the infection is obviously under control, new bone formation is occurring, and the ESR is returning to normal. This is a minimum of six weeks and may extend to six months.

Spinal Epidural Abscess

Introduction.   It is highly unlikely that you will see a cervical epidural abscess. When it appears in the emergency department, you will probably miss it, something that happens 75% of the time.

Demography.   Epidural abscess is predominantly an adult disease, affecting the thoracic-lumbar more than the cervical region (1, 8). As a spontaneous hematogenous event in a normal adult, it is highly unlikely. Most often it occurs after spine surgery and more frequently it appears in debilitated (diabetic or alcoholic) or immunocompromised patients. If you work in an area with high drug abuse, you will see epidural abscess more frequently.

Bacteriology.   The majority of patients will culture out *Staphylococcus aureus;* drug abusers have a higher incidence of gram negative infections such as pseudomonas, but the majority will still grow *S. aureus* (19).

Pathogenesis and Clinical Presentation.   The mass of infective cells in the epidural space may be either granulation tissue or pus. Both occupy space needed for neurological structures. Initially the patient will have local pain (especially nonmechanical nighttime pain). As the mass expands, radicular pain will appear, followed by weakness and, in the end, paralysis. How fast this clinical progression occurs is variable, but the pain to paralysis stage may take but a few hours, making the diagnosis and treatment of epidural abscess an emergency (1).

In the cervical spine, there is no true, only a potential, epidural space. In the thoracic and lumbar spine, there is a posterior epidural space filled with fat. Because of this anatomy, it is easy to understand why epidural abscesses tend to occur posteriorly in the thoracic and lumbar regions. In the cervical spine, they may be anterior or posterior. If they occur after anterior spine surgery or discography, then obviously most epidural collections will be anterior. They may be confined to one segment, but more often the pus or granulation tissue collection occurs over multiple segments.

Diagnosis.   The quickest path to diagnosis is a high index of suspicion in any adult especially debilitated by drugs, disease, or decay, and who presents nighttime neck pain and stiffness with fever. Sometimes, because of immunosuppression, the fever, ESR, and WBC will show minimal change.

Any suspected infectious disease needs immediate identification of the underlying organism through direct abscess culture, blood culture, or culture of a remote but more accessible source, such as an infected skin lesion around the head and neck.

Unless there is associated discitis/osteomyelitis, plain x-rays are likely to be negative. Until the advent of MRI (17, 27), myelography with CT scanning was needed for diagnosis. MRI is now the investigative modality of choice, which avoids all the dangers of subarachnoid puncture in a patient with a spinal infection (Table 9.4).

Treatment.   An epidural abscess is an urgent medical situation. If you are fortunate enough to catch it early, before weakness has occurred, conservative care with the appropriate antibiotic is a choice. Most cases of epidural abscesses require surgical drainage (5) because:

1. The disease is diagnosed late and radicular pain and weakness are present.
2. The time interval between weakness and paralysis can be measured in hours. Some think this is because of venous or arterial thrombosis in the vascular tree of the spinal cord.
3. The lesion is not only a space-occupying lesion in neurological territory, it is an abscess with a necrotic center that may not be reached by antibiotics.
4. The presence of paralysis for more than 36 hours usually results in either no functional recovery or death.

Table 9.4.   MRI Epidural Abscess (Granulation Tissue) Appearance

MRI Sequence	Compared to Spinal Cord	Compared to CSF
T1-weighted Spin Echo	Most often isointense† Sometimes hypointense	Hyperintense
T2-weighted Spin Echo	Almost always hyperintense	Hyperintense
Gradient Echo T2*	Same as T2 SE	Same as T2 SE
Gadolinium enhancement	Hyperintense periphery (granulation tissue) Hypointense core (abscess)	Not routinely done

* T2 is a fast imaging technique that appears somewhat like a T2 spin echo but requires much less time in the machine.
† isotense—same signal intensity
  hyperintense—higher (whiter) signal intensity
  hypointense—lower (grayer) signal intensity

Obviously, the goal of surgery is to evacuate the pus. As with any other spinal condition, the approach is dictated by the location of the pathology. If the pus is posterior, go posteriorly (laminectomy); if it is anterior, go anteriorly (corpectomy or vertebral body excision). Since anterior pathology will usually be associated with osteomyelitis/discitis, two additional demands need to be met:

1. Deal effectively with the osteomyelitis/discitis.
2. Anticipate instability anteriorly and the subsequent necessity for a posterior stabilization procedure.

Epidural abscess extending over multiple segments (three or more) is probably best dealt with posteriorly regardless of where the mass of pus lies. Obviously, all surgeries are done with usual concern for patient positioning, intraoperative monitoring, and appropriate antibiotic coverage.

Discitis in Children

A well-recognized triad of neck pain—torticollis, fever, and disc space narrowing on x-ray—occurs in the first and second decades of life. Laboratory testing reveals the ESR is elevated but the WBC is not. Almost always the blood cultures and disc space cultures are negative, and the child or teenager makes a full recovery with or without antibiotic coverage. Obviously, most physicians would treat such a patient with broad-spectrum antibiotics and a neck collar for comfort. Do not be too quick to operate, because almost all cases resolve spontaneously and quickly over one to two weeks.

Tuberculous Spondylitis (Pott's Disease)

Introduction.   Of all the potential cervical spinal column infections, this is the one you are least likely to see in countries with well-developed medical care systems. Tuberculosis spinal infections are more likely in the thoracic and lumbar spines, in countries where the disease is endemic. With the recent resurgence of TB in America's inner cities, Pott's disease may reappear, but as in the past, it is unlikely to affect the cervical spine.

Pathogenesis.   It is likely that the tuberculous bacillus reaches the spine via the arterioles, which deposit the organism in the anterior metaphyseal region of the vertebral body. From there the infection spreads, but does not affect the disc

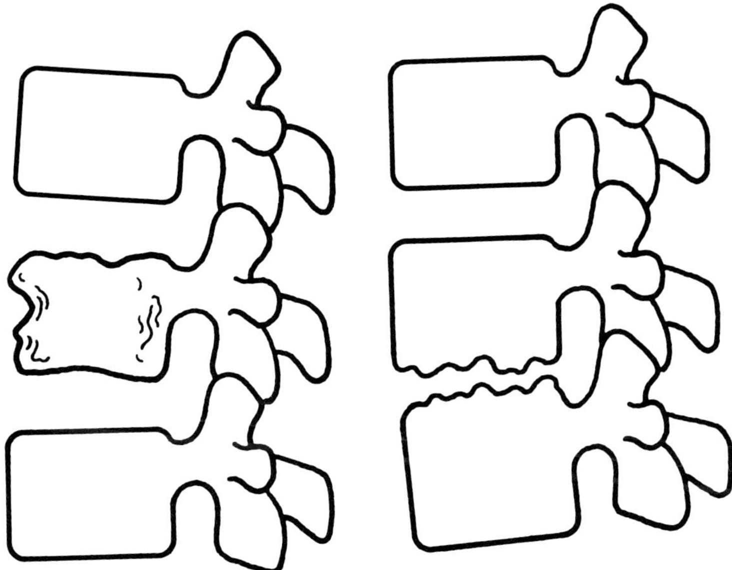

Figure 9.26.   TB (and tumor) characteristically destroy the vertebral body early and the disc space late (*left*) whereas pyogenic infection of the spine destroys the disc space early (*right*).

space. Later in the disease, contiguous vertebral bodies are affected because of anterior subligamentous spread. The end stage in this long insidious course is vertebral body collapse due to the destructive granuloma (Fig. 9.26). The collapse (kyphosis) and mass may compress neurological tissue.

Clinical Presentation.   Tuberculous spondylitis is a long, slow process. Patients may experience local discomfort with loss of movement. More likely, they will have systemic symptoms of fatigue, malaise, weight loss, and night sweats (if you remember to ask about these on functional inquiry!).

Diagnosis.   Since the x-ray appearance may mimic tumor or pyogenic infection, biopsy is necessary to identify the organism. Obviously, the primary focus of infection must be located.

The central area of caseating necrosis and the surrounding rim of Langhans giant cells have a particular MRI appearance.

Treatment.   If the diagnosis is made before neurological compromise, anti-tuberculous medication (streptomycin/isoniazid (INH) and Rifampicin) will usually control the disease. For more resistant organisms, Ethambutol and Pyrazinamide, under the direction of your infectious disease consultant, are available.

Abscess formation, kyphosis, and/or neurological involvement are indications for anterior surgical debridement and bone grafting (22). We mention laminectomy for the treatment of this disease only to condemn it. To prevent deformity, external bracing in a halo-thoracic orthosis is a better approach than internal fixation.

Summary

By now, you must be wondering: if tumors, inflammatory arthritis (RA and AS), and infections of the cervical spine are so rare, why are they included in this book? We have by no means presented a reference-quality discussion of these conditions, but they are included as summary discussions to alert you to other potential conditions as you puzzle over a difficult diagnostic problem in neck pain.

REFERENCES

1. Baker AS, Ojemann RG, Swartz MN, and Richardson EP Jr: Spinal epidural abscess. N Engl J Med 293:463–468 (1975).
2. Bernat JL, Greenberg ER, and Barrett J: Suspected epidural compression of the spinal cord and cauda equina by metastatic carcinoma: clinical diagnosis and survival. Cancer 51:1953–1957 (1983).
3. Bohlman HH, Sachs BL, Carter JR, Riley L, and Robinson RA: Primary neoplasms of the cervical spine. J Bone Joint Surg 68A:483–494 (1986).
4. Calvé JA: Localized affection of spine suggesting osteochondritis of vertebral body, with clinical aspects of Pott's disease. J Bone Joint Surg 7:41–46 (1925).
5. Chamberlain MC, Abitbol JJ, and Garfin SR: Epidural spinal cord compression: treatment options. Semin Spine Surg 2:203–209 (1990).
6. Cooper PR and Epstein F: Radical resection of intramedullary spinal cord tumors in adults. Neurosurg 63:492–499 (1985).
7. Dahlin DC: Bone Tumors. General Aspects and Data on 3,987 Cases. Charles C Thomas, Springfield, IL (1967).
8. Danner RL and Hartmen BJ: Update on spinal epidural abscess: 35 cases and review of the literature. Rev Infect Dis 9:265–274 (1987).
9. DiLorenzo N, Delfini R, Ciappetta P, Cantore G, and Fortuna A: Primary tumors of the cervical spine: surgical experience with 38 cases. Surg Neurol 38:12–18 (1992).
10. Freeman LM and Blaufox MD: Physicians Desk Reference of Radiology and Nuclear Medicine, p 101. Medical Economics, Oradell, NJ (1979).
11. Fornasier VL and Horne JG: Metastases to the vertebral column. Cancer 36:590–594 (1975).
12. Gilbert RW, Kim JH, and Posner JB: Epidural spinal cord compression from metastatic tumor: diagnosis and treatment. Ann Neurol 3:40–51 (1978).
13. Harrington KD: Metastatic disease of the spine. J Bone Joint Surg 68A:1110–1115 (1986).
14. Holder LE: Radionuclide bone imaging in the evaluation of bone pain. J Bone Joint Surg 64A: 1391–1396 (1982).
15. Hollis PH, Malis LI, and Zappulla RA: Neurological deterioration after lumbar puncture below complete spinal subarachnoid block. J Neurosurg 64:253–256 (1986).
16. Kirchner PT and Simon MA: Current concepts review; radioisotopic evaluation of skeletal disease. J Bone Joint Surg 63A:673–681 (1981).
17. Kricun R, Shoemaker EI, Chovanes GI, and Stephen HW: Epidural abscess of the cervical spine: MR findings in five cases. AJR 158:1145–1149 (1992).
18. Krishnamurthy GT, Tubis M, Hiss J, and Blahd WH: Distribution pattern of metabolic bone disease. A need for total body skeletal image. JAMA 237:2504–2506 (1977).
19. Lasker BR and Harter CH. Cervical epidural abscess. Neurology 37:1747–1753 (1987).
20. Li KC and Poon PY. Sensitivity and specificity of MRI in detecting malignant spinal cord compression and in distinguishing malignant from benign compression fractures of vertebrae. Magn Reson Imaging 6:547–556 (1988).
21. Magnusson JE, Brown ML, Hauser MR, Berquist TH, Fitzgerald RH, and Klee GG: In-III-labeled leukocyte scintigraphy in suspected orthopedic prosthesis infection: comparison with other imaging modalities. Radiology 168:235–239 (1988).
22. Medical Research Council Working Party on Tuberculosis of the Spine. Five year assessments of controlled trials of ambulatory treatment: debridement and anterior spinal fusion in the management of tuberculosis of the spine. Studies in Bulawayo (Rhodesia) and in Hong Kong. J Bone Joint Surg 60B:163–177 (1978).
23. Merkel KD, Brown ML, Dewanjee MK, and Fitzgerald RH: Comparison of indium-labeled leukocyte imaging with sequential technetium-gallium scanning in the diagnosis of low-grade musculoskeletal sepsis. J Bone Joint Surg 67A:465–476 (1985).

24. Modic MT, Feiglin DH, Piraino DW, Boumphrey F, Weinstein MA, Duchesneau PM, and Rehm S: Vertebral osteomyelitis: assessment using MR. Radiology 157:157–166 (1985).
25. Modic MT, Pflanze W, Feiglin DHI, and Belhobek G: Magnetic resonance imaging of musculo-skeletal infections. Radiol Clin North Am 24:247–258 (1986).
26. O'Connor MI and Currier BL: Metastatic disease of spine. Orthopedics 15:611–620 (1992).
27. Sandhu FS and Dillon WP: Spinal epidural abscess: evaluation with contrast enhanced MR imaging. AJNR 12:1087–1093 (1991).
28. Schauwecker DS: The scintigraphic diagnosis of osteomyelitis. AJR 158:9–18 (1992).
29. Siegal T and Siegal T: Surgical decompression of anterior and posterior malignant epidural tumors compressing the spinal cord: a prospective study. Neurosurgery 17:424–432 (1985).
30. Siegal T and Siegal T: Current considerations in the management of neoplastic spinal cord compression. Spine 14:223–228 (1989).
31. Subramanian G and McAfee JG: A new complex of ^{99m}Tc for skeletal imaging. Radiology 99:192–196 (1971).
32. Sze G, Krol G, Zimmerman RD, and Deck MDF: Malignant extradural spinal tumors: MR imaging with Gd-DTPA1. Radiology 167:217–223 (1988).
33. Weinstein JN and McLain RF: Primary tumors of the spine. Spine 12:843–851 (1987).

10

Torticollis*

"As knots can, by the conflux of meeting sap, infect the sound pine and divert his grain tortive and errant from his course growth."

—Chaucer

INTRODUCTION

Torticollis, or wry neck, is an abnormal tilting and rotating of the head caused by a contracture or contraction of the cervical muscles or fascia. It is almost always a condition in children and is a symptom and/or sign, not a disease. Usually, the chin is flexed forward and rotated towards the opposite shoulder, making the deformity quite obvious (Fig. 10.1). Torticollis is most frequently produced by intrinsic muscular or bony cervical pathology. On occasion it may be a symptom of lesions quite remote from the neck, as in intracranial lesions or intraspinal pathology. It assumes medical importance when it is involuntary, rigid, recurrent, or painful.

Congenital Muscular Torticollis

Congenital muscular torticollis is the most common cause of torticollis. It is generally not detected before two months of age, occurring as a painless head tilt. It results from scarring and foreshortening of the sternocleidomastoid muscle (1, 2, 8). Consequently, the head is slightly flexed and tilted forward, and the chin is rotated toward the uninvolved shoulder. The severity of deformity is directly related to the degree of the contracture and the age of the patient.

The etiology of this condition is still obscure (8). A number of factors have been indicted, including intrauterine malposition, difficulty with extraction during the birth process, heredity, infection, neurogenic causes, and acquired muscular ischemia (compartment syndrome). A significant number of cases have been associated with breech delivery or difficult forceps delivery. Whether the lesion occurs antepartum or as a consequence of the birth process is still debated. It is seen in caesarean sections, prompting the proponents of antepartum etiology to suggest torticollis might be a product of a facial or brow type of fetal presentation that leads to C-section. That torticollis is a consequence of difficulties in the birth process is supported by studies of human specimens showing similar histological changes in muscle akin to that seen in venous obstruction of muscles in dogs. Support for the traumatic etiology is weakened by the roughly three of four children in whom the lesion is on the right side, and in the 20%–30% of children in whom it is accompanied by congenital dysplasia of the hip.

---

* By Dr. Dennis Weiner, Chief of Orthopaedics, Akron Children's Medical Center, and Professor of Orthopaedics, Northeastern Ohio Universities College of Medicine, Rootstown, Ohio.

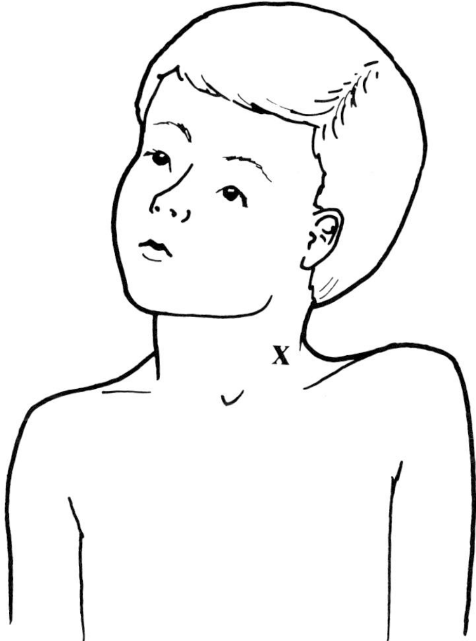

Figure 10.1.   Drawing of a child with torticollis due to shortening of the left (x) sternomastoid. The head is tilted to the left and the chin is rotated to the right.

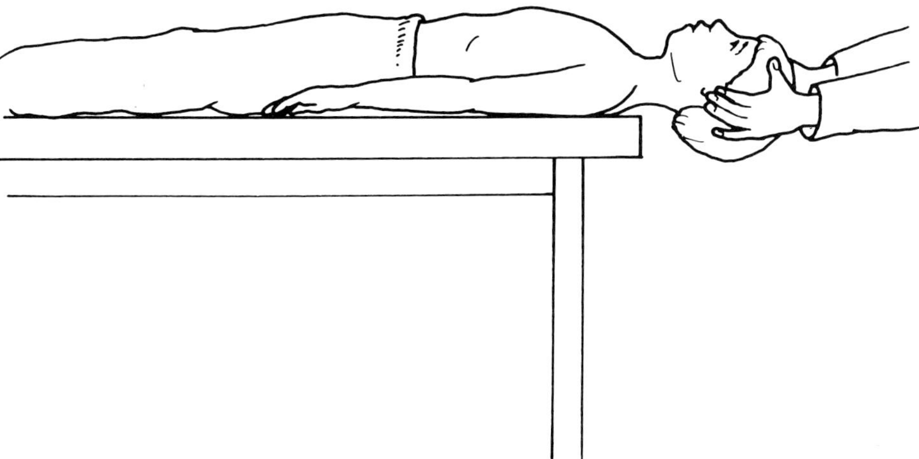

Figure 10.2.   Method of examining a child with torticollis. The examiner can rotate the neck and lateral flex as isolated or combined movements.

Examination is best conducted with the infant's head extended beyond the edge of the examining table, supported by the hands (Fig. 10.2). This facilitates manipulation of the head and neck to determine the degree of muscle tightness and limitation of motion. It is important to stabilize the shoulders against the examining table to prevent thoracic rotation and confusion in determining the arc of passive motion.

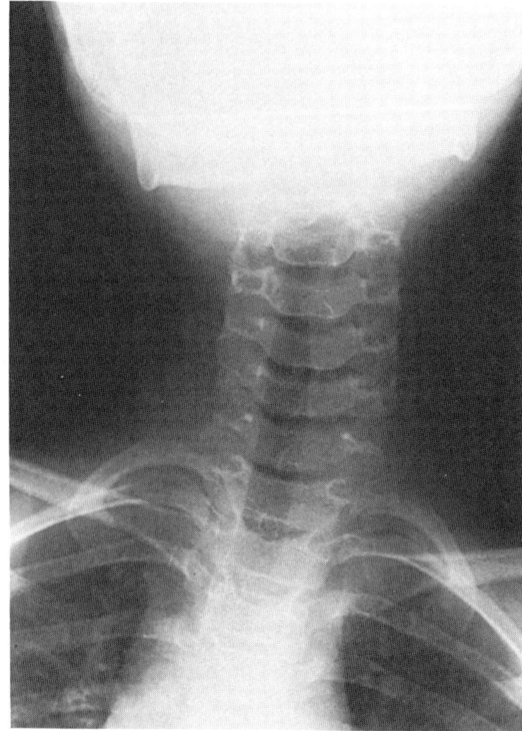

Figure 10.3.   An AP x-ray showing normal vertebral body structure, but the curvature of the torti-collis is evident.

Within the first few weeks of life, a soft nontender mass is frequently palpated within the substance of the involved sternocleidomastoid muscle. The overlying skin and subcutaneous tissue are freely movable and separated from the mass, which generally attains its greatest dimension during the first six weeks of life. Following its appearance, the mass gradually recedes in size and will frequently disappear within four to six months, leaving only the indurated, contracted muscle (5). The mass is frequently overlooked and thus detection requires careful examination.

Routine cervical spine x-rays are normal (Fig. 10.3), but they are necessary to rule out the osseous causes of torticollis as described in the next section.

Although it is clear that some cases may spontaneously resolve, it is generally accepted that progression is the more common path. Facial and skull deformities are a natural accompaniment of the condition, particularly if the torticollis goes untreated. The face can become flattened and underdeveloped on the ipsilateral side, while the parieto-occipital region on the contralateral side of the skull also flattens (plagiocephaly). The degree of facial and skull deformity may become striking, and some evidence of these changes may be present at the time of original diagnosis. If the torticollis is allowed to persist through the early growing years, the facial and skull deformities increase, due to inability of the soft tissues to keep pace with the bony growth of the skull and cervical spine.

The vast majority of children can be treated conservatively. During the first three months, before the child has achieved side rolling, it is of value to position the crib so that the infant will attempt to rotate his or her head in the opposite direction when looking at the rest of the room. In addition to positioning the infant's bed, manual stretching is performed. The parent is instructed in the technique of passively stretching to the opposite position, and this is usually achieved during diaper changes. It is difficult for mothers to stretch the neck of a crying infant. Considerable encouragement and frequent follow-up visits are required to see that conservative care is effective.

Most infants undergoing this regime will improve during the first 18 months of life, leaving less than 10% requiring surgery. Surgery may be indicated for that infrequent case where the disorder was overlooked before one year of age, and for those few cases resistant to conservative management. Surgery for torticollis reaches back to antiquity; it was probably performed as early as the second century, but it is not documented until 1685 (1). Subcutaneous tenotomy was a favorite of practitioners traveling through the fairs of medieval England. The preferred technique of open tenotomy was published more than 200 years ago. The procedure is best performed prior to school age, because the best opportunity for skull and facial remodeling will not have expired. Although some improvement in facial and skull characteristics can be noted after the age of eight, it is generally not significant. The surgical release is either through a longitudinal incision and z-plasty lengthening of the sternomastoid (5) or a transverse incision just above the clavicle, with transection of both the sternal and clavicular attachments (9). Although postoperative techniques vary from surgeon to surgeon, early motion is the hallmark of aftercare. Generally, the results of surgical release are gratifying in regard to the increase in head/neck motion and alterations in cosmetic contours (2, 11).

Congenital Osseous Anomalies (Skeletal Wry Neck)

Lesions of the developing cervical vertebrae that produce asymmetrical growth may result in a fixed tilting of the cervical spine or torticollis. The most common osseous abnormality producing torticollis seen by the orthopaedic surgeon is the Klippel-Feil syndrome (Fig. 10.4) (3, 7). As part of this condition, there is a failure of normal segmentation of the cervical vertebrae from the time of early development, with torticollis occurring in either the congenital muscular form or as a result of irregular osseous maturation of the cervical vertebrae. Patients with this syndrome exhibit a very short, broad neck (brevicollis), a low hairline, and marked restriction of cervical movement, particularly rotation. A high percentage of patients have a myriad of associated problems, such as scoliosis, Sprengel's deformity, and renal abnormalities. It has been estimated that well over one-half of patients will have scoliosis that requires attention, and nearly one-third will have significant renal abnormalities. If the torticollis is clearly secondary to the deformed cervical vertebrae, operative correction is nearly routinely unsuccessful and is not recommended. Occasionally, the severe errors in growth of the cervical thoracic vertebrae or dorsal vertebrae produce a substantial scoliosis that may necessitate early spinal stabilization to preclude severe neurologic sequelae.

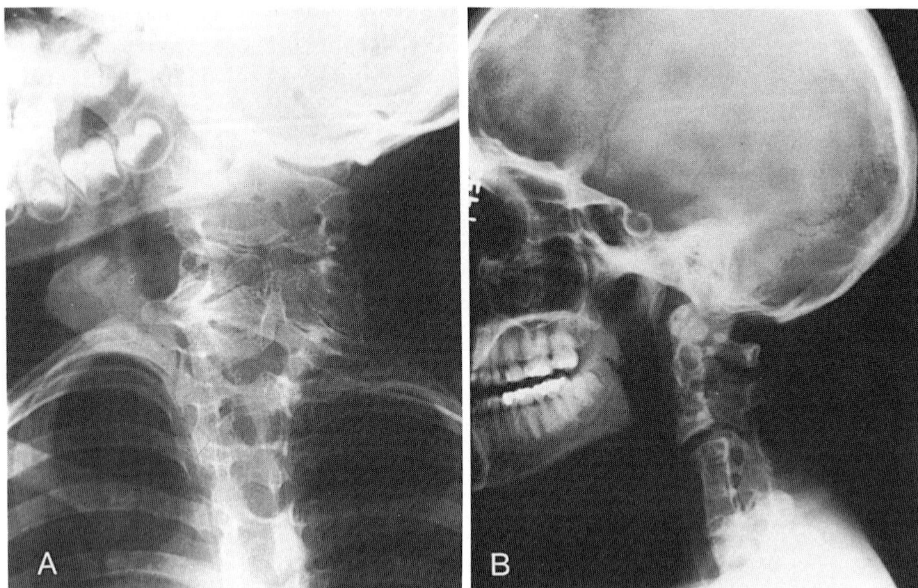

Figure 10.4. An AP (**A**) and lateral (**B**) of the cervical spine in a child showing failure of segmentation or Klippel-Feil syndrome.

Other skeletal anomalies causing wry neck usually affect the upper cervical region (4, 10, 13) and include: unilateral assimilation of the atlas into the skull, asymmetrical facets between the atlas and axis, asymmetrical development of the occipital condyles, and unilateral fusion between the first and second cervical vertebrae. Also seen are basilar impressions, odontoid deformities, and congenital narrowing of the foramen magnum. Some of these conditions may slowly lead to neurological impairment due to the compromised position of the spinal cord. Surprisingly, gross spinal anomalies are not always associated with neurologic manifestations.

The cervical spine itself may assume a rather normal clinically appearing attitude if the vertebrae above and below the defects compensate and allow the head to be maintained directly above the pelvis. The exact nature of the lesions may be quite difficult to demonstrate by conventional radiography because of technical problems in obtaining appropriate radiographs. Proper positioning of a child with either a painful neck or an abnormally rigid neck is most often a challenge for the x-ray technologist. In addition, radiographic interpretations may be quite complicated because of normal variations in the bony architecture and incomplete ossification of the vertebrae in young children. CT scanning for bony abnormalities, and MRI for assessment of neurological tissue, provide the most complete current techniques of evaluation.

Rotary Subluxation of the Upper Cervical Spine

Infrequently in children, rotary subluxation of the atlantoaxial articulation or of the C2-C3 articulation will produce an "acquired" torticollis (6). Characteristically, the child will have neck pain, diminished cervical motion, and neck spasm on passive attempts at motion. The head is generally tilted forward and rotated away from the involved facets. The child can rotate the chin further in the same direction but cannot voluntarily reverse the chin to the opposite side. The history obtained is usually that of a preceding cervical injury during innocuous playtime activities. Neurological manifestations are exceedingly rare. The pathophysiology involves unilateral forward rotational facet locking of the atlas on the axis or C2 on C3. The actual locking mechanism is unclear. Open-mouth odontoid radiographs can be helpful, but are often quite difficult to obtain with proper quality due to the age of the child and associated pain. The tip of the spine of C2 or C3 normally resides on the side opposite the chin when the head is rotated. In a rotary subluxation, the tip of the spine lies on the same side as the chin. Fortunately, there is an almost universal tendency for spontaneous resolution, and everyone should resist the temptation to use aggressive manipulation or operative therapy. Treatment consists of cervical halter traction, physical therapy modalities, and rest. Symptoms will usually resolve in 4–10 days (12).

Inflammatory Cervical Lesions

The association of inflammatory cervical lesions with torticollis is very common. Three major disorders comprise the bulk of cases:

1. Juvenile rheumatoid arthritis and systemic lupus erythematosus
2. Upper respiratory infections
3. Neoplastic conditions that also produce lymphadenopathy of the cervical region

The reason for the torticollis is reflex protective spasm in the cervical strap muscles secondary to a painful focus in the neck. Usually, there is adjacent inflammatory tissue and tender congested lymph nodes that probably induce spasm in the neck muscles manifesting as torticollis. In juvenile arthritis, the inflammatory process may become so prominent as to weaken the supporting ligaments of the cervical vertebrae and jeopardize segmental stability at the C1-C2 junction, resulting in torticollis.

Cervical adenopathy—either secondary to upper respiratory infections, peridental abscesses, tuberculosis, or even leukemia—can produce a reflex "spastic torticollis." Children with this type of torticollis generally present after the second year of life, with peak incidence between two and six years of age.

Direct management of the underlying inflammatory problem will routinely result in relief of the torticollis in a brief period of time. Heat, intermittent cervical traction, and short-term use of a soft cervical collar have been found to be helpful adjuncts in the management plan. The prognosis is generally excellent unless the primary process carries with it a more ominous outcome.

Neoplasms Producing Torticollis

A variety of neoplasms located within the substance of the cervical spine, base of skull, base of brain, and spinal cord may produce a secondary torticollis due to nerve irritation or conductive deficit within the peripheral nerves. Neoplasms such as posterior fossa tumors, gliomas, neurofibromas, neuroblastomas, and teratomas are the most frequent causes. Neoplasms affecting the body or posterior elements of the cervical vertebrae can likewise produce pain with "reflex" torticollis, or they can directly impair the spinal cord and nerve roots that lie

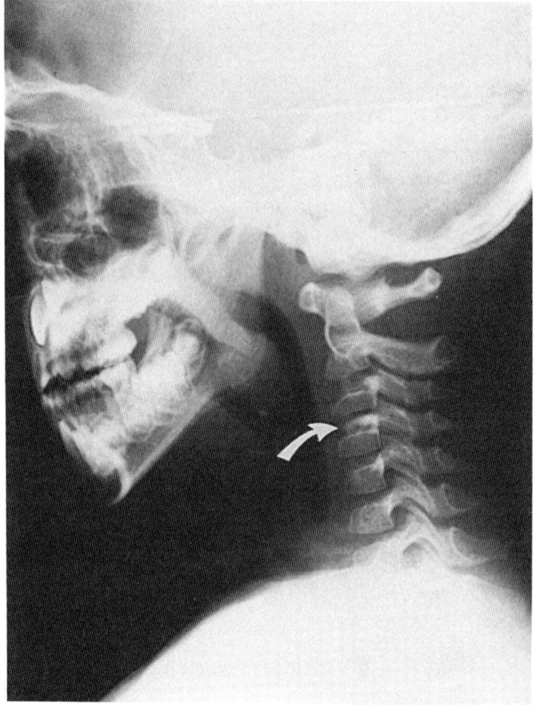

Figure 10.5.   Intervertebral disc calcification (*arrow*) in child.

within and emerge from the cervical vertebrae. Neoplasms generally seen within
the bony parts include osteoid osteoma, osteoblastoma, histiocytosis, aneurysmal
bone cyst, and hemangiomas (see Chapter 9). Obviously, definitive treatment
requires direct attention to the basic etiology of the torticollis.

Uncommon Causes of Torticollis

An assortment of conditions can secondarily induce torticollis, but occur so
infrequently as to warrant but a brief description. Of these uncommon causes,
burn scar contractures are probably the most common today. As a sequela of
third-degree burns in the region of the face and neck, contractures will often
develop within 2–6 months. These are very often relentlessly progressive and
accompanied by eventual soft tissue and bony deformities of the face and neck.
Comprehensive management includes surgical release of the contractures as
soon as the maturity of the cicatrix can be determined. Most often the results are
disappointing. Torticollis is a part of Turner syndrome and pterygium colli,
where the fascial band produces the torticollis.

Ocular disturbances in the form of strabismus may produce a vertical or oblique diplopia as the patient attempts to level his or her eyes. In an effort to
overcome the diplopia, the patient rotates the chin and, with time, this can result
in a postural type of torticollis. Bizarre twisting rotation of the head and neck on
the chest are not uncommonly seen in the extrapyramidal forms of central nervous system dysfunction, particularly the dystonias. Treatment is obviously directed toward control of the basic central nervous system problem.

Intervertebral disc calcification, although rare, is occasionally seen in the cervical spine of children (Fig. 10.5). Vascular channels within the disc space in children are believed to be the source of calcification. The etiology is obscure, but it is probably a nonspecific inflammatory process. The condition consists of neck pain and torticollis, usually in male patients under 10. The symptoms usually last one to two weeks but may persist for one to two years. The nucleus is the site of calcification, and more than one disc may calcify. As time passes, calcification occasionally persists but is more likely to disappear. The progress is generally good and conservative measures (traction, collar, appliances) are beneficial. Disc protrusion is rare.

Psychogenic torticollis can occasionally be seen as a manifestation of severe emotional disturbance. It can occur in the form of an "hysterical conversion reaction," where fixed head rotation on the chest is prevalent, or it may be a periodic phenomenon in the form of intermittent spasmodic episodes. Management is, of course, directed towards the primary etiology.

CONCLUSION

Wry neck is not unusual in a primary care practice. Using age at onset, appropriate examination, and x-rays it is usually easy to reach a quick diagnosis and plan appropriate treatment.

REFERENCES

1. Bratt HD and Menelaus MB: Benign paroxysmal torticollis of infancy. J Bone Joint Surg 74B: 449–451 (1992).
2. Canale ST, Griffin DW, and Hubbard CN: Congenital muscular torticollis. J Bone Joint Surg 64A:810–816 (1982).
3. Dolan KD: Developmental anomalies of C-spine below the axis. Radiol Clin N Am 15:167–175 (1977).
4. Dubousset MD: Torticollis in children caused by congenital anomalies of the atlas. J Bone Joint Surg 68A:178–188 (1986).
5. Ferkel RD, Westin GW, Dawson EG, and Oppenheim WL: Muscular torticollis. J Bone Joint Surg 65A:894–900 (1983).
6. Fielding JW and Hawkins RJ: Atlanto-axial rotary fixation. J Bone Joint Surg 59A:37–44 (1977).
7. Hensinger RN, Lang JR, and MacEwen GD: Klippel-Feil syndrome: a constellation of associated anomalies. J Bone Joint Surg 56A:1242–1253 (1974).
8. Hulbert KF: Congenital torticollis. J Bone Joint Surg 32B:50–59 (1950).
9. Ippolito E, Tudisco C, and Massobrio M: Long-term results of open sternocleidomastoid tenotomy for idiopathic muscular torticollis. J Bone Joint Surg 67A:30–38 (1985).
10. McRae DL: Bony abnormalities in the region of the foramen magnum: correlation of the anatomic and neurologic findings. Acta Radiol 40:335–354 (1953).
11. Morrison DL and MacEwen GD: Congenital muscular torticollis: observations regarding clinical findings, associated conditions, and results of treatment. J Pediatr Orthop 2:500–505 (1982).
12. Phillips WA and Hensinger RN: The management of rotatory atlanto-axial subluxation of children. J Bone Joint Surg 71A:664–668 (1989).
13. Steel HH: Anatomical and mechanical considerations of the atlanto-axial articulations. J Bone Joint Surg 50A:1481–1482 (1968).

Shoulder Pain

11

Anatomy and Biomechanics of the Shoulder Joint

*"A blind man works on wood in the same way as a surgeon
on the body when he is ignorant of anatomy."*
—Chirurigca Magna

In order to understand the loss of function associated with progressive degenerative changes in the shoulder joint, it is necessary to have a clear concept of the anatomy of the shoulder. Detailed studies on the integration of movement of all the components of the "shoulder girdle complex" have been undertaken by many investigators, notably Codman (2), and later by Inman, Saunders, and Abbott (5). As Sir Ashley Cooper (3) stated in 1832 in his preface to *A Treatise on Dislocation and Fractures of Joints*, "I should feel that I was not properly discharging my duty if I omitted to avail myself of all the evidence which might be adduced from those, on whose respectable testimony, I could depend." In this chapter, we hope to summarize the clinically significant work on the anatomy and kinetics of the shoulder.

BONES

How many bones are there in the various joints about the shoulder? Would you believe only nine? Subtract ribs 2–7, which are part of the scapulothoracic joint, and you are down to three key bones: the clavicle, the scapula, and the humerus (Fig. 11.1).

SCAPULA

The scapula is notable for two reasons: its broad flat triangular shape, from which the four important rotator cuff mobilizing muscles of the shoulder joint arise (Fig. 11.2); and its prominences and edges, to which are attached muscles that move the scapula through a tremendous range (Fig. 11.3), contributing to the high degree of mobility of the human upper limb.

The most lateral aspect of the scapula contains the glenoid or proximal half of the shoulder joint (Fig. 11.1).

CLAVICLE

The clavicle (collar bone) is one of the most superficial bones in the body, strutting the gap between the sternum and the scapula. Without it, the scapulohumeral mechanism would collapse into the body and many shoulder muscles would lose their mechanical leverage.

The coracoclavicular ligaments divide the clavicle into a lateral fifth (or less) and a medial four-fifths (Fig. 11.4). More about these important stabilizers later.

252

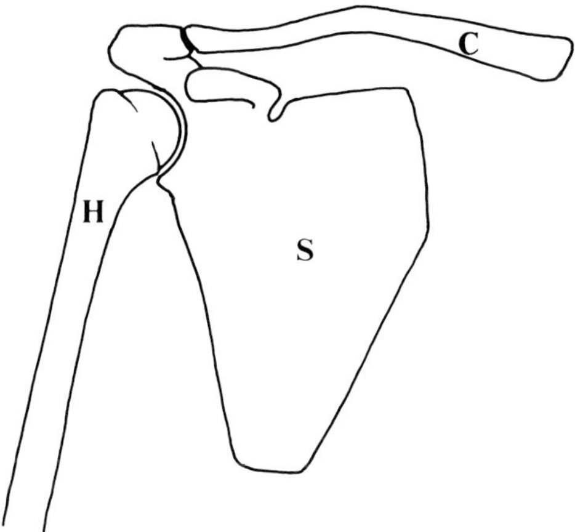

Figure 11.1.   The three major bones of the shoulder joint—the humerus (H), scapula (S), and clavicle (C).

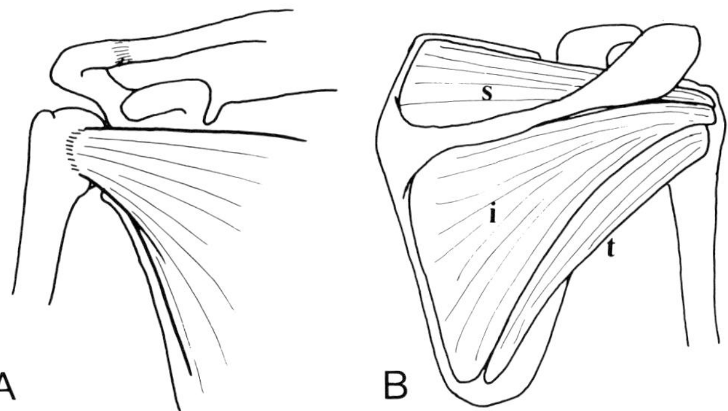

Figure 11.2.   The rotator cuff. (**A**) Anterior view of origin of subscapularis from scapula. (**B**) Posterior view of supraspinatus (s), infraspinatus (i), and teres minor (t).

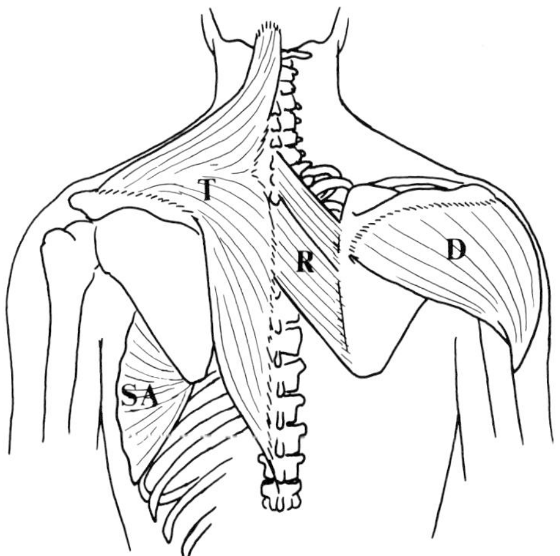

Figure 11.3.   The muscles that rotate the scapula: deltoid (D), rhomboids (R), trapezius (T), serratus anterior (SA).

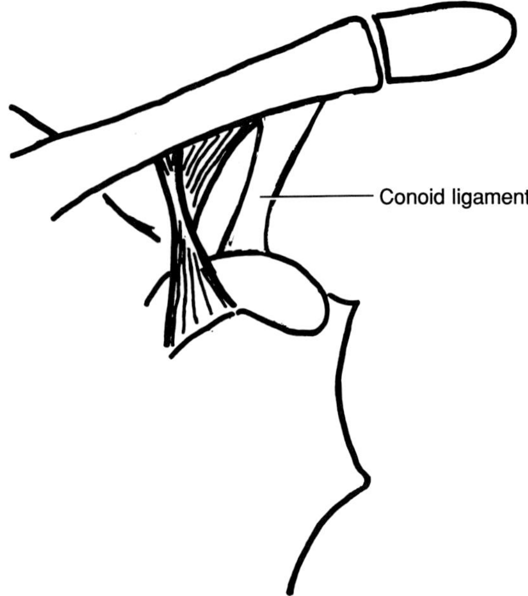

Figure 11.4.   The coracoacromial ligaments. The coracoclavicular ligaments. The conoid is labeled; the trapezoid ligament is unlabeled.

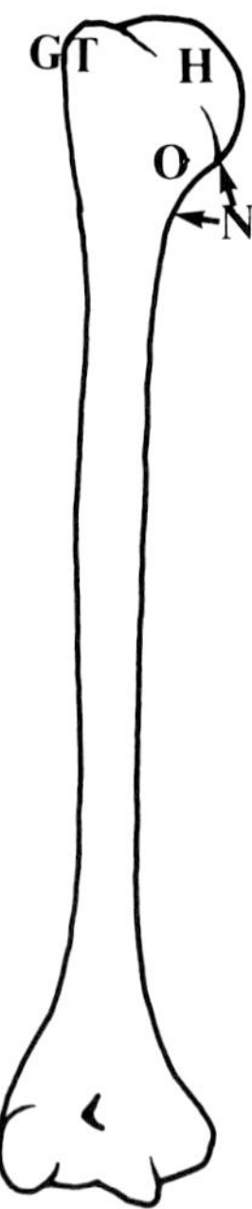

Figure 11.5.   The humeral head (H), neck (N), greater tuberosity (GT), and lesser tuberosity (O). The *upper arrow* points to the anatomical neck (the junction between the head and shaft). The *lower arrow* points to the surgical neck, where all the fractures occur.

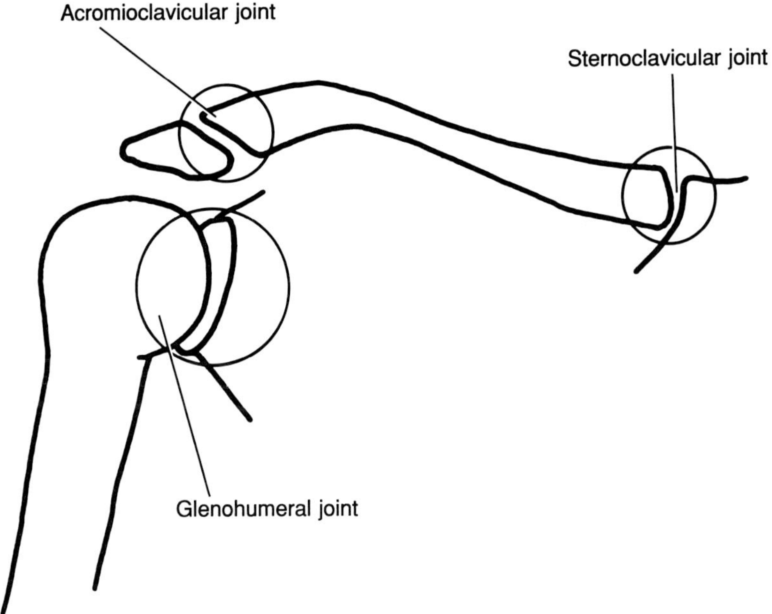

Figure 11.6.   Three of the four joints of the shoulder complex. Which one of the joints is not shown?

HUMERUS

Concentrating on the proximal part of the humerus, note the head, neck, greater tuberosity, and lesser tuberosity (Fig. 11.5). This is a bone with two necks!

Joints of the Shoulder Region

In strict anatomical terms, the shoulder joint consists of the glenohumeral articulation. However, from a practical, clinical point of view, the function of the shoulder depends on a complex of four articulations (Fig. 11.6): the glenohumeral joint, the acromioclavicular joint, the sternoclavicular joint, and the sliding "articulation" between the scapula and the thoracic wall, known as the scapulothoracic joint. The wide range of movement characteristic of the shoulder joint makes it the most mobile joint of the body, the result of the interaction of each of these components.

Glenohumeral Joint

The glenohumeral joint is a ball and socket joint in which the ball and socket are modified to allow a greater range of movement at the expense of intrinsic stability. Compare it to its lower extremity mate, the hip joint (Fig. 11.7). The humeral head is slightly greater than a third of a sphere and faces medially upward and posteriorly. It is retroverted about 40°. The glenoid fossa is shallow, pear-shaped in outline, and faces anterolaterally. Although the shallowness of the glenoid is slightly compensated for by the presence of a condensed fold of the capsule, known as the glenoid labrum, the articular surface is only one-half as

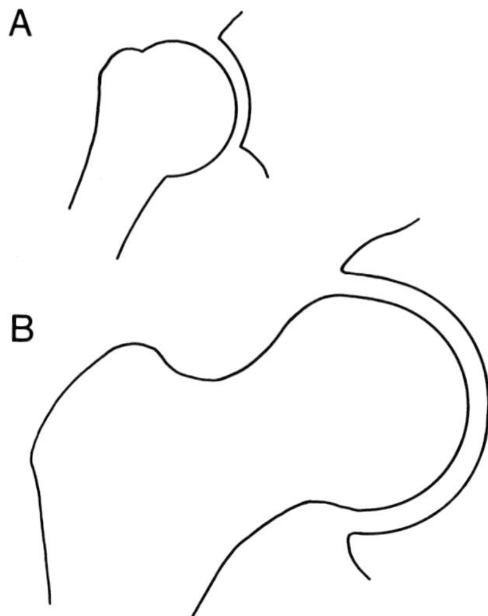

Figure 11.7.   The shallow shoulder joint articulation (**A**), with little inherent stability compared to the deep-set bony articulation of the hip joint (**B**).

long and one-third as broad as the corresponding articular surface of the humeral head.

There is a common misconception that the glenoid labrum is a triangular fibrocartilaginous ring acting like a "snap-fit" washer, maintaining contact between the humeral head and the glenoid. Detailed dissections have shown that the labrum has been the source of recurrent dislocations of the shoulder; in routine cadaveric dissection, it has been repeatedly noted that detachments of the anterior labrum are common in the elderly—an age when recurrent dislocations of the shoulder are excessively rare. It is also noteworthy that, in any anterior dislocation of the glenohumeral joint, the humeral head dislocates anterior to the glenoid labrum. It rarely passes through a tear between the labrum and the glenoid rim, although these conditions may coexist (1).

Capsule and Ligaments of the Shoulder Joint

The capsule is lined by the synovia, which has named prolongations (Fig. 11.8): one extending medially through the foramen of Weitbrecht, passing under the base of the coracoid to lie in front of the subscapularis; a second (infraspinatus bursa) lying inferiorly (Fig. 11.9), forming an important recess to accommodate the head of the humerus when the arm is fully abducted; and a third passing beneath the transverse humeral ligament, forming a synovial sheath for the emerging long head of the biceps in the fibro-osseous canal. It is important to realize that the long head of the biceps does not pass through the synovial cavity. It is extrasynovial, passing through the tube made by invagination of the synovial sheath.

The re-enforcing ligamentous structures are both capsular and extracapsular. The so-called capsular ligaments are really thickenings of the capsule forming the superior, middle, and inferior glenohumeral ligaments (Fig. 11.10). These ligaments extend from the glenoid lip to the lesser tuberosity of the humerus. Fur-

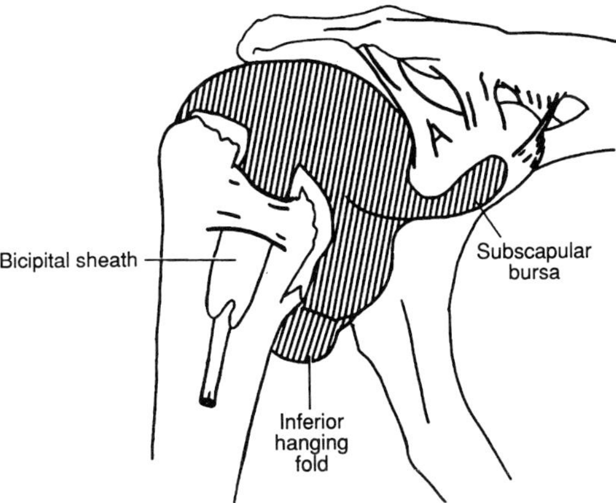

Figure 11.8. The synovial lining of the capsule with its extensions. The letter "*A*" is superimposed on the coracoid.

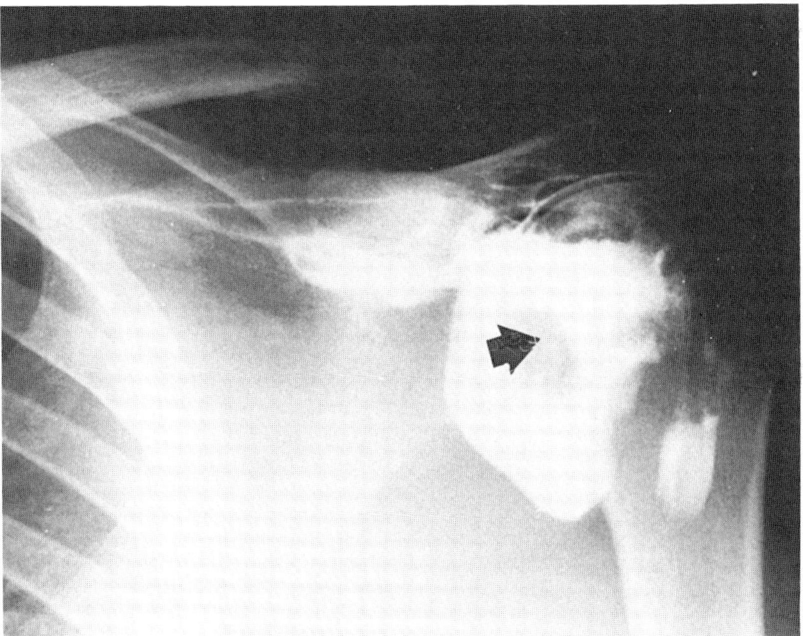

Figure 11.9. Normal shoulder arthrogram showing the subscapular bursa (*arrow*).

ther stability is contributed by the intracapsular portion of the long head of the biceps, which passes superiorly across the head of the humerus.

The coracohumeral ligament (Fig. 11.11) is attached to the lateral border of the coracoid process below the coracoacromial ligament and lies between the supraspinatus and the subscapularis, attached inferiorly to the greater and lesser tuberosities. It is a suspensory ligament. In some cases, it would appear to be a prolongation of the tendon of pectoralis minor and, in such instances, it passes between the two limbs of the coracoacromial ligament. This would be a confusing

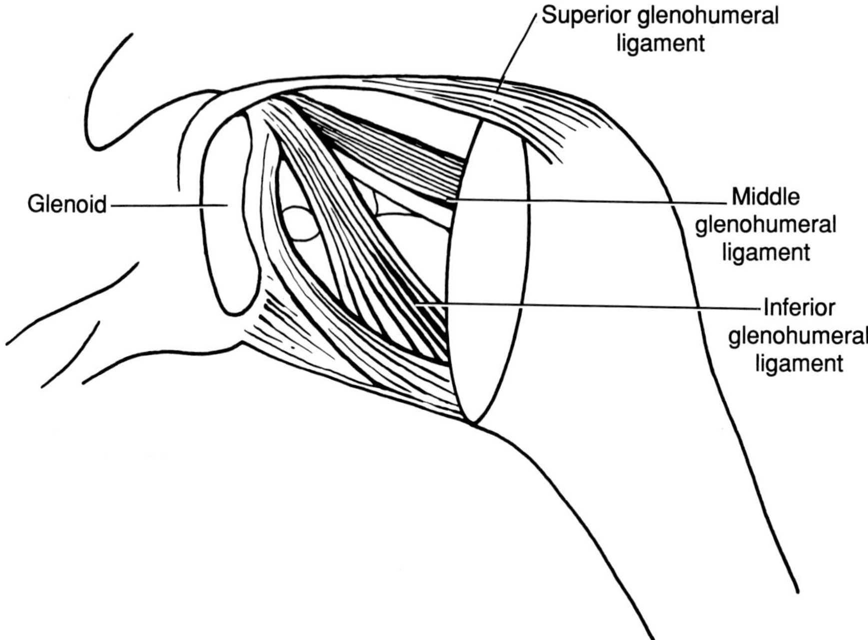

Figure 11.10.   The reinforcing ligamentous structures that contain the synovial lining.

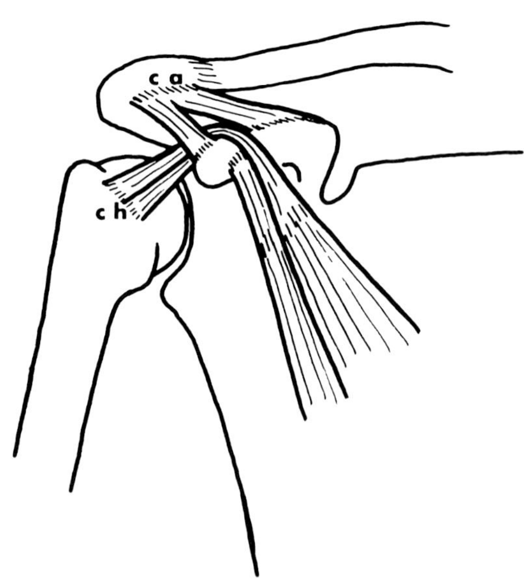

Figure 11.11.   The coracohumeral ligament (*ch*) and the coracoacromial (*ca*) ligament.

anatomical structure if found unexpectedly during the operative procedure of division of the coracoacromial ligament.

The coracoacromial ligament is a strong extracapsular ligament. Medially, it is attached by two arms to the lateral surface of the base of the coracoid and extends to the anteromedial aspect of the acromion. This ligament, with the coracoid and acromion process, forms the coracoacromial arch (Fig. 11.11). Its function has not been determined but it may resist forces tending to produce superior displacement of the humeral head. The supraspinatus tendon passes under the coracoacromial ligament to reach its point of insertion. Impingement of a degenerating rotator cuff against the sharp anterior edge of this ligament may be a source of shoulder discomfort (7). The pressure that can be produced by the knife-like edge of the ligament may be readily demonstrated if, on exposing the shoulder joint, the surgeon places the tip of his or her index finger under the coracoacromial ligament and an assistant then abducts the patient's shoulder. The pain that the surgeon will experience will be a constant reminder of this potential source of discomfort in patients with the so-called impingement syndrome.

Innervation Around the Shoulder Joint

By anatomical law (Hilton's), the nerves innervating muscles that exert action on a joint contribute to the innervation of that joint. The glenohumeral joint is, therefore, supplied by articular branches derived from the suprascapular nerve (supraspinatus and infraspinatus), the axillary nerve (teres minor and deltoid), the medial and lateral pectoral nerves (pectoralis minor), the musculocutaneous nerve (biceps and coracobrachialis), the radial nerve (triceps), and branches of that nerve to the subscapularis. The individual contributions vary widely and have a reciprocal relationship. After piercing the capsule, the nerve fibers form a plexus that can be roughly divided into superior, anterior, and posterior groups.

From a clinical point of view, the important nerves are the axillary nerve and the musculocutaneous nerve. The axillary nerve arises from the posterior cord of the brachial plexus and, in company with the posterior circumflex humeral vessels, exits from the axilla through the potential quadrangular space bounded by the teres minor, the long head of the triceps, the teres major, and the humerus. It passes around the surgical neck of the humerus. It is in this position that it can be damaged by anteroinferior dislocations of the glenohumeral joint (Fig. 11.12).

The musculocutaneous nerve arises from the lateral cord of the brachial plexus and, after coursing distally and laterally across the anterior wall of the axilla, it enters the body of the coracobrachialis approximately 2 cm or 3 cm distal to its origin from the coracoid process. In this part of its course, it is exposed to potential injury during deltopectoral approaches to the shoulder joint, especially if an osteotomy of the coracoid process is performed and the coracobrachialis is retracted distally, pulling with it the rough edge of the tip of the coracoid.

Blood Vessels Around the Shoulder Joint

The blood supply of the shoulder is of interest to the surgeon, not only because of the danger of damage to major vessels as a result of trauma but also because the profuse vascular bed and the anastomotic chain of blood vessels, on occasion, will cause a bloody mess during surgical exposure. It might, therefore, be of some help to describe the anatomical disposition of the major vessels and the surgically significant branches (Fig. 11.13).

The vessels encountered directly in the surgical exposure of the shoulder joint are those derived from the axillary artery. Of these, the acromiothoracic trunk,

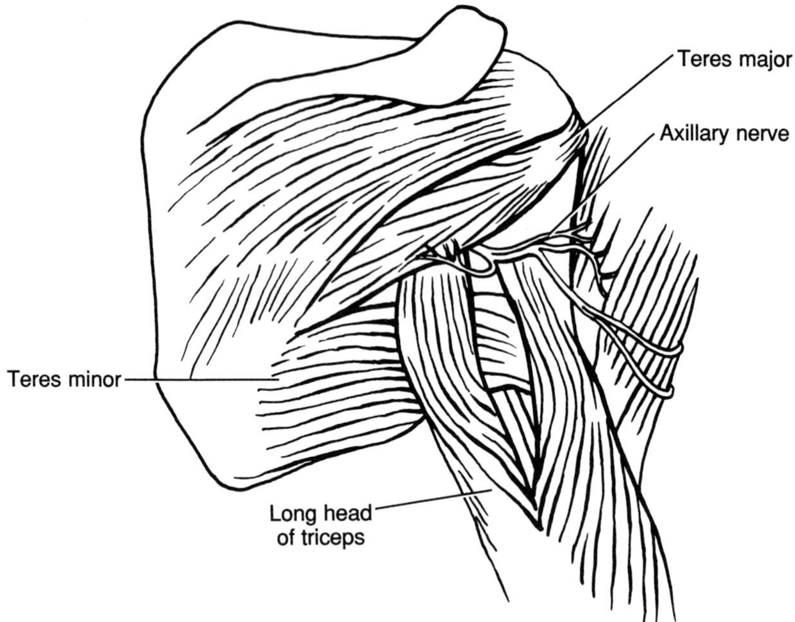

Figure 11.12. The axillary nerve and the posterior circumflex humeral artery exiting the axilla through the quadrangular space.

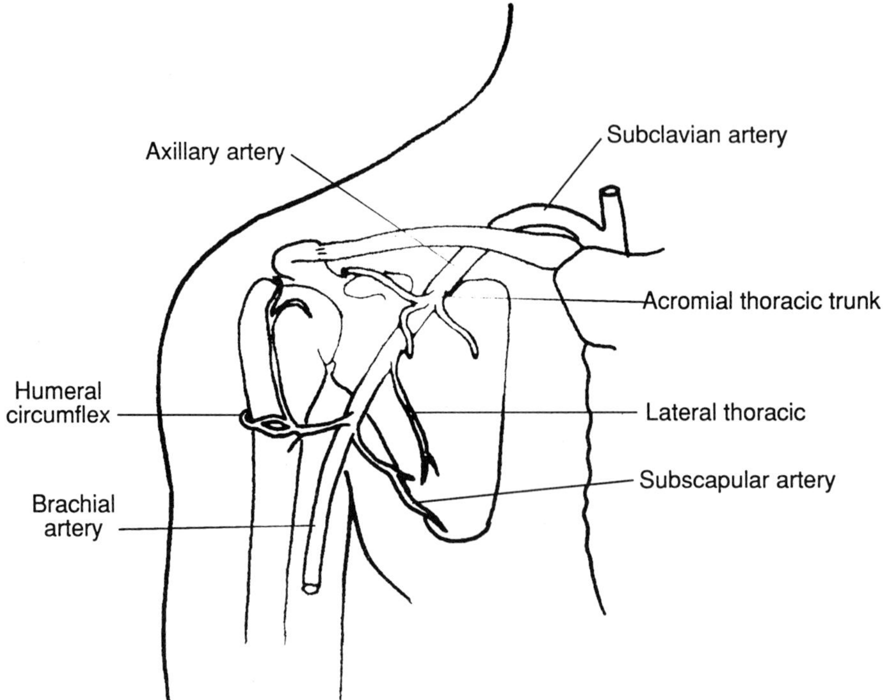

Figure 11.13. The major arteries and branches around the shoulder joint.

the anterior and posterior circumflex arteries, and the subscapular artery are the most important:

1. The acromiothoracic trunk arises at the medial border of the pectoralis minor and, after piercing the clavipectoral fascia, divides into four radiating branches: the pectoral, deltoid, acromial, and clavicular arteries. The branches of this trunk are responsible for the troublesome bleeding so commonly encountered in exposure of the medial portion of the attachment of the deltoid to the clavicle.
2. The posterior circumflex artery is larger than the anterior circumflex and leaves the axilla through the quadrangular space in company with the axillary nerve and passes around the neck of the humerus.
3. The subscapular artery is the largest branch of the axillary artery. It follows the lower border of the subscapularis to the medial wall of the axilla. Its presence in this region may come as an unpleasant surprise during mobilization of the subscapularis in the treatment of recurrent anterior dislocations of the shoulder. The surgical importance of the subscapular artery is that, by means of the anastomosis of the terminal branches of this vessel on the scapula and the chest wall, the first part of the subclavian artery and the third part of the axillary artery are placed in communication.

Some veins make useful landmarks. The cephalic vein delineates the deltopectoral groove (Fig. 11.14). Most surgeons try to preserve it, but frequently the decision to preserve it depends on whether the surgeon ties the vessel at the beginning of the operation or at the end! A constant leash of well-defined veins runs along the inferior border of the subscapularis (veins of Galen) (4) and is of great value in identifying the lower boundary of the muscle in operations requiring transection of the subscapularis.

Acromioclavicular Joint

The acromioclavicular joint is the articulation between the distal end of the clavicle and the scapula at the medial and anterior end of the acromial process. The plane of the articular surface is usually inclined from inferiorly and medially to superiorly and laterally, but shows considerable variation (Fig. 11.6). The acromial aspect usually faces upward and medially, whereas the clavicular aspect usually faces downward and laterally. This anatomical point is to be remembered when attempting to inject the acromioclavicular joint, whether diagnostically with local anesthetic or therapeutically with steroids.

The articular surfaces are separated by a small fibrocartilaginous meniscus which contributes to the stability of the joint by virtue of its attachment superiorly to the clavicle and inferiorly to the acromion, thereby restraining the tendency for the clavicle to rise superiorly and laterally over the acromion. With increasing age, the meniscus degenerates, and it is rarely functional after the fourth decade. Although the capsule of the acromioclavicular joint is relatively strong, the stability of the joint is dependent primarily on the conoid and trapezoid ligaments that pass from the coracoid process below, upward, and outward to the conoid and trapezoid tubercles on the undersurface of the outer one-fifth of the clavicle (Fig. 11.4). They are the main reins holding the clavicle in its normal relationship to the scapula.

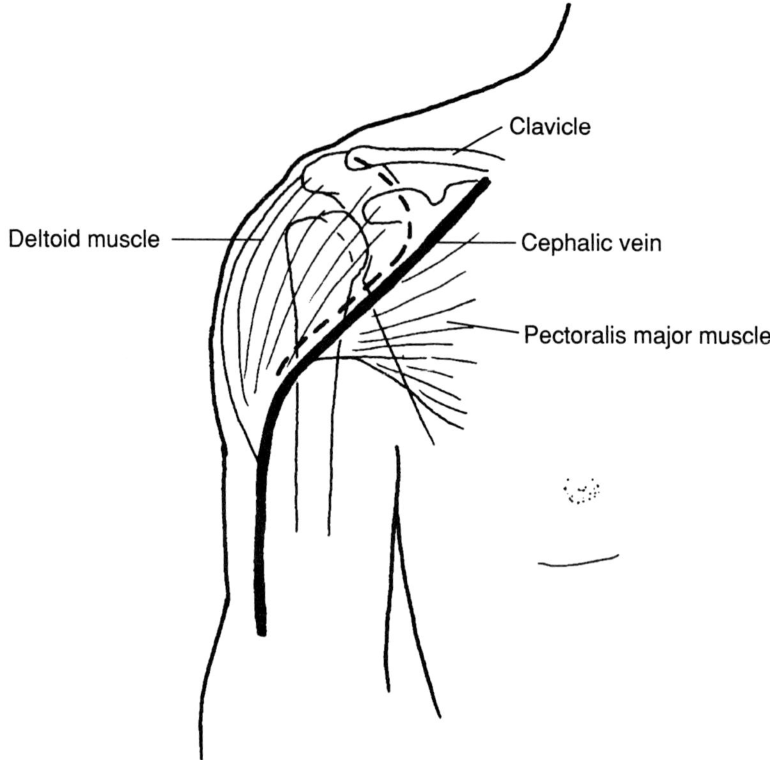

Figure 11.14. The cephalic vein divides the deltoid muscle (laterally) from the pectoralis muscle (medially). (The *broken line* is the usual deltopectoral skin incision.)

Sternoclavicular Joint

The sternoclavicular joint represents the only true articulation of the shoulder complex with the axial skeleton. The point of articulation is between the medial end of the clavicle and the manubrium sterni (Fig. 11.6). This joint also possesses an intra-articular disc which, by virtue of its attachment inferiorly to the manubrium and superiorly to the clavicle, resists superior displacement of the clavicle. Detachment of the intra-articular meniscus as a result of trauma may produce symptoms.

The joint has a strong fibrous capsule but is largely dependent for its stability on the strong costoclavicular ligament which passes from the inferior surface of the clavicle to the first rib. This ligament acts as a fulcrum around which the axis of rotation of the sternoclavicular joint occurs during elevation and depression of the shoulder. It is a crucial restraint that holds the medial end of the clavicle within the articular fossa of the manubrium sterni.

Scapulothoracic "Articulation"

This component of the shoulder girdle complex is an anatomical curiosity because it is an example of a bone that moves by simple displacement. It lies on the posterior thoracic wall and, by virtue of its muscle attachments (Fig. 11.3), can move in any direction, although only in one plane. The scapula is bound to the

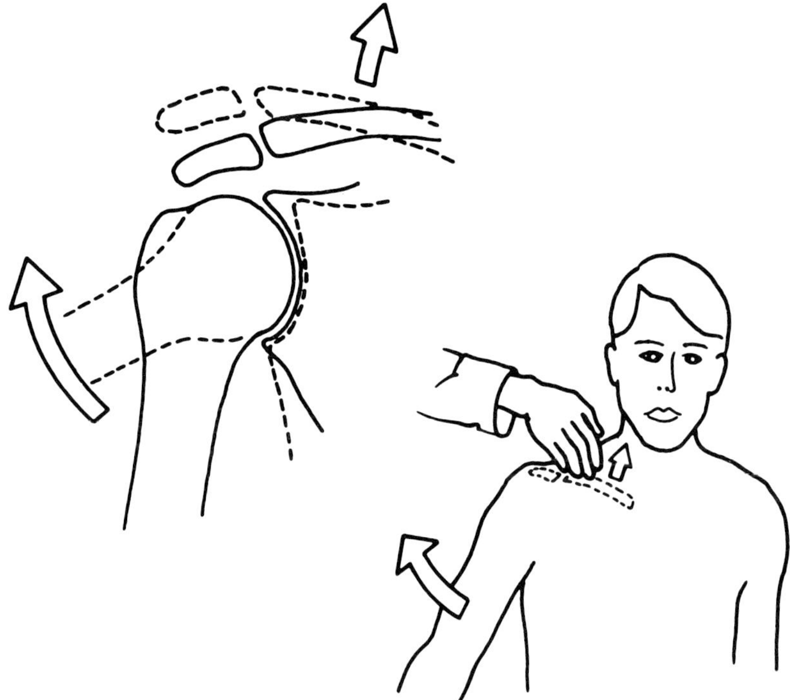

Figure 11.15.   Shoulder adduction puts a significant strain on the a-c joint, which can be palpated.

thoracic wall by extensive muscular attachments to all its borders, both processes, and both ventral and dorsal surfaces. The scapula is suspended from the axial skeleton by its attachment to the clavicle by the acromioclavicular and coracoclavicular ligaments.

Lesions involving the acromioclavicular joint will tend to restrict movement between the scapula and clavicle, and will thereby restrict the range of scapulothoracic glide. Conversely, when glenohumeral movement is restricted by any lesion, movements of the shoulder girdle as a whole are achieved by an excessive degree of scapulothoracic glide (6). This demands an increased range of movement of the acromioclavicular joint, which may lead to articular breakdown and painful degenerative changes (Fig. 11.15).

KINETICS

Biomechanics and kinetics are commonly regarded as tedious subjects. However, with the shoulder joint, the complex integration of movements may well provide us in later years with the key to the development and persistence of mechanically induced shoulder pain. In an attempt to stimulate your interest, let us remind you of Codman's paradox (Fig. 11.16) (2). Test Codman's observations on yourself. First of all, stand erect with the palms of your hands flat against the outer sides of your thighs. Now, without pronating or supinating the forearms, flex your arms forward 90° so that your palms are now facing one another. Now, without pronating or supinating your forearms, swing your arms backward, assuming the "spread eagle" position, with your palms facing forward. Finally,

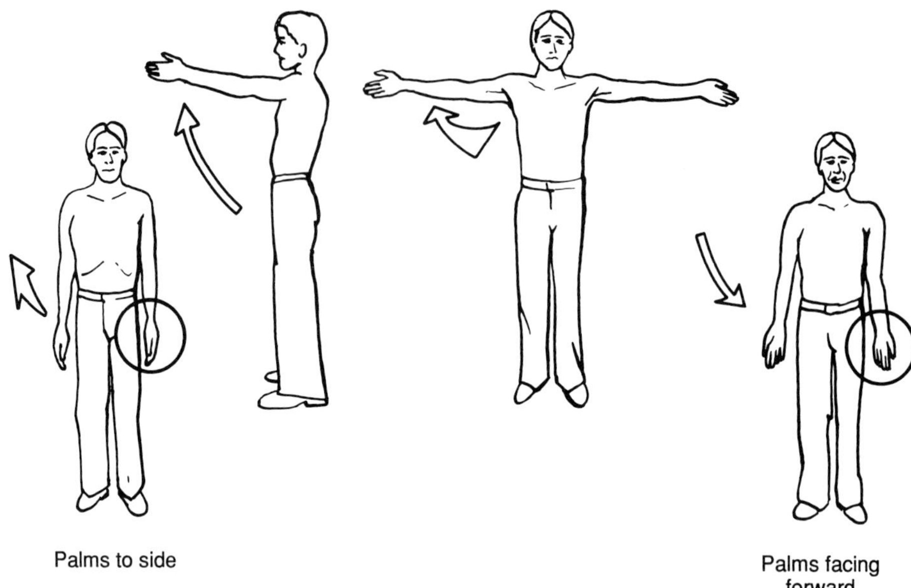

Figure 11.16.   Codman's paradox. See text for description of the exercise.

bring your arms slowly to your sides without pronating or supinating your fore-arms. You will find that the palms of your hands are now facing forwards. When you started this set of movements, they were flat against the sides of your legs. Your shoulder has rotated externally 90° in spite of your trying not to let it happen!

It would not be helpful to describe the multitude of experimental investigations that have been carried out analyzing the components of shoulder girdle movement. However, a brief description may be of help in the clinical evaluation of patients with restricted motion and decisions concerning the operative procedures that are indicated.

Movements of the Shoulder Girdle

Flexion and Extension

In an anatomical sense, these movements occur in the sagittal plane and range from 60° of extension to 180° of full flexion (Figs. 11.17 and 11.18). The movement occurs at the glenohumeral joint around the transverse axis and is combined with displacement of the scapula. Movement of forward flexion from 0°–60° may take place at the glenohumeral joint alone. From 60°–120°, glenohumeral movement is complemented by elevation and abduction of the scapula, thereby placing the glenoid in an upward and forward position. Although this is the theoretical sequence of movements, in actual fact the range of movement from 0°–120° involves a combination of glenohumeral and scapulothoracic movements from the onset, and they cannot be broken down in this simple manner. It should be noted that the articular surfaces of the acromioclavicular joint describe a crescentic configuration that allows the acromion to swing around the outer end of the clavicle during forward flexion and extension of the arm.

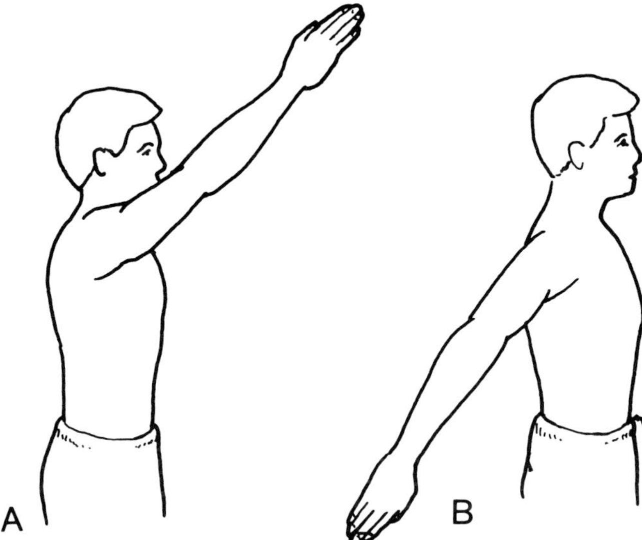

Figure 11.17.   Flexion (**A**) and extension (**B**) of the shoulder joint.

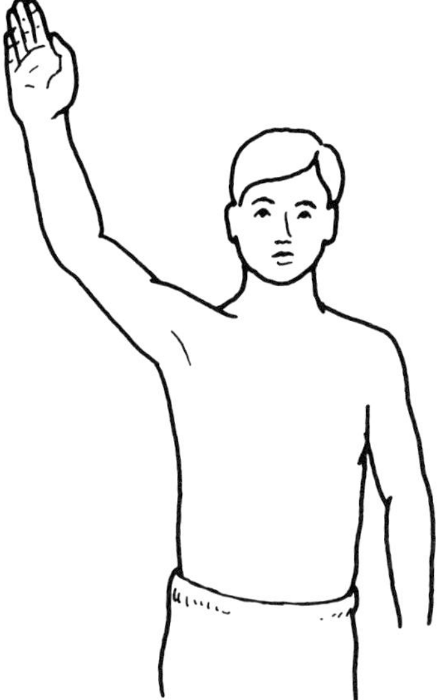

Figure 11.18.   Shoulder elevation, a range-of-movement exam favored by clinicians. It is predominantly abduction but occurs in a slightly flexed position.

From 120°–180°, all the muscles continue to rotate the scapula and elevate the humerus. The muscles are aided in the last few degrees of movement of forward flexion by contraction of the paraspinal muscles of the opposite side which, by producing a lateral flexion of the spine, elevate the point of the shoulder.

As the scapula glides forward, the clavicle must also glide forward and, indeed, during the full range of movement, the clavicle describes an arc of 35°–40° at its outer end along a horizontal plane. In addition to this, the clavicle moves vertically around the fulcrum formed by the costoclavicular ligament and, as it does, it rotates around its long axis.

When the arm is extended from neutral to the fully extended position, the range of movement is achieved by rotation at the glenohumeral joint carried out simultaneously with adduction and rotation of the scapula.

Rotation

The clinically permitted range of rotation of the shoulder is demonstrated in Figure 11.19*A*. External rotation would appear to take place exclusively at the glenohumeral joint. However, scapulothoracic glide plays a significant role in the amount of rotation that can be achieved. Starting from the military position (Fig. 11.19*B*), flex the elbows 90° and then externally rotate the forearms so that the palms are facing forward (Fig. 11.19*C*). The degree of outward rotation achieved is the clinical measure of external rotation. From this position, drop your hands to the side without allowing any rotation. You are now in the anatomical position and have just repeated Codman's paradox. Also note that external rotation is initiated by adducting the scapula and allowing it to glide backward so that the glenoid now faces laterally. External rotation is then initiated and controlled by the rotator cuff muscles, with the final 30°–40° achieved by maximally adducting the scapula, thereby permitting the glenoid to face posterolaterally. This combination of glenohumeral and scapulothoracic movement is found in reverse when the arm is taken from full external rotation to full internal rotation (Fig. 11.19*D*).

Abduction

This is the most important movement of the shoulder joint and, functionally, it almost always occurs with flexion (Fig. 11.18). Analyzing it as a separate movement from a position of maximum adduction (the anatomical/military position), the shoulder joint is moved by simultaneous abduction of the humerus at the glenohumeral joint and displacement of the upper tip of the scapula posteriorly toward the midline. From the neutral (military) position, abduction is initiated by contraction of the supraspinatus and other rotator cuff muscles (Fig. 11.20). The fixed glenohumeral joint then acts as a fulcrum for the action of the deltoid. Further abduction to 110° is achieved by the supraspinatus and the deltoid muscles combined with rotation of the scapula. Scapular rotation is produced by the action of the upper portion of the trapezius and the lower slips of the serratus anterior. The final 30° of abduction is assisted by inclination of the spine toward the opposite side.

The acromioclavicular joint is of vital importance because it permits the scapula to pivot around the outer end of the clavicle during the early and later stages of the abduction arc. This role is enhanced by the clavicle's rotation. This rotation functionally lengthens the coracoclavicular ligaments, thereby permitting greater motion between the clavicle and the acromion.

Let us now consider the action of the deltoid muscles. Contracting the deltoid alone will just pull the arm vertically until it abuts against the acromion. This type of translocation of the humerus is found in chronic ruptures of the supraspinatus tendon. For the deltoid to act as an abductor, the humeral head of the humerus must be held firmly against the glenoid by the rotator cuff, allowing the glenoid to act as a fulcrum of movement (Fig. 11.21).

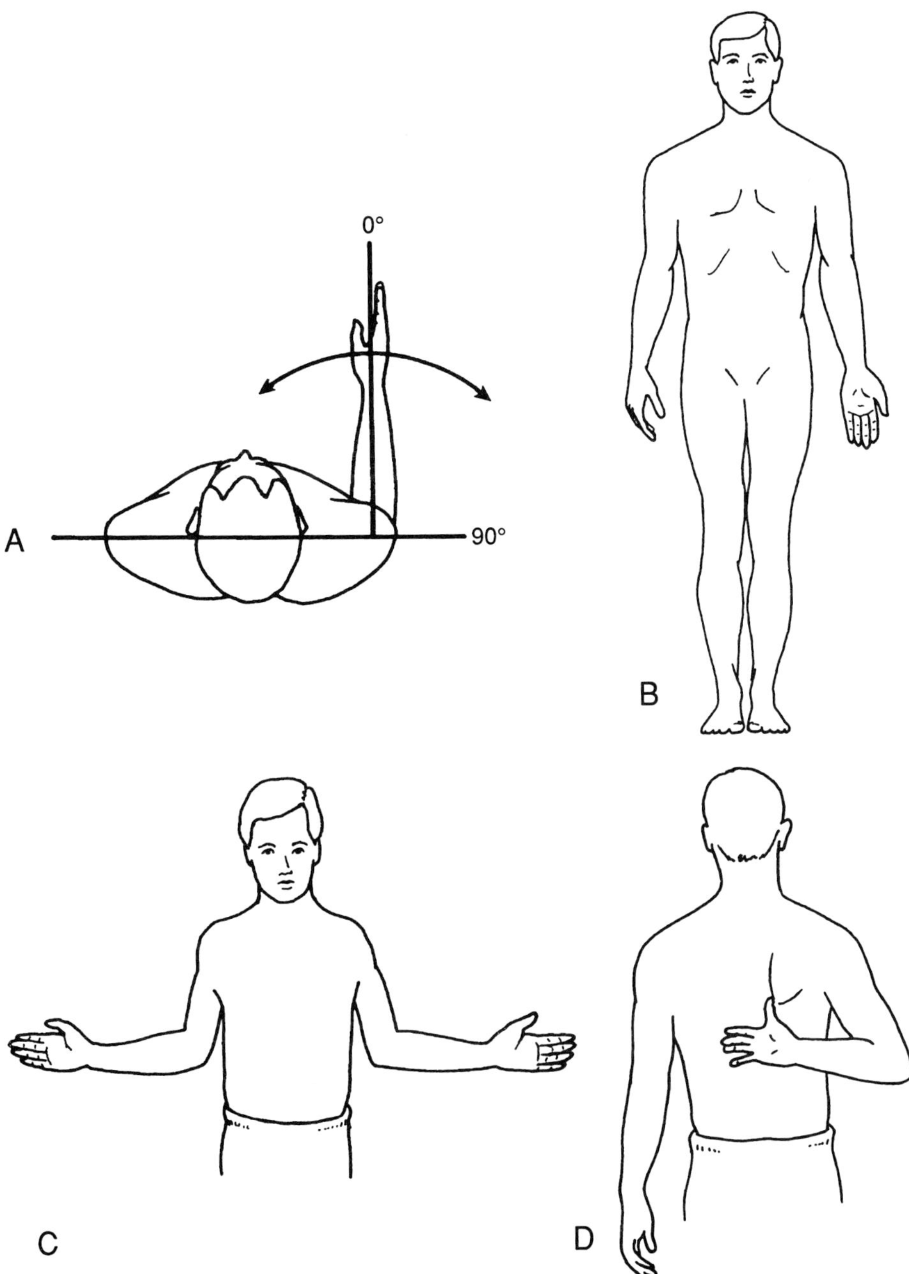

Figure 11.19.   **A,** internal and external rotation from 0°. **B,** The anatomical position—on the left the forearm and hand are supinated; the right forearm and hand are pronated and in the military position. **C,** external rotation from the military position. **D,** the range of internal rotation is described by how high the thumb can be placed up the spine, measured from the sacrum.

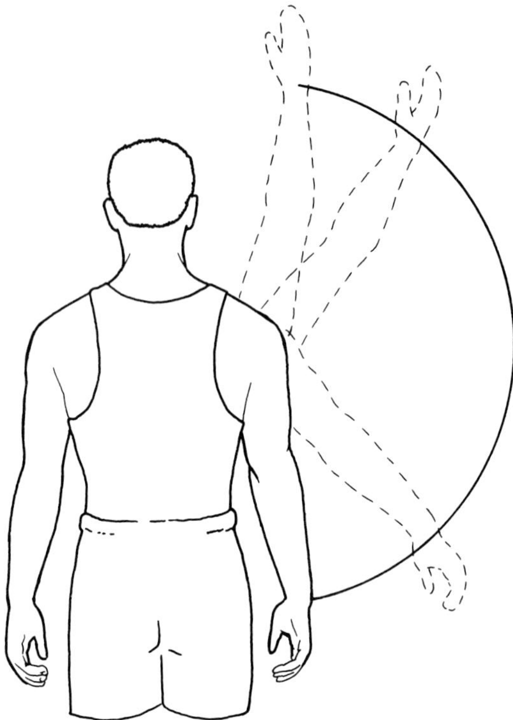

Figure 11.20.   Abduction from the military position. The lowest *broken line* represents about 45° of abduction, the highest 170° of abduction.

Even so, after the deltoid has abducted the humerus through 90°, the deltoid becomes relatively shortened with a subsequent marked decrease in its muscular efficiency. Scapular rotation will now restore the relative length of the deltoid and its muscular efficiency (Fig. 11.22).

At 90° of abduction, there are two further factors limiting movement. First, the greater tuberosity impinges against the acromion, blocking further glenohumeral movement. Second, the head of the humerus has nearly run out of articular cartilage. However, external rotation of the humerus will swing the greater tuberosity away from the acromion and restore articular contact (Fig. 11.23) (6). The infraspinatus is a powerful external rotator and of vital importance in abduction at the glenohumeral joint.

The long head of the biceps also plays an important role. On exposure of the long head of the biceps at operation, it can be seen that the tendon does not move in its groove on passive flexion and extension of the elbow or on pronation and supination of the forearm. Motion of the tendon in the bicipital groove occurs only on passive movement of the glenohumeral joint. On abduction and external rotation, the biceps tendon moves downward, with the result that the head of the humerus is depressed in relation to the glenoid.

When the supraspinatus is ruptured on contraction of the deltoid, the head of the humerus tends to be pulled vertically upward (Fig. 11.21*B*). This movement is resisted by the biceps tendon, and it is very interesting to note that, in long-

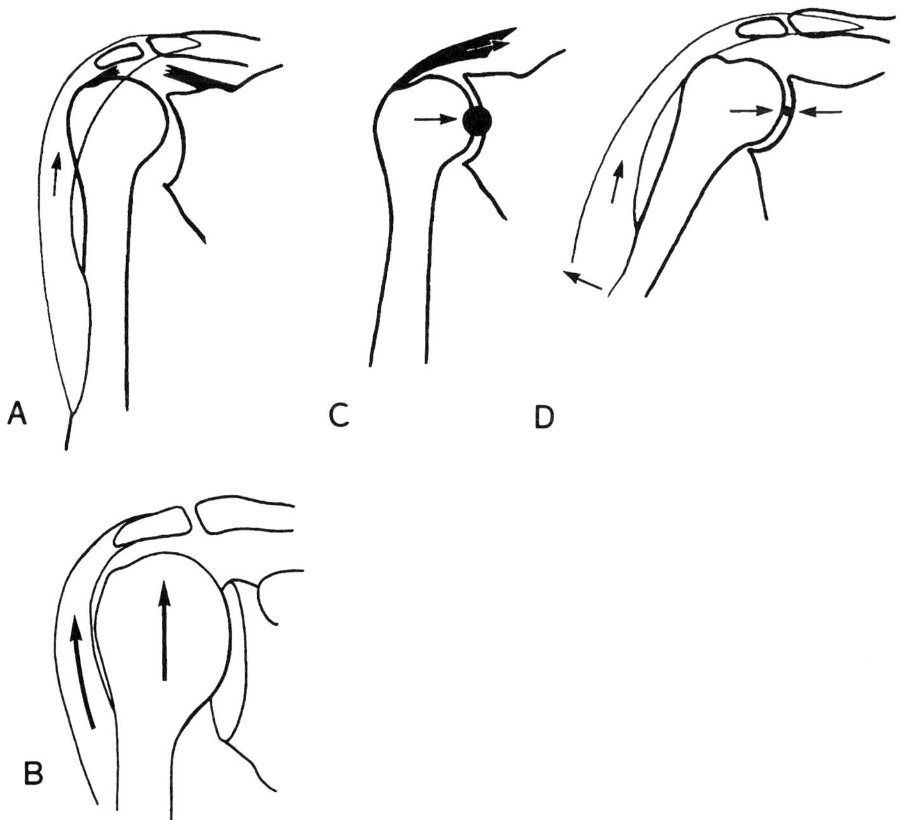

Figure 11.21.   A, torn rotator cuff; humeral head elevates during shoulder abduction. Complete tear of rotator cuff is shown in (**B**). With an intact rotator cuff (**C** and **D**) humeral head is firmly fixed in the glenoid for proper abduction of the shoulder.

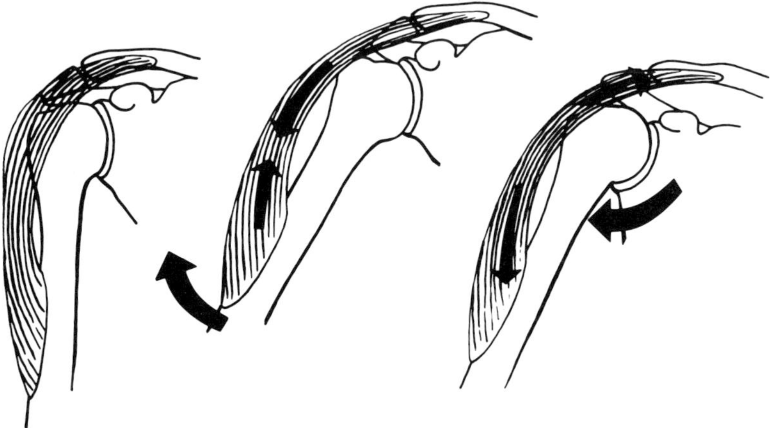

Figure 11.22.   Rotation of the scapula is an integral part of shoulder abduction.

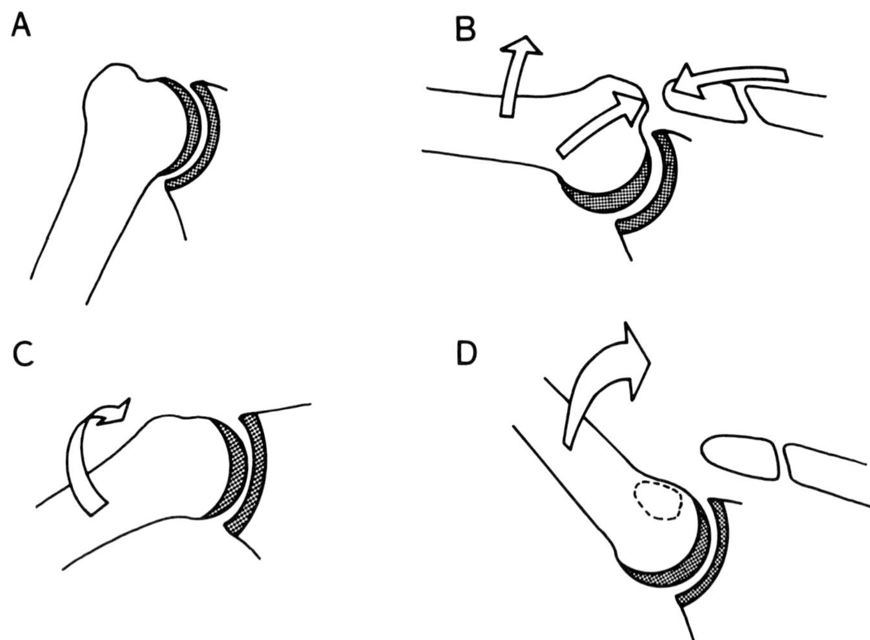

Figure 11.23.   Pure abduction from resting position (**A**) is hampered by the greater tuberosity impinging on the acromion (**B**), and compensated for by external rotation of the humerus (**C** and **D**).

standing ruptures of the supraspinatus, the biceps tendon is frequently flattened and is more than twice its normal width.

Inman, Saunders, and Abbott (5) have analyzed the role played of various articulations in the shoulder joint complex during the action of abduction. Their findings may be summarized as follows: during the initial 30°, the scapula moves into a position to provide stability for the glenohumeral joint—the so-called setting stage. Thereafter, glenohumeral and scapular motion hold a ratio of 2° of glenohumeral movement to every 1° of scapulothoracic movement. Movement at the sternoclavicular joint reaches its maximum in the 45°–90° range and diminishes from 90°–180°. It is estimated that, up to 90°, there are 4° of elevation of the clavicle for every 10° elevation of the arm.

Circumduction of the Shoulder

Although three basic movements of the glenohumeral joint—flexion/extension, abduction/adduction, internal/external rotation—have been described, movements around the shoulder girdle are more often than not a combination of basic movements (e.g., abduction and flexion to reach a high shelf). These combined movements, involving all the joints of the shoulder girdle, give the upper extremity of man a tremendous versatility.

Surgical Approaches to the Shoulder Joint

Anterior Approach

The classic surgical approach to the shoulder joint has been the anterior deltopectoral approach (Fig. 11.14). This exposes the subscapularis tendon, which can

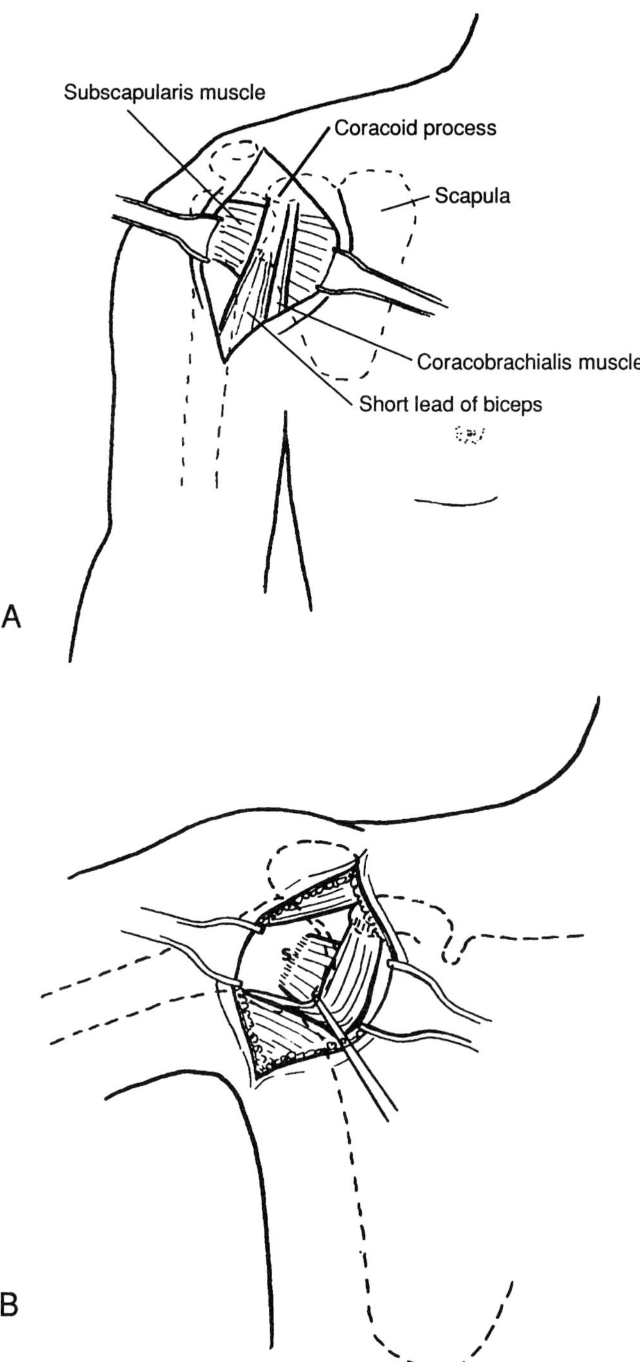

Figure 11.24.   A, after opening the deltopectoral groove, the coracoid process and the attached short head of biceps and coracobrachialis are seen. **B,** lateral to these muscles is the safe route to the subscapularis (*s*) muscle and joint capsule. Medial to these muscles lies the axillary/brachial artery and brachial plexus—a potential surgical disaster.

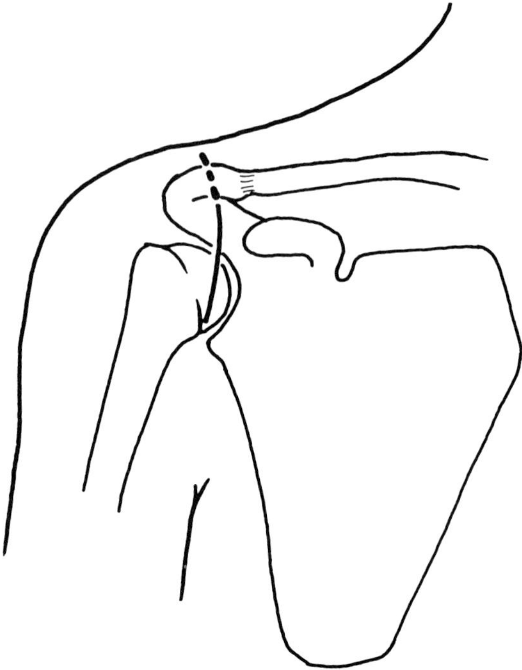

Figure 11.25.   The transdeltoid muscle splitting approach for impingement surgery. The incision can be extended to reach the a-c joint.

be transected to enter the shoulder joint (Fig. 11.24). This approach is usually used for anterior instability operations and total shoulder procedures.

Transdeltoid Approach

The classic approach and Neer's modification are shown in Figure 11.25. This approach is most useful for subacromial decompressions and/or rotator cuff repairs.

Posterior Approach

This approach is a little more difficult because the axillary nerve (Fig. 11.12) limits how much the deltoid can be retracted. The approach is used for posterior repairs (Fig. 11.26).

Axillary Approach

This is the most cosmetically acceptable approach (Fig. 11.27) but more tedious and less expansile than the deltopectoral approach.

CONCLUSION

Anatomy is the foundation of any clinical understanding, and it is the essential road map for successful surgical exposure.

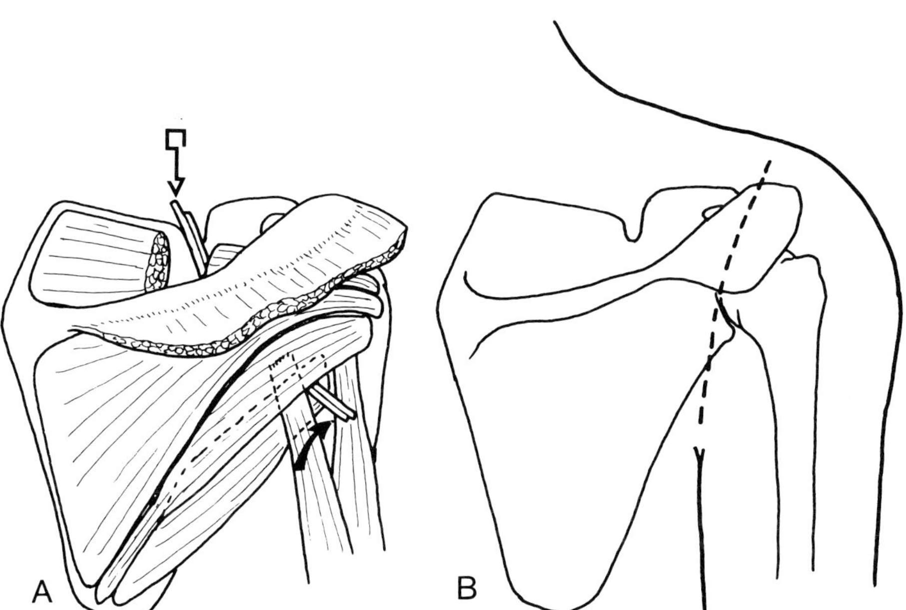

Figure 11.26. **A,** important anatomy when contemplating the posterior approach. Note the suprascapular nerve (*open arrow, top*) going deep to the supraspinatus and infraspinatus. Note the axillary nerve (*curved arrow*) exiting the axilla through the quadrangular space defined by the teres minor muscle superiorly and the teres major muscle inferiorly. From here it enters the deltoid and limits retraction of that muscle. **B,** the incision for the posterior approach. First, split the deltoid inferiorly no more than 4 cm from the acromion so that the muscle is not denervated. Second, find the interval between infraspinatus and teres minor. The posterior capsule of the shoulder joint can be exposed by elevating the infraspinatus from its inferior border or splitting the infraspinatus vertically or horizontally, staying lateral to the suprascapular nerve (Fig. 11.26*A*).

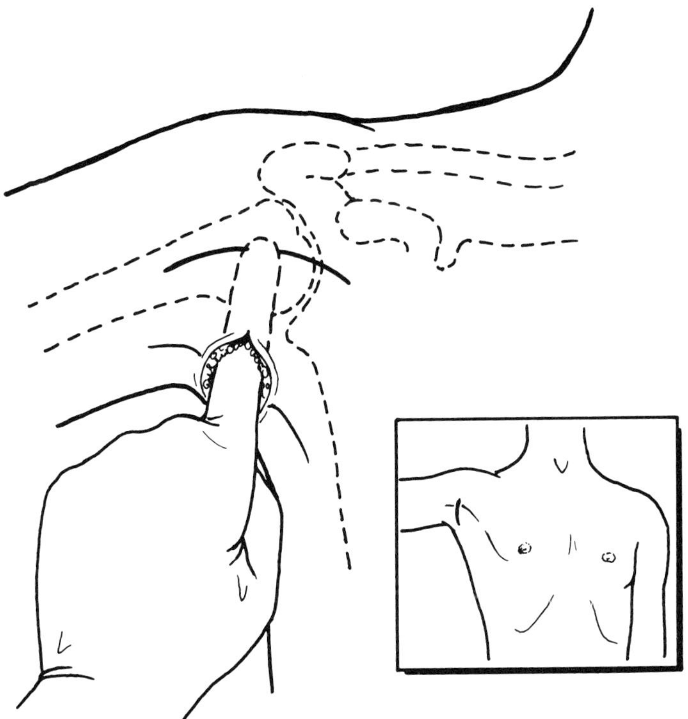

Figure 11.27. The incision for the axillary approach. From here the anatomy is the same as Figure 11.24.

REFERENCES

1. Bankart A: Recurrent or habitual dislocation of the shoulder joint. BMJ 2:1132–1133 (1923).
2. Codman EA: Rupture of the Supraspinatus Tendon and Other Lesions in or About the Subacromial Bursa. Thomas Todd Co., Boston (1934).
3. Cooper A: A Treatise on Dislocation and Fractures of Joints, 2nd American ed. from 6th London ed. Lilly, Wint, Carter and Hendee, Boston (1832).
4. Galenus: On the Usefulness of the Parts of the Body, vol. 2. Ed and trans: May MT. Cornell University Press, Ithaca, NY (1968).
5. Inman VT, Saunders JB, and Abbott LC: Observations of the function of the shoulder joint. J Bone Joint Surg 26A:1–30 (1944).
6. Macnab I: The Frozen Shoulder: Recent Advances in Orthopaedics. Churchill Livingstone, Edinburgh (1979).
7. Neer CS II: Anterior acromioplasty for the chronic impingement syndrome in the shoulder. A preliminary report. J Bone Joint Surg 54A:41–50 (1972).

12

Classification of Shoulder Disorders and Assessment of Shoulder Function

"Where a man feels pain; there is put his hand."
—Anonymous

CLASSIFICATION

Because shoulder lesions are so common, we will start with rotator cuff disorders (Table 12.1). Closely related to these are osteoarthritic conditions of the glenohumeral joints, which occur in the final stages of shoulder degeneration. There are also miscellaneous inflammatory and infective conditions of the glenohumeral joint.

Understanding instability is an ever-evolving part of shoulder dysfunction and is covered in Chapter 17. Finally, for completeness, injuries (fractures and dislocations) and tumors are included here. Consistent with the purpose of this book—written primarily for residents and primary care doctors trying to understand neck and shoulder disorders—this chapter is a summary. This book contains in-depth descriptions of neck disorders; it is also essential to have a clear understanding of shoulder disorders to adequately assess problems the reader will encounter.

ASSESSMENT OF SHOULDER FUNCTION
History

It can't be overemphasized: good old-fashioned history and physical examination yield more positive diagnoses than fancy investigations that lack specificity (a high yield of false-positives) and carry high costs.

There are two primary shoulder complaints:

1. Pain
2. Instability

Table 12.1. A Classification of Shoulder Disorders

1. Rotator cuff tendinitis, tears, and other soft tissue lesions
2. Osteoarthritic degeneration
3. Miscellaneous inflammatory conditions and infections
4. Instability syndromes
5. Injuries around the shoulder joint complex
   • Fractures and dislocations
6. Tumors around the shoulder

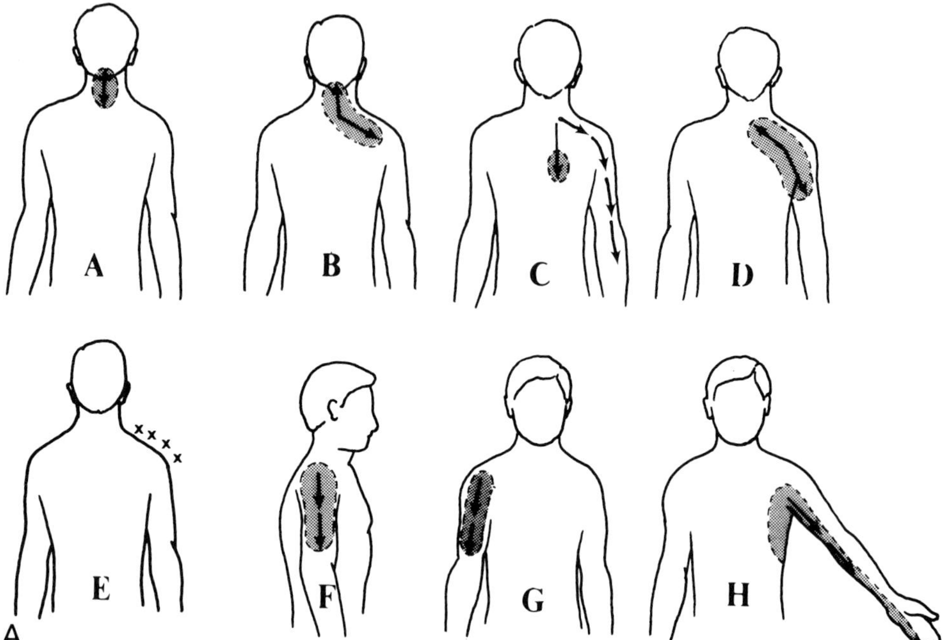

Figure 12.1.   A, location of pain about the neck and shoulder. Axial neck (**A**). Axial neck and referred shoulder (**B**). Neck—radicular and parascapular (**C**). Shoulder—with proximal referral (**D**). Acromioclavicular joint (**E**). Shoulder (**F**). Shoulder (**G**). Lower brachial plexus lesions (**H**).

Sometimes it is hard to distinguish between the two. Secondary symptoms, such as stiffness, clicking, and weakness are also common when taking the history.

If pain is the major complaint, standard questions regarding location (Fig. 12.1), type, onset, duration, aggravation, relief, and response to treatment are documented. The pattern of nighttime pain needs to be established, an important clue to rotator cuff problems and frozen shoulder.

Instability is more difficult to assess. A young man with a previous traumatic dislocation from a football injury may readily say, "My shoulder goes out," when he is in the abducted, externally rotated position. This is obvious instability. More difficult are patients with no history of injury, and who, because of overuse or joint laxity, have a subluxating shoulder associated with pain. If possible, the direction of instability (anterior, posterior, or multidirectional) should be determined, along with the position of the arm when the sudden sensation of subluxation ("dead arm") occurs.

A Word About Psychogenic Pain

Throughout this text, nonorganic or psychogenic pain is frequently mentioned. For good reason! So many patients, especially patients in motor vehicle accidents and other insurance settings, have a nonphysical component to their disability that is easily missed.

First of all, you must remember that you are treating a patient and not a disease. Coventry (2) has pointed out that certain patients, particularly those

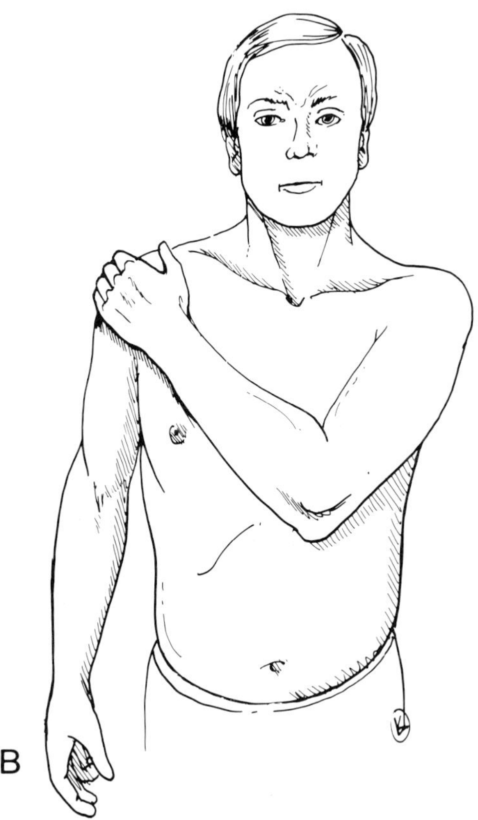

Figure 12.1.   B, with his hand, patient shows the typical location of pain for conditions within the shoulder (glenohumeral) joint.

with diffuse capsulitis, have what he termed a "periarthritic personality." Many of these patients are timid, have a low pain threshold, and are terrified to do anything that may produce pain. These traits may prolong their symptoms.

Characteristically, they relate their history as someone struggling to remember a dream. They may present the clinical signs commonly seen in patients with a psychogenic magnification of disability—most frequently, tenderness on lightly pinching the skin. This is a trap for unwary clinicians, whose fingers prod too deeply before they explore the possibility of skin tenderness. No statement can be made about the significance of deep tenderness in the presence of superficial skin tenderness.

Over the area of maximum pain, these patients may show areas of hypoesthesia to pinprick—a condition known as anesthesia dolorosa. Other areas of hypoesthesia may cross anatomical dermatomal boundaries. These patients demonstrate discrepant motor weakness, that is, they have greater weakness on initiating a movement than on maintaining it. They frequently have dissociated weakness—weakness remote from the damaged area (7).

This type of response is found in hysterical states and in depression. The clinician must be careful to distinguish between a patient with hysterical personality who reacts "hysterically" to any pain and the more seriously ill patient with a psychogenic magnification of disability, hysterical in nature. The depressed patient is not sad or disconsolate—the overriding response is concealed or overt anger. Characteristically, these depressed patients find they are more easily provoked to anger or tears, and they tend to vent their spleen on those closest and dearest to them—even the dog. They feel tired all the time, and they awaken early in the morning. Sleep does not refresh them. They do not want to go out and they hate staying in. All in all, they have lost their sense of fun. If such patients develop a painful lesion, it is very easy and understandable for them to attribute their inability to succeed to the pain from which they are suffering.

It must be remembered that there are no words in the English language that describe pain. Patients, therefore, seek medical advice because of the disability caused by the pain. For example, the patient may say, "I cannot do the vacuum cleaning because of the pain in my shoulder; I cannot make the beds; I cannot carry in the groceries." They are not describing the pain—they are describing their reaction to the pain, and a patient's reaction to any pain varies enormously, according to his or her emotional state. Occasionally, the pain is less noticeable because of an emotional event. For example, one can imagine a farmer walking home across the fields; he sprains his ankle severely by stepping in a gopher hole. He continues home, limping badly. Suddenly, a bull appears in the meadow and the farmer starts to run without any limp. What has changed? Has the pain changed or has the farmer changed? Unfortunately, most emotional stresses and breakdowns usually have the reverse effect. In better emotional health, such patients would probably not seek medical attention, but because of an uncontrollable breakdown in their emotional strength, the pain becomes devastating and prevents them from carrying on the normal activities of daily living.

Pain and disability are synonymous. A patient with marked psychogenic magnification of disability will not benefit from physical or drug therapy directed solely at the lesion from which he or she is suffering. The anxious patient needs reassurance as much, if not more than, drugs. Depressed patients are difficult to manage, and psychotropic drugs must be carefully titrated against the patient's need by someone skilled in the drug's use.

Assess the patient first. With a clear picture of the patient who has pain, the clinician can then spend time considering the pain the patient has. Because changes in the cervical spine are a common source of pain in the shoulder, special attention must always be given to examination of the neck, a topic dominating Chapters 1–10.

Examination

There are basically three parts to the examination of the shoulder—look, feel, and move. Obviously it is essential to look at the patient's general health and carefully assess the neck. For now, let us confine our discussion to the shoulder joint.

Inspection

Most importantly, compare the two shoulders for symmetry. Start by looking for roundness or fullness of the shoulder. Roundness is lost with an anterior dislocation or atrophy of the deltoid (Fig. 12.2). Atrophy of the supraspinatus and infraspinatus will leave hollows in the supraspinatus and infraspinatus fossae

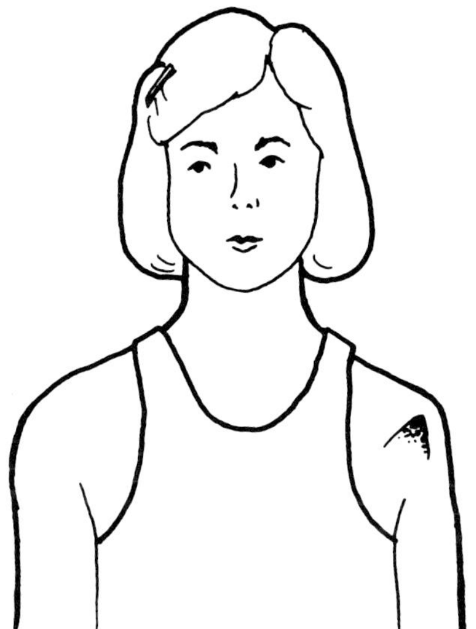

Figure 12.2. Loss of deltoid fullness (*left*) due to dislocation of shoulder.

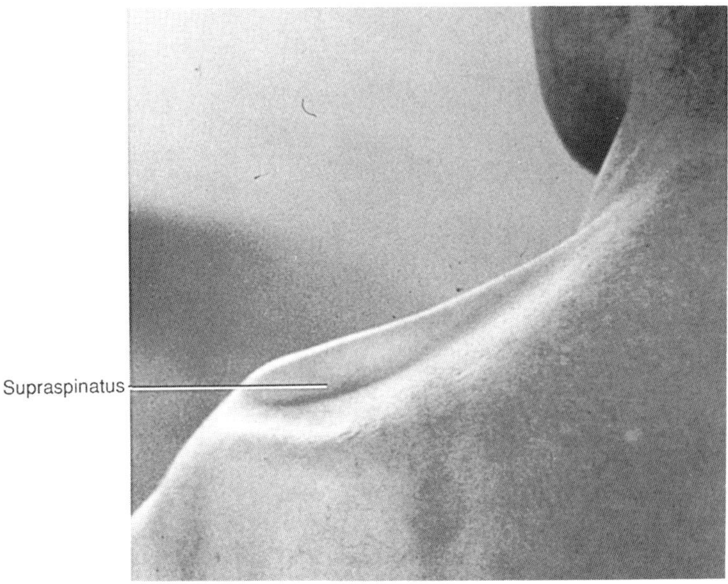

Figure 12.3. Significant wasting of the supraspinatus muscle, left shoulder (note fullness of supraspinatus region left in Figure 12.4).

(Fig. 12.3). Muscle weakness is sometimes detected as easily on inspection as on specific testing.

Rhomboid weakness does not permit such a marked winging of the scapula as do weakness of the trapezius or serratus anterior (Fig. 12.4). Trapezius paralysis allows the scapula to migrate downward and outward, whereas serratus anterior palsy permits migration of the scapula upward and inward. With marked weak-

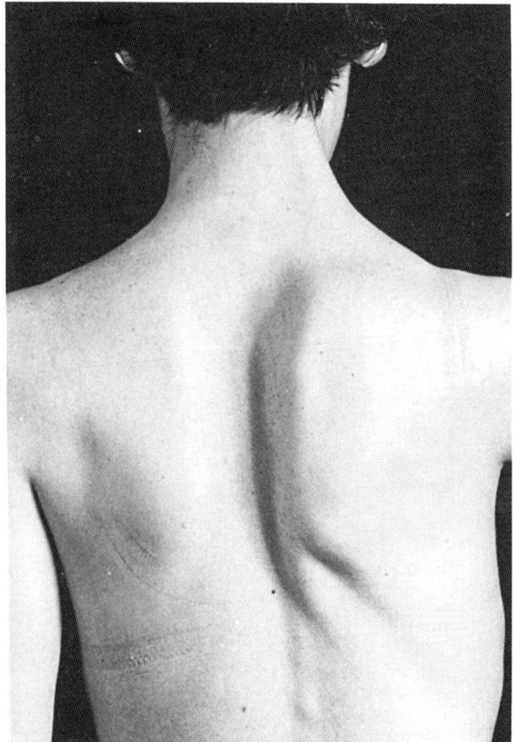

Figure 12.4. Winging of the right scapula evident with the patient pushing with the right arm. Because of its paralysis, the serratus anterior cannot keep the scapula flat to the thorax.

ness of the serratus anterior, the shoulder girdle can be passively lifted so that the acromion is at a level opposite the patient's chin—the so-called loose shoulder. A prominent outer edge of clavicle suggests a dislocation of the a-c joint.

Palpation

On palpation, the most important finding is the demonstration of tenderness, its location, and its type. The presence of superficial tenderness elicited by pinching the skin lightly should be determined first. After this, feel for bony subluxations at the sternoclavicular and acromioclavicular joints, and their associated tenderness. Next, palpate deeply for rotator cuff tenderness, felt at the anterior edge of the acromion with the shoulder extended. Also palpate for biceps tendon tenderness.

There are several zones of nonspecific tenderness constantly present around the shoulder girdle—areas of "myotatic irritability": the trapezius, the superomedial border of the scapula, the insertion of the deltoid, and the tip of the coracoid process (Fig. 12.5).

These areas are tender in everyone, but become more tender in the presence of any painful lesion in the neck. They have no significant localizing value whatsoever, and indeed their presence may be confusing. Pain referred from the C5-C6 segment will be associated with tenderness on squeezing the pectoralis major or on pressure over the points of origin of the pectoralis major from the rib cage.

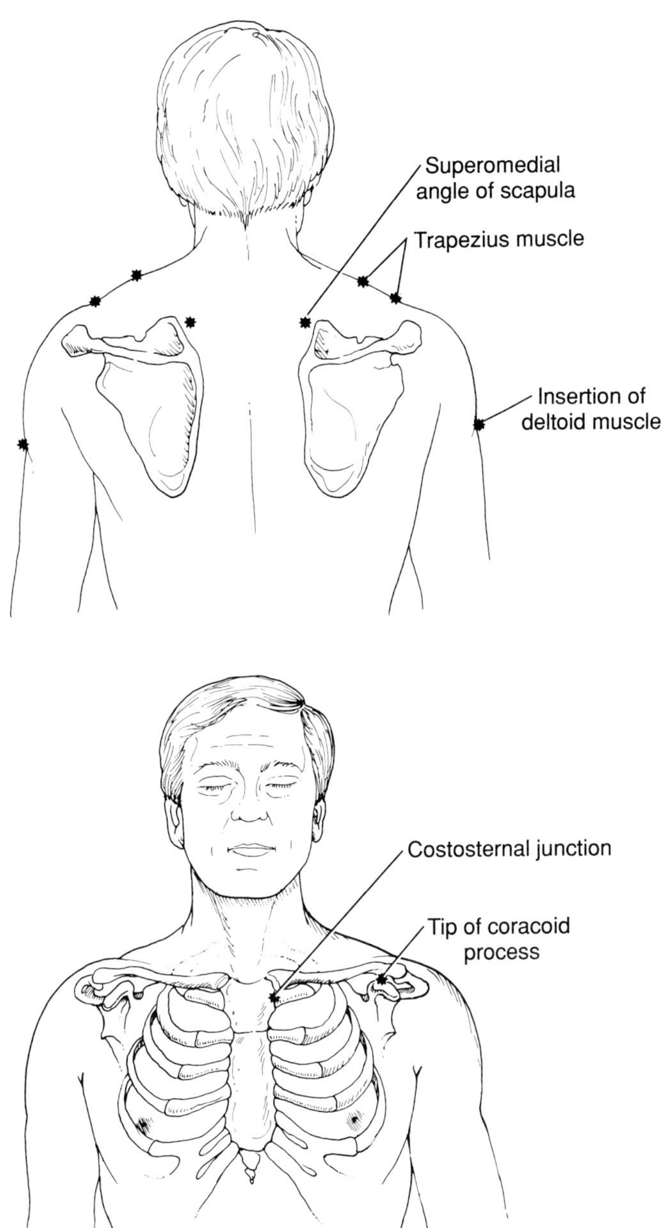

Figure 12.5.   Areas of "myotactic irritability"—sometimes called trigger points if excessively tender. Be sure that simply palpating the skin in these areas does not demonstrate superficial tenderness.

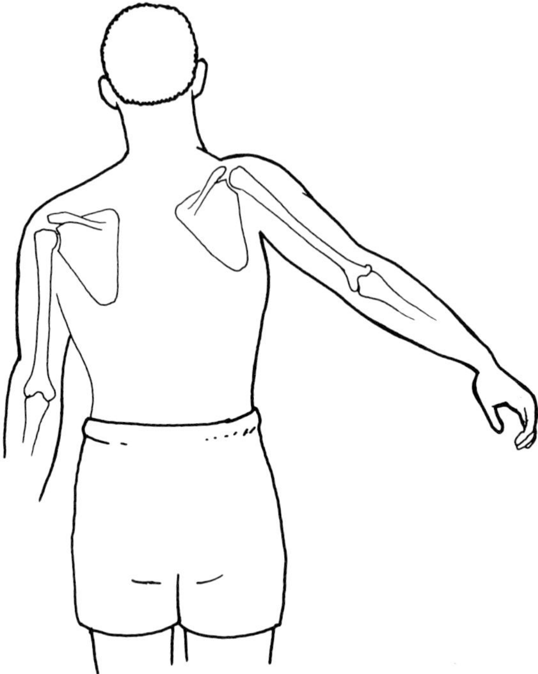

Figure 12.6. Watch not only the degree of abduction but also synchrony. During normal abduction, the scapula moves late; with a rotator cuff tear, active abduction most likely will start with a "shrug" as the deltoid pulls the humerus up into the acromion, followed by limited abduction of the arm and scapula as one unit.

This referred tenderness may mimic costochondritis (Tietze syndrome). Tenderness may be elicited on squeezing the biceps muscle belly. The triceps are tender on pressure when there is a painful lesion involving the C6-C7 segment (the C7 root).

Movements

Both active and passive movements need to be assessed. Active movements of the shoulder may be viewed when the patient is removing his or her shirt. More specifically, overall elevation (Fig. 11.18) and the synchrony of abduction should be determined (Fig. 12.6).

Next on the list is the passive ROM determination for flexion-extension, abduction, and internal/external rotation. The scapulothoracic component of these movements is most easily detected if the examiner stands in front of the patient and places two fingers on the patient's clavicle. As soon as the clavicle moves, the scapula is gliding. Although there is some academic significance in the differentiation of glenohumeral and scapulothoracic movement, from a practical point of view the movement to be recorded is the combined movement.

When assessing forward flexion, the forearm may be supinated or pronated (Fig. 11.17).

Active abduction is measured from the side; the patient externally rotates the shoulder and attempts to touch the ceiling with his or her fingertips (Fig. 11.20 and Fig 12.6).

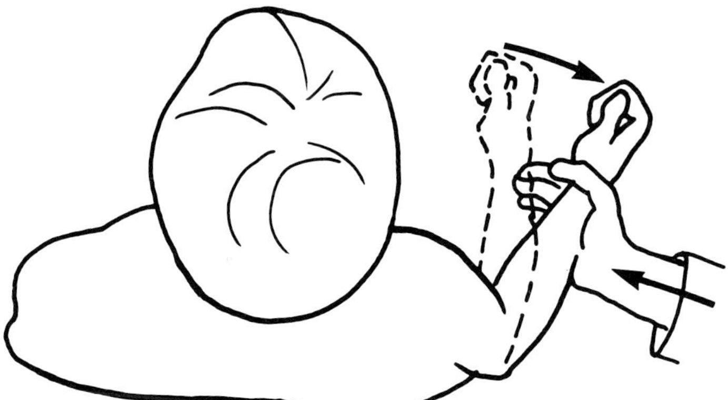

Figure 12.7.   Testing external rotation strength.

External rotation may be difficult to assess accurately because the patient tends to take his or her arm away from the side. The examiner must hold the patient's arm against the chest wall. External rotation can also be assessed with the shoulder abducted to 90°. At this stage of examination, the strength of the external rotators must be assessed to determine the possibility of a rotator cuff tear (Fig. 12.7).

As suggested by Neer and Welsh (4), internal rotation is best recorded by noting the relationship of the tip of the patient's thumb to his hip or lumbar spine (Fig. 12.8).

Above all, an accurate record must be kept, detailing the results of the evaluation of the shoulder function.

Weakness.   Weakness (and associated wasting) will be tested as part of a neurological exam. However, problems intrinsic to the shoulder joint may cause weakness in flexion (palm-up test for bicipital tendinitis, Fig. 12.9), and abduction/internal rotation (in rotator cuff disorders, Fig. 12.10).

Instability Tests.   It is important to decide, in the face of "giving way" or instability complaints, the direction of instability. This can be anterior, posterior, or inferior. Also be aware of the patient with multidirectional instability. The classic instability or "apprehension" test is for anterior shoulder subluxations (Fig. 12.11). Other tests for posterior instability and inferior instability are shown in Figure 12.12. The drawer test for multidirectional instability is shown in Figure 12.13.

Impingement Tests.   The original impingement test was active abduction to demonstrate the painful arc (Fig. 12.6). Neer and Welsh have modified this to a passive test (Fig. 12.14*A*). A further refinement in this passive impingement test is to inject local anesthetic into the subacromial bursa (Fig. 12.14*B*) to relieve the pain and prove that the lesion is a local shoulder problem (usually in the supraspinatus tendon).

Neurological Examination.   The potential for cervical disc disease causing pain around the shoulder joint is so great that every patient presenting with shoulder-centered pain merits a full neurological assessment as outlined in Chapter 3.

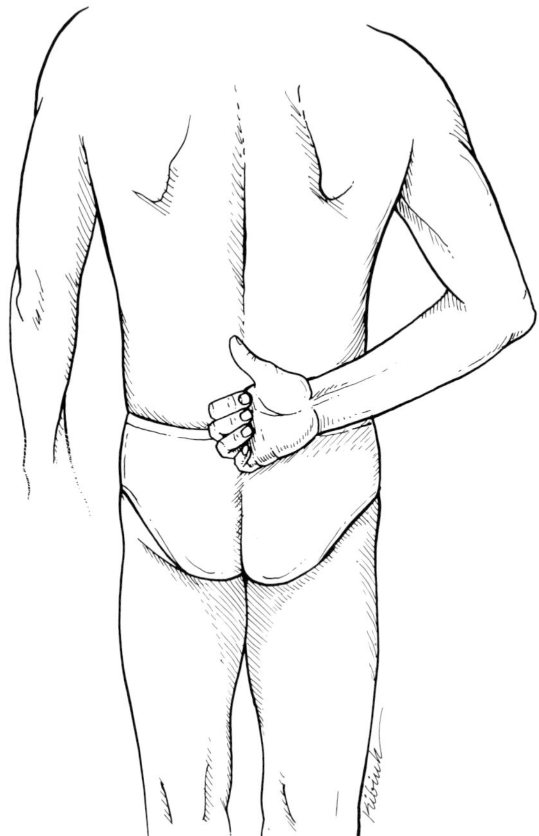

Figure 12.8.   The extent of internal rotation is recorded as the thumb level relative to the spine. This example shows internal rotation to about lumbar three.

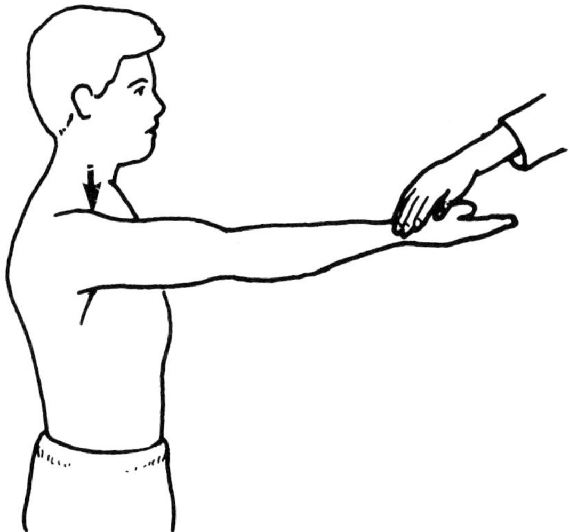

Figure 12.9.   "Palm-up" test or Speed's test for bicipital tendinitis. With the patient's palm up (supination), elevation against resistance will produce pain in the region of the inflamed biceps tendon (*arrow*).

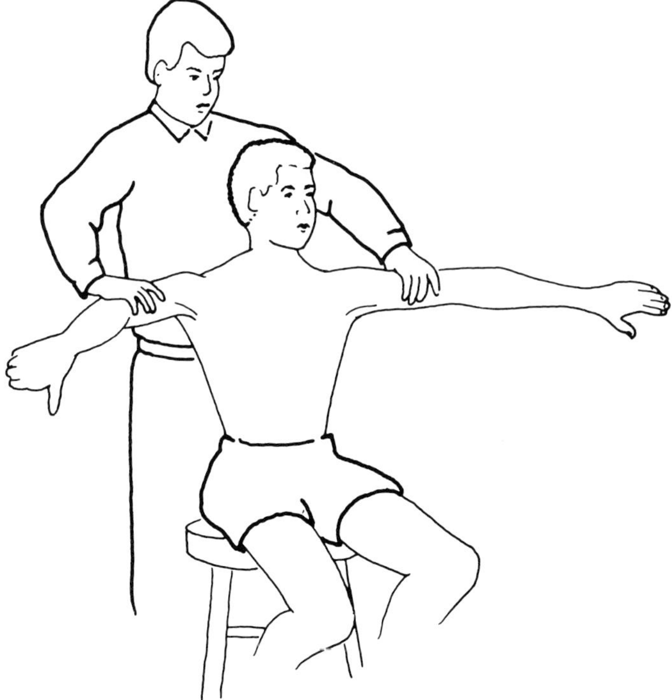

Figure 12.10.   Abduction against resistance in internal rotation. Compare strength of the two shoulders. This test specifically focuses on the supraspinatus tendon.

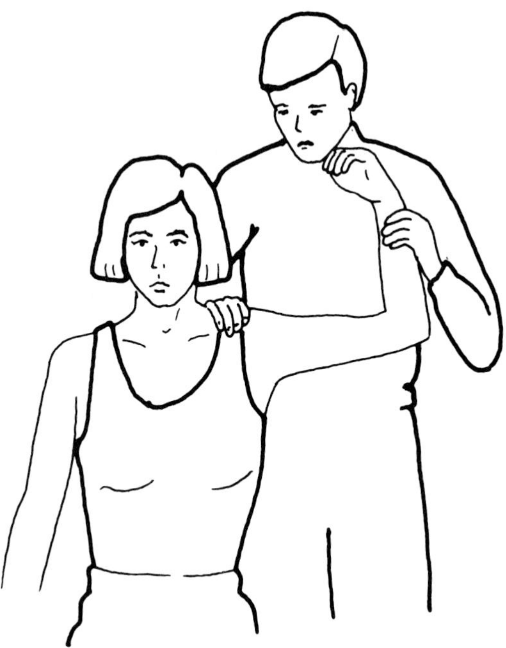

Figure 12.11. The "apprehension" test for anterior shoulder subluxations. The examiner moves the arm into abduction and external rotation (which may produce apprehension) or he adds (with his right hand) pressure posteriorly inward to try and dislocate the shoulder.

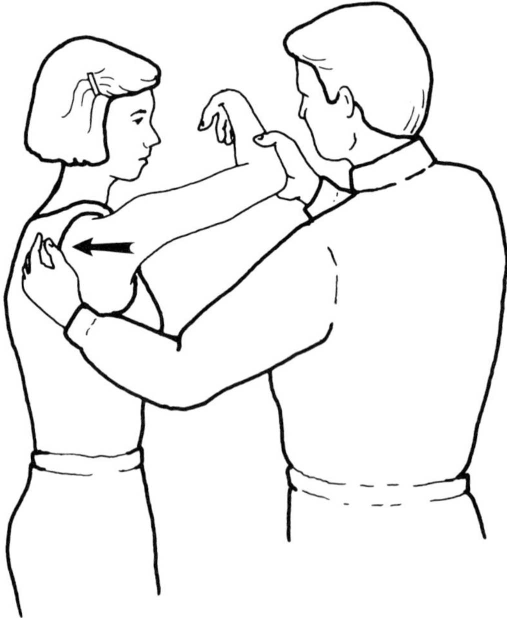

Figure 12.12. Test for posterior instability. With the arm in flexion adduction and internal rotation, the examiner tries to dislocate the shoulder posteriorly.

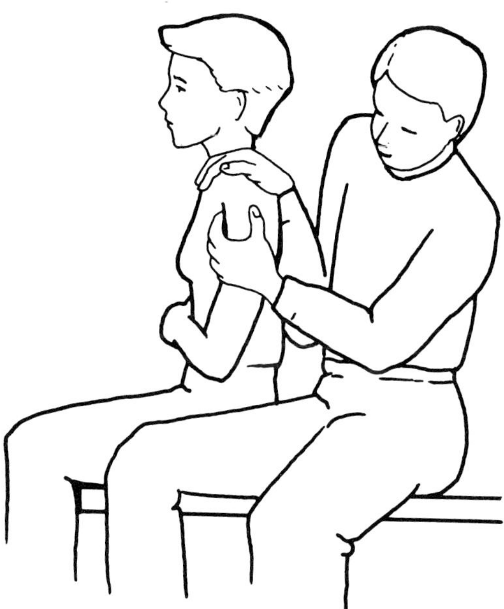

Figure 12.13.   Test for multidirectional instability. From behind, the examiner tries to dislocate the shoulder anteriorly and posteriorly.

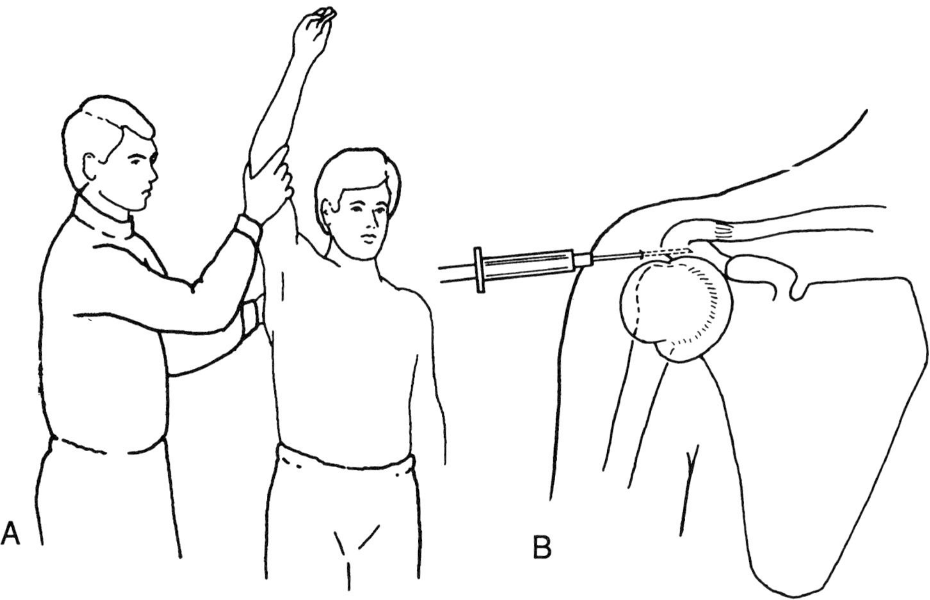

Figure 12.14.   **A**, the passive impingement test. In abduction and various phases of internal rotation (shown here) or external rotation, the examiner attempts to reproduce discomfort. **B**, abolition of the pain with an injection of local anesthetic in the subacromial bursa.

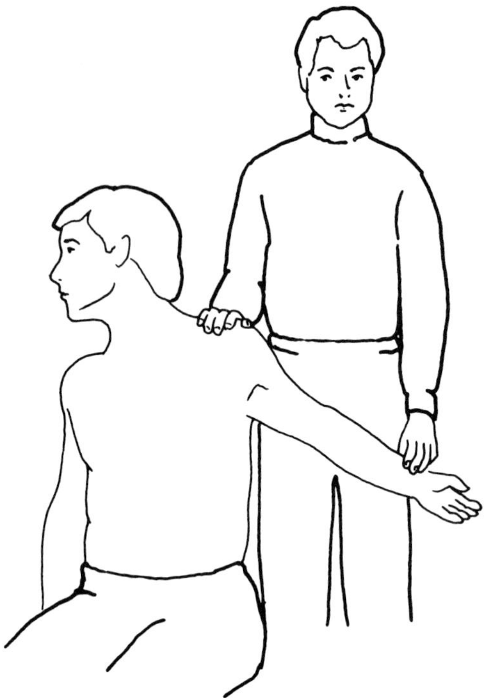

Figure 12.15.   This is Adson's test as originally described. The head is turned away from the side being examined, the neck is extended, and the patient inspires. At the same time, the arm is extended and two observations are made:
1. Does the radial pulse obliterate?
2. Does the maneuver reproduce the patient's symptoms?

Vascular Assessment.   For those who feel thoracic outlet syndrome is a common clinical problem, the Adson's maneuver is an important test (Fig. 12.15).

Radiological Assessment of the Shoulder Girdle

The classic teaching in orthopaedics is that every x-ray is a minimum of two views (usually AP and lateral) that are perpendicular to each other. Another classic rule is that every long bone x-ray must show the joints at either end. Because of the multiple joints that make up the shoulder girdle, and the awkward location of the shoulder joint close to the trunk, it is necessary to take extra steps to assure the adequacy of a shoulder x-ray exam.

The senior author (I.M.) is indebted to his instructors in radiologic techniques: Dr. Brailsford of Birmingham University; Dr. Golding of the Middlesex Hospital; and particularly Dr. Rockwood and Dr. Green, whose excellent section on "Radiology of the Shoulder Joint," published in volume 2 of the second edition of *Fractures in Adults*, proved invaluable in describing positioning of the shoulder joint for various x-ray projections (5).

Anteroposterior View of the Glenohumeral Joint

Because of the obliquity of the scapula on the chest wall, a projection taken in a "true" anatomical anteroposterior plane will show foreshortening of the glenoid fossa and superimposition of the humeral head upon the glenoid (Fig. 12.16). To

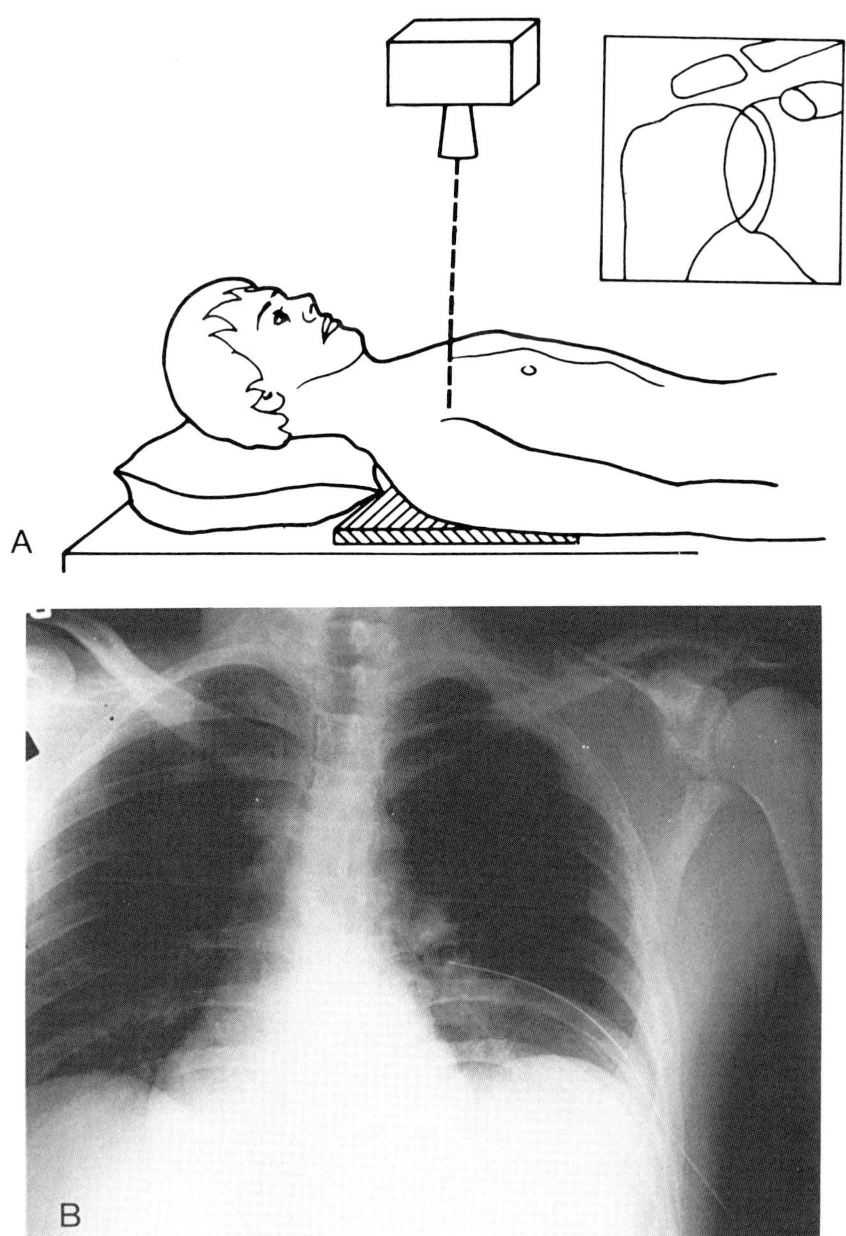

Figure 12.16.   **A**, simple AP of the shoulder will produce an x-ray (*insert*) with overlap of the humeral head on the glenoid. **B**, chest x-ray delivers a "simple AP" of the shoulder. Notice the overlap of the humeral head on the glenoid. Did you notice the fractured scapula?

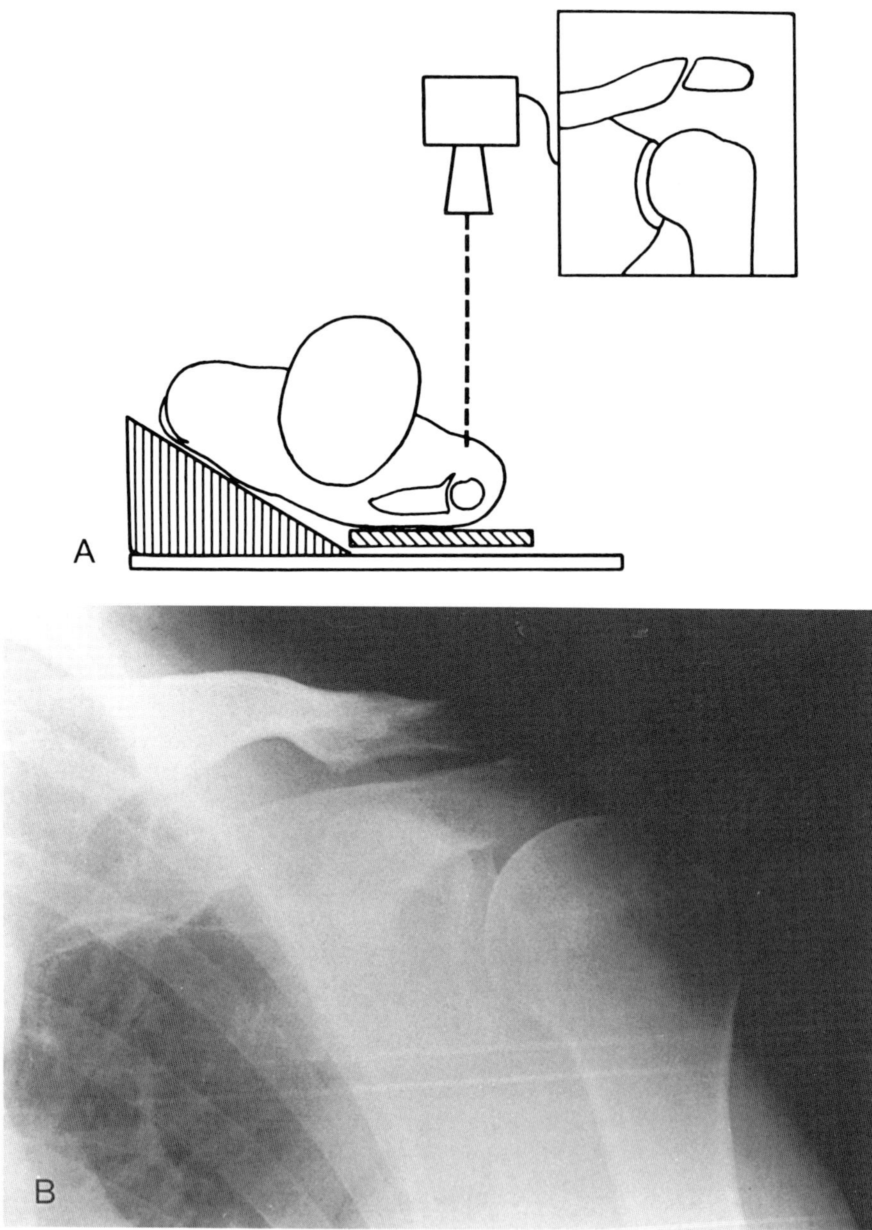

Figure 12.17.   Proper AP of the shoulder (glenohumeral joint) taken as shown in Figure 12.16.

avoid this, place the patient in the position that allows the scapula to lie parallel to the x-ray cassette, thereby permitting the central ray to pass through the glenohumeral joint. This is accomplished by rotating the trunk of the patient toward the affected shoulder through an angle of about 45°. The arm is held in slight abduction, and in the degree of rotation required, to reveal the appropriate anatomical features (Fig. 12.17).

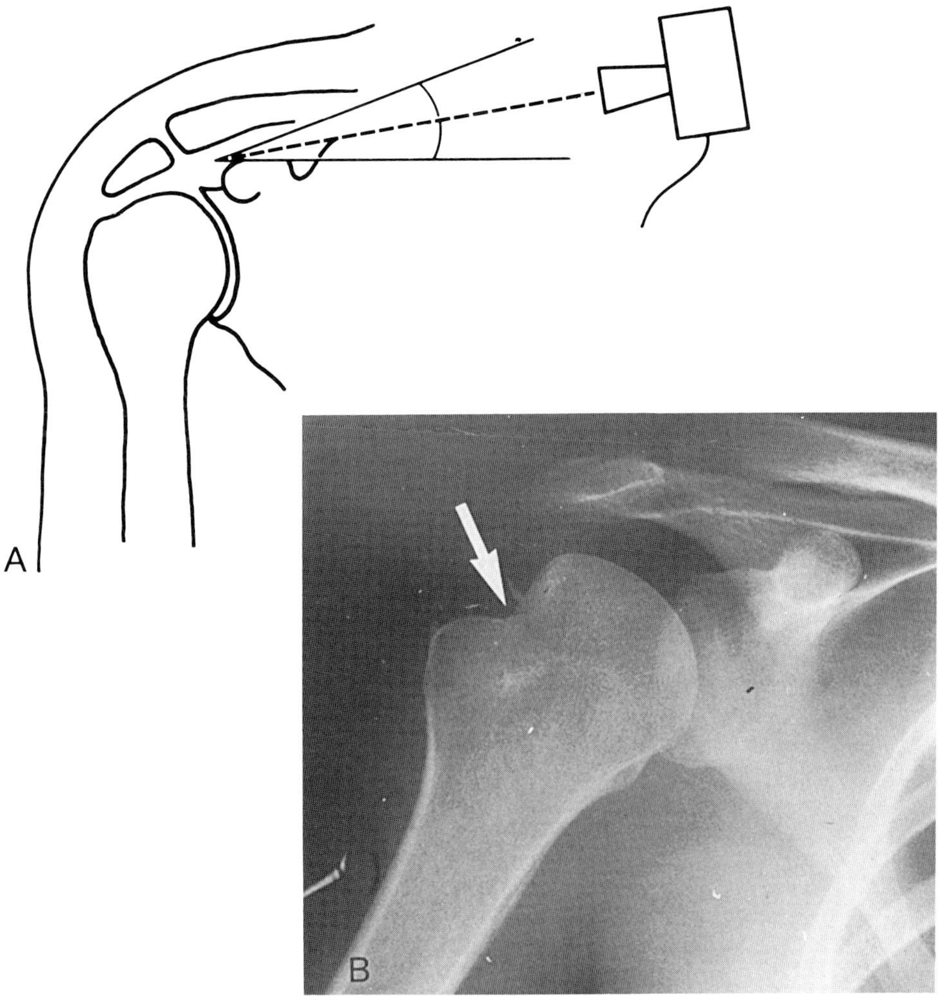

Figure 12.18.   **A,** method of x-ray assessment to open up the subacromial space. **B,** Hill-Sachs lesion (*arrow*).

In order to demonstrate the subacromial space clearly, the beam must be tilted ±20° caudally and centered 2 in. medial to and 2 in. distal from the point of the shoulder (Fig. 12.18*A*). This technique clearly demonstrates the subacromial space, the glenohumeral joint, and the greater tuberosity. By internally rotating the arm, a tangential view of the greater tuberosity is obtained and the lesser tuberosity is seen medially, either superimposed on the glenoid or just inferior to it. Positioning the patient in this manner will permit radiological demonstration of the Hill-Sachs lesion (3), commonly noted in recurrent anterior dislocations of the glenohumeral joint (Fig. 12.18*B*). A variant of this anteroposterior projection is a view taken with the glenohumeral joint held in abduction by asking the pa tient to place the palm of his or her hand on the occiput. This exposure may be taken with the patient seated or lying supine, with the trunk rotated 45° (Fig. 12.19).

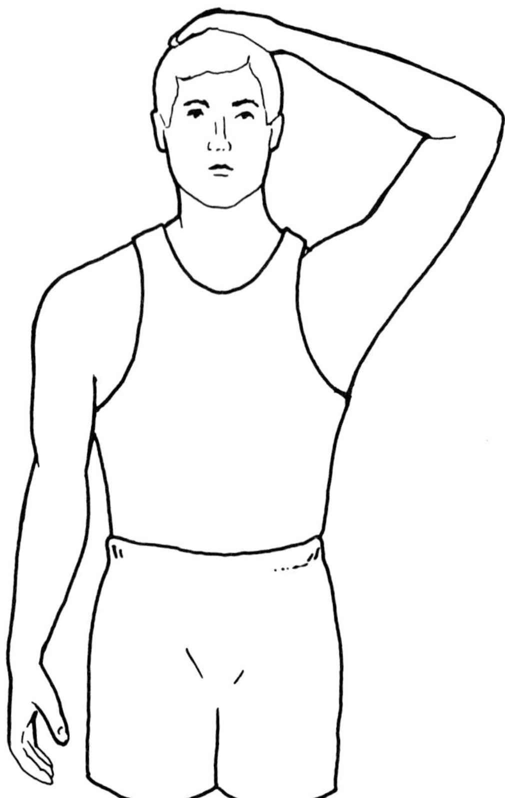

Figure 12.19.   Anterior-posterior view with the arm in abduction.

Lateral Views of the Glenohumeral Joint

Axillary View.   With the patient lying supine, the arm is placed in external rotation and abducted as near as possible to a right angle with the forearm and hand resting beside the patient's head. The cassette is placed above the shoulder and is pressed against the patient's neck as firmly as possible. The central ray is directed horizontally through the apex of the axilla (Fig. 12.20).

If the patient cannot abduct the shoulder to 90°, the cassette is placed under the axilla, sometimes with a gap of several inches between the axilla and cassette. The central ray is directed just posterior to the acromioclavicular joint, with an inclination of 5° in the sagittal plane (Fig. 12.21). It is sometimes of value to use a malleable cassette (6).

Patients suffering from recurrent subluxations of the shoulder without frank dislocation frequently demonstrate bony fragmentation on the anteroinferior glenoid rim. Rokus (5) and his colleagues demonstrated bony abnormalities at the anterior glenoid rim in patients whose histories suggested recurrent anterior subluxation of the glenohumeral joint (Fig. 12.22).

Transthoracic Projection.   The involved extremity is placed against the cassette, parallel to the sagittal plane. The other arm is elevated, with the forearm resting against the vertex of the skull while the neck and head are held erect (Fig. 12.23). The cassette is centered on the surgical neck of the humerus, and

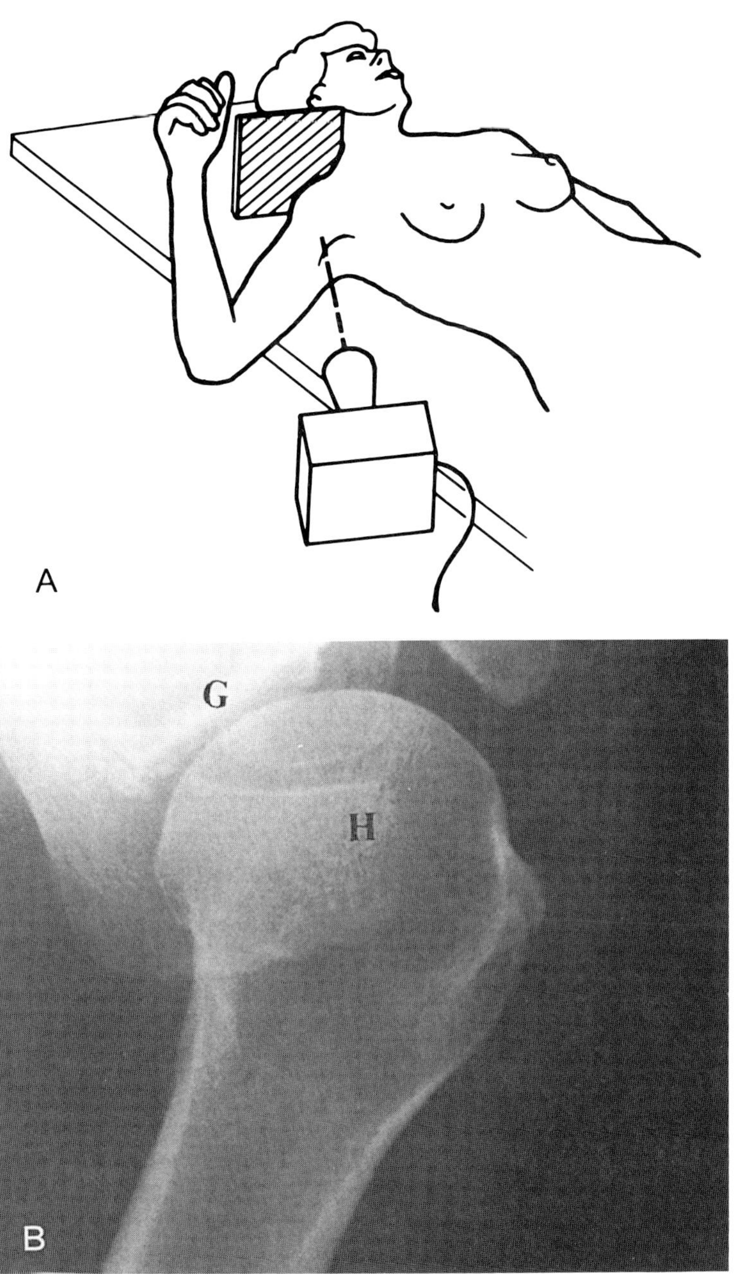

Figure 12.20.   **A,** method of obtaining an axillary view. **B,** axillary view: the humeral head (*H*) and glenoid (*G*).

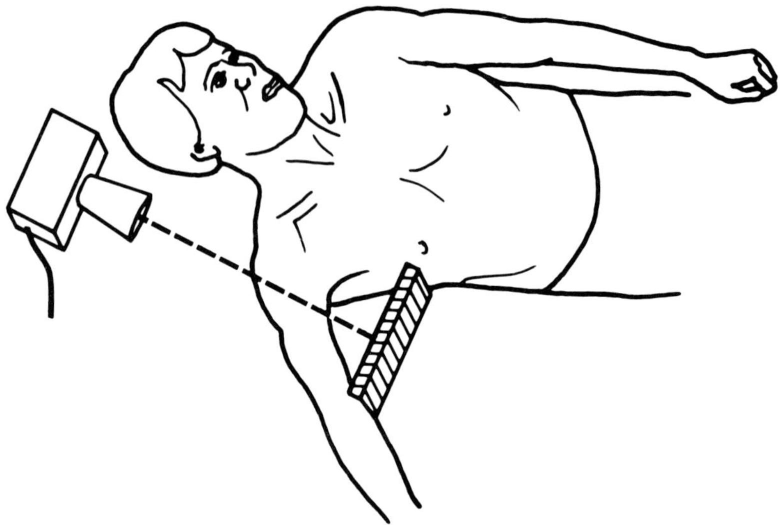

Figure 12.21.   Reversed method of taking an axillary view in patients with limited abduction.

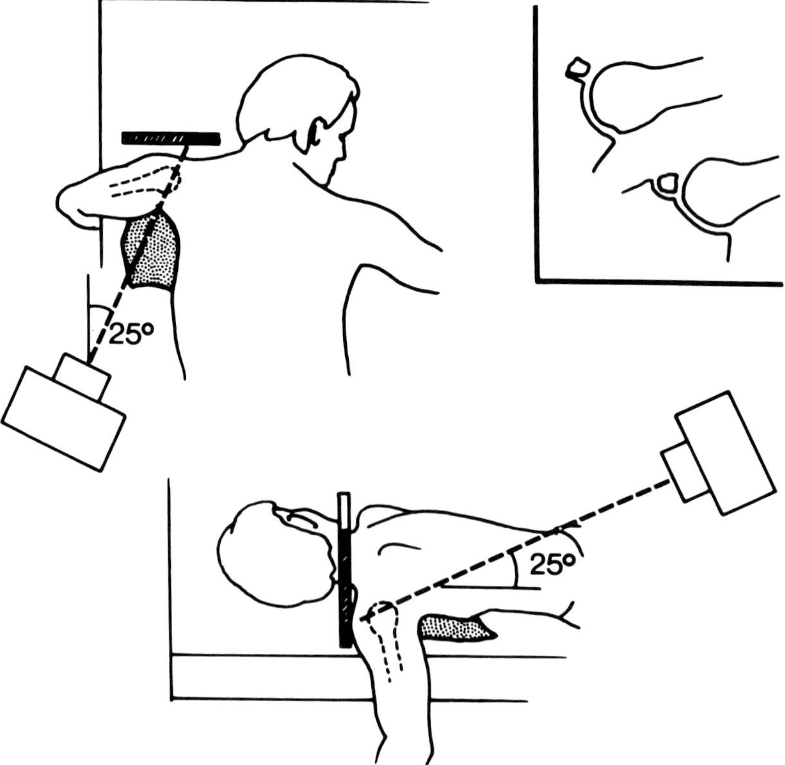

Figure 12.22.   Rokus modification of the West Point view that shows bony abnormalities at the anterior glenoid rim (*inset*).

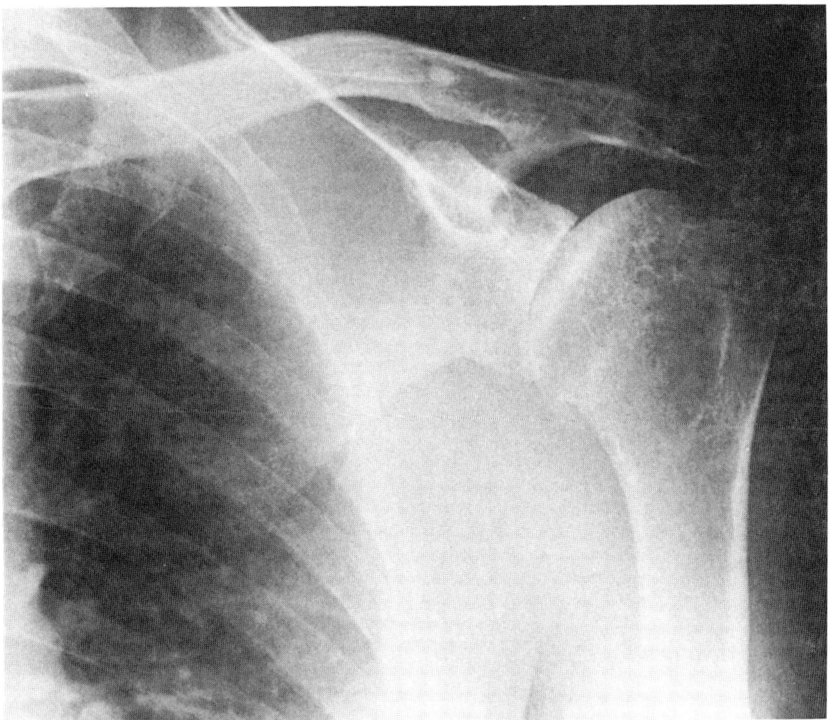

Figure 12.25.   The transthoracic view of the scapula.

Special X-ray Views of the Glenohumeral Joint

Bicipital Groove.   X-rays of the bicipital groove are not commonly required, but may be used to demonstrate calcification of the long head of the biceps or to demonstrate spur formation. The patient is positioned either sitting or standing, leaning over the end of the table with the forearms resting on the table in the supinated position. The palms of the hands press against the cassette. The patient leans forward, thereby angling the humerus 10°–15° from the vertical. After palpating the bicipital groove, the collimated beam is directed through it perpendicular to the film. This projection allows a clear view of the bicipital groove, occasionally overlapped by the tip of the acromion (Fig. 12.26).

West Point Axillary Lateral.   This view is especially useful for examining the anterior aspect of the glenoid rim for the Bankart lesion (Fig. 12.22).

Special Views for Posterior Dislocation.   Although posterior dislocation accounts for only 1%–3% of dislocations, it is easily missed if special views (Fig. 12.27) are not done (1). A good rule is this: if a patient cannot externally rotate the shoulder at least 5°–10°, you have a posterior dislocation until proven otherwise by these special x-ray views.

AP 30° Caudal Tilt View.   This was described in the section on AP view (Fig. 12.18A) and is useful to evaluate the undersurface of the acromion in impingement syndromes.

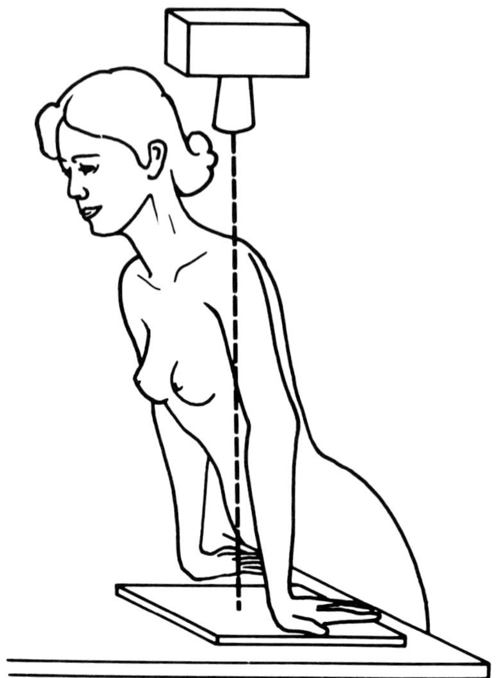

Figure 12.26.   The bicipital groove view.

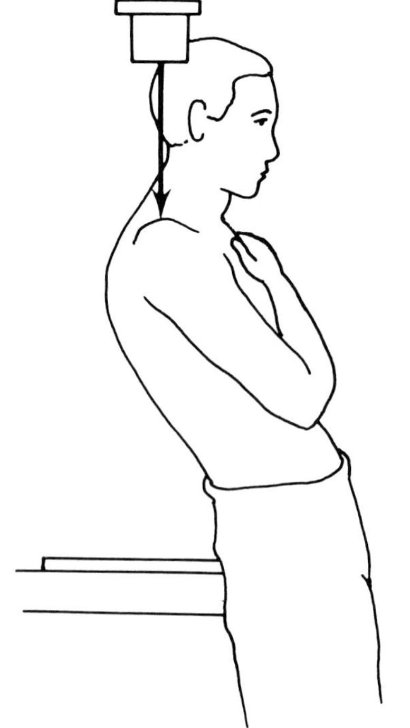

Figure 12.27.   The Bloom/Obata axillary lateral view for posterior dislocation.

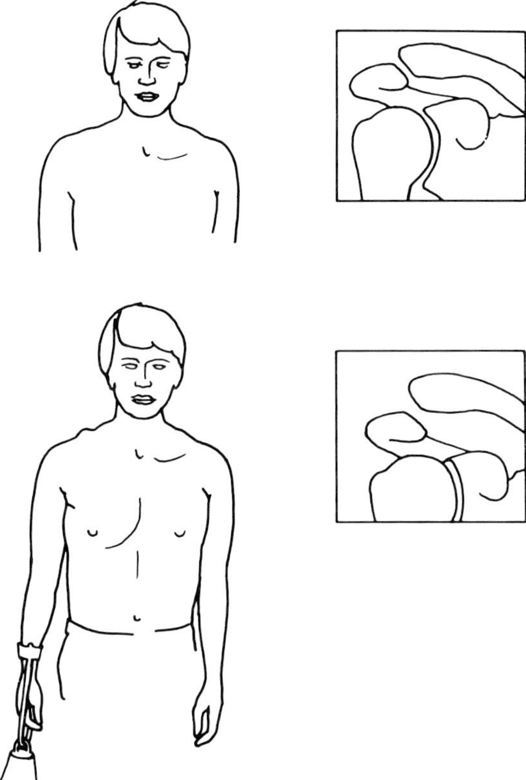

Figure 12.28.   *Upper*: nonweighted views of a-c joint (*inset*). *Lower*: weighted views of a-c joint (*inset* showing separation of joint surfaces).

Acromioclavicular Joint

These joints are demonstrated well on standard anteroposterior projections. In the radiological diagnosis of acromioclavicular subluxations and dislocations, special techniques may be indicated. If possible, both shoulders should be included on the same plate to allow for comparison. The patient is placed in the neutral AP position in front of a vertical cassette so that the midpoint of the film lies at the level of the acromioclavicular joint. The central ray is then directed at right angles to the body at the acromioclavicular joint level. Two exposures are taken: first, with the arms hanging by the sides; second, with the patient supporting sandbags weighing about 25 kg. It is important that the weights be allowed to hang rather than have the patient lift them. For this reason, it is better to tape the weights to the wrists so they hang correctly (Fig. 12.28).

In the analysis of those views, certain anatomical features must be remembered. Because of inaccuracy in position or even individual variation, the width of the acromioclavicular joint space may vary. Gross disparity of the two sides does not necessarily establish a diagnosis of joint disruption. Of equal or greater importance is the observation of a soft tissue swelling in relation to the affected joint. Probably the most significant finding is the alignment of the inferior bor-

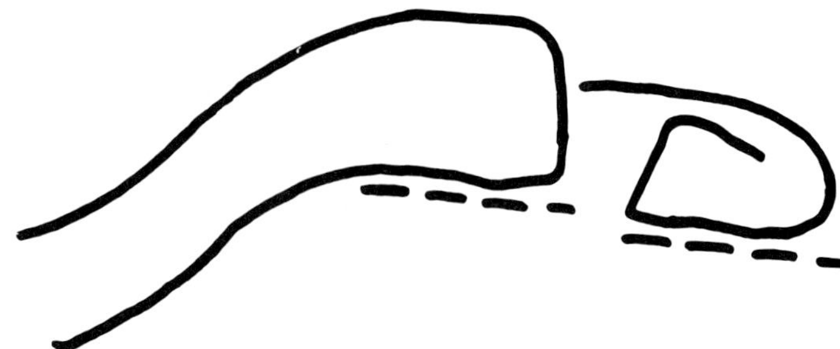

Figure 12.29.   Examine the lower margin of clavicle, relative to lower border of the acromion.

der of the acromion with respect to that of the outer edge of the clavicle (Fig. 12.29). When the integrity of the acromioclavicular joint is disturbed, this line is broken as the acromion is dragged inferiorly by the weight of the extremity and the clavicle is held elevated by the sternomastoid and trapezius muscles.

Clavicle

Two projections are used, with both clavicles being demonstrated, if possible, on one film.

The first projection is a true anteroposterior view. Patients lie supine with arms held by their sides. The x-ray is taken with the central ray centered on the midline. If it is not possible to get both clavicles on the same film, then the beam is centered through the middle of the clavicle.

The second view is obtained simply by altering the direction of the central ray to an angle of 35° cephalad, which provides a clear view of the clavicle—free of superimposition of the thoracic cage (Fig. 12.30).

Sternoclavicular Joint

This joint is difficult to visualize radiologically because of the superimposition of the neighboring structures, but an adequate demonstration is possible using anteroposterior and oblique views.

For the anteroposterior view, the patient is placed supine. The central ray is perpendicular to the body at the level of the manubrial notch or the spinous process of T2. The exposure is made at full expiration to obtain uniform density. The oblique view is obtained with the patient lying with his or her body rotated 45° so that the involved joint is closest to the film. This rotates the vertebral column away from the sternoclavicular joint. The central ray, perpendicular to the film, is centered at T3—4 in. from the midline. A variation of this oblique view is to project the central ray obliquely through the manubrium at 40° (Fig. 12.31).

Arthrography

For years, the shoulder arthrogram has been the mainstay of investigation for rotator cuff pathology and glenoid rim detachments in instability. The shoulder joint proper is injected with water soluble contrast material, with or without air (Fig. 12.32).

Adding CT post-contrast injection (CT/arthrography) is especially useful in instability syndromes. The CT with contrast will show glenoid lesions anteriorly

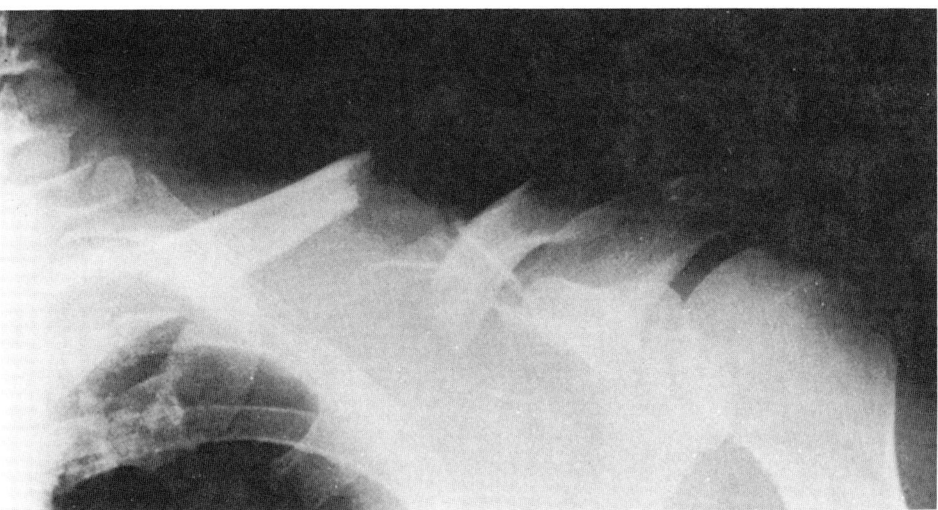

Figure 12.30. Upshot view of a fractured clavicle.

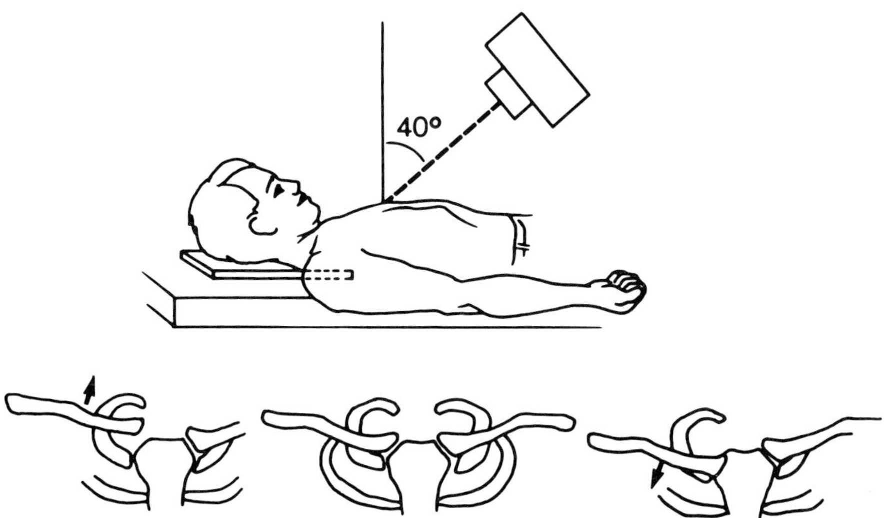

Figure 12.31. Technique for x-ray assessment of the manubriosternal joint, showing a superior dislocation (*left*) and inferior dislocation (*right*).

or posteriorly, and sometimes will help sort out the young athlete with impingement syndrome (no glenoid labrum lesion) from the young athlete with recurrent anterior dislocation (positive contrast CT for glenoid lesion). Note that both these conditions can be associated with pain and/or apprehension in the abducted, externally rotated position.

Ultrasonography of the Rotator Cuff

With the move away from invasive diagnostic tests (arthrography), rotator cuff ultrasonography fills the bill. It is noninvasive, can compare both shoulders

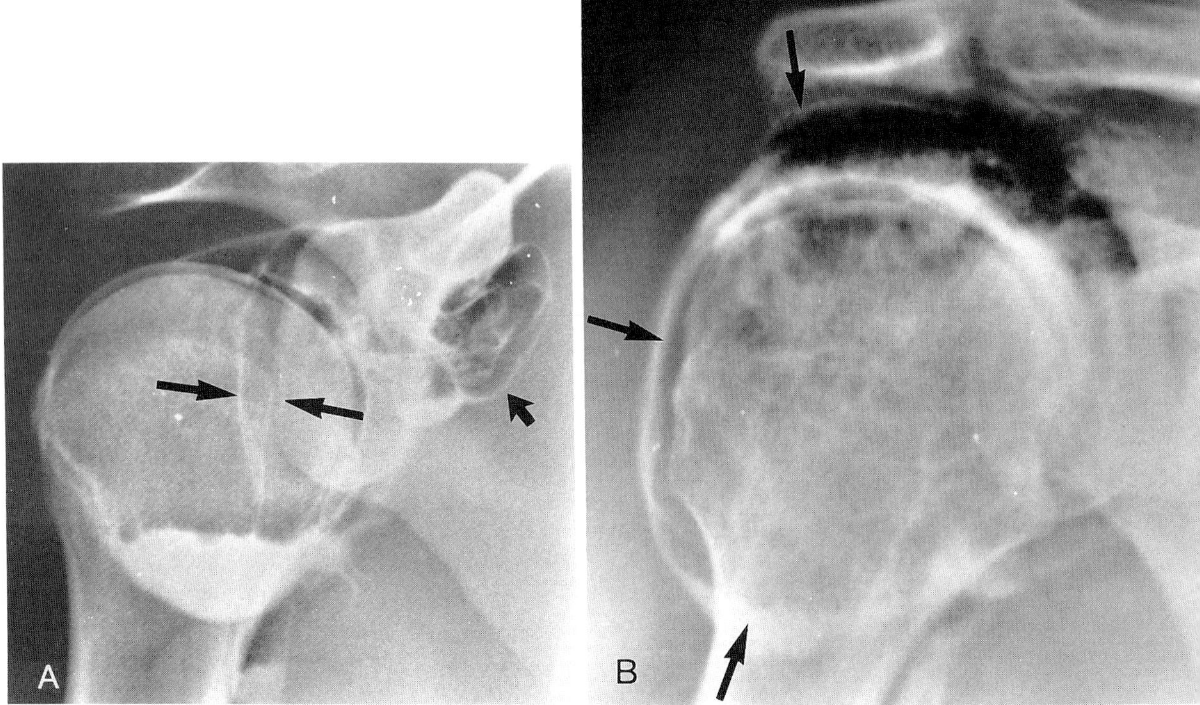

Figure 12.32.   A, normal shoulder arthrogram. **B,** rotator cuff tear (arrow).

readily, and examines both sides of the rotator cuff (the shoulder joint side and the bursal side). It is especially attractive to the patient because it is nonpainful and relatively inexpensive (Fig. 12.33). The only problems are:

1. It is technically difficult to obtain consistently good scans.
2. Scans are difficult for orthopedic surgeons to read with a high degree of sensitivity for location and extent (partial or full thickness) of the rotator cuff tear. Because of poor spatial resolution, it is truly an exercise in "shadowboxing" that requires much hands-on experience on the part of the surgeon to make it a useful tool in the surgical game plan.

Magnetic Resonance Imaging (MRI) of the Shoulder

Just as ultrasonography was making inroads as a noninvasive procedure, along comes MRI of the shoulder. Admittedly, it is a more expensive and longer procedure than ultrasonography, and a claustrophobic procedure for a few patients. On the other hand, the spatial resolution for soft tissue disorders is so much better than ultrasonography that many orthopaedic surgeons are switching to MRI to reduce shadowboxing and increase the value of the presurgical game plan.

The physics of magnetic resonance imaging cannot be explained in a few pages but can be summarized as follows:

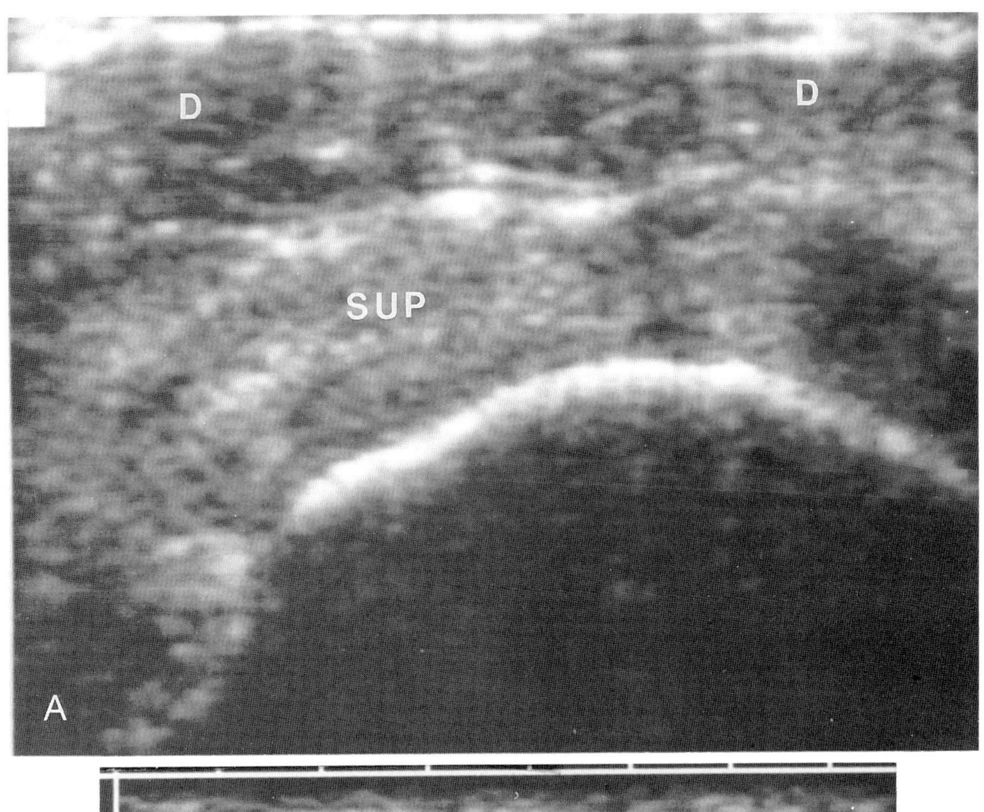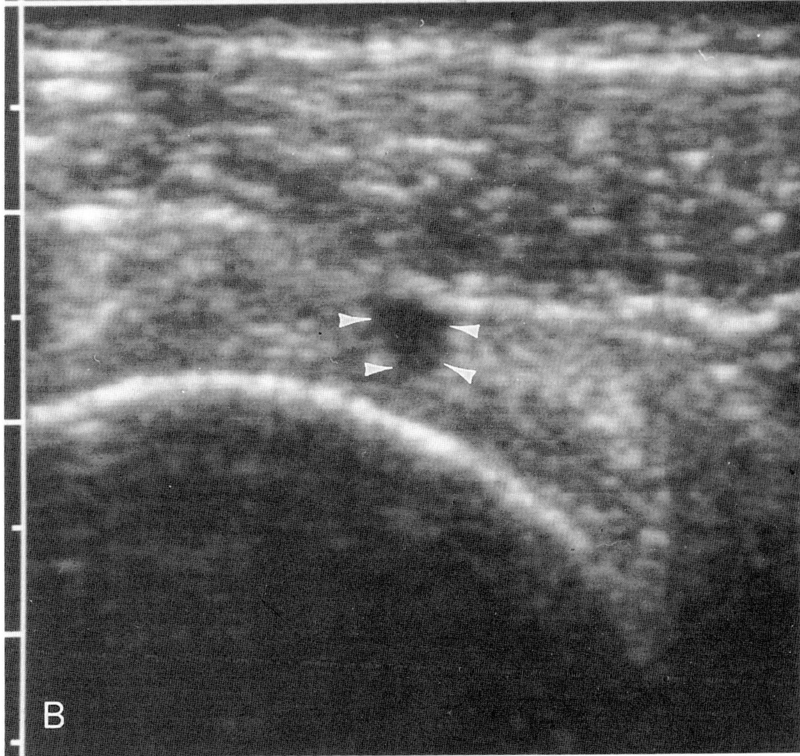

Figure 12.33. Ultrasound of a rotator cuff tear (*arrowheads*).

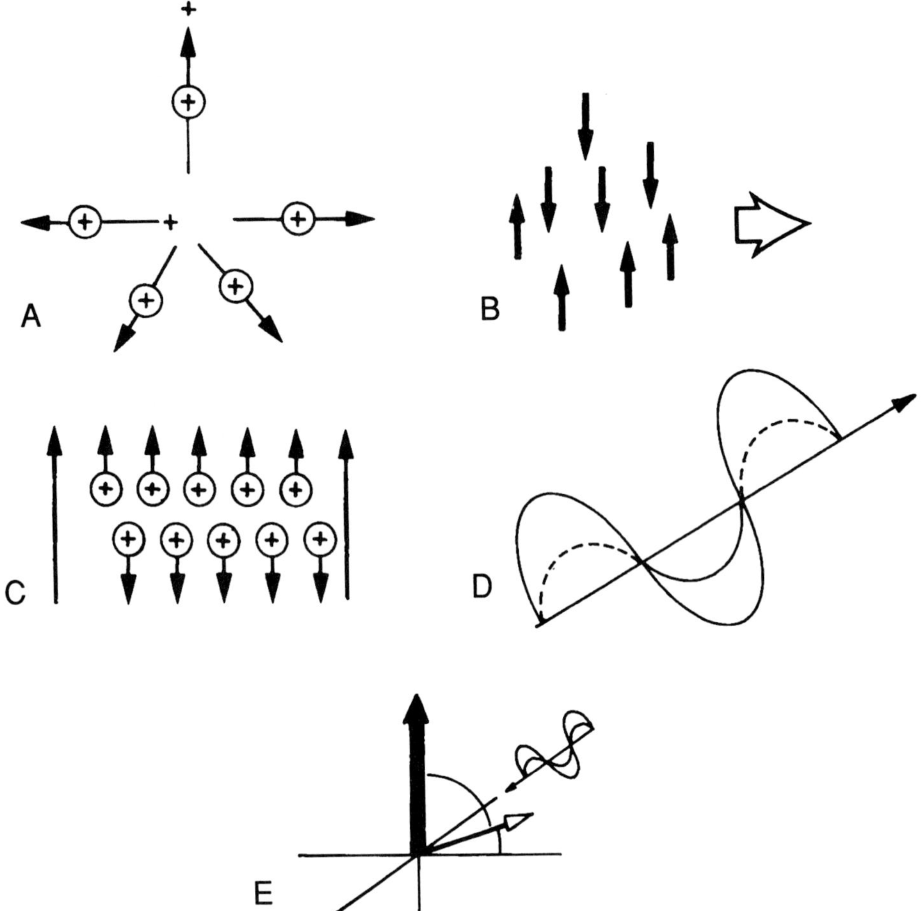

Figure 12.34.   *A*, outside of magnetic influence, the H$^+$ atoms are randomly arranged with no force vector. *B*, inside a powerful MRI magnet, the atoms are forced to reorient themselves. *C*, atoms line up with the magnetic force (high-energy level) or against the magnetic force (low-energy level). *D*, pick a radio-frequency that is specific for the resonating hydrogen ion and broadcast it into the patient lying in the scanner with his or her hydrogen ions "lined-up." *E*, the radio-frequency wave energy will be absorbed by the hydrogen atoms, which will be deflected away from their magnetized position. These deflected atoms are in a much higher energy state and result in the vector depicted by the *open-ended arrow*. Now shut off the wave. What happens? Read the text!

1. The body is loaded with trillions of minor internal magnets (elements with odd numbered protons, e.g., H$^+$) that are randomly arranged (Fig. 12.34) until placed under the influence of a giant external magnet (the gantry of the MRI machine).
2. Under the influence of the external magnet, the protons dutifully line up with the external magnetic field. They have no choice because of the power of the external magnet (Fig. 12.34).
3. In this lined-up position, they are bombarded by a radio-frequency wave that displaces the magnetic vector of the proton from its lined-up or home position.

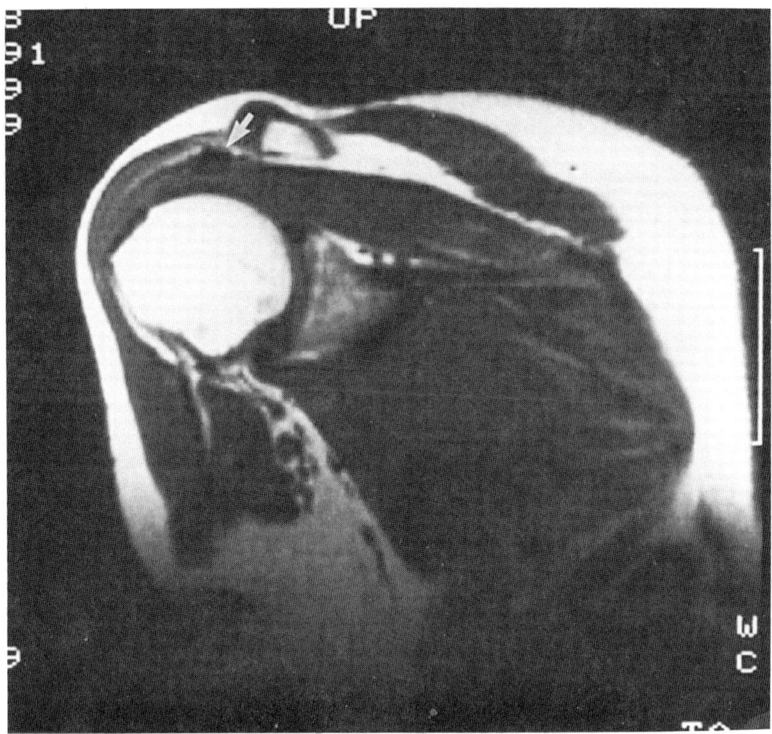

Figure 12.35. MRI showing low signal intensity (*black*) from a calcific deposit in the rotator cuff (*arrow*).

4. This displaced position of the protons (as measured by a vector) is said to be a "high-energy" position because the atom has absorbed energy from the radio-frequency wave.
5. When the radio-frequency wave is shut off, the displaced protons run for home, having no choice because of the powerful external magnet.
6. As they run for home, they throw off the excess energy as a radio-frequency wave that can be picked up just as your radio picks up a signal from a broadcast station.
7. The amount of energy thrown off will vary in different areas of the shoulder, depending on the amount of H^+ protons in the water and fat.
8. This variation in signal intensity is digitalized and spatially interpreted by banks of computers.
9. The information is then converted to a gray scale (white to black) and printed on x-ray film (Fig. 12.35).

Many look at an MRI film and describe it as a wonderful x-ray depiction of soft tissue anatomy, when in fact no x-ray has been used. MRI's greatest weakness is in detection of bone lesions, because there are no freely mobile H^+ protons in bone to be manipulated by the magnet and the radio-frequency waves. Bone therefore is of low signal intensity (black).

More detailed explanations of the physics and the pros and cons of MRI should be sought in other texts. It is sufficient to say that MRI is increasingly the imag-

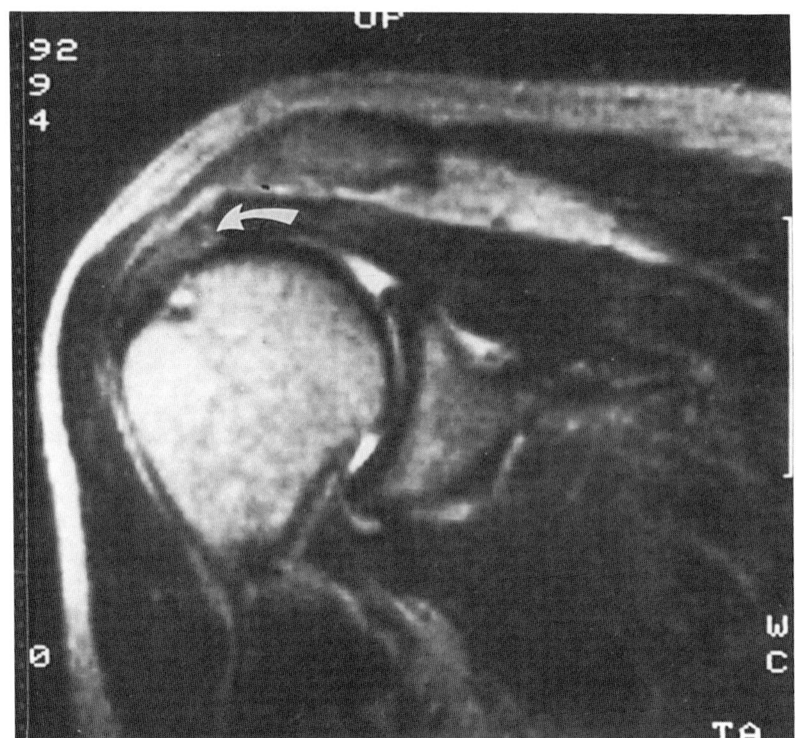

Figure 12.36. MRI showing a rotator cuff tear (*arrow*).

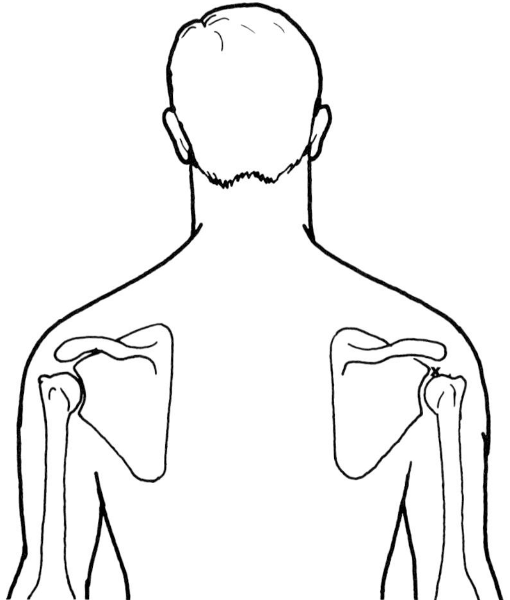

Figure 12.37. The usual portal to enter the shoulder arthroscopically is posterior (*X*). An anterior portal is used to distend the shoulder with saline.

ing modality of choice to study soft tissue disorders, such as rotator cuff tears (Fig. 12.36) and instability syndromes.

Diagnostic Arthroscopy

Throughout this book, you will read about shoulder arthroscopy. Originally used as a diagnostic technique, it was invasive and required a general anesthetic—quite a big step to establish a diagnosis. Arthrography and ultrasound have largely usurped that role, while shoulder arthroscopy has moved into the realm of actual surgical repair of labral tears, rotator cuff tears, subacromial impingement syndromes, and an ever-expanding group of shoulder disorders.

MRI is further reducing indications for diagnostic shoulder arthroscopy, but we mention arthroscopy for completeness. The procedure is done under general anesthesia with endotracheal intubation, which in itself carries a complication rate and high expense.

The usual portal of entry is posteriorly, 3 cm inferior and slightly medial to the acromial angle (Fig. 12.37). Using maximum distention of the joint with saline via an infusion pump, the arthroscope is inserted to view the joint. Anterior portals can also be used to view other areas of the shoulder. Eventually, the glenohumeral joint, the entire glenoid labrum, and the undersurface of the rotator cuff can be viewed.

REFERENCES

1. Bloom MH and Obata WB: Diagnosis of posterior dislocations of the shoulder joint with use of the Velpeau axillary and angle-up roentgenographic views. J Bone Joint Surg 49A:943–949 (1967).
2. Coventry MB: Problems of a painful shoulder. JAMA 151:177–185 (1953).
3. Hill SA and Sachs MD: The grooved defect of the humeral head: a frequently unrecognized complication of dislocations of the shoulder joint. Radiology 3:690–700 (1940).
4. Neer CS II and Welsh RP: The shoulder in sports. Orthop Clin North Am 8B:583–591 (1977).
5. Rokus quoted by Rockwood and Green. Fractures in Adults, 2nd ed., vol. 2. JB Lippincott, Philadelphia (1984).
6. Tietge RA and Ciullo JV: CAM axillary x-ray. Exhibit at meeting of American Academy of Orthopedic Surgeons (AAOS). Orthop Trans 6:451 (1982).
7. Walters JA: The psychogenic regional pain syndrome and its diagnosis. Ford Hospital Symposium. Eds: Knighton and Dinkle. Little, Brown and Co., Boston (1966).

13

Pathogenesis of Rotator Cuff Tendinitis and Tears

"The life of a man is too short to allow him, even with the greatest industry and zeal and with the most advantageous opportunities, to witness all the varieties of accident or disease."

—Sir Ashley Cooper

The rotator cuff is made up of the tendinous insertions of the muscles that rotate the shoulder: the subscapularis, the infraspinatus, the supraspinatus, and, to some extent, the teres minor. These tendinous insertions blend intimately with each other and with the capsule of the shoulder joint, forming an epaulet (Fig. 13.1). These tendons all lie under an arch formed by the acromion, the acromioclavicular joint, and the coracoacromial ligament. The rotator cuff is pushed up into the arch by the action of the humerus, an effect that is cushioned by the subacromial or subdeltoid bursa (Fig. 13.2). The biceps tendon emerges through the rotator cuff to reach the bicipital groove (Fig. 13.1).

VASCULAR THEORY OF ROTATOR CUFF TENDINITIS AND TEARS

Although the tendinous insertions of the muscles forming the rotator cuff appear to be avascular structures, microangiographic studies reveal a relatively profuse blood supply (Fig. 13.3) which, as the lateral sections show, runs through each tendon from the muscle belly to its point of insertion (Fig. 13.4). Each of the tendons has a characteristic microvascular pattern: a coarse railway distribution in the subscapularis, a fine filigree pattern in the teres minor, and a rapid arborization of vessels in the infraspinatus (16).

The supraspinatus demonstrates a constant area of hypovascularity near its point of insertion (Fig. 13.5*A*). This area of decreased vascularity, also seen on the lateral view (Fig. 13.5*B*), probably relates to the passage of the supraspinatus over the head of the humerus to reach its insertion; the prominence of the head of the humerus compresses the vessels in this area (Fig. 13.6). It is in this zone of relative avascularity that degenerative changes are first seen and, indeed, it is tempting to theorize that these changes are related to the impoverished vascularity in this area. This is the so-called critical zone of Codman (3).

To investigate this possibility further, the histological changes associated with rotator cuff degeneration were studied (12). On histological examination of the normal rotator cuff, it can be seen that the collagen fascicles demonstrate a regular wavy pattern (Fig. 13.7). This waviness probably accounts for the inherent elasticity of the tendons. On electron microscopy, the individual fibrils and the fascicles themselves can be seen to be surrounded by a sheath,

309

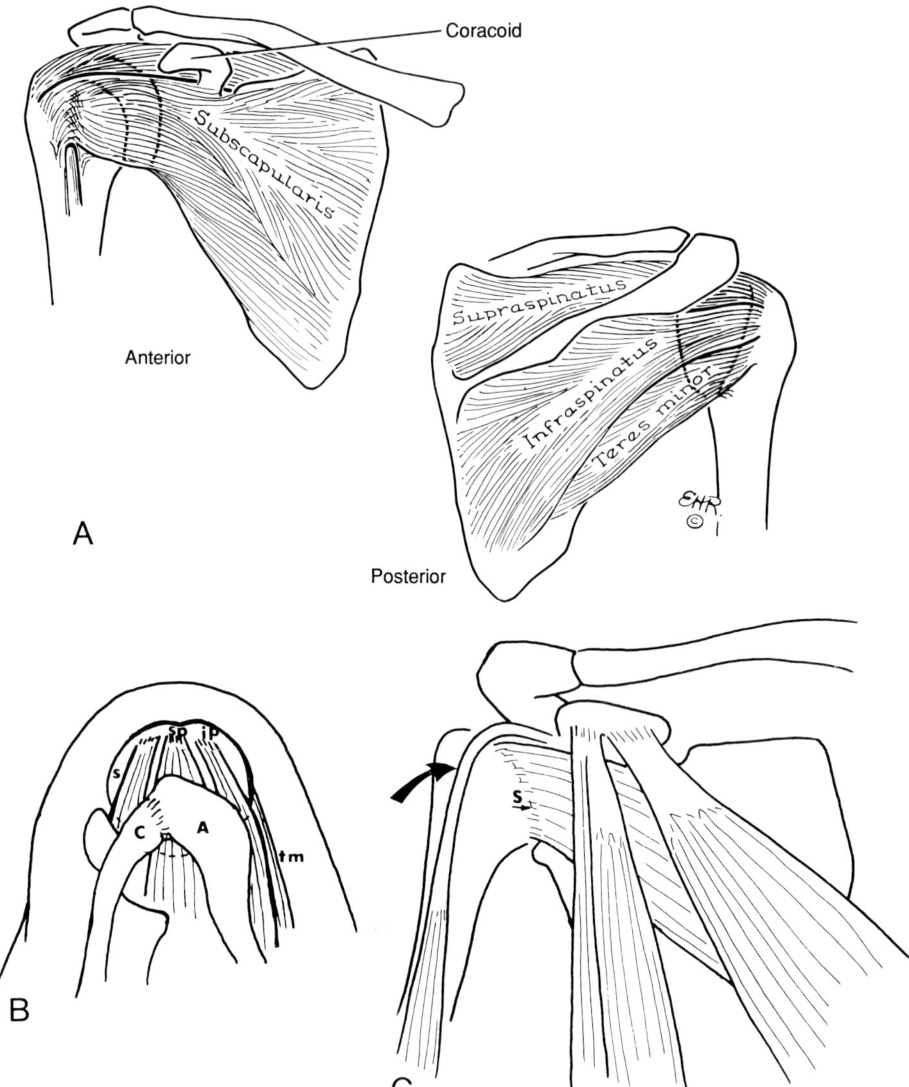

Figure 13.1.   A, the muscular anatomy of the rotator cuff. **B,** looking down on the epaulet of the rotator cuff as it inserts into the tuberosities of the humerus (A = acromion, C = clavicle, s = subscapularis, sp = supraspinatus, is = infraspinatus, tm = teres minor). **C,** the biceps tendon (*arrow*) emerges through the rotator cuff posterior and superior to the subscapularis (*s*). Posterior to the biceps tendon is the supraspinatus tendon.

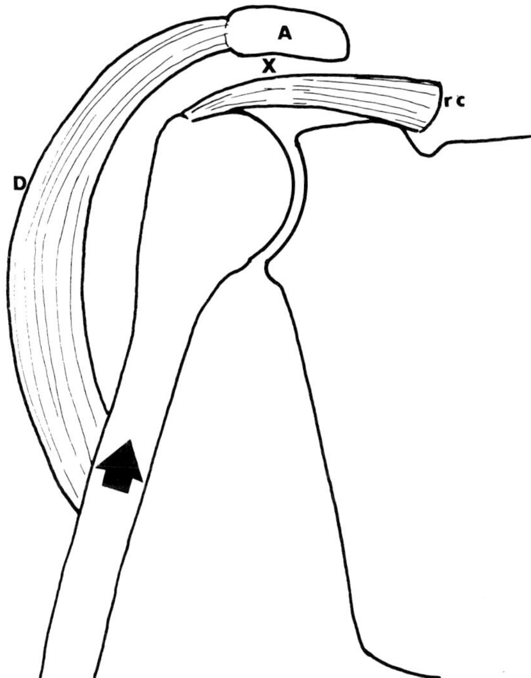

Figure 13.2. The humerus is pulled up by the action of the deltoid (*D*), pushing the rotator cuff (*rc*) into the acromion (*A*). The rotator cuff is protected by the subacromial bursa (*X*) that occupies the intervening space.

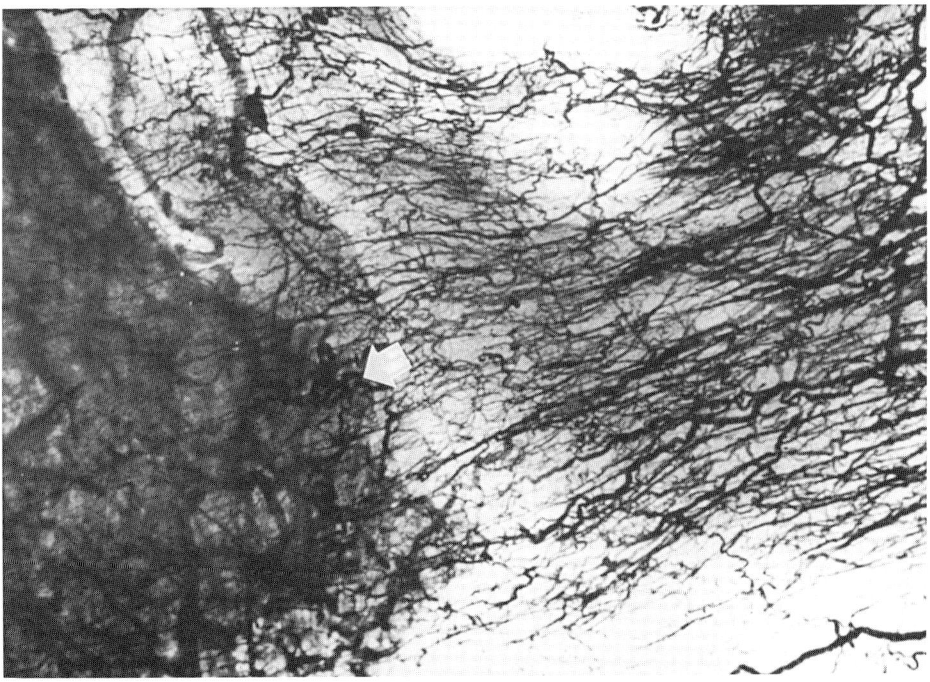

Figure 13.3. Microradiography of the tendons shows a profuse blood supply which runs from the muscles to the point of insertion (*arrow*).

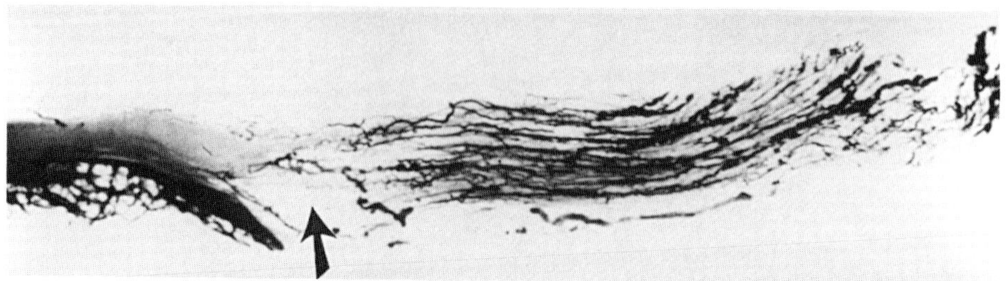

Figure 13.4.   Microangiographic study depicting the vascularity of the tendon at its point of insertion (*arrow*).

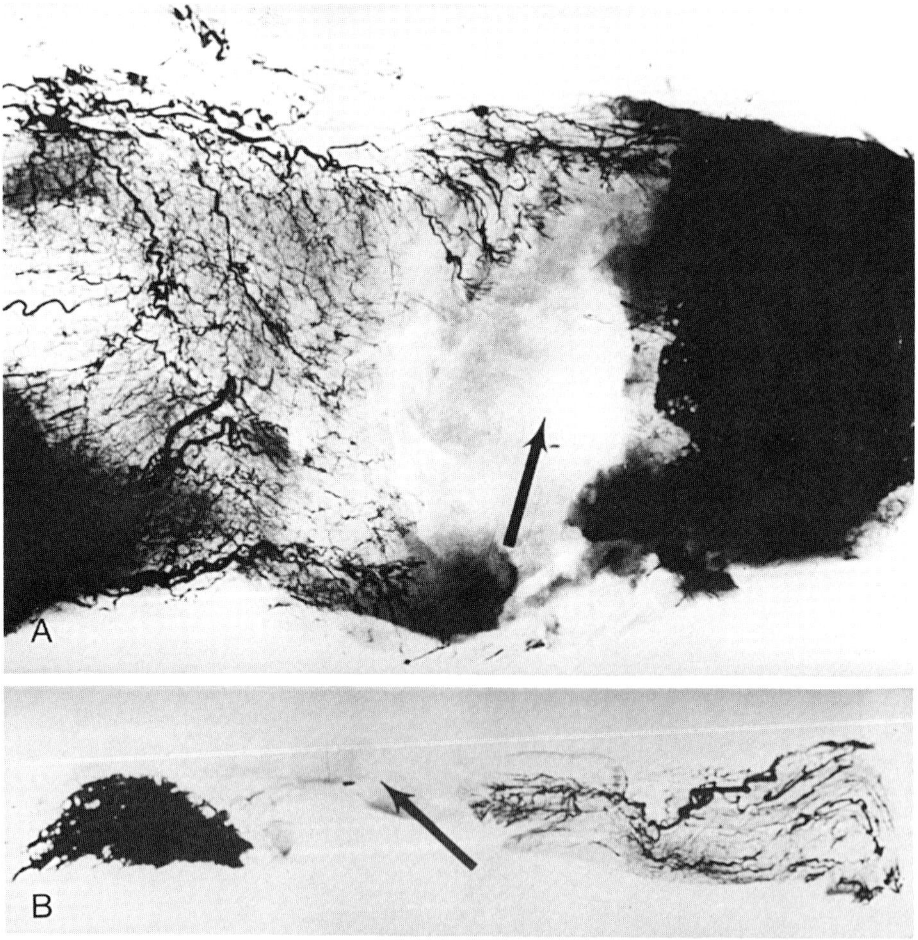

Figure 13.5.   **A,** AP and **B,** lateral view of the supraspinatus tendon with *arrows* depicting hypovascular area at its point of insertion.

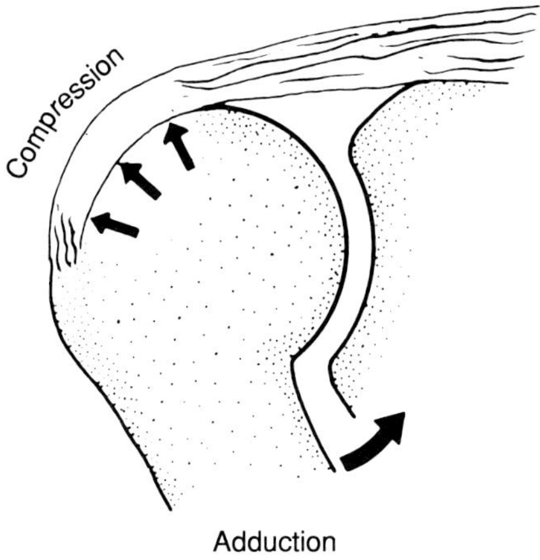

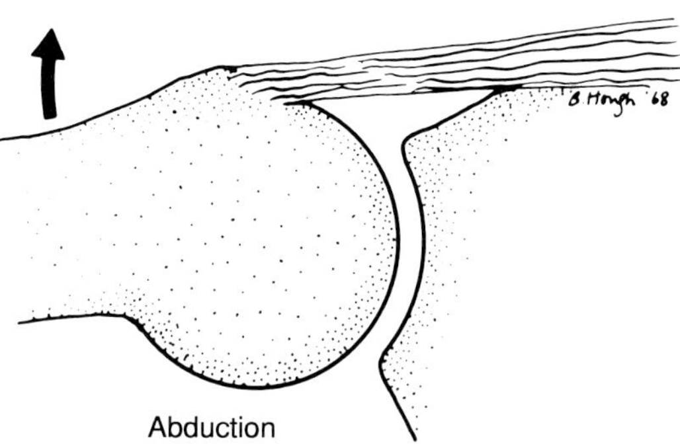

Figure 13.6. The head of the humerus presses firmly on the undersurface of the tendon of the supraspinatus when the shoulder joint is held in adduction.

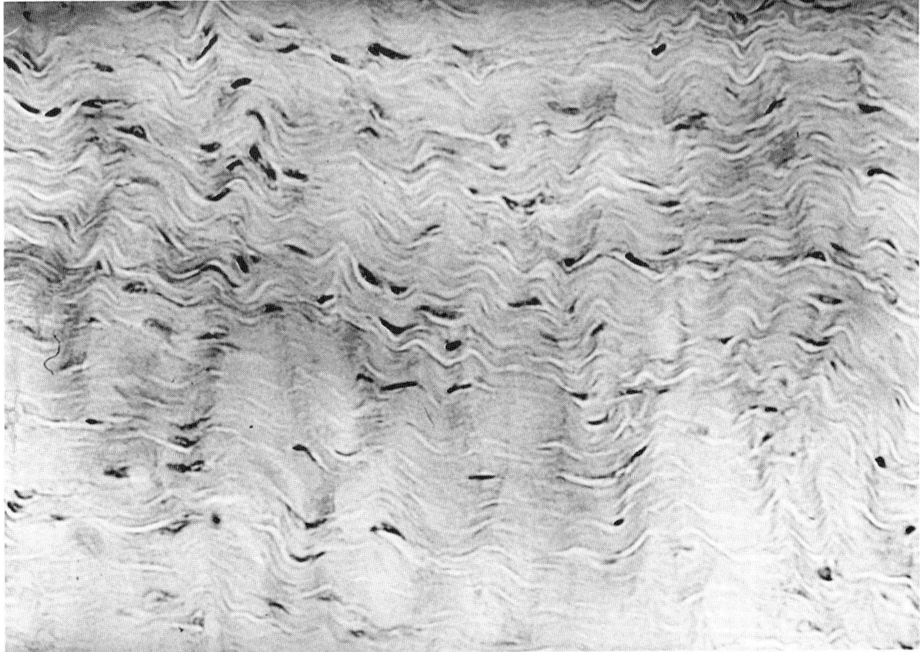

Figure 13.7. Histology of a normal rotator cuff. The wavy fibers are collagen, the cells are fibroblasts, which maintain the collagen.

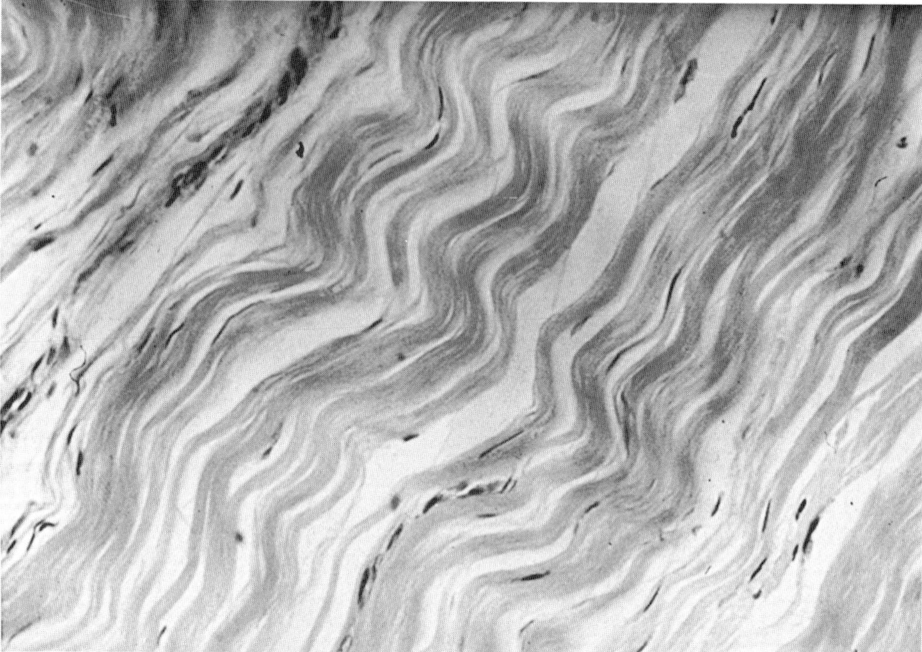

Figure 13.8.   Early degeneration of the rotator cuff includes separation of the collagen fascicles.

probably a proteoglycan. The tenocytes, compressed between the fascicles, are regularly spaced with the elongated deeply staining nuclei. One of the earliest breakdown changes is separation of the collagen fascicles (Fig. 13.8). As the process continues, the individual strands of collagen become widely separated and acellular, and later they become fragmented (Fig. 13.9). It is possible that these collagen strands, separated from the tenocytes that lie freely in the proteoglycan envelope, cannot be continuously reconstituted. This results in their breakdown under stress.

Although it is impossible to state that these histological changes are caused by impaired vascularity, experimental deprivation of the blood supply of tendons resulted in similar histological breakdown patterns. In an experimental study (18), a mound of plastic fixed in position under the Achilles tendon of a rabbit produced a partial deprivation of the blood supply in a manner comparable to the devascularizing effect of the pressure exerted on the supraspinatus by the head of the humerus (Fig. 13.10).

The sequential histological changes were identical with those seen in rotator cuff degeneration. After 30 days, marked disorganization had occurred in the center of the tendon. The observation that the changes occurred first in the center of the tendon is of interest. A similar distribution of degenerative changes was seen in the human tendons studied. The central portion of the tendon showed breakdown changes first, and the superficial portions were the last to be involved. This may be a significant observation in view of the commonly held belief that friction of the tendon against the free edge of the coracoacromial ligament is the cause of degenerative changes in the supraspinatus. If mechanical

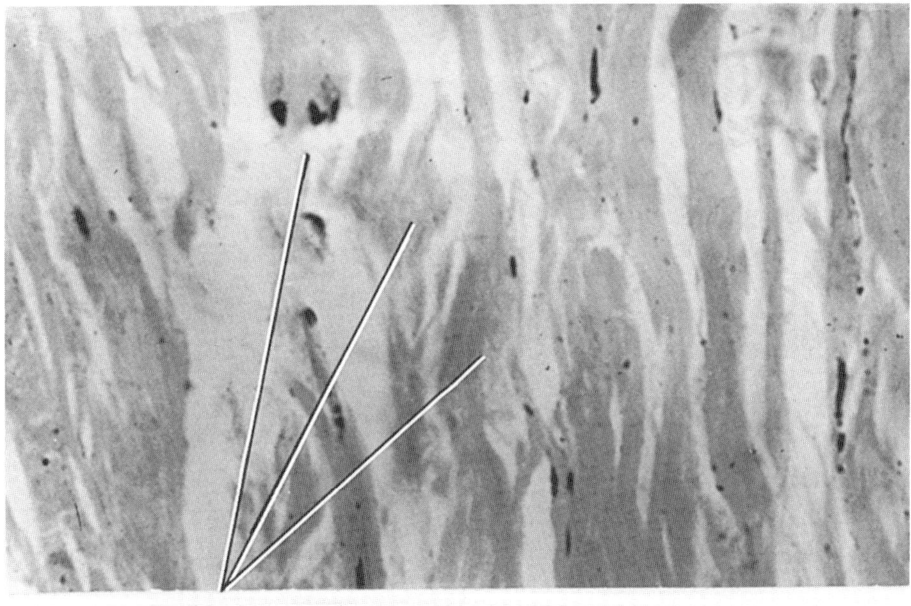

Figure 13.9.   Late degeneration includes fragmented collagen fascicles, with few cells intervening (compare to Fig. 13.7).

attrition of this type were indeed the major etiological factor, then early changes should be found on the superficial aspects of the tendon.

These experimental observations in a study of the histological changes associated with rotator cuff tendinitis lead to the following hypothesis: because of the anatomical disposition of the supraspinatus tendon around the head of the humerus, there is an area of impoverished vascularity near the point of insertion of the supraspinatus tendon. Here, cells depend for their survival on the ability of tissue fluids to diffuse through the tendon. With the tendon's increasing age, diffusion may become increasingly difficult and portions of the tendon may die. This is the basic lesion—cell death—which may be local or diffuse. This area of cell death may invoke an inflammatory "foreign body" response, which can be termed a tendinitis. This in turn produces a bursitis. The dead portion of the tendon may calcify (Fig. 13.11). Fatty degeneration was frequently seen in the human tendons studied, with globules of fat strung out in the interfascicular spaces, often in close proximity to the blood vessels. The calcification occasionally associated with tendinitis may result from calcification of fatty soaps. It was interesting to note that the calcific deposits, when first seen—and before they coalesced—were found in relation to small vessels. In the tendon mound experiments in rabbits, calcification occurred in the degenerate tendon after the mound was removed, thereby allowing partial revascularization. This observation may explain why calcification is rarely seen at the site of a complete avulsion of the rotator cuff. Complete avulsions of the rotator cuff occur most commonly in areas of total avascularity.

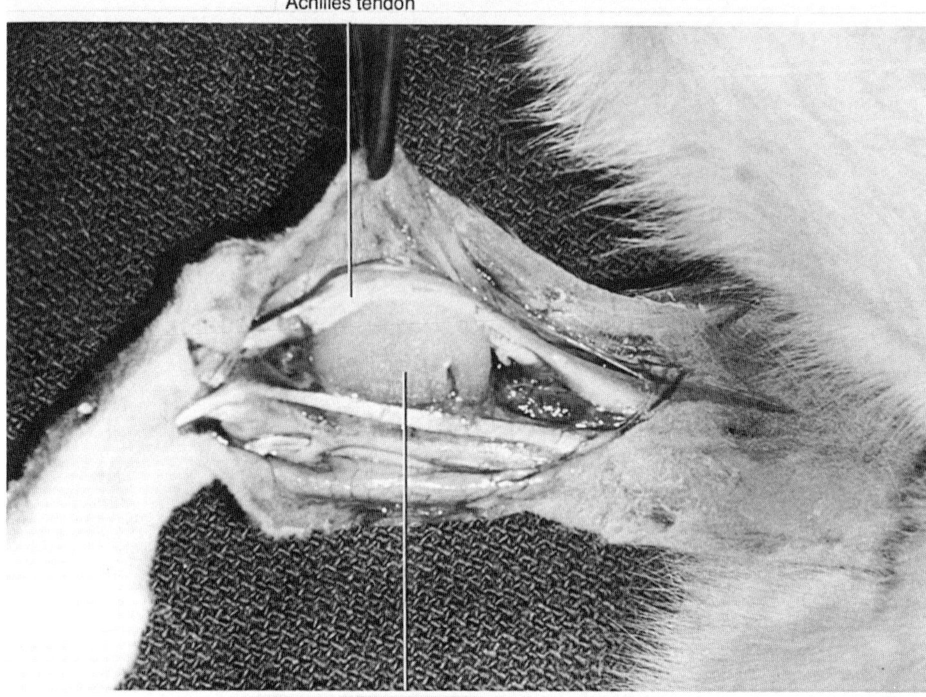

Figure 13.10.   Mound of plastic placed underneath the Achilles tendon of a rabbit, thereby applying pressure to the tendon in a manner comparable to the head of the humerus applying pressure on the supraspinatus tendon.

MECHANICAL THEORY OF ROTATOR CUFF TENDINITIS AND TEARS

Rupture of the supraspinatus tendon is common. In order to understand the pathomechanics of rupture of the supraspinatus tendon, muscle-tendon-bone preparations from the hind limb of a rabbit were subjected to loads applied at varying rates using an Instron bench testing machine (18). A normal tendon never broke; either a small flake of bone broke off at its point of insertion or the muscle fibers tore. If the tendon itself was placed in the jaws of the machine, then the tendon broke at the point of clamping. The point of clamping is an area of stress concentration. If a lateral force was applied while the tendon was stretched, a greater degree of stress concentration occurred at the point of clamping and the tendon ruptured more readily at this point. These experimental findings are of interest when one considers that the pressure of the humerus against the supraspinatus tendon will therefore increase the stress concentration at the point of insertion of the tendon, the common site of rupture.

A similar zone of stress concentration is seen in relation to any defect. Experimentally, if a small nick was made in a tendon prior to stretching, this defect became the focus of stress concentration. When a load was applied to the tendon, the notch was found to open up and, when the tendon ruptured, it ruptured at the site of the notch.

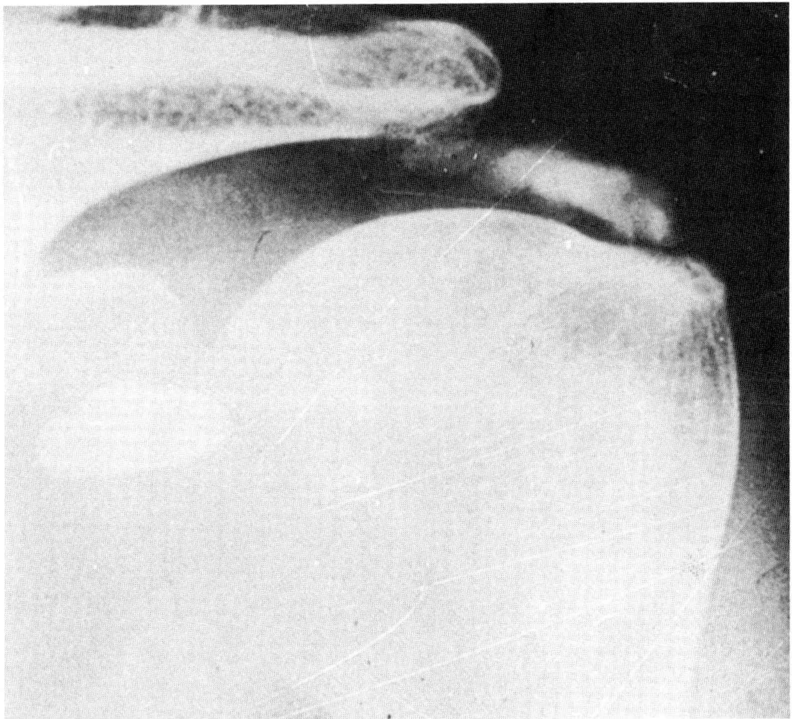

Figure 13.11.   Calcific tendinitis.

Although a normal tendon will only break at an area of stress concentration, such as a point of clamping or at the site of a notch cut in the tendon, tendons with experimentally produced degenerative changes ruptured at the site of degeneration at much lower loads. As mentioned before, one of the earliest histological changes associated with tendon degeneration is fasciculation with separation of the collagen bundles. The weakening effect of fasciculation can be easily demonstrated on a model. When sheaves of paper are bonded together by pins driven through them, they can support a weight. When the pins are removed, the sheaves of paper can glide on each other and the paper will bend under the load (Fig. 13.12).

Summary of Vascular and Mechanical Theories

Several factors, therefore, predispose the rupture of a supraspinatus tendon (8). First, a short tendon disrupts more easily than a long tendon of equal dimensions. Second, hypovascularity predisposes degenerative changes and the resulting fasciculation decreases the tensile strength of the tendon. Third, the vice-like compression effect of the head of the humerus against the acromion increases the degree of stress concentration at the point of insertion of the tendon. A partial tear commonly seen in the examined specimens produces an "izod notch" effect, which by itself will cause an area of stress concentration, predisposing the tendon to complete disruption on strain.

In Neer's classic articles (11, 12), the mechanical impingement was localized to the anterior edge and undersurface of the anterior third of the acromion and the

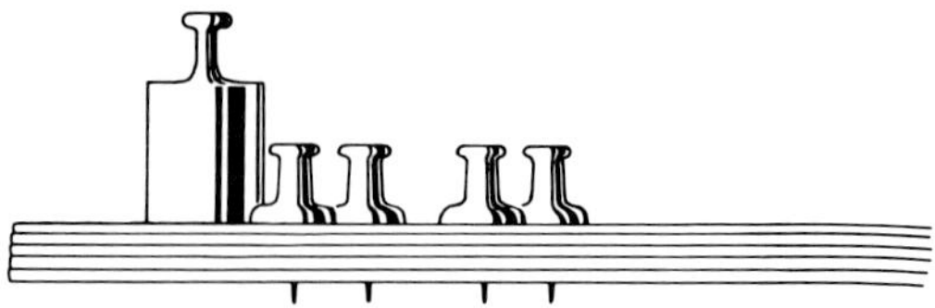

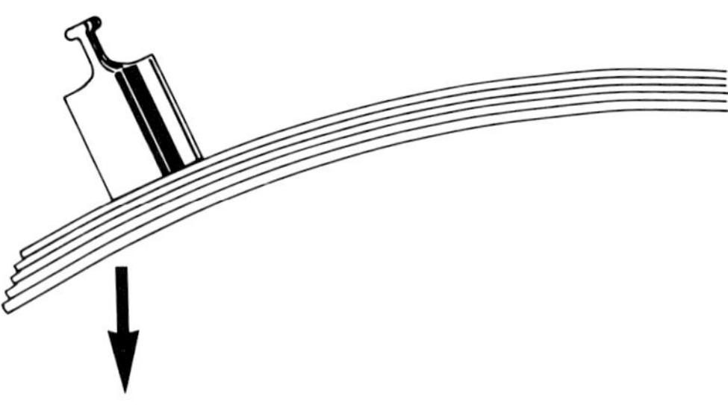

Figure 13.12. Sheaves of paper bonded together by pins driven through can support a weight. When pins are removed the sheaves of paper glide and bend under the load.

coracoacromial ligament. At times, osteophytes on the inferior surface of the acromioclavicular joint impinge on the rotator cuff. This observation by Neer has reduced almost all rotator cuff decompressive procedures to the anterior undersurface of the coracoacromial joint.

Single traumatic episodes, such as a fall in a middle-aged worker or a dislocation in an older patient, may rupture the supraspinatus tendon. These are infrequent injuries mentioned only for completeness. The bulk of rotator cuff tendinitis and tears relates to a combination of repeated microtrauma to a tendon with established vascular impairment.

Overuse Syndrome

Neer and Welsh (13) initially described the repetitive microtrauma of the competitive athlete, who performs repetitive tasks at near maximum tolerance. This usually involves overhead motion, with the best North American example being baseball pitchers. Repetitive microtrauma also occurs in racket sports and swimming. The work of mechanics, plumbers, and carpenters may include a lot of forced overhead activity, which also traumatizes the rotator cuff. The early phases of microtrauma in the overuse syndrome are associated with pain (see Chapter 19).

Neurological Considerations

The nerve supply of the rotator cuff has been studied (16). Although nerve fibrils could be constantly demonstrated in the subscapularis, the infraspinatus, and the teres minor, such nerve fibers were only found in healthy, normal supraspinatus tendons (Fig. 13.13) and were never found in specimens showing

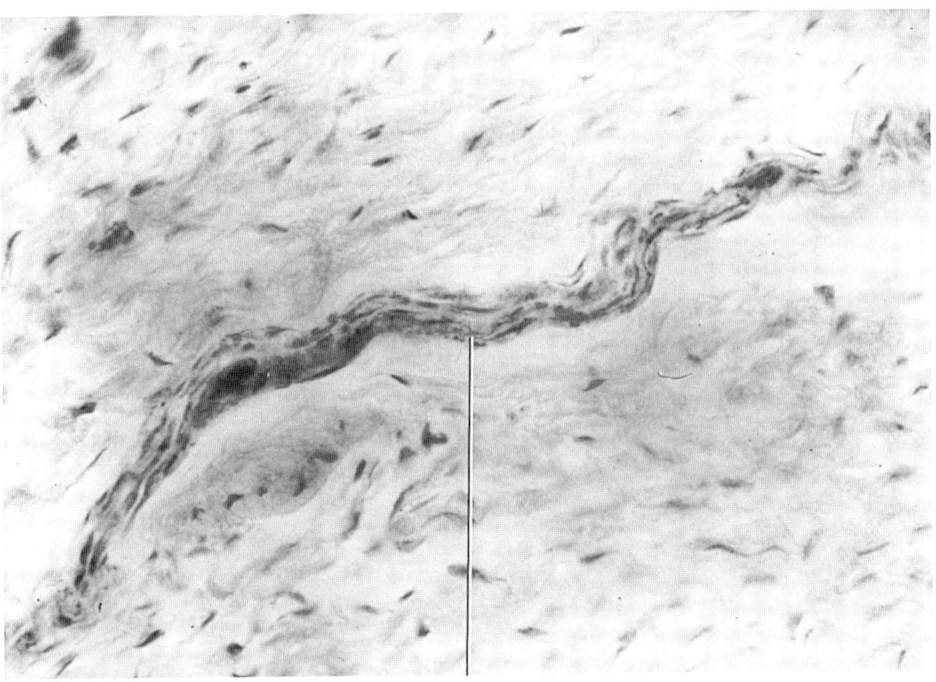

Figure 13.13.   Nerve fibrils found in healthy supraspinatus tendons.

marked degenerative changes with extensive avascularity. It is possible that interference with the blood supply in this area—of sufficient degree to cause collagen breakdown—also caused degeneration of the nerve fibrils, particularly in view of their higher oxygen demand.

The loss of nerve supply to the degenerative avascular area of the supraspinatus tendon brings in the possibility of another interesting mechanism in the production of rotator cuff tears. Because of the loss of nerve fibers, the tendon loses proprioceptive feedback and therefore has little muscular protection against sudden adduction forces. This feedback mechanism is important in the protection of all tendons in the body.

Summary

The interrelationship of these various anatomical, physiological, pathological, and mechanical factors account for the remarkable frequency of tendinitis and ruptures of the supraspinatus tendon, when compared with other tendons in the body.

Under such circumstances, marked degeneration caused by avascularity of the supraspinatus tendon could be painless. However, the other tendons comprising the rotator cuff maintain their blood supply, and when a diffuse capsulitis occurs, they have the potential of invoking a painful response.

It is noteworthy that, when nerve fibers were demonstrated in the supraspinatus tendon, they lay mostly in the superficial layers of the tendon and in the floor of the subacromial bursa. It is possible, therefore, that although surface

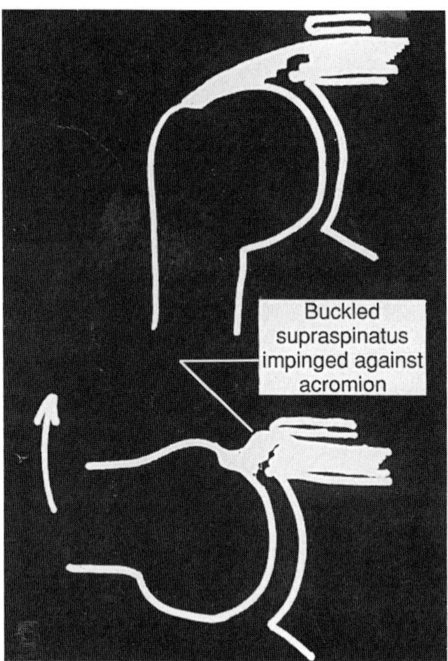

Figure 13.14.   Buckling of the supraspinatus tendon at the level of a deep tear.

changes might give rise to pain, degenerative changes occurring in the center of the tendon might not evoke a painful response.

A chronic tear generally starts on the deep surface of the tendon (10), gradually extending through the tendon substance until it reaches the superficial surface.

Partial ruptures not extending to the surface of the tendon were frequently encountered in autopsy specimens. The ruptures could not be seen on inspection of the tendon, but were demonstrated by the buckling of the tendon that occurred on abduction of the arm (Fig. 13.14). On occasion, when this buckling occurred, the rotator cuff impinged against the coracoacromial ligament. The resulting impingement may act as a source of symptoms of rotator cuff tendinitis. Even more important, impingement may be produced by an osteophyte developing on the anteroinferior edge of the acromion (12).

Therefore, as a result of minor trauma, a degenerate tendon may rupture and the resulting tear may be small or may be a complete avulsion of the rotator cuff at its attachment to bone. Rotator cuff tendinitis, subacromial bursitis, calcific tendinitis, and rotator cuff tears are, then, all varying manifestations of the underlying basic pathological lesion of focal cell death (Table 13.1) from repeated microtrauma in a tendon with vascular impairment.

Because the biceps tendon runs over the head of the humerus, the vascular bed of the tendon may be wrung out by the prominence of the bone. Degenerative changes invariably occur first at this relatively avascular area of the biceps tendon, and this is a common site of rupture. Focal cell death may become diffuse and spread to involve the whole capsule of the shoulder, giving rise to a diffuse capsulitis.

Table 13.1.   Classification of Subacromial Impingement Lesions

Stage	Age	Pathology	Cuff Tear	Residual After Appropriate Treatment
1. Early Stage	Tend to be less than 25 years old	Edema Inflammation Hemorrhage	No	None if appropriate conservative treatment instituted
2. Mid Stage	Tend to be 25–40 years old	Same as above plus fibrosis Subacromial bursal thickening	Early fiber dissociation but no tear	Fibrosis = permanent impairment that can be lessened by subacromial decompression
3. Late Stage	Usually 40 + years	Same as above plus tears in rotator cuff Spurs on undersurface of acromion Bony changes occur in greater tuberosity	Partial or full thickness Small or large tears	Permanent impairment of shoulder function, even with surgical repair and subacromial decompression

If the initial precipitating lesion of supraspinatus tendinitis is focal cell death resulting from microtrauma and partial avascularity, it is difficult to understand why the lesion should spread to involve other tendons normally well vascularized. In the rabbit mound experiment (18), it was noted that after 30 days, even when there was marked disorganization at the center of the tendon, the outer fibers remained relatively normal. However, this relatively healthy tendon surrounding the central area of necrosis was infiltrated with round cells. It was impossible to determine whether this was a tissue response to the contained degenerate denatured tendon or an early histological change associated with impending tendon breakdown. To study this further, the response of a viable tendon to an implanted avascular tendon was observed. A portion of degenerate tendon was excised and buried inside an adjacent healthy tendon. This buried avascular fragment of tendon became mummified and the host became infiltrated with round cells. Morphologically, these round cells appeared to belong to the lymphoid series and, when stained with the Unna Pappenheim stain, showed the characteristic rose-red cytoplasm of pyroninophilic lymphoid cells. Although these cells are in no way specific, the presence of them in large clusters suggests the possibility of a cellular immune response, mediated through the lymphatic system.

In this type of immune response, the antigen is transported to the regional lymph nodes, where it invokes an antibody response. The antibodies are now transported in cells—the pyroninophilic cells—back to the site of antigen production, and there they give rise to a local antigen-antibody response.

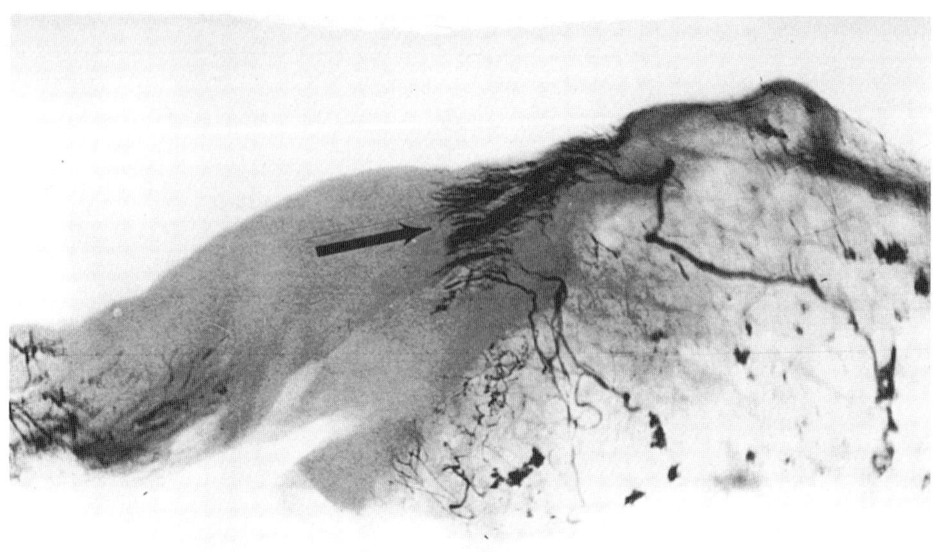

Figure 13.15.   Microangiography showing tufts of vessels in areas of granulation tissues.

This was readily observed because, in the rabbit, the lymphatics of the hind foot drain into a single node in the popliteal fossa. Four days after implantation of a tendon fragment into the Achilles tendon, the normal histology of the popliteal lymph node, characteristically loaded with basophilic lymphocytes, changed and numerous pyroninophilic cells appeared. Two days later, rose-red pyroninophilic lymphoid cells were seen in the host tendon around the implant.

When implantation of a fragment of tendon was repeated in another rabbit after removal of the popliteal lymph node, the implanted tendon did not evoke any response in the host; it was well-tolerated and there was no round cell infiltration.

In order to evoke an autoimmune response, vascular or lymphatic contact must occur with abnormal proteins, which in these instances are presumably the products of proteoglycans.

In this regard, it is interesting to note that, in studies of the rotator cuff of the human shoulder, there is frequently a vascular reaction around the area of tendon degeneration. Brush-like vascular tufts are frequently seen, corresponding to areas that histologically resemble granulation tissue (Fig. 13.15). Under such circumstances, a small infarcted portion of the supraspinatus tendon could theoretically initiate an autoimmune response, with a cellular reaction occurring in all the adjacent tendons comprising the rotator cuff. Surgical division of the subscapularis in the treatment of frozen shoulders has provided opportunity for examination of portions of the rotator cuff in this lesion. Histological examination has consistently demonstrated infiltration of the tendon of the subscapularis with pyroninophilic lymphoid cells, showing the distinctive and characteristic rose-red cytoplasm.

Obviously, this is not the sole mechanism of the complex changes that occur in diffuse rotator cuff tendinitis, but it is suggested that changes of this type may play a significant role in the production of histological changes that do occur and the clinical symptoms associated with them. The weakness of the autoimmune theory is the need to explain how a system universal to all body tissues can target only a single joint for tendinous degeneration.

Towards a Classification of Rotator Cuff Problems

A plethora of terms has been used to describe the clinical syndromes resulting from rotator cuff degeneration: supraspinatus tendinitis, rotator cuff tears, calcifying tendinitis, bursitis, periarthritis, frozen shoulder, capsulitis, etc. This is unfortunate because these terms cloud the pathogenesis of the symptoms and tend to lead to empirical treatment. To conduct treatment along rational lines, it is important to recognize the relationship of these symptom complexes to underlying pathological processes. The basic lesion is cell death and the "inflammatory" response to this change may lead to supraspinatus tendinitis which, in turn, may evoke subacromial bursitis. The necrotic portion of the tendon may calcify or, as the result of a minor repeated injury, the tendon may rupture. The changes may spread to involve the whole rotator cuff or, indeed, the initial pathology may be diffuse, producing what may best be termed a capsulitis (14).

Classification

With the drift away from acute tendon ruptures, and the establishment of repeated microtrauma to vascularly impaired tendons as the dominant factor in rotator cuff tendinitis and tears, the terminology now used for this group of disorders has been classified by Neer and others into various stages (Table 13.1).

One word of caution: It is becoming more evident that a third factor of shoulder instability may join with microtrauma and impaired vascularity to produce these lesions. By re-examining failed subacromial decompressions, Jobe (6) noted an element of instability that was missed preoperatively (see Chapter 17).

In the last few pages, you have seen the term "capsulitis." Because of the marked restriction of movement of the glenohumeral joint, this syndrome is frequently referred to as a "frozen shoulder." In 1896, Duplay (5) was the first to describe this clinical syndrome and introduced the term "scapulohumeral periarthritis." He felt that the initiating lesion was an obliteration of the subdeltoid bursa. From a study of postmortem specimens, Meyer (10) felt the initiating lesion was a breakdown of the intra-articular portion of the biceps tendon. His observations were supported by Pasteur (15), Lippman (7), and, more recently, by DePalma (4).

It was McLaughlin (9) who was the first to stress the importance of contracture of the subscapularis in the development of the syndrome, and Neviaser (14) noted that in this lesion the inferior hanging fold was obliterated, thereby limiting abduction. In an anatomical study of over 100 instances of frozen shoulder, it was impossible to substantiate Bateman's suggestion that the lesion was caused by intra-articular adhesions (1).

The multiple diagnoses support Caillet's (2) statement that "frozen shoulder was a term widely used and poorly understood." It is fairly reasonable to presume, however, that a frozen shoulder represents an idiopathic diffuse rotator cuff tendinitis, resulting in a gross limitation of movements of the glenohumeral joint in all planes.

Because of marked restriction of movement of the glenohumeral joint associated with a diffuse capsulitis, the patient can only move the shoulder by swinging the scapula around the chest wall. This necessitates excessive movement of the acromioclavicular joint, which may eventually break down and become symptomatic. Similarly, with marked restriction of glenohumeral movement on forward flexion of the humerus as the scapula is swung anteriorly around the chest wall, traction is applied to the suprascapular nerve and may produce a suprascapular nerve neuropathy.

Calcific Tendinitis

Historically, calcification of a rotator cuff tendon has been ascribed to cell death and dystrophic deposit of calcium crystals. More recently, Uhthoff et al (17) noted that the calcific deposit has a tendency to undergo spontaneous resorption, followed by complete healing of the tendon. Because of this evolution, they call the process "reactive" rather than dystrophic.

The location of the calcification is usually near the insertion of the supraspinatus tendon (Fig. 13.11) and not in the subacromial bursa. It is unusual to see tendon rupture with calcification, and usual to see spontaneous resorption—both phenomena requiring good blood supply. This is another reason to consider the process reactive rather than dystrophic (occurring in "dead cells").

Shoulder-Hand Syndrome

Finally, a diffuse rotator cuff tendinitis may lead to an ill-defined symptom complex, the so-called shoulder-hand syndrome (see Chapter 21).

CONCLUSION

Starting with the simple concepts of "focal or diffuse cell death," it is easy to understand the basis of the symptom complexes associated with rotator cuff tendinitis; the painful arc syndrome associated with supraspinatus tendinitis; the impingement syndrome; the pseudoparalysis found with massive tears; the anterior shoulder pain of biceps tendinitis; the frozen shoulder produced by a diffuse rotator cuff tendinitis, and its sequelae—acromioclavicular strain, degenerative changes involving the acromioclavicular joint, suprascapular neuropathy, and, finally, the shoulder-hand syndrome. This is truly a spectrum of clinical conditions.

REFERENCES

1. Bateman JE: The Shoulder and Neck, 2nd ed. WB Saunders, Philadelphia (1978).
2. Caillet R: Shoulder Pain, 2nd ed. FA Davis Co., Philadelphia (1969).
3. Codman EA: Rupture of the Supraspinatus Tendon and Other Lesions in or About the Subacromial Bursa. Thomas Todd Co., Boston (1934).
4. De Palma AF: Surgery of the Shoulder, 3rd ed. JB Lippincott, Philadelphia (1983).
5. Duplay S: De la perianthrite scapulo-humeral. Rev Frat Trav Med 53:236 (1896).
6. Jobe FW and Jobe CM: Painful athletic injuries of the shoulder. Clin Orthop 173:117–124 (1983).

7. Lippman RK: Frozen shoulder, periarthritis, bicipital tenosynovitis. Arch Surg 47:283–296 (1943).
8. Macnab I: Rotator cuff tendinitis. Ann R Coll Surg Engl 53:271–287 (1973).
9. McLaughlin HL: Lesions of the musculotendinous cuff of the shoulder. J Bone Joint Surg 26A: 31–51 (1944).
10. Meyer AW: Chronic functional lesions of the shoulder. Arch Surg 35:646–649 (1937).
11. Neer CS: Anterior acromioplasty for the chronic impingement syndrome in the shoulder. A preliminary report. J Bone Joint Surg 54A:41–50 (1972).
12. Neer CS: Impingement lesions. Clinic Orthop 173:70–77 (1983).
13. Neer CS and Welsh RP: The shoulder in sports. Orthop Clin North Am 8:583–591 (1977).
14. Neviaser JS: Adhesive capsulitis of the shoulder. J Bone Joint Surg 27A:211–222 (1945).
15. Pasteur F: Sur une forme nouvelle de perianthralogie et d'lankylose de l'epaule. J Radiol Eletrol 18:327 (1934).
16. Rathbun JB and Macnab I: The microvascular pattern of the rotator cuff. J Bone Joint Surg 52A: 540–543 (1970).
17. Uhthoff HK, Sarkark, and Maynard JA: Calcifying tendonitis. Clin Orthop 118:164–168 (1976).
18. Welsh P and Macnab I: Biomechanical studies of rabbit tendons. Clin Orthop 81:171–177 (1971).

14

Rotator Cuff Tendinitis and Related Clinical Syndromes and Their Diagnosis

"Immediate revelation is a much easier way for men to establish their opinions and regulate their conduct, than the tedious and not always successful labor of strict reasoning."
—John Locke

When discussing the pathogenesis of rotator cuff tendinitis, it has been suggested that the initiating factor is probably cell death, secondary to repeated microtrauma in a vascular-deficient tendon.

This induces an inflammatory response that can be focal, that is, localized to one small area and giving rise to tendinitis. Or, it can be diffuse and produce capsulitis, involving the whole capsule of the shoulder joint, including all of the tendons that constitute the rotator cuff.

Each of these clinicopathologic lesions merges with the others and can present a confusing array of symptoms and signs. However, at the risk of sounding dogmatic, it is perhaps best to describe each as a specific entity.

ROTATOR CUFF TENDINITIS AND THE IMPINGEMENT SYNDROME

Neer (11, 12) has proposed that anterior mechanical impingement of the rotator cuff occurs between the humeral head inferiorly and the coracoacromial arch superiorly, and is of greater cause for rotator cuff lesions than vascular impairment. Neer has described a continuum of conditions as a result of this impingement—from bursitis, to tendinitis, to partial rotator cuff tears, and finally to complete tears of the rotator cuff (Table 13.1).

When a patient presents a painful shoulder, it is very important, as mentioned previously, to ask the patient to demonstrate the site of the pain. Obviously, pain derived from the neck is intensified by movements of the neck, particularly extension. Glenohumeral pain is aggravated by any movements of the shoulder, particularly external rotation. The shoulder of the dominant extremity is the one most frequently involved. There is usually an underlying history of repetitive overhead activity at work (e.g., carpentry and painting) or play (e.g., racquet sports and swimming). Rarely will a specific injury be the cause of these syndromes.

The pain may be severe at night in bed, particularly if the patient rolls over onto the painful side. Sometimes the pain is more severe during the first hour after arising.

On examination, the patient is usually between the ages of 35 and 45. Onset may be earlier in diabetics or in people with a family history of diabetes. The

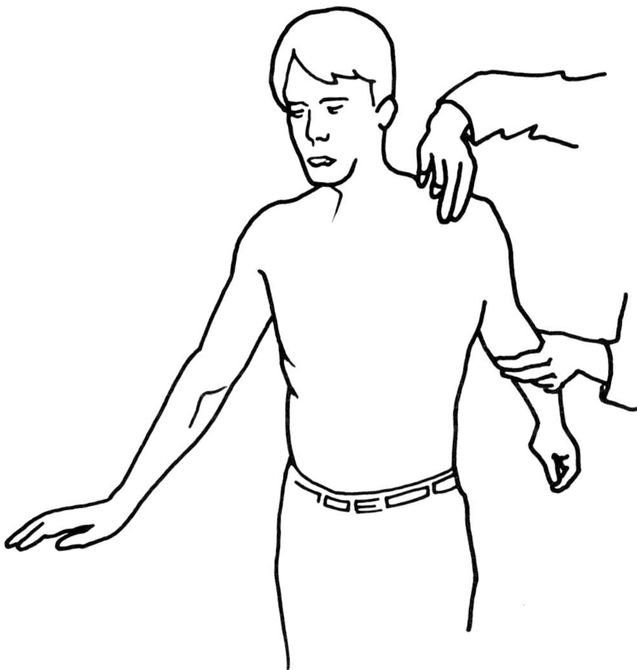

Figure 14.1.   With the shoulder extended, palpate the rotator cuff for tenderness in front of the acromion.

supraspinatus tendon is the most common tendon involved, because it is impinged in the common movement of shoulder elevation in the flexed internally rotated position.

There is tenderness on palpation immediately anterior to the edge of the acromion. If the shoulder is extended passively to its full extent, the insertion of the supraspinatus becomes palpable immediately in front of the anterior border of the acromion, and deep pressure applied here may feel exquisitely tender (Fig. 14.1). When assessing active movement of the shoulder, active abduction can usually be performed relatively painlessly from 0°–60°. Movement from 60°–120° is much more painful. In the early stages, abduction from 120°–180° can be done easily. The patients, then, characteristically have a painful arc of abduction from 60°–120°, and this has been termed the painful arc syndrome (Fig. 14.2). Final support for the diagnosis comes with abolition of the pain on injection of lidocaine (10 ml/1%) into the subacromial bursa (Fig. 14.3).

The explanation for the painful arc is a combination of impingement of the rotator cuff, especially in partial flexion and internal rotation, and the fact that the greatest strain taken by the tendon of the supraspinatus is through the range of 60°–120° of abduction (1).

In cadaveric studies (9), it can be shown that, on passive abduction of the shoulder, the supraspinatus does not abut the acromion until flexion and internal rotation occur. In pure abduction, impingement will occur when there is a deep tear in the tendon on its humeral surface. In the presence of such a tear, the

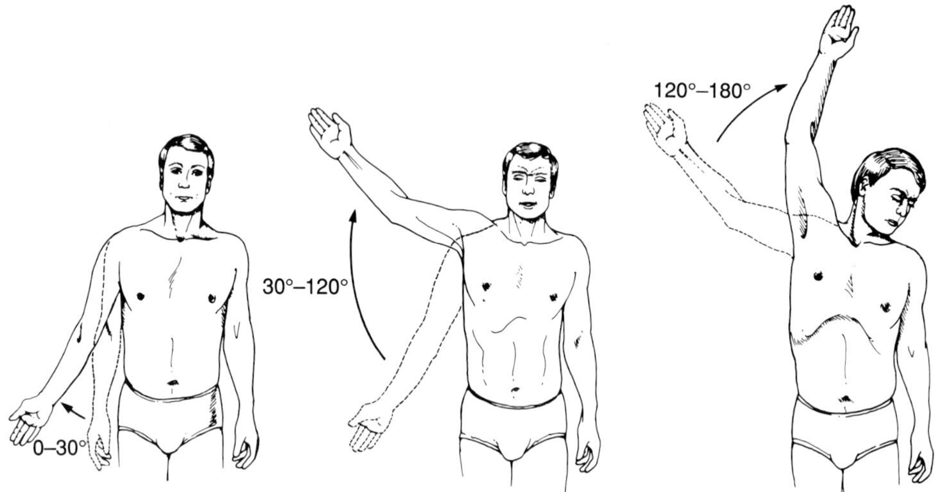

Figure 14.2. The painful arc of abduction from 60°–120°.

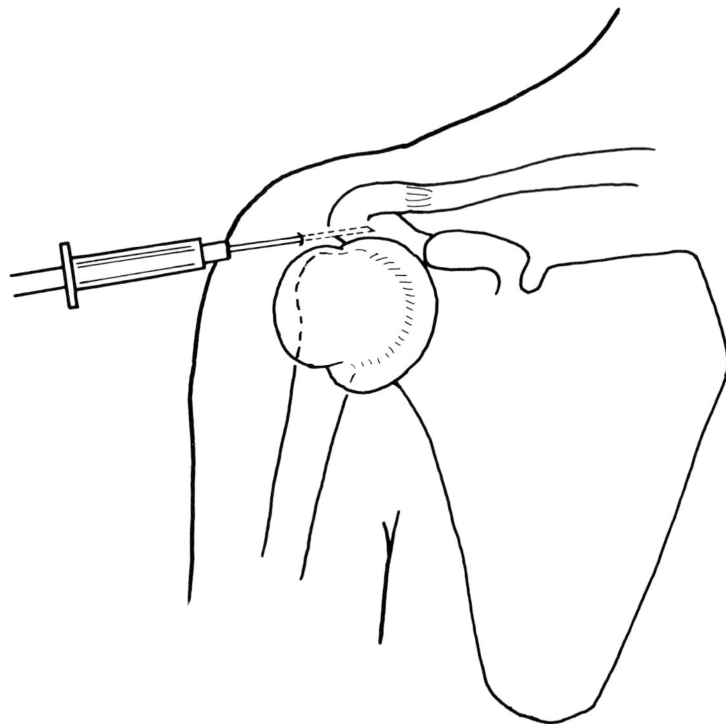

Figure 14.3. It is often useful to see if you can abolish the painful arc with an injection of local anesthetic into the subacromial bursa (not into the shoulder joint!).

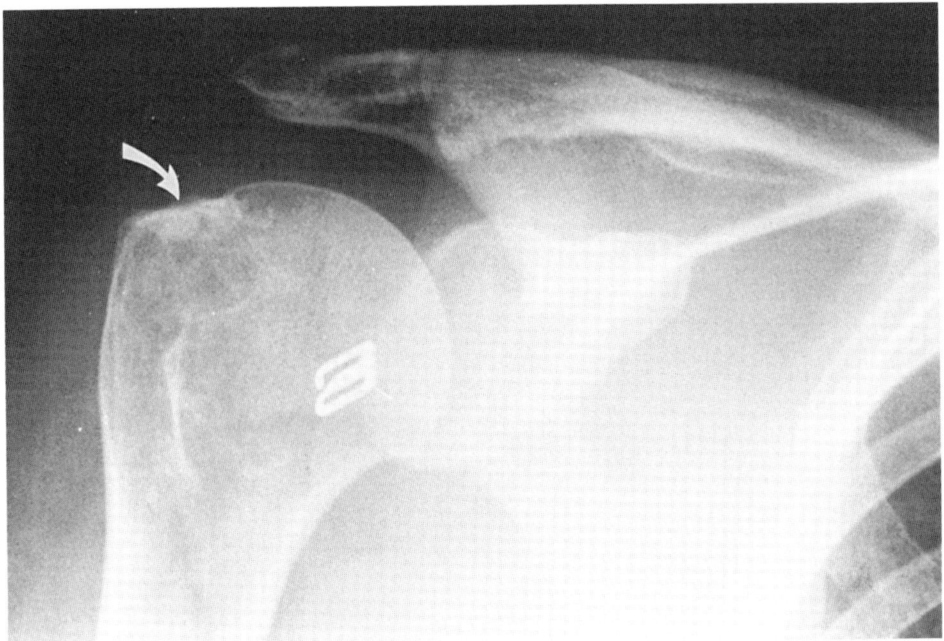

Figure 14.4.   Sclerosis (*arrow*) at sight of insertion of supraspinatus.

tendon buckles on abduction at the site of the tear and impinges against the acromion or the coracoacromial ligament.

X-rays of the shoulder usually do not show any significant changes, except for the occasional sclerosis or cystic changes of the superior portion of the greater tuberosity at the site of insertion of the supraspinatus (Fig. 14.4).

Treatment

The most important aspect of treatment is passive: rest the shoulder from the aggravating activity, and observe the patient over time. During the weeks of observation, active treatment in the form of pain relief (analgesics) and/or nonsteroidal anti-inflammatory medication is useful. It is important to maintain shoulder mobility during this observation period and, when the pain settles, to start a rehabilitation program of strengthening exercises (Appendix).

The analgesic should be one that patients know they can tolerate, and it should not be given on demand—patients should not be permitted to pop pills for pain. If patients are told to take an analgesic "when necessary," they may postpone taking the analgesic for as long as possible. By this time, the discomfort has reached a level where the analgesic dosage is not sufficient to stop the pain.

Patients understandably tend to double the dosage, and then they are on the way to habituation. Analgesics must always be given on a time-dependent basis. Severe isolated episodes of pain, as from an unexpected twist or an unanticipated lift, are best controlled by icing rather than by increasing the dose of analgesic. Attention must be paid to a history of gastric disturbances before prescribing anti-inflammatory drugs.

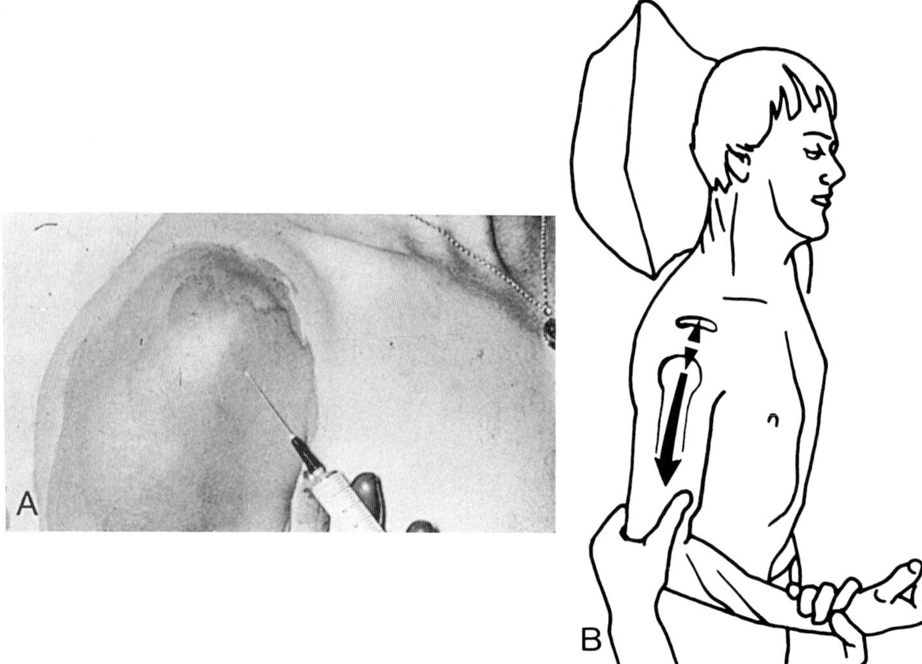

Figure 14.5.   To help inject the subacromial bursa, have an assistant pull down on the shoulder joint.

If the patient does not show any response to this routine within two or three weeks, or shows evidence of gastric irritation from nonsteroidals, it is best to treat the lesion by injecting one of the local steroid suspensions, such as hydrocortisone (Fig. 14.3). The cortisone suspension must be injected into the subdeltoid bursa, never into the tendon. Intratendinous injections, apart from being exquisitely painful, run the serious risk of causing tendon rupture.

If help is available, the injection is greatly facilitated by having someone pull vertically downward on the humerus (Fig. 14.5). This increases the subacromial space and makes it much easier to insert the needle into the subdeltoid bursa by avoiding all bony obstruction.

There should be no resistance to the injection. If there is resistance, the needle has probably been inserted into the tendon. The needle must be partly withdrawn and redirected. It is helpful on occasion to inject .5 ml of air. If the needle is correctly placed in the bursa, then the air in the syringe enters easily. If the tip of the needle is imbedded in tissue, even the injection of air will be resisted.

It is also important to remember that other areas around the shoulder joint are frequently tender on pressure, particularly the insertion of the deltoid and the tip of the coracoid process. Although the origin of the coracobrachialis occasionally develops tendinitis, this is relatively uncommon. These tender areas, though commonly demonstrated, do not denote other sites of "tendinitis"—they are areas of "referred" tenderness or areas of myotatic irritability. There is never any indication whatsoever to inject steroids into these sites.

There is some controversy about the use of steroid injections to treat this and other joint disorders. Many investigators (8, 15) have shown deleterious effects from repeated intra-articular or intratendinal injections. Others (20) have shown no advantage of intra-articular injections in double-blind studies with saline, while Valtonen (18) has shown no difference between gluteal and subacromial injections of steroids.

The use of intrabursal or intra-articular steroid injections in these conditions should probably be limited to strict indications and few repeats. Someday, when newer, more effective, and less toxic NSAIDs become available, injections may be abandoned altogether.

Failure of Conservative Care

No one has yet defined the correct period of conservative care. The pressures on defining this length of time is one thing for the star high school quarterback and another for the carpenter unhappy with his work and facing a seasonal lay-off. Obviously, the duration of conservative care will vary with the individual. Usually, surgery should not be considered until six to eight weeks have elapsed, and no more than six to eight months should pass before surgery is undertaken.

Surgical Intervention for Impingement Syndromes

Neer (12) is credited with localizing impingement to the anterior acromial region and describing the subacromial decompression, also known as anterior acromioplasty. This usually includes excision of the undersurface of the anterior-inferior third of the acromion, and resection of the coracoacromial ligament (Fig. 11.25). If osteophytes are present on the undersurface of the acromioclavicular joint (Fig. 14.6), they are excised along with the outer edge of the clavicle. The debridement part of this procedure was initially described as an open procedure, but is increasingly done as an arthroscopic procedure.

High expectations for return to competitive sports or overhead labor activities following acromioplasty have not been supported by detailed follow-up studies (7, 16). Part of the reason lies in associated conditions, such as instabilities and rotator cuff tears.

Obviously, surgery is not a panacea for impingement syndromes. This has led to the opinion that exercise and job modification should precede acromion modification.

Exercise Rehabilitation

Whether or not surgery is performed, exercise ultimately becomes the backbone of rehabilitation. Two basic programs are used. The first restores a normal range of movement, the second restores normal strength. Both programs are outlined in the Appendix.

Calcifying Tendinitis

If we accept that calcification of the rotator cuff is usually reactive (17) rather than dystrophic into degenerating or dead tissue, why should we include the condition in this chapter? There is no easy answer, except that its presentation is no different than other impingement syndromes.

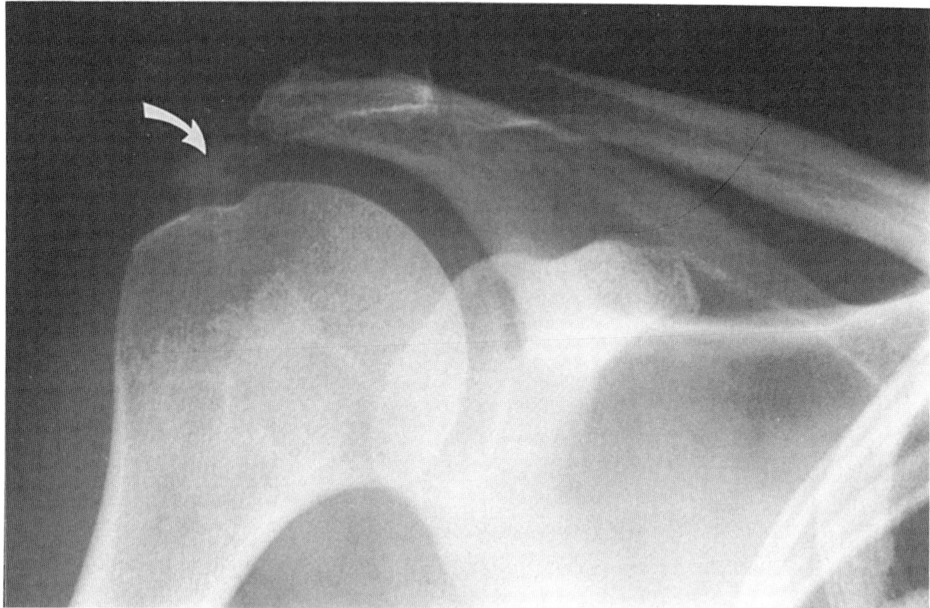

Figure 14.6.   Obvious calcification of rotator cuff (*arrow*).

Calcific tendinitis may be symptomatic or asymptomatic. If it is symptomatic, it usually occurs in middle-aged females and usually causes chronic grumbling pain. Its presentation is not unlike the impingement syndromes, and diagnosis will not be evident until an x-ray is obtained (Fig. 14.7). Almost all deposits will be in the supraspinatus tendon (90%), and are located .5 in. from its insertion. This is the "critical blood supply zone" of Codman (2).

The natural history of calcifying tendinitis is very cyclic, with the mass varying in size, and symptoms varying in extent, in the same patient. Eventually, most patients experience spontaneous disappearance of impingement symptoms along with the calcific mass.

In deciding on treatment alternatives, divide your patients into acute or chronic symptoms. The few patients with acute pain will have a virtually paralyzed shoulder because of pain, and are best treated with rest, strong analgesia and NSAIDs. Skilled orthopedic surgeons can often aspirate the calcific deposit via needle lavage, although this is not a widely accepted technique (2). Most patients will have chronic symptoms and need encouragement to be "patient patients". ROM and strengthening exercises, along with mild NSAIDs, are the standard treatment.

Rarely does a patient with calcifying tendinitis require surgery. Occasionally, a patient with chronic impingement symptoms will not accept the prolonged interference in overhead activities—in spite of adequate conservative care—and will require surgery. The surgical approach is a simple deltoid splitting approach and evacuation of the deposit (Fig. 11.25). If the subacromial space is impinged at surgery, Neer's (11) anterior acromioplasty is indicated. Surgery should not be considered in the acute phase since it represents the body's attempt to resorb the mass. The only invasive procedure useful in the acute phase is a double nee-

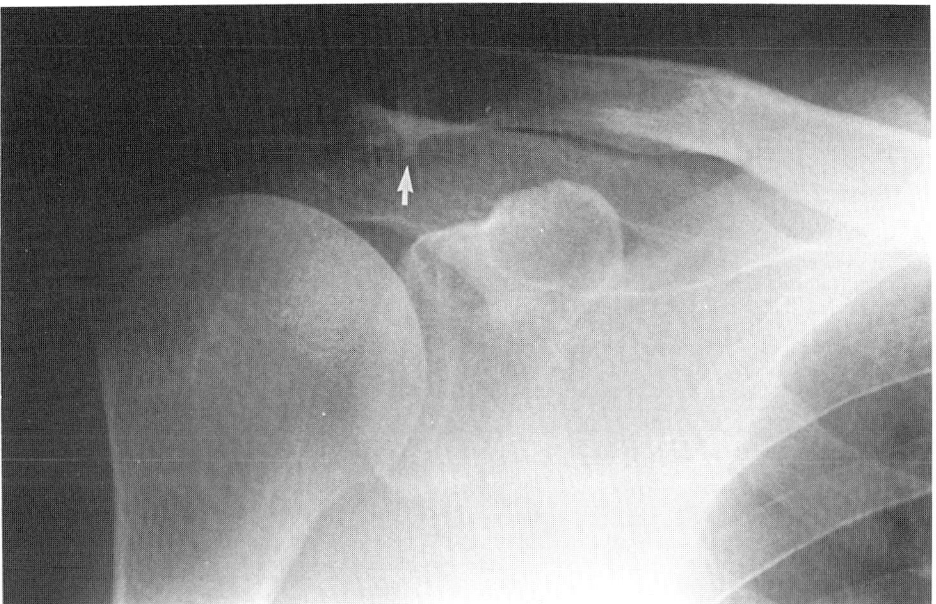

Figure 14.7.   An osteophyte on the undersurface of the acromioclavicular joint, that needs to be excised.

dle attempt at lavage. Follow any surgery for this condition with an immediate, aggressive exercise program.

On infrequent occasions you will see patients with actual dystrophic calcification in rotator cuff tears or osteoarthritis. This phenomenon is obviously secondary to the primary tear of arthritic degeneration and is a poor prognostic sign for any form of treatment.

Bicipital Tendinitis

The poor old biceps tendon! What is its action on the shoulder joint? Is bicipital tendinitis as common as believed in the past? Neer (12) believes most patients with the diagnosis of bicipital tendinitis have a primary impingement syndrome with secondary involvement of the biceps tendon.

Anatomy

The long head of the biceps tendon originates along the superior edge of the labrum and traverses the shoulder joint as an "extra-synovial" structure (Fig. 14.8). In the arm, it joins with the short head of the biceps and is inserted into the biceps tubercle of the radius and the bicipital aponeurosis. Its action on the elbow is obvious: it is a supinator (its strongest action being from the forearm pronated position) and an elbow flexor. Its action on the shoulder is less obvious: it probably serves as a mildly passive humeral head stabilizer.

Proximal to the surgical neck of the humerus, it is an intimate part of the rotator cuff, separating the subscapularis from the supraspinatus. Distal to the surgical neck and capsular insertion, it lies in the bicipital groove, a bony trough. This groove separates the lesser tuberosity from the greater tuberosity. In the

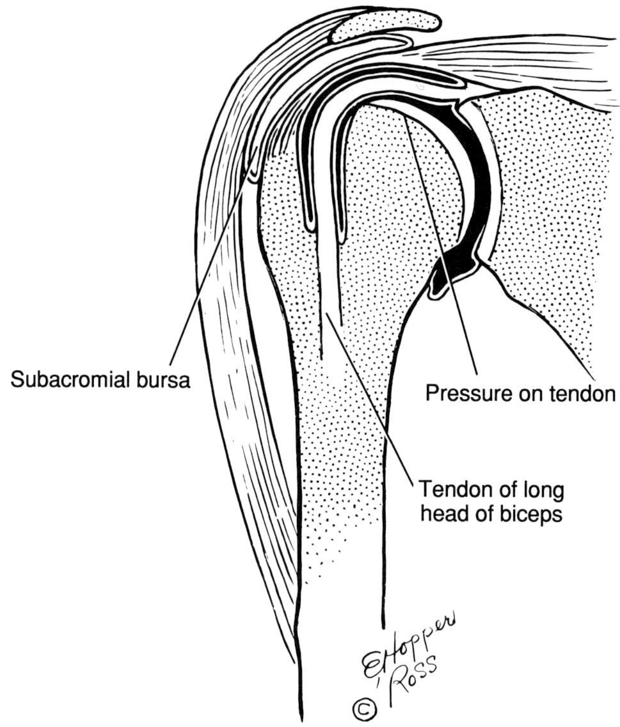

Figure 14.8.   Note that the biceps tendon traverses the shoulder joint as an "extra synovial" structure.

groove, the biceps tendon is lined with synovial tissue and is held in place by the transverse humeral ligament.

It is hard to imagine that a tendon moving in a bony groove, restrained by ligaments and lined by synovia, cannot become inflamed and painful. Bicipital tendinitis may occur as an isolated lesion, or it may occur in association with a diffuse capsulitis, rheumatoid arthritis, or osteoarthritis. The pathogenesis of these changes within the biceps tendon is probably the same as in supraspinatus tendinitis. The biceps has to run over the hump of the head of the humerus to reach the bicipital groove. It has been shown in microangiographic studies that the vascular bed is wrung out at the area of maximum pressure. It is in this zone that degenerative changes first appear and are most extensive. Pain is experienced over the anterior aspect of the shoulder and is aggravated by general use of the arm.

The pain in bicipital tendinitis is located over the tendon in the groove and is mechanical in nature, aggravated by shoulder movements. Neer has suggested that it is virtually indistinguishable from impingement syndromes on history.

On examination, there is tenderness on palpating the tendon anteriorly; this can best be demonstrated by the examiner placing the tips of his or her fingers over the biceps tendon in the groove as the shoulder is elevated (Fig. 14.9). Keeping the fingers in the same place, the shoulder should then be placed in the anatomical position, and internally and externally rotated a few degrees. By rotating the humerus, the biceps tendon is taken away from the pressure of the

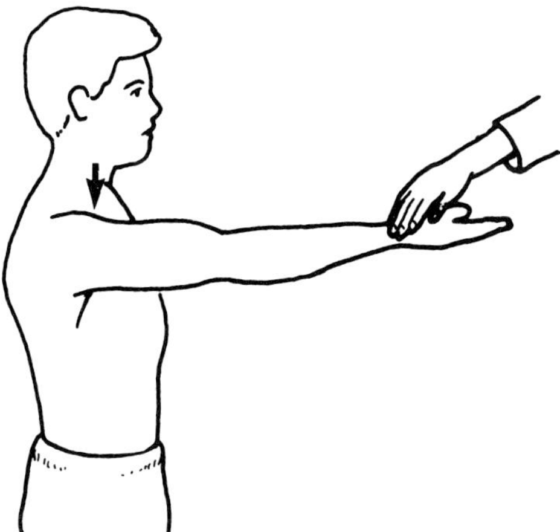

Figure 14.9.   Speed's test for bicipital tendinitis. Elevation of the arm increases shoulder pain in the region of the bicipital tendon (*arrow*).

examiner's fingers, and the tenderness goes away, only to return when the humerus is rotated in the opposite direction (Fig. 14.10). This specificity of pain localization is the physical finding that distinguishes bicipital tendinitis from the more diffuse conditions of bursitis and from impingement syndromes. The pain experienced is frequently increased on forced extension of the glenohumeral joint. The best diagnostic test for bicipital tendinitis is local infiltration of the tendon sheath with anesthetic and, for treatment, steroid occasionally is included.

In many, the pain will subside on oral nonsteroidal anti-inflammatory drugs and rest. For those in whom the pain persists, further infiltration of the biceps tendon sheath with steroid may be of value. There are two things to remember if you are going to inject steroid. First, you are injecting into a very tight space (compared to the subacromial bursa) and have a good chance of injecting directly into the tendon, contributing to subsequent tendon rupture. Second, if the patient has that much pain persisting over a long time and interfering so much with function, it is probably better to operate.

Some cases of bicipital tendinitis are very refractory to conservative treatment. This is probably because of mechanical constriction of the tendon as it glides through the intertubercular groove on movement of the shoulder joint. In these patients, an impingement decompression is indicated and, if a frayed tendon is found, a bicipital tenodesis may be of value (dividing the biceps tendon and suturing it to the sides of the intertubercular groove). When conservative care fails, also be aware of other diagnoses, such as Neer's subacromial impingement syndromes (11).

Rupture of the Biceps Tendon

At times, bicipital tendinitis will persist to the point of tendon attrition and rupture. The most common site of rupture is just proximal to the intertubercular groove at the point of maximum convexity of the head of the humerus. Rupture at this site commonly occurs without provocative trauma. If pain was present in the shoulder, it generally subsides when the tendon ruptures. Following rupture

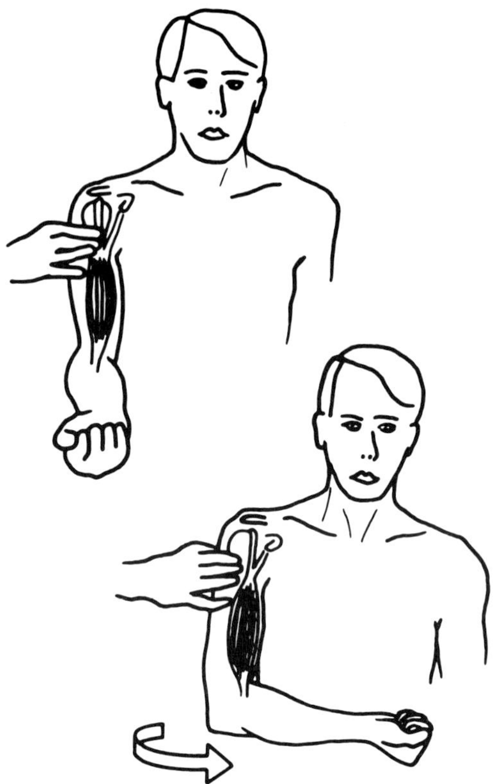

Figure 14.10.   Internal and external rotation, with palpation over the biceps tendon, takes the tendon in and out of the "range of local tenderness."

of the long head of the biceps, it is unusual for the patient to complain of significant weakness on flexion of the elbow or on supination of the forearm. However, to maintain the shoulder abducted and externally rotated to 90° with the elbow flexed is extremely difficult, because the head of the humerus has to be stabilized in this position by the long head of the biceps. In certain occupations, such as waiting tables, the inability to hold the arm in this position may interfere with the waiter's capacity to work.

In young, active athletes and in workers needing sustained arm strength, repair is often entertained. With older patients (55 and up), simply reassure them that nothing terrible is amiss, that their old pain will now be gone, and that they will be happy with their activity level. More often than not, surgery becomes part of an overall impingement and rotator cuff repair procedure. The prominence of the biceps muscle following rupture of the long head of the biceps produces a significant cosmetic defect frequently distasteful to women who have the condition. This can be overcome by suturing the tendon to the bicipital groove. It is wise to combine this with excision of the intra-articular portion of the tendon.

If the rupture occurs near the distal insertion of the biceps, surgical repair is mandatory. Otherwise, there will be a significant loss of power in flexion of the elbow and supination of the forearm.

Rupture of the Rotator Cuff

It must be remembered that a normal, healthy tendon never breaks. If the tendon is normal, forced adduction results in an avulsion fracture of the greater tuberosity. Partial or complete tears of the rotator cuff need pre-existing pathology (tendinitis, impingement) to weaken the tendon over a long period of time. When this happens, two situations prevail: the patient does a lot of overhead activity at play or at work, and he or she does it over a long enough time to develop wear and then tear of the rotator cuff. Tears seldom occur before the age of 40 and may follow trivial injury, generally a resisted abduction strain of the shoulder.

The injury may be trivial as, for example, in the "lonely skier syndrome," in which the head of the family waits at the bottom of the slopes for the kids to have their last few runs before the chair lifts close for the day. An enthusiastic, if not skillful, skier comes schussing down the hill and hits the older man mightily on his side. The "lonely skier" falls, putting out his arm to break his fall, and sustains a forced adduction strain of the shoulder joint. This may result in a rupture of the supraspinatus tendon at its point of insertion to the humerus.

More often, a minor injury initiates a partial tear, followed by an accumulation of repeated abduction stresses that enlarge the tear to full thickness lesions and/or massive tears. The tendon most commonly involved is the supraspinatus.

The primary symptom is deltoid pain in the 40 + athletic individual or overhead worker. The pain is aggravated by abduction elevation of the shoulder—the painful arc (Fig. 14.2). With time, the pain becomes more constant and wakes the patient when he or she rolls onto the shoulder at night.

On examination, inspection may reveal wasting of the muscle attached to the nonfunctioning torn tendon (supraspinatus). Palpation for a gap in the tendon, or local tenderness in the tear, is rarely successful. The typical physical finding is asynchronous active abduction with a shrug (Fig. 14.11) and weakness in abduction against resistance (Fig. 14.12). For some unknown reason, patients with rotator cuff tears maintain a good passive range of movement in the shoulder and may even have a good active range of movement.

In acute cases, a fairly accurate assessment of the size of the tear can be obtained by measuring the induced intra-articular pressure (Fig. 14.13). If the rotator cuff is intact, the intra-articular pressure increases proportionately as fluid is injected into the joint. If the defect is small, the intra-articular pressure rises initially and then reaches a plateau. If there is a massive avulsion, there is little if any increase in the pressure on increasing the volume injected. In practice, three diagnostic methods may be combined. Local anesthetic is first injected into the joint to assess whether the inability to abduct the arm is because of pain or loss of the stabilizing action of the supraspinatus. If the patient is still unable to abduct the arm after the intra-articular injection of local anesthetic, a radiopaque dye is injected in an attempt to confirm the presence of a defect in the rotator cuff. If the dye is found to escape, then the glenohumeral joint is distended with 50 cc of saline and the needle is connected to a pressure transducer. It is sometimes technically easier to fill the joint to its maximum pressure and then measure the rate of degradation. With a complete avulsion of the rotator cuff, the pressure falls rapidly.

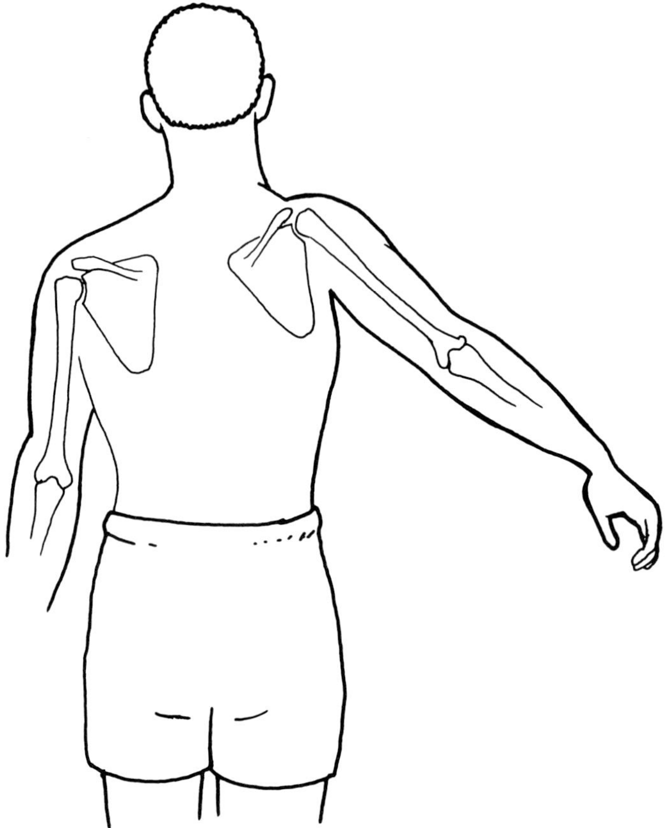

Figure 14.11. Note the asynchronous shrug of abduction on the right, due to inability of the weak/painful rotator cuff to fix the humeral head in the glenoid.

X-ray Findings

Nonspecific x-ray changes, such as degeneration in the acromioclavicular joint, sclerosis at the insertion of the rotator cuff (Fig. 14.4), and elevation of the humeral head (Fig. 14.14) are often present (19).

The gold standard for diagnosis is arthrography (Fig. 12.32*B*) and ultrasound (Fig. 12.33). Quickly, these standards are being replaced by MRI (Fig. 14.15).

Treatment—Conservative

A small tear that is not interfering significantly with work or play should be rested and medicated. Strengthening and stretching exercises are then used to rehabilitate the patient into an acceptable activity program. Occasionally, a conservative treatment program can be boosted with a subacromial injection of local anesthetic and steroid (do it late in conservative care and not too often!).

Treatment—Surgical

Massive tears, acute traumatic tears, and smaller tears that interfere with work or play should be surgically repaired. Operative (open) repair with subacro-

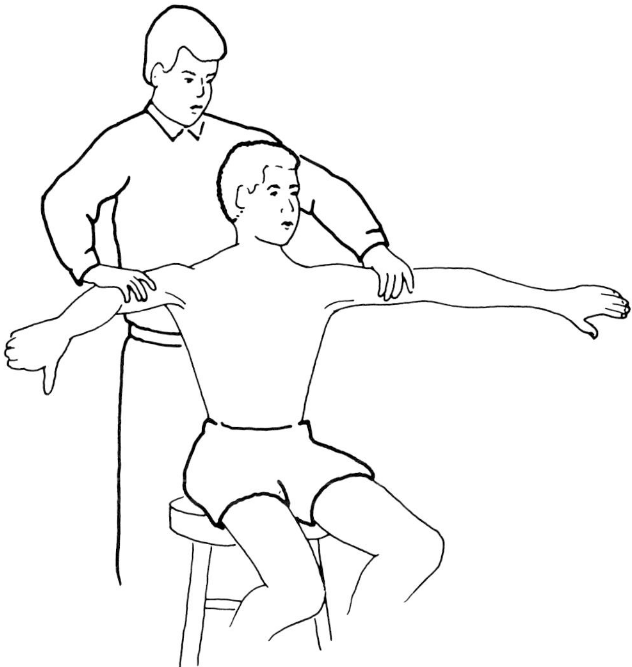

Figure 14.12.   Testing abduction against resistance, in various phases of internal and external rotation, will detect painful impingement.

mial decompression is the treatment of choice (Fig. 14.16). In proposing such treatment, remind patients that they will achieve improvement in shoulder function but will not return to the level of "world-class weekend sports" (7).

Wherever possible, early repair is preferable, avoiding the difficulties encountered when attempting a repair with the humeral head superiorly displaced and the ruptured tendon densely adherent to the supraspinous fossa.

Early Repair.   Two points distinguish the repair of fresh traumatic tears from delayed repairs. First, it is easy to mobilize the recently torn tendon to obtain firm apposition of the components of the tear. Second, it is not always necessary to combine the repair with an acromioclavicular arthroplasty.

Late Repair.   Late repair should be combined with a subacromial decompression and, if acromioclavicular arthritic changes are present, with an excision of the outer .5 in. of the clavicle. This excisional arthroplasty of the acromioclavicular joint is carried out to facilitate acromiothoracic movement, thereby enhancing the degree of postoperative functional recovery. Excision of the outer .5 in. of the clavicle, combined with a subacromial decompression (acromioplasty and excision of the coracoacromial ligament), also improves the ability to see the retracted portion of the rotator cuff.

Although the methods of repair that have been described are legion, two major principles are common to all:

1. The integrity of the deltoid muscle must be maintained.
2. The repair of the tendon must be completed without tension.

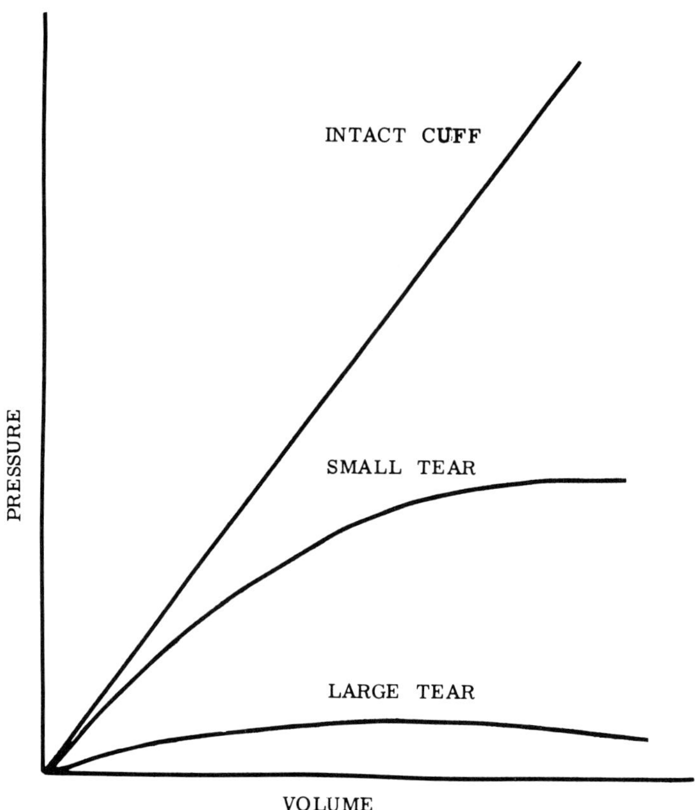

Figure 14.13.   Determination of the presence of a rotator cuff tear can be made by measurement of intra-articular pressure following injection of saline into the shoulder joint. If the rotator cuff is intact, intra-articular pressure increases proportionately in relation to the amount of fluid injected into the joint. If there is a massive avulsion, there is little if any increase in the pressure on increasing the volume of fluid injected.

Surgical details are described in order to enable the practitioner to explain to the patient the reasons for the timing of the operation and the difficulties attending surgical repair. An incision is made along the spine of the scapula to the edge of the acromion and extended down over the deltoid 2 in. The incision is deepened and the superior portion of the muscle is freed from the spine of the scapula. The incision in the deltoid is made in this plane so that the trapezius and deltoid remain as a single sheath. The combined trapezius and deltoid are now dissected off the acromioclavicular joint. The outer inch of the clavicle is removed to provide good access to the coracoacromial ligament. When the coracoacromial ligament and the subjacent bursa are excised, full internal rotation and extension of the glenohumeral joint will demonstrate the supraspinatus very clearly.

The supraspinatus tendon must be mobilized by making a longitudinal incision to separate it from the subscapularis. The incision will be made parallel to the biceps tendon. It is frequently necessary to separate the supraspinatus from the infraspinatus with another incision in the rotator cuff made parallel to the first. This second incision extends posteriorly along the base of the spine of the scap-

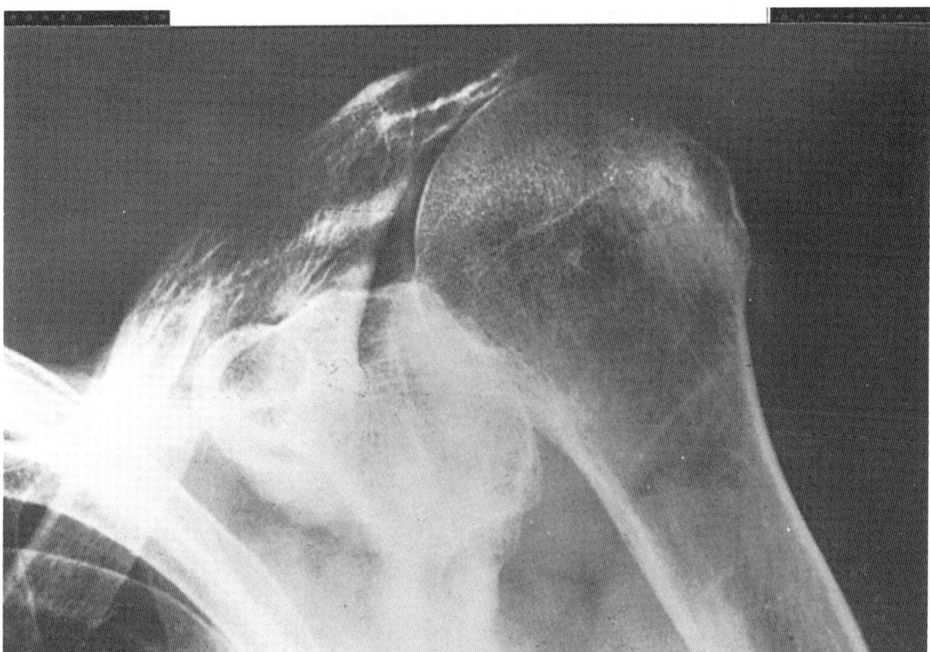

Figure 14.14.   When the rotator cuff is ruptured, the head of the humerus is not held against the glenoid, and contraction of the deltoid merely displaces the head superiorly. This represents an obvious case.

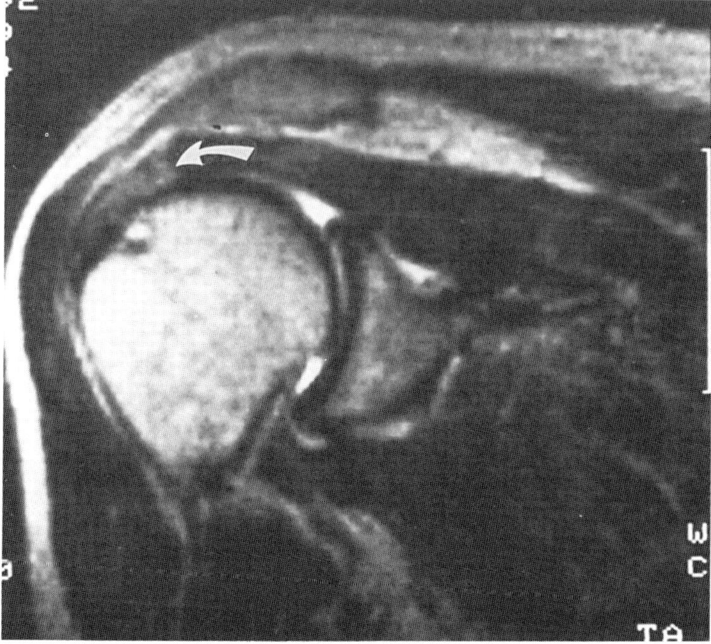

Figure 14.15.   MRI showing a rotator cuff tear (*arrow*).

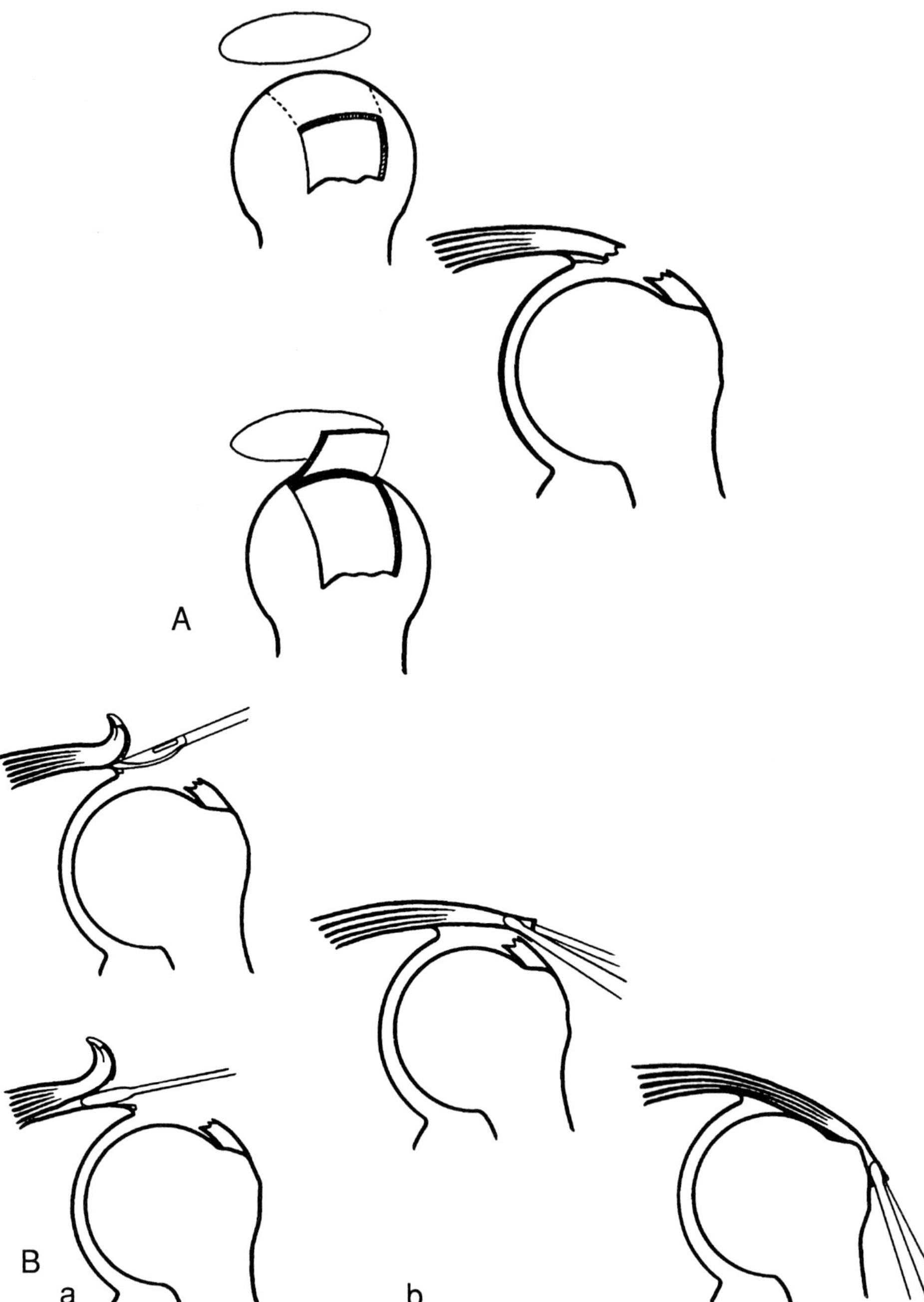

Figure 14.16.   A, the supraspinatus is separated from the infraspinatus by a vertical incision in the rotator cuff made parallel to the biceps tendon. A flap of the supraspinatus is now raised to expose the superior portion of the glenoid labrum. **B,** once the tendon has been mobilized, it is sometimes possible to repair the tear by end-to-end suture (*a*) or by fixing the distal end of the supraspinatus to a trough cut in the bone immediately proximal to the tuberosity of the humerus and holding it in this position with a staple (*b*).

ula. A flap of the supraspinatus is now raised to expose the superior portion of the glenoid labrum (Fig. 14.16*A*). A cut is made through the labrum to the rim of the glenoid, and the muscle belly of the supraspinatus is dissected by blunt dissection from the supraspinous fossa. Once the tendon has been mobilized, it is sometimes possible to repair the tear by end-to-end suture reinforced by suturing the supraspinatus side-to-side with the subscapularis and infraspinatus (Fig. 14.16*B*). More frequently, however, it is necessary to suture the torn end of the supraspinatus into a trough cut in the bone immediately proximal to the tuberosity of the humerus. Reinforce the repair by suturing the infraspinatus to the flap of the supraspinatus.

Postoperative rehabilitation usually consists of brief splinting (a period of days), then passive range-of-movement exercises daily for the first week and active assisted exercises subsequently. Gradually, resistance is added when the active range of movement can be performed comfortably—generally about eight weeks after surgery.

Irreparable Avulsion

The superior migration of the head of the humerus associated with longstanding avulsions of the rotator cuff has already been described (19). This superior displacement of the humeral head may make it technically impossible to effect any repair of the rotator cuff. Fortunately, in many patients the articulation between the head of the humerus and the undersurface of the acromion provides an adequate fulcrum, and these patients regain a useful range of active abduction of the shoulder. In some, however, this false joint may become painful. An operation popularized in Toronto used a metal spacer inserted between the undersurface of the acromion and the head of the humerus (Fig. 14.17) (2). Most surgeons prefer a debridement of the tuberosity and cuff remnant, coupled with an acromioplasty to control pain symptoms. Little improvement in function should be anticipated.

Frozen Shoulder (Adhesive Capsulitis)

Adhesive capsulitis may be considered the end stage of the progressive inflammatory and degenerative conditions described in the past few pages (13). Some consider it an enigmatic entity, unrelated to degeneration. The term specifically excludes lost shoulder movement caused by rheumatoid or osteoarthritic affliction of the shoulder joint.

In the early stages of this syndrome, the synovial membranes show hypertrophy and increased vascularity. At this stage, the synovial linings of the inferior hanging fold may adhere to each other. The synovial extensions, which normally pass behind the subscapularis and around the biceps tendon, become obliterated. The biceps tendon commonly demonstrates marked degenerative changes, which are related to interference with its vascular bed as it passes over the head of the humerus. It appears that the changes in the biceps tendon are secondary to the diffuse rotator cuff tendinitis and capsulitis, and these are an effect and not the cause, as suggested by Meyer (10) and Pasteur (14).

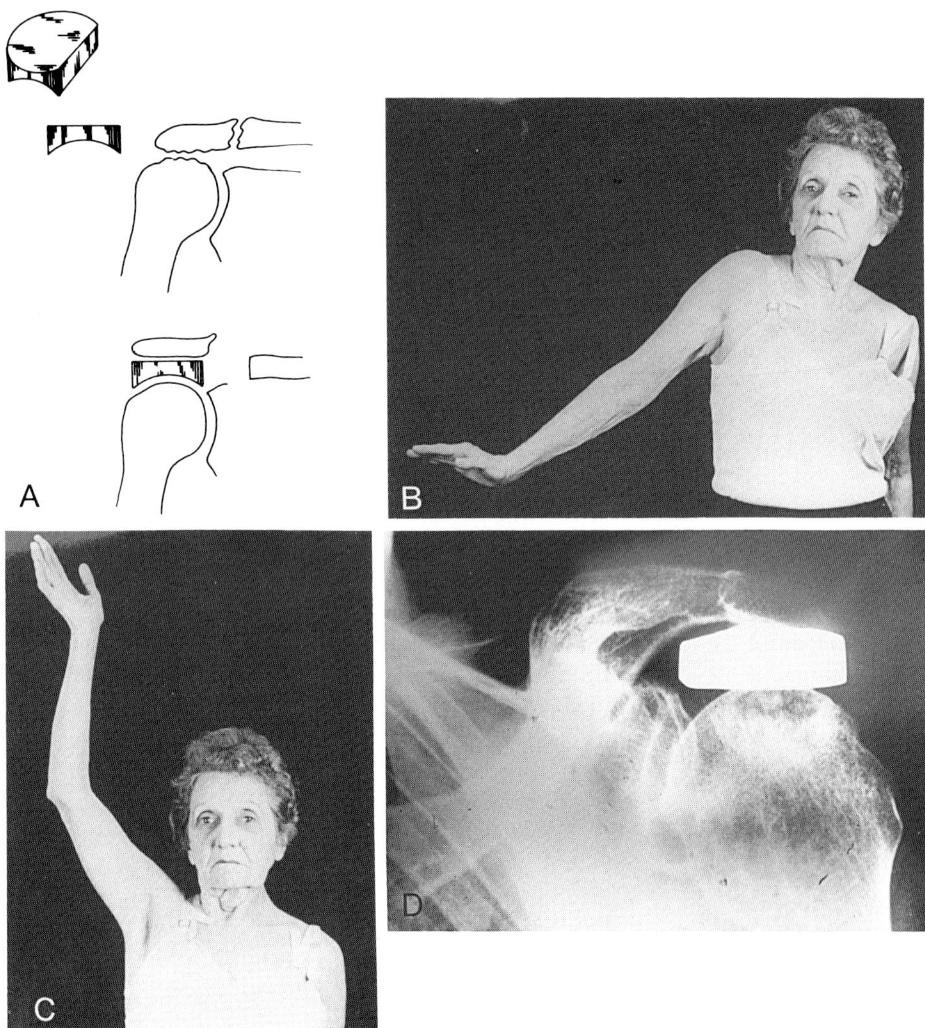

Figure 14.17.   A rarely used and occasionally successful way of treating a massive rotator cuff tear by insertion of a spacer—an old MacIntosh knee prosthesis (**A**). Preoperative abduction (**B**); postoperative abduction (**C**); x-ray of shoulder showing metal spacer in place (**D**).

Development of the Clinical Picture

Frequently without provocative trauma, a patient—usually over the age of 50—becomes conscious of a dull aching pain in the shoulder, experienced mostly over the deltoid. Although movements of the shoulder will aggravate the pain, initially the patient presents a full range of active and passive movement. Later, during the inflammatory stage, active and passive movements are limited by protective muscle spasm induced by the pain. Many patients are extremely apprehensive, and they are reluctant to move the shoulder or permit any passive movement. Noting this, several authors have suggested that the apprehension reflects the character of the patient rather than the severity of the pain (3). During the initial stage, the patient finds pain a constant companion, aggravated and intensified by normal daily activity. The most disabling aspect of the pain is that it is frequently worse at night, interfering markedly with the patient's sleep.

In the final stage, all movements of the glenohumeral joint are restricted by contracture of the capsule. Pain is experienced only if passive movement is forced. It is to this last stage that the term "frozen shoulder" is applied. On examination, the spinatii and the deltoid present a varying degree of atrophy, which in some instances may be very marked indeed. The most notable clinical feature, of course, is the inability of the patient to externally rotate or abduct the arm. When the patient is asked to take the arm away from the side, he just shrugs his shoulder. Contraction of the deltoid alone will just pull the humerus vertically until it abuts against the acromion. It should be noted that, in the normal shoulder, after 60° of abduction the articular surface of the head of the humerus faces inferiorly. Thereafter, to maintain articular contact between the humerus and glenoid, the humerus must externally rotate. This helps in understanding how contracture of the tendon of the subscapularis and the coracohumeral ligament result in gross restriction of external rotation. When external rotation is grossly limited, abduction will be prevented by impingement of the greater tuberosity against the acromion.

In a normal shoulder, when the glenohumeral joint is adducted, the inferior capsule is lax and hangs down as a free fold. On abduction, the slack is taken up as the head of the humerus drops into this pocket. With the development of a diffuse capsulitis, this fold is frequently obliterated; on abduction, the prominence of the head of the humerus cannot be accommodated, thereby limiting further glenohumeral movement (Fig. 14.18).

In the absence of glenohumeral movement, abduction can be achieved by rotating the scapula around the chest wall (Fig. 14.18). The excessive amount of scapulothoracic glide necessary to achieve movement of the arm results in an abnormal degree of acromioclavicular joint movement, eventually resulting in articular breakdown. The pain associated with acromioclavicular arthritis is characteristically felt at the point of the shoulder, and it radiates up the trapezius to the mastoid process. Pain derived from degenerative changes in the acromioclavicular joint is frequently a factor interfering with the progress of a physiotherapy program designed to mobilize the glenohumeral joint.

With a frozen shoulder, when the arm is swung forward and toward the opposite side of the chest, the movement of the scapula around the chest wall may put a marked traction strain on the suprascapular nerve, particularly if the nerve is tethered by the suprascapular ligament as it passes through the suprascapular notch. The onset of suprascapular nerve neuropathy markedly increases the pain, and gross wasting of the supraspinatus and the infraspinatus develops. The muscles are exquisitely tender on palpation. The diagnosis of suprascapular nerve entrapment must be confirmed by an electromyogram (EMG) study. Marked entrapment of the suprascapular nerve demands division of the suprascapular ligament to permit free gliding of the nerve on movement of the scapula. This point must be remembered when considering operative intervention in the treatment of a frozen shoulder that has resisted all forms of conservative therapy. It is necessary to look for signs of suprascapular nerve entrapment and,

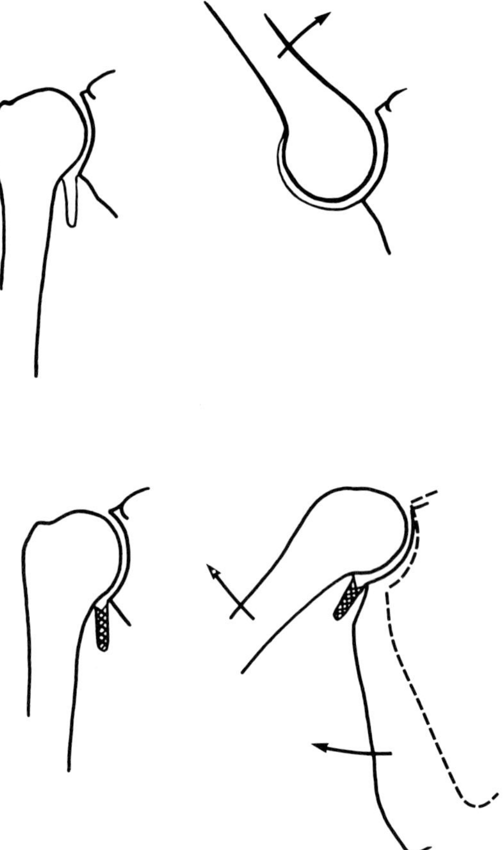

Figure 14.18.   On abduction of the shoulder, the head of the humerus drops into the inferior hanging fold. When this is obliterated, the prominence of the head of the humerus cannot be accommodated and glenohumeral movement is limited. In the absence of glenohumeral movement, abduction can be achieved by rotating the scapula around the chest wall.

if present, to include division of the transverse ligament in the operative procedure.

In the later stages of development of a frozen shoulder, the range of scapular glide is decreased. This is because the points of origin and insertion of the deltoid appear to be reversed. The force exerted by contracting the deltoid rotates the scapula and tends to swing the inferior angle towards the midline, and because of this the range of external scapulothoracic glide is markedly decreased.

Radiographic examination shows osteoporosis resulting from disuse and, occasionally, superior migration of the head of the humerus. Arthrography shows obliteration of the synovial pouches, but the cartilage space of the glenohumeral joint is maintained (Fig. 14.19).

Neviaser (13) clearly defined the pathology as a thickened joint capsule and a contracted synovial membrane with decreased synovial fluid in the joint. The only sign of inflammation was in the subsynovial layer of the capsule.

In almost every patient, the natural history is one of spontaneous resolution with loss of pain and restoration of movement within 18 months. Once the lesion

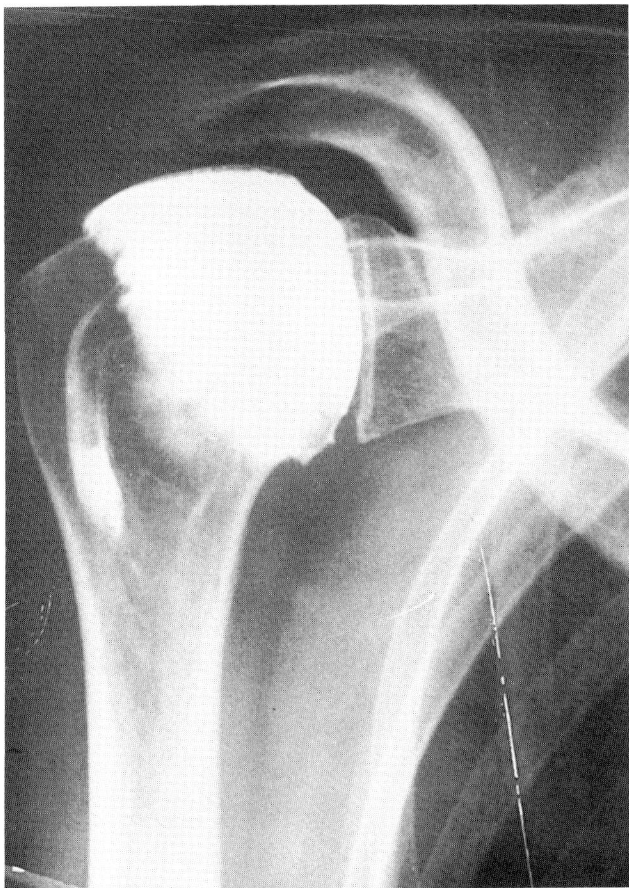

Figure 14.19. Arthrography of a frozen shoulder showing contracture of the capsule, although the cartilage space of the glenohumeral joint is maintained.

has resolved, it does not recur. A few patients, however, may have symptoms persisting for several years. De Palma (5) observed two groups of patients. The first group, although afflicted with significant pain, found it tolerable and could cooperate in an exercise program. These patients recovered within six months of onset. In the second group, the patients were much more disabled, either because of the severity of the pain or because of excessive reaction to it. These patients could not or would not engage fully in a supervised exercise program. It was in this group that protracted disability was observed. In the treatment of patients with a frozen shoulder, it is important, therefore, not only to assess the amount of pain the patient is suffering from; it is also important to assess the patient who has the pain.

Treatment

Treatment is primarily directed towards shortening the duration of the pain. With a diffuse capsulitis, injection of steroids into the subacromial bursa or even into the shoulder joint itself is rarely of value. Patients respond more favorably and more rapidly to a brief course of systemic steroids.

During the inflammatory phase, it is best to rest the arm and attempt to maintain the few degrees of motion still remaining in the glenohumeral joint by gentle exercises with gravity eliminated—pendulum exercises, skateboard exercises, and exercise in a therapeutic pool. Ice is far more useful than heat in this phase.

As the pain and spasms subside, the exercise program is increased to include assisted active movement with an emphasis on increasing the range of external rotation. If the patient progresses well, with loss of pain associated with an increase in active movement, then he or she may be started on a full shoulder rehabilitation program and continue the exercises at home. As this progresses, heat becomes more useful than ice.

On occasion, and regrettably too often, despite adequately supervised physiotherapy, the patient reaches a plateau in recovery. Movement is limited in all ranges and is painful only when forced. The following line of treatment may then be followed.

Hydraulic Distention. Hydraulic distention of the glenohumeral joint is controversial but may be used on occasion to "stretch" the capsule by hydraulic pressure. The glenohumeral joint is anesthetized by injecting lidocaine, and then a hydraulic manipulation is done by injecting saline. Considerable pressure has to be employed, and it is suggested that a metal and glass syringe be used. The amount of distention possible is usually determined by the production of severe discomfort. At the conclusion of hydraulic distention, the joint is aspirated and 2 cc of prednisolone or its equivalent should be injected to minimize traumatic inflammatory response produced by stretching of the capsule.

Manipulation. Manipulation of the shoulder joint under general anesthesia has frequently been employed and is often followed by a gratifying degree of success. However, it must be remembered that blind manipulation does not restore a range of movement by virtue of tearing a mythical "intra-articular adhesion" or stretching the tightened structures around the joint. During an operation, if a frozen shoulder is manipulated with the capsule exposed, it can be found that various structures will tear. First of all, the subscapularis tears across the musculotendinous junction as the arm is externally rotated forcibly. The inferior capsule of the shoulder will frequently tear when the arm has been abducted beyond 60°.

Most surgeons have experienced two separate and distinct responses during the process of manipulating a frozen shoulder. Occasionally, with relatively minimal force, the shoulder suddenly "gives" and a full range of passive movement is regained. There is no explanation for this phenomenon. Patients who present sudden release on manipulation can start an active exercise program immediately, covered by a short course of systemic steroids. The results are usually gratifying.

In other patients, increasing resistance is experienced as the arm is flexed, abducted, and externally rotated. As further pressure is applied, there is a tearing sound similar to the crunch of treading on fresh snow. In these patients, tissue is being torn. The organization of the inevitable hematoma in the torn tissues results in further contractures. These patients are rarely helped by manipulation. If, on manipulating the shoulder, the surgeon hears a sound similar to the snap of a whip, an immediate x-ray appraisal of the situation is mandatory. The humerus is osteoporotic, and it is readily fractured! To avoid such a catastrophe, the surgeon must remember that, during the abduction phase, the humerus forms a long lever. The surgeon should steady the shoulder by placing one hand over the top of the shoulder. The manipulation is performed with the surgeon's other hand grasping the patient's arm just distal to the axilla while resting the patient's upper arm on the surgeon's forearm.

The radial nerve traverses from the axilla to the posterior aspect of the humerus by passing through the triangular space formed by the deep and long heads of the triceps, anteriorly, and the teres major, superiorly (Figs. 11.12 and 11.26A). In the presence of diffuse rotator cuff tendinitis, the radial nerve may adhere to the teres major. If the shoulder is manipulated to 180° of abduction, a radial nerve palsy may result. Manipulation should stop with the shoulder abducted to 90° and externally rotated to 45°.

Surgical Release.   Manipulation of the kind just described is rather a blunderbuss type of therapy. It is probably preferable, therefore, to expose the shoulder operatively and divide the tightened structures to a limited extent under direct vision (9). Before doing so, you have the patient's informed consent. Before consenting to surgery, the patient should know that, if treated only with medication, support, ice and/or heat, most frozen shoulders will spontaneously resolve. The only problem is the months of time needed for this to occur. Most patients are impatient, largely because of the intolerable pain that is especially disruptive to sleep, and they opt for surgical intervention.

A decompression acromioplasty is performed. The tendon of the subscapularis is separated from the underlying capsule, which is then released along the anatomic neck, freeing it anteriorly and inferiorly. The coracoacromial ligament is released at the same time. The shoulder is then moved through a full range of movement before the subscapularis is replaced anatomically.

One of the most gratifying features of this type of procedure is the immediate relief of discomfort. Despite the inevitable pain associated with operative exposure, patients are grateful that the dull, nagging shoulder discomfort has left them. After surgical release of a frozen shoulder, the patient must continue with an exercise program. Although 90% of abductions of the shoulder are usually rapidly restored postoperatively, it may be another three or four months before the patient regains a full range of painless movement.

Shoulder-Hand Syndrome (Reflex Sympathetic Dystrophy)

Patients who develop the shoulder-hand syndrome are similar in their emotional make-up to those who develop Sudeck's atrophy. They are generally timid and afraid of hurting themselves. They give the impression of having a low pain threshold and they are unduly fearful of doing anything that may aggravate their discomfort and prolong their disability. These patients tend to nurse their painful members; their hands are carried as if covered with oil—as if a touch of their hands would soil their clothes or their furniture. This syndrome has been aptly described as "ocular palmar palsy" (W.R. Harris, personal communication). These patients sit around all day, looking at their poor, painful upper limbs.

Like beggars in the bazaars of the Far East, who deliberately hold their hands at their sides for two or three days, these patients develop swollen, painful hands (6). Blood will not run uphill. It has to be pumped back to the heart from the arm. This is done by clenching the fist, flexing the arm, and extending the wrist and elbow. If this is not done because of pain or fear of pain, the resulting venous stasis produces edema. With persisting edema, eventually a pericapsular fibrosis will develop, with resulting pain and stiffness on moving the joints of the hand. Once this additional pain is added, it is easy to see how a vicious circle develops.

Obviously, this is not the only source of this poorly understood syndrome, which may occur in association with other lesions, such as a myocardial infarction. However, in patients with a frozen shoulder, holding the hand in the sling position and the arm motionless certainly play a significant role in perpetuating discomfort that ensues (see a further discussion of this entity in Chapter 21).

Treatment

With very marked stiffness of the fingers, a retrograde intravenous anesthesia is of great value. With their hands anesthetized, patients are more capable of following instructions in regard to mobilization of their fingers. Robin De Andrade (4) demonstrated on himself that, when vital green was injected intravenously at the elbow, the whole of the extremity below the tourniquet, including the hand, became discolored with the injected dye. The dye was not just concentrated around the restricting cuff.

With evidence of possible retrograde flow from an intravenous injection, it was rational to use this route to administer intravenous steroids and get a high concentration in the affected area. One of the major advantages of this technique of retrograde regional anesthesia is that patients can see that their own fingers are capable of moving under their own direction. The tourniquet is maintained for one hour and then slowly and intermittently released. Although this technique can be repeated at weekly intervals, it does not substitute for a vigorous physiotherapy program in which discomfort is mollified, to some extent, by neuromodulation of pain by percutaneous electrical stimulation.

Patients must be given a very detailed program of physical therapy at home. This program should include specific exercises that are performed for 15 minutes of every hour. A daily check of progress in the physiotherapy department is mandatory. Patients must be encouraged almost to the point of flagellation!

Summary

The impingement syndrome as a manifestation of rotator cuff disease may represent several clinical entities, such as rotator cuff tendinitis, subacromial bursitis, biceps tendinitis, or rotator cuff tears (partial or complete). These symptom complexes are readily identified and each demands a specific type of therapy.

The more diffuse clinical entities, adhesive capsulitis and the shoulder hand syndrome, continue to prove a challenge to both understanding and management. Although this is an oversimplification of a poorly understood problem, it is hoped that presenting it in this manner will help direct treatment along rational lines.

REFERENCES

1. Caillet R: Shoulder Joint Pain. Philadelphia, F.A. Davis Co. (1969).
2. Codman EA: Rupture of the Supraspinatus Tendon and Other Lesions in or About the Subacromial Bursa. Thomas Todd Co., Boston (1934).
3. Coventry MB: Problems of a painful shoulder. JAMA 151:177–185 (1953).
4. De Andrade R: Personal communication.
5. De Palma AF: Surgery of the Shoulder, 3rd ed. Philadelphia, JB Lippincott (1983).
6. Gilcreest EL and Albi P: Unusual lesions of muscles and tendons of the shoulder girdle and upper arm. Surg Gynecol Obstet 58:322–339 (1934).
7. Hawkins RJ, Chris AD, and Kiefer G: Failed anterior acromioplasty. Paper presented at American Shoulder and Elbow Society, San Francisco (1987).
8. Kennedy JC and Willis RB: The effects of local steroid injections on tendons: a biomechanical and microscopic correlative study. Am J Sports Med 4:11–21 (1976).
9. Macnab I: Rotator cuff tendinitis. Ann R Coll Surg Engl 53:271–287 (1973).
10. Meyer AW: Chronic functional lesions of the shoulder. Arch Surg 35:646–649 (1937).
11. Neer CS: Anterior acromioplasty for the chronic impingement syndrome in the shoulder. A preliminary report. J Bone Joint Surg 54A:41–50 (1972).
12. Neer CS: Impingement lesions. Clin Orthop 173:70–77 (1983).
13. Neviaser TJ: Adhesive capsulitis. Orthop Clin North Am 18:439–443 (1987).
14. Pasteur F: Sur une forme nouvelle de perianthralogy et de'ankylose de l'epaule. J Radiol Eletrol 18:327 (1934).
15. Salter RB, Gross A, and Hall JH: Hydrocortisone arthropathy: an experimental investigation. Can Med Assoc J 97:374–377 (1967).
16. Tibone JE, Jobe FW, Kerlan RK, Carter VS, Shields CL, Lombardo SJ, and Yocum LA: Shoulder impingement syndrome in athletes treated by anterior acromioplasty. Clin Orthop 198:134–140 (1985).
17. Uhthoff HK, Sarkark, and Maynard JA: Calcifying tendonitis. Clin Orthop 118:164–168 (1976).
18. Valtonen EJ: Double acting betamethasone (celestone) in the treatment of supraspinatus tendinitis: a comparison of subacromial and gluteal single injections with placebo. J Int Med Res 6:463–467 (1978).
19. Weiner DS and Macnab I: Superior migration of the humeral head. J Bone Joint Surg 52B:524–527 (1970).
20. Withrington RH, Girgis FL, and Seifert MH: A placebo-controlled trial of steroid injections in the treatment of supraspinatus tendinitis. Scand J Rheumatol 14:76–78 (1985).

15

Osteoarthritis of the Shoulder Complex

*"The work of science is to substitute facts for appearance
and demonstration for impression."*
—John Ruskin

Since the shoulder is not a weight-bearing joint, significant functional limitation due to osteoarthritis is not as common as in the hip and knee. Still, patients exhibit pain, loss of shoulder movement, and crepitus around the shoulder complex. This signals that something is amiss, either in the form of osteoarthritis of the glenohumeral joint or osteoarthritis of the acromioclavicular joint.

GLENOHUMERAL JOINT

Osteoarthritis degeneration of the glenohumeral joint may be primary or, more likely, secondary to previous injury to the humeral head, untreated recurrent dislocations, avascular necrosis, or old sepsis (Table 15.1). Poor outcomes to complicated three-part and four-part humeral head fractures are now recognized (1). The more aggressive, immediate total shoulder approach to treatment is replacing nonoperative treatment or open reduction and internal fixation, which often failed because of multiple fragments, the devascular nature of the injury, and the high incidence of osteoporotic bone.

On examination of the osteoarthritic glenohumeral joint, note the patient's painful loss of range of movement and palpable crepitus. The loss of ROM may be severe, to the point that the patient has lost all overhead function and/or is unable to complete perineal hygiene. Swelling and tenderness is notable because both are minor and diffuse.

Assessment of muscle strength is essential, since surgical success is so dependent on integrity of all soft tissues—strong functioning of the rotator cuff and deltoid are most important. Loss of strength, sensory upset, and reflex alteration that fit a radicular distribution should also alert you to the likelihood that some or all of the pain and functional limitation has its origin in the neck and not

Table 15.1. Causes of Glenohumeral Arthritis

1. Primary osteoarthritis
2. Secondary osteoarthritis
   - Old fractures of humeral head or glenoid
   - Recurrent (untreated) dislocations
   - Avascular necrosis
   - Old sepsis

the shoulder. If there is any doubt about the source of weakness, perform EMG and nerve conduction testing.

Investigation

Obviously, plain x-rays, including a true AP and a lateral of the glenohumeral joint (Fig. 15.1) form the basis of evaluation. Note the degree of cartilage loss, osteophytes, sclerosis, and subluxation.

After history, physical exam, and plain x-rays, rarely is there any doubt about diagnosis and treatment options. Occasionally, it is necessary to aspirate the joint to reaffirm the absence of infection, checking in these situations that the cell count is below 10,000 WBC, and that there is no bacterial growth.

Look for all potential causes of neck and shoulder pain, as outlined in Chapter 21.

Treatment

If the functional disability is mild, conservative treatment in the form of rest, exercise therapy, and NSAIDs may be sufficient.

Because the joint is not weight-bearing, patients tend to suffer a little longer before seeking medical care, and they usually have reached a stage where only surgery will relieve pain and return acceptable function.

Principles of Surgical Treatment

There is usually only one surgical option: replacement of the glenoid and humeral head surfaces with artificial materials—the so-called total shoulder arthroplasty (TSA). Nearly always, the best choice is a plastic (polyethylene) glenoid with or without metal backing, and a metal (cobalt-chrome) humeral head (Fig. 15.2). Almost all total shoulder arthroplasties are of the nonconstrained type, with the most popular being the Neer prosthesis (Fig. 15.3). The semiconstrained Macnab-English prosthesis is not commonly used. Constrained TSA models are available for poorly functioning muscles, but there is such a high component failure rate—usually involving loosening of the glenoid component—that very few constrained prostheses are used today.

The indications for total shoulder arthroplasty are arthritic degeneration of the glenohumeral joint from any cause (Table 15.1) that (1) significantly interferes with function because of pain and lost movement, and (2) does not respond to conservative nonoperative care. Because this is not a weight-bearing joint, total shoulder arthroplasty does not have the minimum age limitation that applies to the hip and knee.

Contraindications to TSA include recent or remote sepsis that could be reactivated, painless loss of shoulder function from any neurological disorder, and poor soft tissues—specifically, a weak deltoid or a nonfunctioning rotator cuff.

Total shoulder arthroplasty is a much more difficult operation than total knee or total hip arthroplasty. It is as much a soft tissue procedure as it is a bony procedure. It is absolutely vital to good postoperative function to view the prosthesis as an interposition for maintaining soft tissue integrity and serving as a fulcrum for the functioning of the deltoid and rotator cuff. For the rotator cuff to function, it must be attached to the prosthesis and proximal humerus. Failure to re-establish the integrity of the soft tissues will result in failure of the surgery.

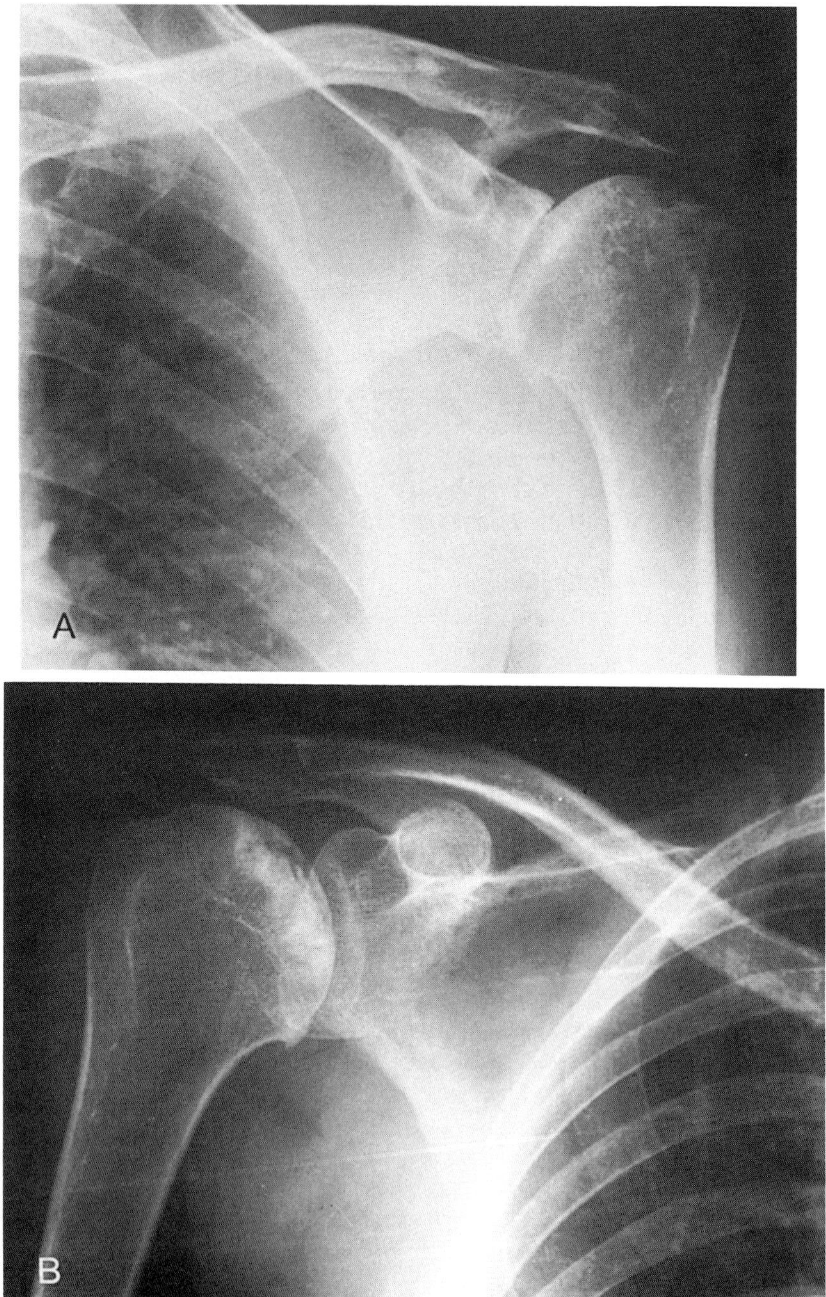

Figure 15.1.   **A,** AP showing osteoarthritis of the glenohumeral joint. **B,** AP showing avascular necrosis of the humeral head.

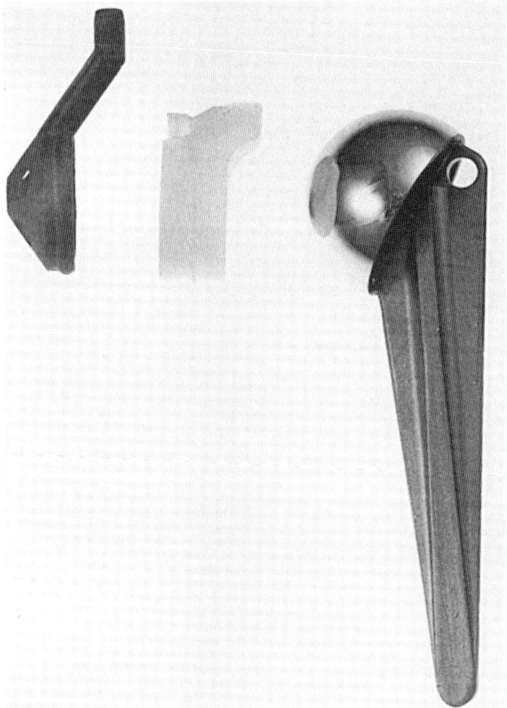

Figure 15.2.   The English-Macnab prosthesis, metal humeral head, and polyethylene glenoid.

The internal and external rotation you end up with on the operating table will not be improved by postoperative exercise. This is another soft tissue principle, and it may mean resection of the posterior capsule and release of the subscapularis.

Finally, don't forget to address the acromioclavicular joint. Most often, it is arthritic in nature, with osteophytic impingement of the subacromial space. If this is the case, an excision of the outer end of the clavicle and an acromioplasty must be part of the total shoulder arthroplasty.

Surgery.   The surgical approach is the anterior deltopectoral approach (Fig. 15.4). The first part of the procedure is excision of the humeral head, saving as much bone stock as possible, especially the greater and lesser tuberosities (Fig. 15.3). The humeral head naturally faces 40° posteriorly; thus, the humeral head cut must follow this angle.

Next, assess the soft tissues for integrity and the need for repair or release. If there is a poorly functioning or nonexistent rotator cuff, a constrained prosthesis may be selected.

On occasion, especially in the primary treatment of humeral head fractures, the glenoid cartilage will be intact and the operation can be confined to a unipolar (humeral head only) prosthesis, with no necessity to implant the glenoid component (the bipolar arthroplasty).

The most difficult part of the operation is cutting the trough in the glenoid to receive the keel of the glenoid prosthesis.

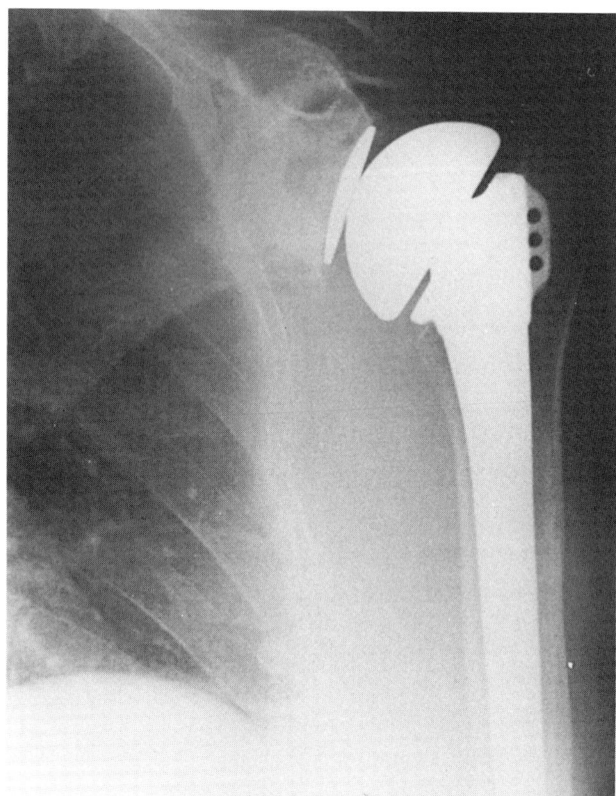

Figure 15.3.   The most popular prosthesis (Neer). Note the preservation of as much humeral bone stock as possible.

The next step in the procedure is to select the size of humeral prosthesis that maintains the functioning length of the deltoid. It is better not to cement the humeral prosthesis in place, but poor (osteoporosis) or short (recent fracture) bone stalk may mandate cementing.

Finally, repair the rotator cuff and assure its attachment to the proximal humerus and prosthesis. Examine internal and external rotation, and complete any z-plasty lengthening of the subscapularis muscle to achieve at least 50° of external rotation.

Rehabilitation

The postoperative rehabilitation (exercise) program is every bit as important as the surgery. The longer it is delayed, the poorer the outcome. Within a few days of surgery, pendulum exercises are initiated. These are followed by gentle passive ROM and active strengthening exercises. Within a few weeks of surgery, the patient is on the way to a good ROM, with minimal use of a sling.

There is usually immediate relief of the arthritic pain, and most patients should achieve a good functional result that allows for a high level of function in daily activities—even a return to noncontact sports, such as golf, swimming, tennis, and bowling.

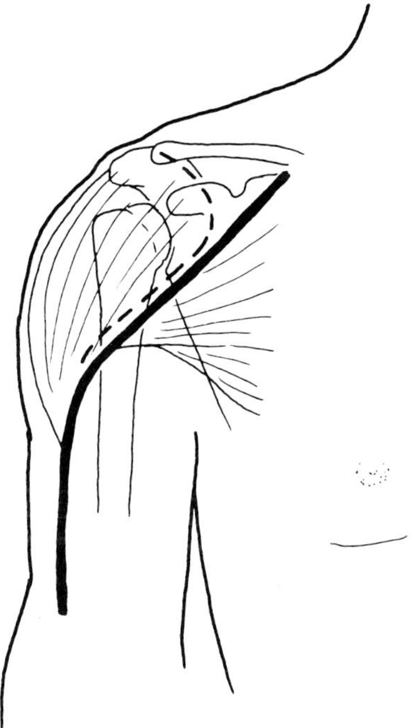

Figure 15.4.   The anterior deltopectoral approach for total shoulder arthroplasty (TSA).

Complications, in the hands of the skilled surgeon, are rare. The main concern is a less than 1% septic rate. As in all implanted joints, late sepsis from a remote bacteremia (e.g., dental work, genitourinary manipulation) should be prevented with prophylactic antibiotics.

Aseptic (Mechanical) Loosening

Aseptic (mechanical) loosening is a rare cause of failure when strict indications and technique are followed. The newer unconstrained (Neer) prosthesis has an excellent track record with virtually no implant breakage (4).

Conclusion

Neer and his prosthetic design have brought hope and good results to patients with osteoarthritis of the shoulder joint. Since the joint is not weight-bearing, a wide variety of problems in a broader age group can be treated by total shoulder arthroplasty. There are still some situations where a TSA will not work and arthrodesis needs to be considered.

Arthrodesis of the Glenohumeral Joint

Arthrodesis of the glenohumeral joint was frequently undertaken in the days when it was not uncommon for a child to develop either tuberculous arthritis of the shoulder or a flail shoulder as a result of poliomyelitis. The indications for arthrodesis of the shoulder are now largely limited to paralytic lesions of the shoulder joint, low grade infections, or failure of total shoulder arthroplasty. It may also be indicated following tumor resection. Post TSA fusion may be needed for prior multiple procedures involving loss of soft tissue prosthetic support (rotator cuff), sepsis, and prosthetic loosening or breakage.

Following glenohumeral fusion, movement of the humerus depends on scapulothoracic glide that is motored by the trapezius, levator scapula, and serratus anterior. As a prerequisite for fusion, therefore, the patient must have a stable scapula with powerful muscles controlling its movement. If the fusion is to be performed in a child, it should be delayed until 12 to 15 years of age, when enough cancellous bone is present in the humeral head, and the operation can be undertaken without danger of interfering with growth of the arm.

The optimum position for fusion has been the subject of much debate, but certain premises must be observed. They include:

1. The hand must be able to reach the face and the midline of the body in front and behind.
2. Painful winging of the scapula, when the arm is lying by the side, must be avoided. This depends on the plane of resection of the humeral head.
3. The patient must be able to use the arm for lifting and pushing.

The optimum position for fusion is one that allows the hand to be placed against the symphysis and allows the elbow placed at the level of the umbilicus in front of the abdomen. Richards and Kostuik (2) have recommended the 30-30-30 position: 30° of abduction (arm relative to thorax), 30° of forward flexion, and 30° of internal rotation.

Many techniques of arthrodesis have been described; those most commonly utilized now employ rigid internal fixation, thereby obviating the unpleasant necessity for postoperative immobilization in a shoulder spica. The authors feel that, because most arthrodesis techniques necessitate an acromioclavicular excisional arthroplasty to maintain and increase scapulothoracic glide, an arthrodesis of the shoulder should be performed in two stages. Stage one should be confined to an excisional arthroplasty of the acromioclavicular joint. Sometimes, the increase in movement and the freedom from pain that follow this simple procedure are extraordinary. Movements of the shoulder are subsequently dependent on scapulothoracic glide, without putting much stress on the glenohumeral joint. Many patients are very happy with what they achieve and do not wish to proceed to the second stage of a glenohumeral fusion.

If the fusion must then be done, we recommend the technique described by Richards et al. (2, 3). They use the 30-30-30 position and try to obtain bone contact between the humeral head and both the glenoid and the undersurface of the acromion. They use a malleable pelvic reconstruction plate, passing three screws through the plate and humeral head into the glenoid (Fig. 15.5). The patient is immobilized in a abduction splint for a minimum of six weeks, after which gentle range-of-movement exercise is permitted until union appears on x-ray. Return to strenuous activity is delayed until at least four months.

Acromioclavicular Joint Arthritis

Isolated arthritic degeneration of this joint may occur as the result of an old injury to the joint, or as part of a generalized osteoarthritic process. With aging, all joints in the body deteriorate by variable amounts, but seldom is this the cause of symptomatic arthritis of the acromioclavicular joint.

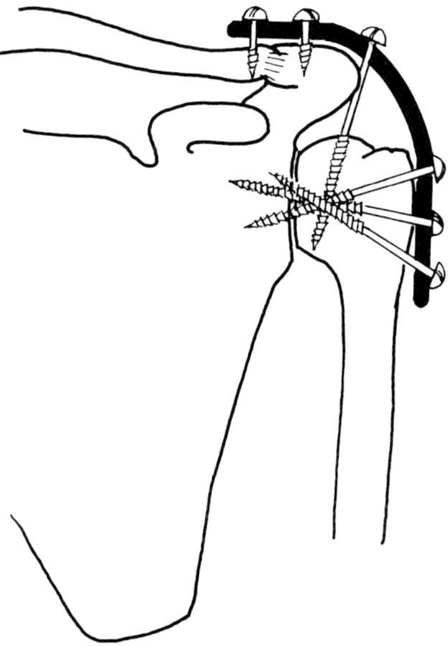

Figure 15.5. A method of fusion of the glenohumeral joint.

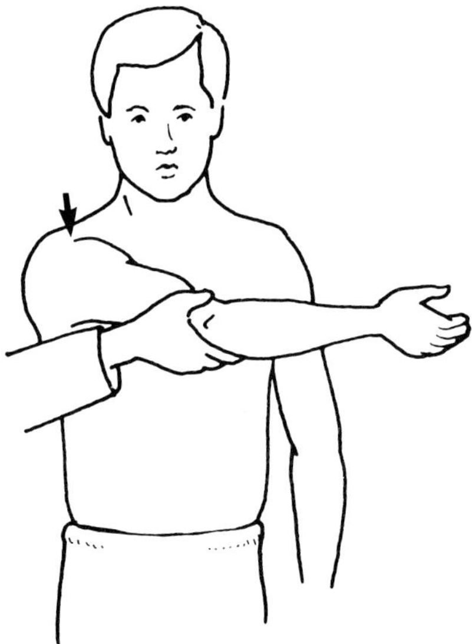

Figure 15.6. Increased pain in an arthritic a-c joint (*arrow*) is the result of forced shoulder adduction.

Posttraumatic degeneration is the most common cause of symptoms in the joint. Patients exhibit pain, swelling, and tenderness over the joint. The pain is increased by forced adduction of the flexed shoulder (Fig. 15.6).

If the symptoms and functional limitation are mild, an intra-articular injection of cortisone may be useful. More often, symptomatic arthritis of the a-c joint requires excision of the outer .5–.75 in. of the distal clavicle for relief of symptoms. Be especially aware that degeneration of the a-c joint is usually part of a more diffuse process, such as cuff tears, rather than an isolated condition.

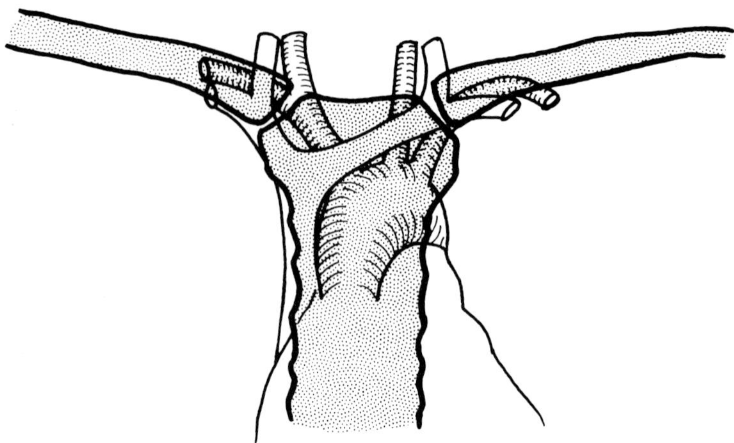

Figure 15.7.   The sternoclavicular joint is directly anterior to the great vessels.

Sternoclavicular Joint Arthritis

Arthritis of the sternoclavicular joint is rare. The spontaneous occurrence of pain and swelling over the s-c joint should immediately raise the suspicion of some underlying problem, such as tumor, infection, or a generalized arthritic state.

Isolated arthritis of the s-c joint is often mild and can be treated with physical therapy, modalities, NSAIDs, and, occasionally, careful injection of steroids. For the rare case in which the joint becomes very painful, excision of the inner edge of the clavicle, and tendinous stabilization of the remaining clavicle to the first rib, have been recommended. However, the sternoclavicular joints lie directly anterior to the great vessels of the root of the neck (Fig. 15.7), and any procedure in this area must be undertaken with great care. Failure to stabilize the inner end of the clavicle in such surgery may leave the patient worse off than before, a reason most surgeons do not recommend this procedure.

REFERENCES

1. Cofield RH: Comminuted fractures of the proximal humerus. Clin Orthop 230:49–57 (1988).
2. Richards RR and Kostuik JP: Shoulder arthrodesis: indications and techniques. In: Surgical Disorders of the Shoulder. Ed: Watson MS. Churchill Livingstone, London (1991).
3. Richards RR, Sherman RM, Hudson AR, and Waddell JP: Shoulder arthrodesis using a pelvic-reconstruction plate. J Bone Joint Surg 70A:416–421 (1988).
4. Wilde AH, Borden LS, and Brems JJ: Experience with the Neer total shoulder replacement. In: Surgery of the Shoulder. Eds: Bateman JE and Welsh RP. BC Decker, Philadelphia (1984).

16

Miscellaneous Inflammatory and Infective Conditions

"Life is a disease; and the only difference between one man and another is the stage of the disease at which he lives."
—George Bernard Shaw

INTRODUCTION

Before gaining an understanding of the clinical presentation of septic arthritis of the shoulder, it is necessary to know a little about the inflammatory conditions that debilitate not only the shoulder joint, but the patient's general health. It is rare that septic arthritis appears de novo in a healthy adult; almost all cases appear in debilitated patients, especially those with arthritic involvement.

Rheumatoid Arthritis

Rheumatoid arthritis is the classic model for inflammatory joint disorders. It is more likely to affect the peripheral joints, such as hands, wrists, and feet. Late in the disease process, it may affect the axial skeleton and the shoulders. When it does produce symptomatic shoulder disease, this is usually in a clearly diagnosed and long-treated rheumatoid patient. Both shoulders are usually affected, producing pain and stiffness. If there is significant synovial proliferation, the joint will appear swollen and feel boggy. The pain of rheumatoid shoulder involvement is especially bothersome at night—the reverse of pain and stiffness in the wrists and hands, which occurs on awakening in the morning.

There are no specific x-ray features that distinguish rheumatoid arthritis of the shoulder (Fig. 16.1). Laboratory diagnosis with elevated sedimentation rate and rheumatoid factor has usually been made.

Treatment is similar to other joints and includes rest for acute episodes, strengthening exercises for resolving episodes, and varying doses and types of NSAIDs. The occasional use of intra-articular water insoluble corticosteroids is beneficial. Rarely does a rheumatoid patient with shoulder disease arrive at a point where a shoulder arthroplasty will make a big difference in function. The reason is that shoulder affliction occurs so late in the disease process that shoulder arthroplasty will make little functional difference. In addition, it would be difficult to have a successful outcome because of the rheumatoid destruction of essential soft tissues.

Gout

The next classic arthritic model (aside from osteoarthritis, discussed in Chapter 15) is gout. Like rheumatoid arthritis, gout rarely affects the shoulder joint,

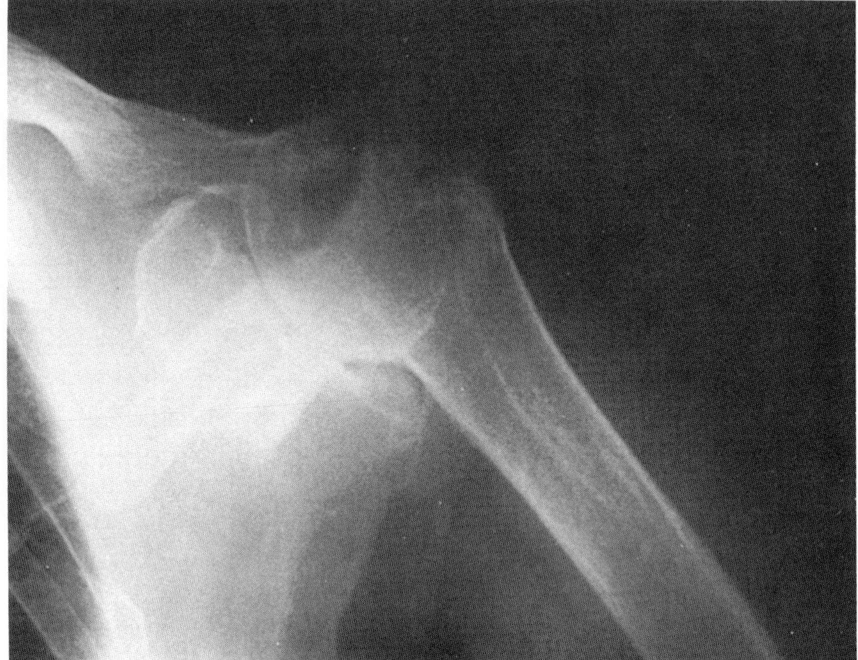

Figure 16.1.   Rheumatoid arthritis affecting the shoulder joint. This is a destroyed joint, but nothing distinguishes it as rheumatoid arthritis.

except late in the disease process and almost always in conjunction with other obvious gouty joint involvement.

Symptoms are initiated by the deposit of uric acid crystals in tophetic collections in the synovia. After surgery, trauma, or some other precipitating event, these crystals are released. The leukocytes, in turn, gobble up the crystals, taking on more than they can digest. This leads to rupture of the leukocytes and release of toxins into the shoulder joint, precipitating the acute arthritic episode. Involvement of the shoulder is most often unilateral, and the pain is very severe.

Aspiration of the joint fluid will yield uric acid crystals visible on polarized light microscopy.

Treatment employs colchicine and/or anti-inflammatories (especially indomethacin) for the acute attacks and uric acid inhibitors (allopurinol) for prophylaxis.

Pseudogout

Pseudogout, causing unilateral shoulder pain, is far more common than gout. With aging, calcium pyrophosphate crystals are deposited on cartilage (Fig. 16.2).

The acute inflammatory episode occurs just as in gout. The crystals are released into the synovial fluid of the joint, followed by leukocytic ingestion, then by cell rupture and the release of toxic substances.

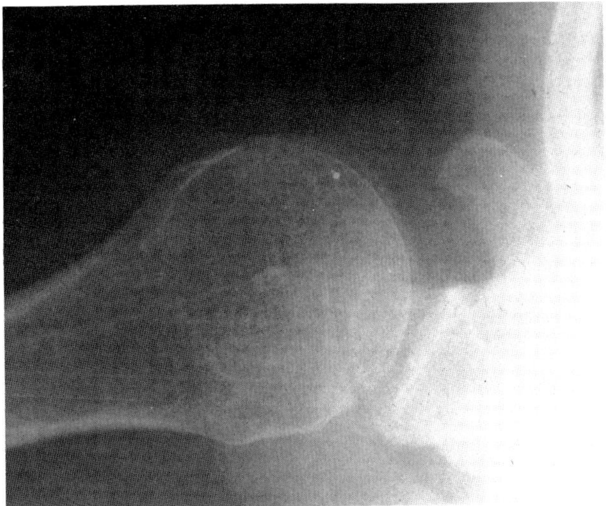

Figure 16.2.   Pseudogout, with calcification forming a halo in the cartilage.

The diagnosis is usually obvious when linear, stippled calcification is seen on x-ray, and the calcium pyrophosphate crystals are seen under the polarized light microscope. Treatment is by long-term anti-inflammatory medicine.

Septic Arthritis

The classic teaching is that joint sepsis produces an acute clinical state with severe pain, high fever, and a very sick-looking patient. Septic arthritis of the shoulder joint is a much more indolent condition, often superimposed on the previously noted arthritides and taking on the clinical appearance of any one of the previously described conditions (5, 7, 8). Add to this its rarity, and you see what a particularly vexing problem septic arthritis of the shoulder can be. The usual outcome, in terms of shoulder joint function, is often disastrous.

Incidence and Underlying Factors

Leslie et al. (8) managed to gather 18 cases of septic arthritis of the shoulder over an 18-year span seen at two large hospitals in Boston. Almost all of their cases appeared in the older population (average age: 65) with associated debilitating diseases. These included chronic generalized diseases (diabetes mellitus, renal disease), a debilitated joint (rheumatoid arthritis, gout) or chronic abuse of drugs and/ or alcohol. Repeated intra-articular injections of steroids into the shoulder of such a patient carries a greater risk of subsequent septic arthritis.

Classically, it is taught that bacterial seeding in a joint occurs through:

- Hematogenous spread;
- Direct spread from an adjacent infected source (e.g., osteomyelitis);
- Invasion of the joint via trauma, injection, or surgery.

Hematogenous spread is the most common route of infection in the adult, but it rarely occurs in the healthy adult shoulder because of excellent blood supply and adequate host defenses.

Organisms

Staphylococcus aureus is still the most common organism, isolated in about 60% of cases (8). Other gram-positive cocci, such as hemolytic streptococcus, will appear in 20% of cases, and gram-negative organisms, such as *E. coli*, *Proteus*, and *P. aeruginosa* will be cultured in another 20%.

Clinical Presentation

Because most of these patients have additional debilitating factors, the diagnosis of septic arthritis is usually missed for a number of days or weeks. The pain, local tenderness, and minor reduction in range of movement may be no different than what you would expect to see in a rheumatoid shoulder. Only when the pain relentlessly increases and the patient becomes more systemically ill should you investigate the possibility of sepsis.

Investigation

If the patient's defense mechanisms rally, a fever, leukocytosis, and an elevated sedimentation rate will be present. Often enough, no fever or elevation of the WBC appears, and the patient's debilitating disease has already elevated the ESR, making the diagnosis very elusive.

Proof of the clinical condition obviously rests with bacteriology. Blood cultures and cultures of a remote infected sight are less valuable than an aspiration of the joint, with Gram stain and culture. The fluid is usually turbid and has a high WBC count (just like rheumatoid arthritis). The higher the WBC count, the more likely infection is present. Counts between 50,000 and 100,000 mm3 are probably due to joint infection; counts above 100,000 mm3 are certainly due to infection. Most of the cells will be polymorphonuclear leukocytes. Counts below 10,000 mm3 are more likely to be associated with a noninfected inflammatory reaction. Glucose in the synovial fluid aspirant is also reduced in both conditions, but to a much greater extent in septic arthritis (most consider this a useless observation!).

Gram stain will tell you the organism in 80% of cases. Subsequent cultures will reveal the organism in most patients, except those who have had antibiotic therapy instituted before the cultures.

X-ray Changes

X-rays are notoriously unreliable early in the disease process, because other disease changes (e.g., rheumatoid arthritis) are present. Within a few days, undiagnosed septic arthritis will reduce whatever joint space is left, through cartilage destruction (Fig. 16.3).

A bone scan may be nonspecific because of associated conditions (Fig. 16.4), and because technetium will not light up joint exudate. CT will show early bone defects before these erosions are evident on plain x-ray. MRI is most useful (Fig. 16.5).

Differential Diagnosis

Because septic arthritis usually appears in the debilitated adult, it is usually missed on presentation. Other conditions, such as rheumatoid arthritis, gout,

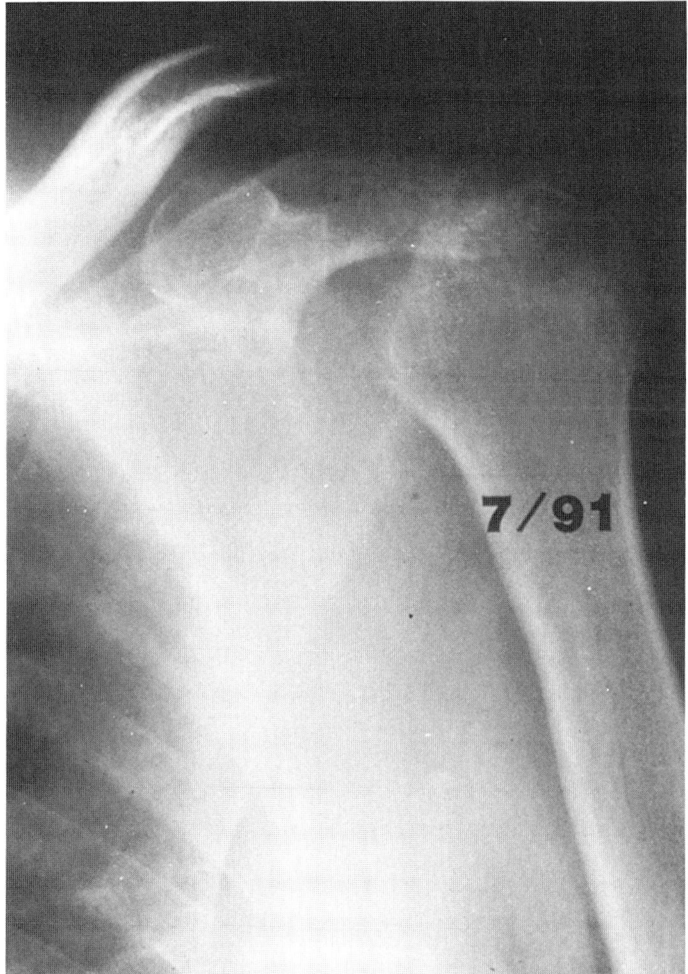

Figure 16.3.   A septic shoulder, with loss of cartilage space and erosion of the humeral head.

and pigmented villonodular synovitis are usually considered before septic arthritis.

Treatment

Pus kills cartilage (3, 4). It is imperative that pus be removed from the shoulder joint as soon as possible. Some choose needle aspiration, others arthroscopic lavage (6). Most orthopaedic surgeons would use open drainage and lavage of the joint through an anterior deltopectoral approach (Fig. 15.4).

Before the infecting organism is known, and after cultures have been taken, IV broad spectrum antibiotics are used (2). A common regimen is first-generation cephalosporins (e.g., Cefazolin) and an aminoglycoside (Gentamycin). Once cultures and sensitivities are available, appropriate IV antibiotics can be instituted for two to four weeks. Total antibiotic coverage should extend for four to eight weeks and beyond if the infection has not been eradicated.

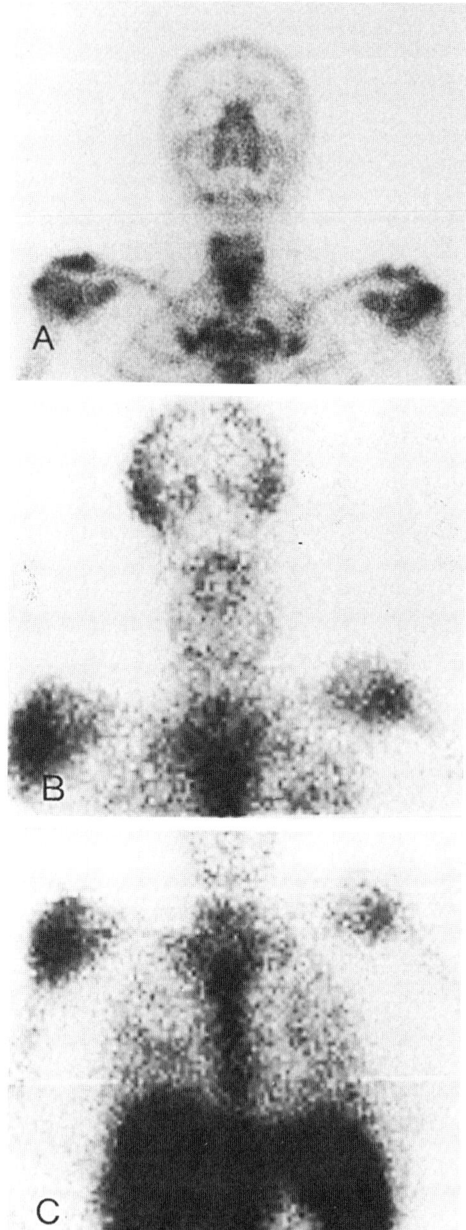

Figure 16.4. **A,** technetium bone scan in bilateral osteoarthritis of the shoulders. **B,** technetium bone scan in bilateral septic arthritis of shoulders—not very different from Figure 16.4*A*. **C,** indium scan from the same patient as in Figure 16.4*B*.

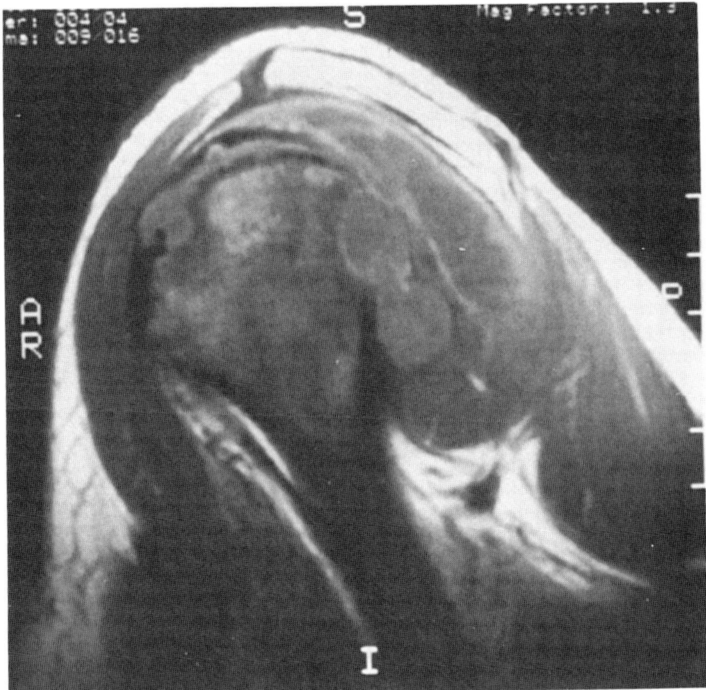

Figure 16.5.   MRI of septic arthritis. This is tuberculosis with granuloma formation (T1 spin echo).

The shoulder should be rested in a sling and binder until the infection is brought under control, usually in 10+ days. At that time, gentle exercises can begin, leading to a more vigorous rehabilitation program. Unfortunately, most of these patients, for one reason or another, end up with a poorly functioning shoulder joint.

Septic Arthritis in Children

You are more likely to see septic arthritis of the shoulder in children than adults (1, 9). The specific age group is usually infants with irritability and fever. It is necessary to carefully examine each bone and joint in these infants, because they won't point to the sore joint! Unlike adults, these children have high temperatures, increased WBC counts, and a high sedimentation rate.

The route of infection is either hematogenous or it has spread from an adjacent metaphyseal osteomyelitis. Aspiration of the joint is mandatory and will usually yield hemolytic streptococcus in infants and *S. aureus* in the older child.

X-rays again are unreliable in diagnosis. Bone scanning, especially with indium-labeled WBC (Fig. 16.4), will pinpoint the foci of infection.

Treatment

Pus kills cartilage. It is mandatory, to save joint function, to aspirate the joint either with a large bore needle or open surgery. Surgeons obviously prefer the open route to guarantee complete joint lavage at the earliest possible moment. Obviously, antibiotic coverage, along the same principles as for adults, is used.

If the diagnosis is made early and swift definitive treatment is instituted, there is little need for rehabilitation and a high likelihood that a normal joint will result.

REFERENCES

1. Borella L, Goobar JE, Summitt RL, and Clark GM: Septic arthritis in childhood. J Pediatr 62: 742–747 (1963).
2. Clawson DK and Dunn AW: Management of common bacterial infections of bones and joints. J Bone Joint Surg 49A:164–182 (1967).
3. Curtiss PH Jr and Klein L: Destruction of articular cartilage in septic arthritis. I. In vitro studies. J Bone Joint Surg 45A:797–806 (1963).
4. Curtiss PH Jr and Klein L: Destruction of articular cartilage in septic arthritis. II. In vitro studies. J Bone Joint Surg 45A:1595–1604 (1965).
5. Gelberman RH, Menon J, Austerlitz MS, and Weisman MH: Pyogenic arthritis of the shoulder in adults. J Bone Joint Surg 62A:550–553 (1980).
6. Goldenberg DL, Brandt KD, Cohen AS, and Cathcart ES: Treatment of septic arthritis. Comparison of needle aspiration and surgery as initial modes of joint drainage. Arthritis Rheum 18: 83–90 (1975).
7. Kelly PJ, Martin WJ, and Coventry MB: Bacterial (suppurative) arthritis in the adult. J Bone Joint Surg 52A:1595–1602 (1970).
8. Leslie BM, Harris JM III, and Driscoll D: Septic arthritis of the shoulder in adults. J Bone Joint Surg 71A:1516–1522 (1989).
9. Schmitt D, Mubarak S, and Gelberman R: Septic shoulders in children. J Pediatr Orthop 1:67–72 (1981).

17

Instability of the Shoulder Joint

"If everyone believes a thing it is probably untrue."
—Sir W. Arbuthnot Lane

INTRODUCTION

Glenohumeral instability has many faces—from the instantly recognized acute traumatic dislocation in the high school tackle, to the voluntary multidirectional instability in the loose-jointed young girl. A classification of shoulder instability is presented in Table 17.1. The most common shoulder dislocation is acute traumatic anterior dislocation. Another common shoulder problem is chronic atraumatic multidirectional subluxation in the loose-jointed growing female. As you can see from Table 17.1, there are a multitude of combinations of shoulder instabilities; only the common garden varieties are presented here.

Incidence

The shoulder is the most commonly dislocated major joint in the body. The bulk of these are anterior dislocations; less than 2% of dislocations occur in a posterior direction.

Acute Traumatic Anterior Dislocation

Incidence and Mechanism

This is a young person's injury and the most common large joint dislocation you will see in the emergency department (9). As designated, it is traumatic in

Table 17.1. Classification of Shoulder Instability

1. Chronology	Acute
	Chronic
	Recurrent
2. Etiology	Traumatic (involuntary)
	Atraumatic (voluntary)
3. Direction	Anterior
	Posterior
	Inferior
	Multidirectional
4. Degree	Partial—subluxation
	Complete—dislocation
5. Miscellaneous	Neuromuscular
	Congenital
	Extreme joint laxity

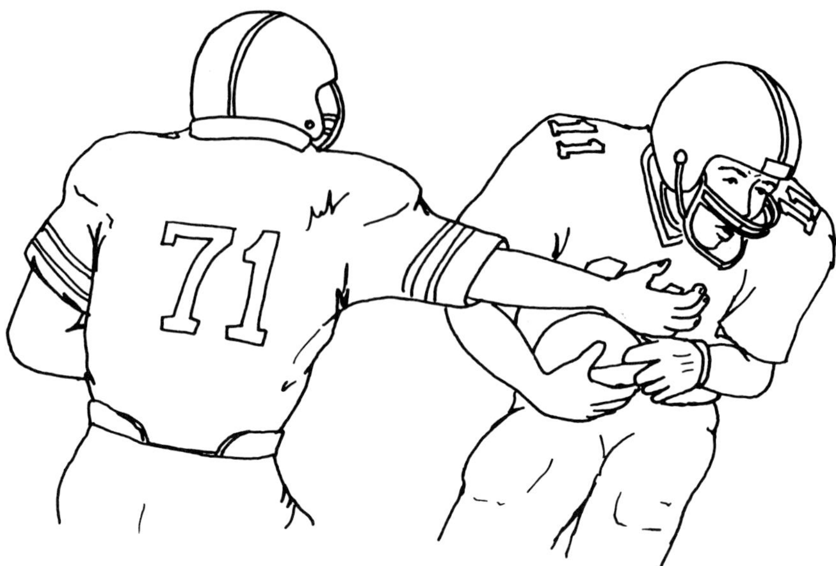

Figure 17.1.   The player carrying the ball is being "arm tackled." The outstretched arm will be suddenly abducted and externally rotated, which could lead to a dislocation.

origin and usually occurs in the athletic male—the football player who "arm tackles" (Fig. 17.1) and the skier who falls on his or her outstretched arm. Because of forced abduction and external rotation, the humeral head is forced against the weak anterior capsule, resulting in separation of the capsule from the anterior glenoid labrum and injury to the bony structure of that portion of the labrum (Bankart lesion) (1) (Fig. 17.2).

Now that we have mentioned an eponym, let us remind you of another: the Hill-Sachs lesion (7) (Fig. 12.18*B*).

Presentation

More often than not, you will meet this patient in a sporting uniform, sitting in a classic tilted position with the arm firmly held to the side (Fig. 17.3). Muscle spasm and heightened pain will increase with the length of time the dislocation has been present (measured in hours). Patients can usually describe the mechanism of injury and the actual sensation of dislocation. This is the moment when the arm becomes completely useless—the so-called "dead arm" sensation.

On examination, you will note a loss of deltoid fullness to the afflicted shoulder (Fig. 17.4). The most common location of an anterior dislocation is subcoracoid (Fig. 17.5,) which takes it away from the acromion, leaving the acromion prominent. If you are gentle, you may palpate the humeral head fullness anteriorly.

X-ray Assessment

You live by two basic rules in all orthopaedic fracture problems:

1. The injured area requires a minimum of two views at 90° angles to each other.
2. The joints above and below the injured extremity must be seen on x-ray.

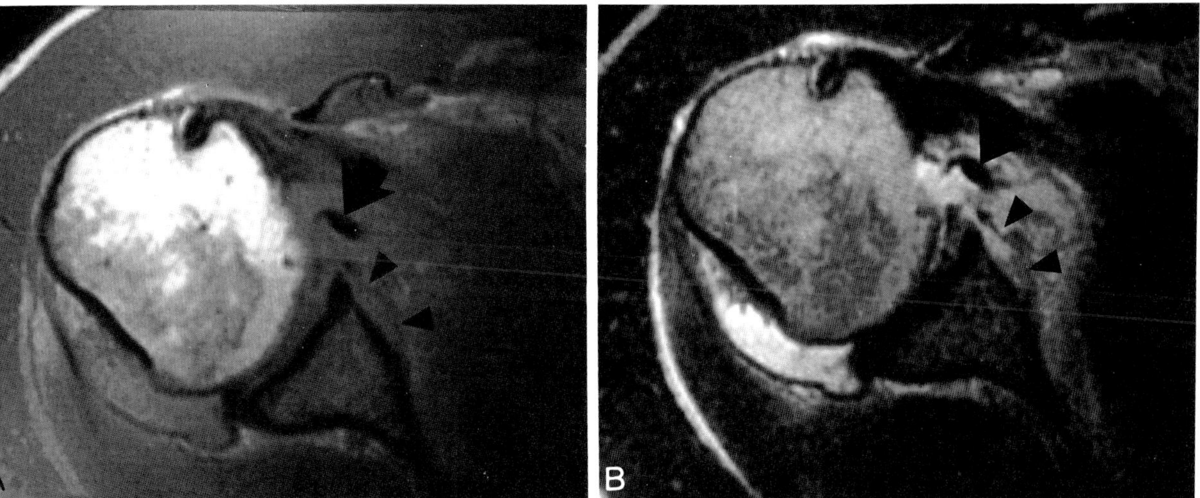

Figure 17.2.   Bankart lesion. Axial double-echo images (A = SE 1500/15, B = 1500/80). The anterior labrum (*arrow*) is detached from the bony glenoid. A portion of the anterior capsule (*arrowheads*) is seen floating in the large effusion. Note edema in subscapularis muscle along its scapular border.

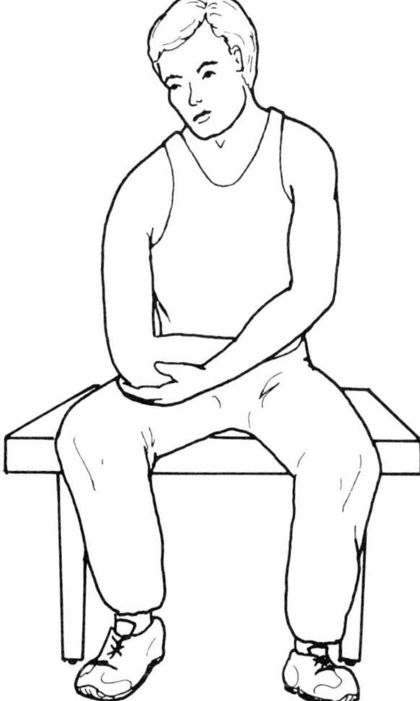

Figure 17.3.   Classic posture of a patient in emergency room with a shoulder dislocation.

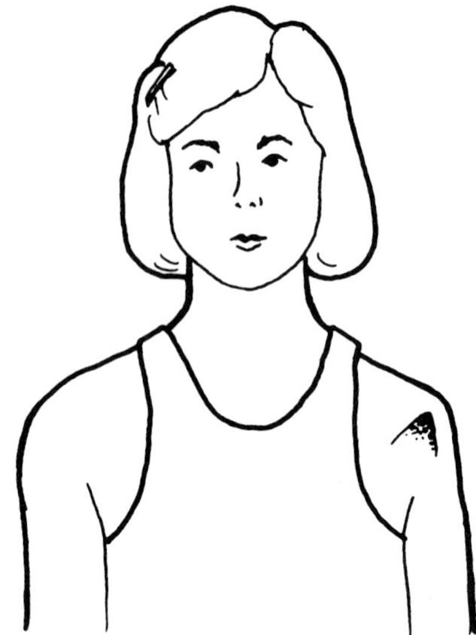

Figure 17.4.   Note the flattening of deltoid fullness on the dislocated side (*left*).

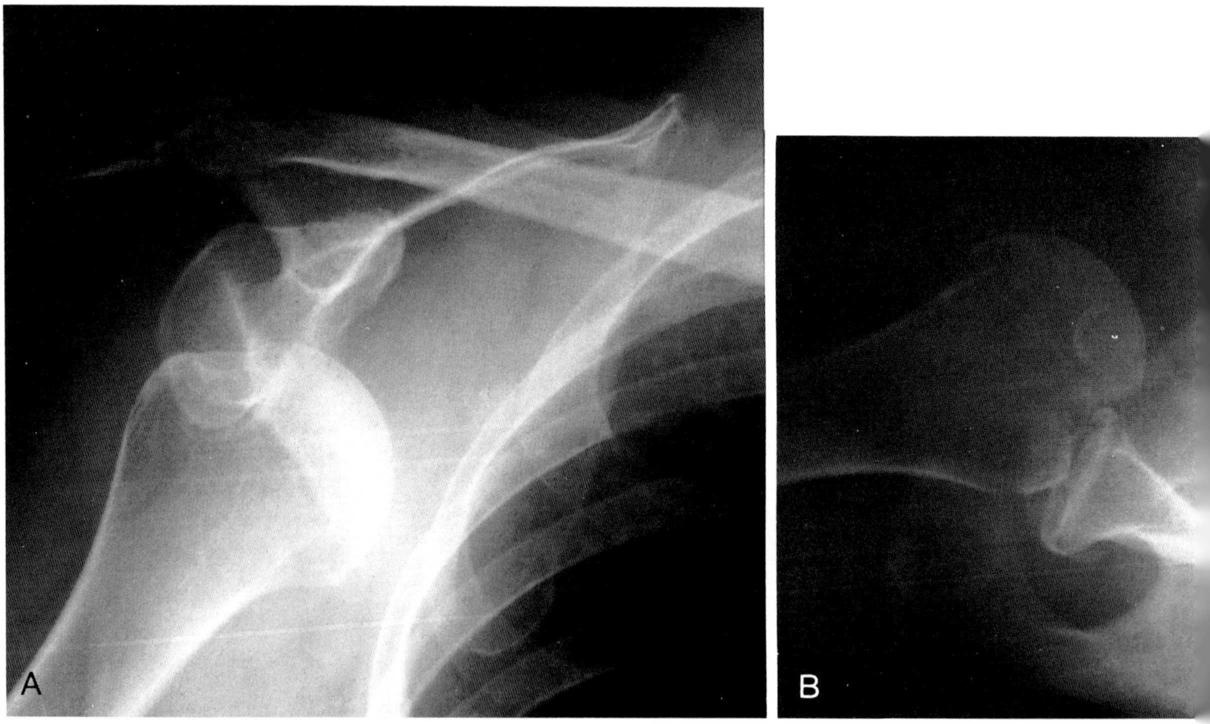

Figure 17.5.   Infraglenoid anterior dislocation. *A*, anteroposterior view. *B*, axillary view discloses the mechanism of compression fracture of the posterolateral aspect of the humeral head by the anteroinferior rim of the glenoid. This results in a Hill-Sachs defect.

The second rule does not bear too much on a dislocated joint, but be mindful that the neck and elbow should not be ignored, requiring at minimum a careful clinical exam.

How do you follow the first rule? A true AP is easy to obtain (Fig. 17.5). A transthoracic view is easy to obtain (Fig. 12.23). An axillary view is more difficult, but Figure 12.20 and Figure 12.21 show how it can be done.

There are other special views that have been described over the years, but they are beyond the scope of this discussion. If you are still in doubt after obtaining routine AP, transthoracic, and axillary views—or if you cannot obtain adequate views—sedate the patient and do a CT scan. This step has largely replaced special views requiring complicated patient positioning that is often unfamiliar to emergency x-ray technologists. A CT can be more informative than double-contrast shoulder arthroscopy.

Treatment

The essence of treatment is a reduction—as quickly and gently as possible. Take the following steps:

1. Know the precise position of the humeral head after history, physical exam, and x-ray.
2. Know your complication. The younger the patient, the less likely it is that a complication will be present. Above 20 years, and especially over 40 years, look for the following complications:
   a. Ten percent of older patients (and a few younger ones) will have nerve injury—axillary nerve neurapraxia manifested by deltoid paralysis and numbness over the area of the deltoid insertion.
   b. Less than 2% of older patients will have arterial injury. If you are too vigorous with your reduction, you may produce a vascular lesion in this patient.
   c. The more inferior the dislocation (Fig. 17.6), and the older the patient, the greater the possibility of a rotator cuff tear. Obviously, you will not make that determination until after reduction.
   d. Watch out for the fractured greater tuberosity or surgical neck in the older patient.
   e. Occasionally, you will overlook that you are dealing with a chronic dislocation–one that has been present and unrecognized for days or weeks. You will rarely reduce a chronic dislocation with the treatment described below (10). It is embarrassing to make the diagnosis of an anterior shoulder dislocation and try a failed reduction, only to have the unreliable or intoxicated patient mention in passing that the injury might have occurred a few weeks ago!

How do you reduce an uncomplicated acute anterior shoulder dislocation?

Step 1. Be gentle; if you have a complication or a difficult first attempt at reduction, quickly switch to a general anesthetic.
Step 2. Most traumatic acute anterior dislocations can be reduced in the emergency room under IV sedation. If you are a team doctor at the site of the injury and are sure of an anterior dislocation, you may even achieve a reduc-

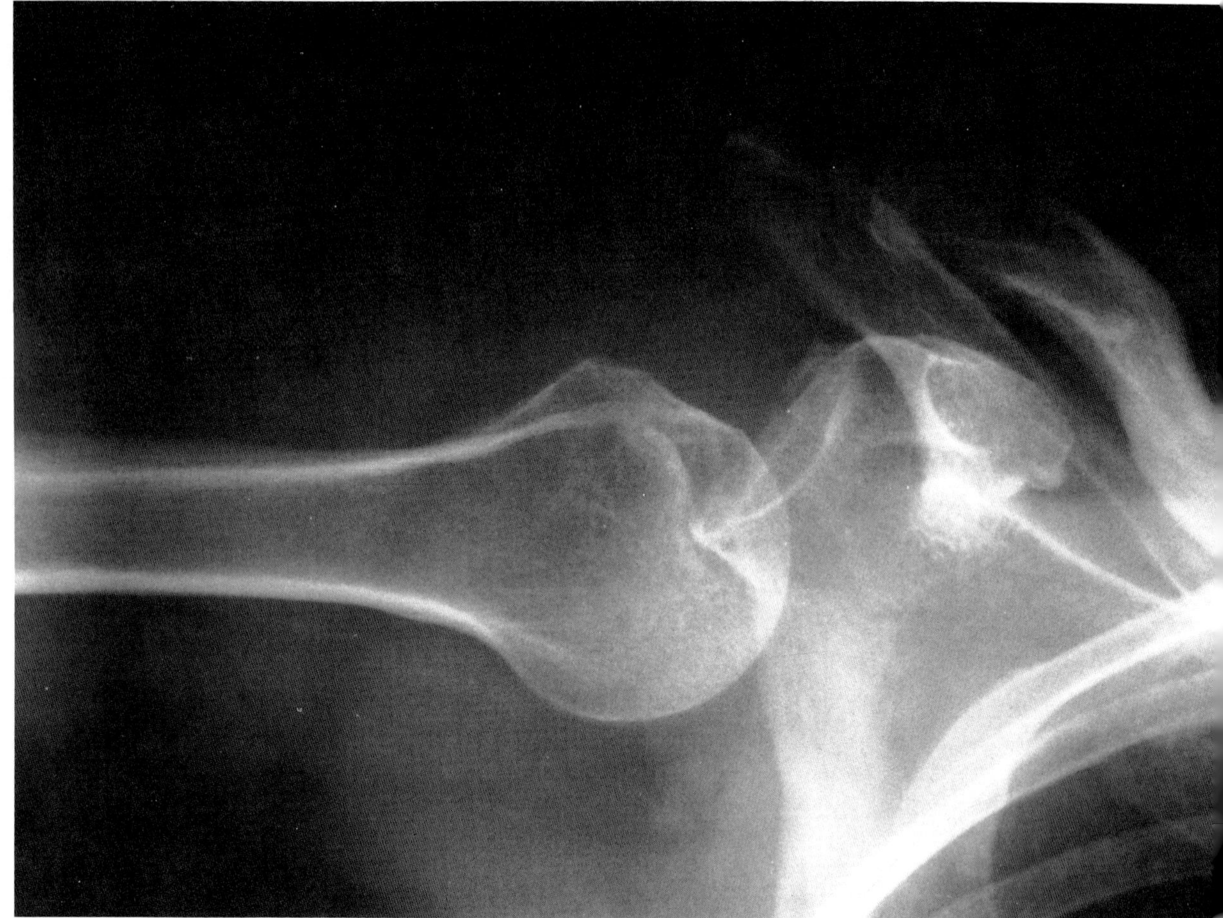

Figure 17.6.   Inferior dislocation (luxatio erecta). Anteroposterior view shows the characteristic abduction and elevation of the arm.

tion immediately after injury, without any anesthesia. In emergency, most patients require some form of IV sedation and relaxation.

Step 3. Pick one of three maneuvers:

   a. Traction (Fig. 17.7)

   b. Manipulation (Fig. 17.8)

   c. Prone Passive Traction (Fig. 17.9). If you are unable to reduce the shoulder in this fashion, place the patient under general anesthesia, at which time the shoulder usually spontaneously reduces.

Step 4. Reassess the patient's clinical state—are the neurovascular structures still intact? It is mandatory to obtain an x-ray post-reduction to be sure that no unrecognized complications, such as a fracture, have occurred, and that a reduction has been achieved.

Post-Reduction Immobilization

The length of immobilization post-reduction is decided as follows:

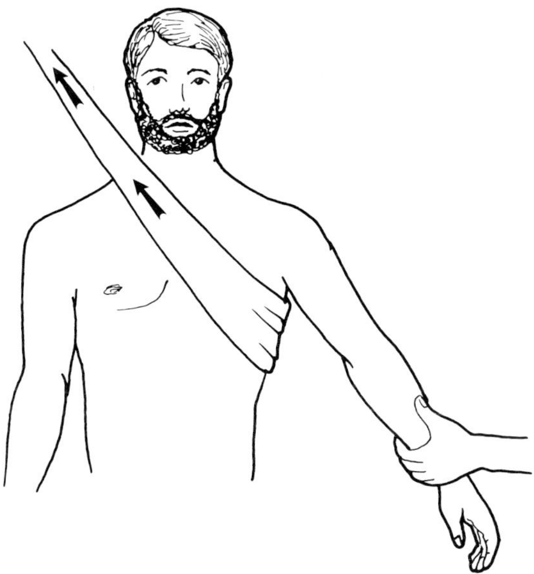

Figure 17.7.   Reduction of anterior shoulder dislocation with traction against countertraction. The position is one of slight abduction and external rotation—to unlock the Hill-Sachs lesion.

1. The younger the patient, the longer the immobilization. Below age 20, immobilize at least three weeks; above age 40, immobilize less than one week.
2. If you are sure of a significant degree of trauma and a first-time dislocation, immobilize for a longer period. If the trauma was minimal and you are possibly dealing with a recurrent dislocation, limited immobilization is indicated.

Rehabilitation

Exercise rehabilitation starts on day one. Have the patient do isometrics (abduction, flexion, and extension) a number of times per day (Appendix). At least once per day, the sling should come off and the elbow is extended. As you come to the end of the period of immobilization, start pendulum exercises (Fig. 17.10). As movement is regained, institute strengthening exercises and, finally, start functional activities, such as an overhead swing for racquet sports.

Usually, full function is obtained within three months from the time of injury. If things are moving slowly, you are missing something—a fracture, loose bodies, or a rotator cuff tear. Reassess the patient.

Recurrent Anterior Subluxation or Dislocation

The most common complication of an acute traumatic anterior dislocation is recurrent dislocation. The younger the patient is at the time of the acute traumatic anterior dislocation, the more likely a recurrence within two years. Recurrence figures range as high as 90% for teenagers who have an acute traumatic dislocation.

Why?

The glenoid fossa is a shallow socket for the humeral head; add to that an anterior capsular tear and glenoid damage (Bankart lesion) and a defect in the

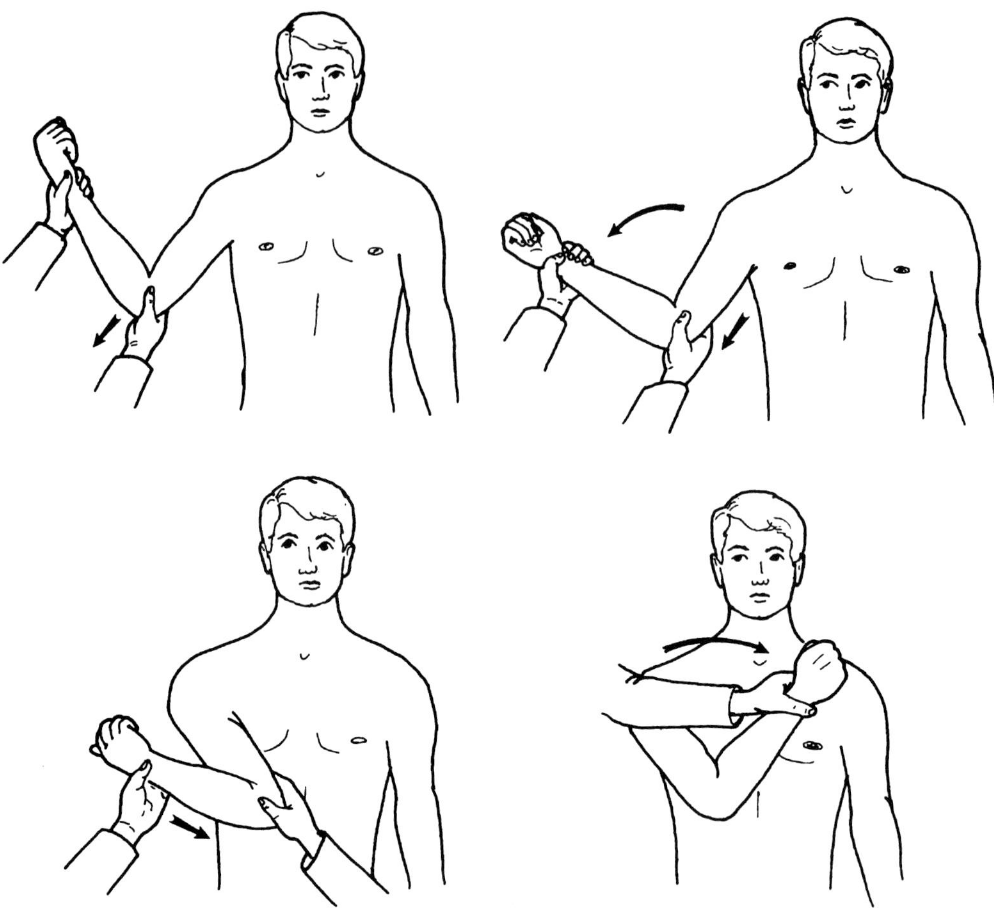

Figure 17.8. Reduction of an anterior shoulder dislocation with manipulation (Kocher maneuver). Step 1: apply longitudinal traction to the humerus with the shoulder in some abduction. Step 2: externally rotate the shoulder. Step 3: adduct the shoulder by moving the elbow across the front of the trunk. Step 4: rotate the shoulder internally.

humeral head (Hill-Sachs lesion), and you have perfect conditions for recurrence when the arm goes into abduction and external rotation (Fig. 17.11).

Subluxation or Dislocation?

Subluxation (partial, temporary joint dislocation) is just as common as frank dislocation. It is known as the "dead arm syndrome" because the partial dislocation and spontaneous reduction paralyzes the arm with pain and the patient is momentarily unable to use the extremity. Patients often state that, during the moment of subluxation, the arm "went dead."

A dislocation will often present as such—a dislocated shoulder—with the following characteristics (which distinguish it from an acute traumatic anterior dislocation):

1. The trauma that produced this dislocation was minor.

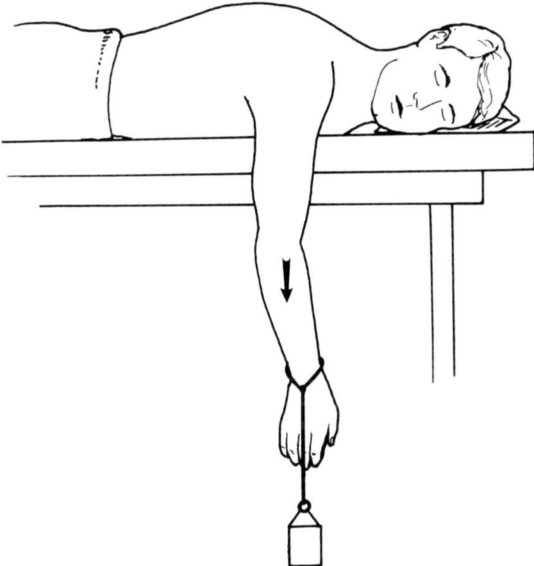

Figure 17.9.   Prone traction method of reduction. This is useful in a busy emergency room using a 5–10-lb weight for 5–10 minutes. (Don't get too busy and forget the patient!)

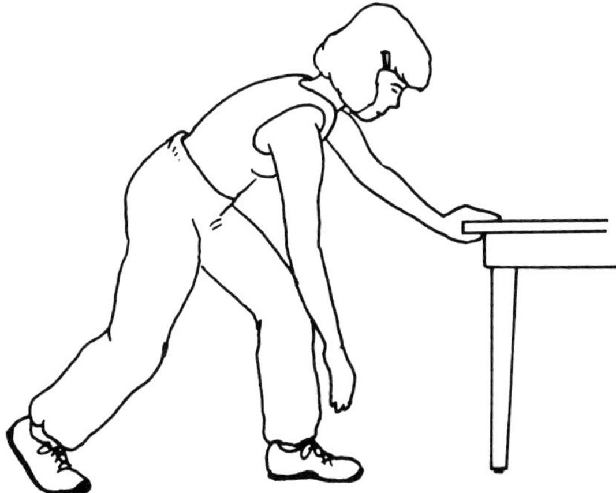

Figure 17.10.   Classic pendulum exercise. In this position, the patient passively moves the shoulder in a "circular pendulum" motion using movement of the trunk.

2. There was an initial dislocation in the past, produced by significant trauma, that required manipulative reduction. Afterwards, the arm hurt for a few weeks.
3. If you are lucky, you will be able to obtain pre- and post-reduction x-rays from the initial event that clearly establish the diagnosis.

Diagnosis

The diagnosis is often easy—you see the patient with a history of prior dislocations, or an existing dislocation that was the result of minimal trauma ,and you easily reduce the shoulder.

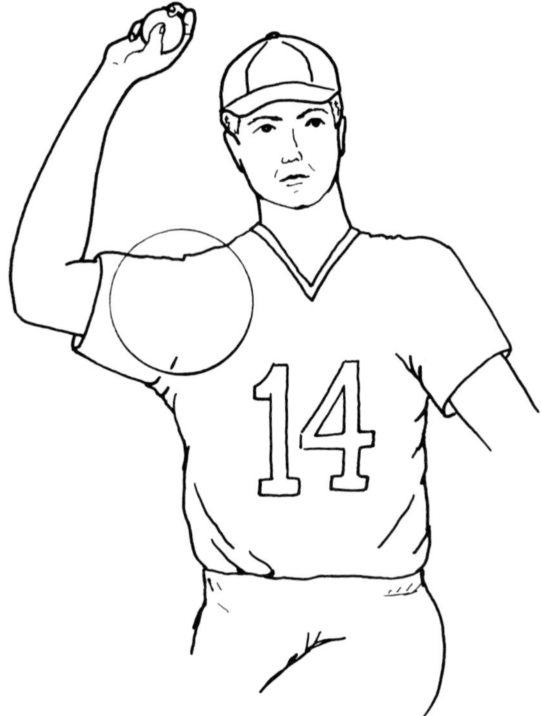

Figure 17.11.   The pitcher or football player, in the act of throwing, has the shoulder in the abducted externally rotated position of redislocation.

Other times, reduction occurs so easily the patient will present a story of a shoulder that gives way or deadens with certain movements (abduction and external rotation), and you have to turn detective.

Question 1.   What is the arm position when the sensation of instability or deadening occurs?

Question 2.   Can I stress the arm to reproduce some apprehension on the part of the patient (Fig. 17.12)? Are there any signs of impingement using the Neer and/or Hawkins tests (Fig. 17.13)?

Question 3.   Are there any clues on x-ray of a prior dislocation (Fig. 12.18*B*)?

Treatment of Recurrent Anterior Dislocations

The younger the patient and the more frequent the dislocations, the more likely continuing untreated dislocations will result in arthritis of the glenohumeral joint. More than two dislocations within two years of each other become the indication for surgery.

Before operating, be sure of your diagnosis through careful history, physical diagnosis, and well-documented x-rays. This may include double-contrast arthrography to show the Bankart lesion (Fig. 17.14).

Surgery for Recurrent Anterior Dislocations

Surgical repair requires a balance between range of movement and stability (14). It is possible to surgically tighten down soft tissues so much that no future

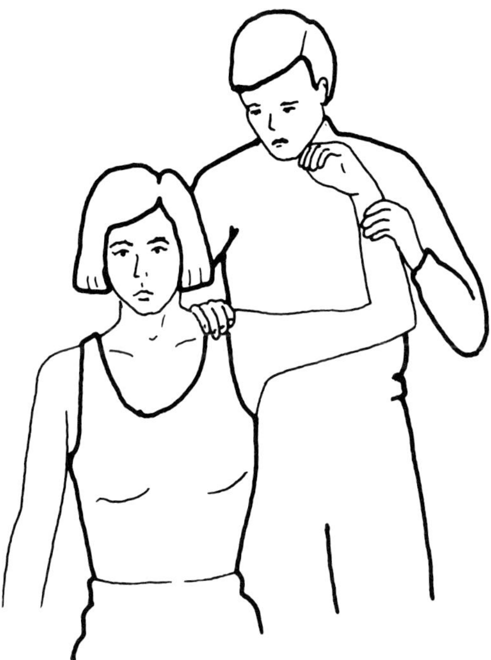

Figure 17.12.   Apprehension test. The examiner attempts to put the shoulder into abduction and external rotation, which will cause apprehension, guarding, and resistance as the patient feels the shoulder begin to sublux.

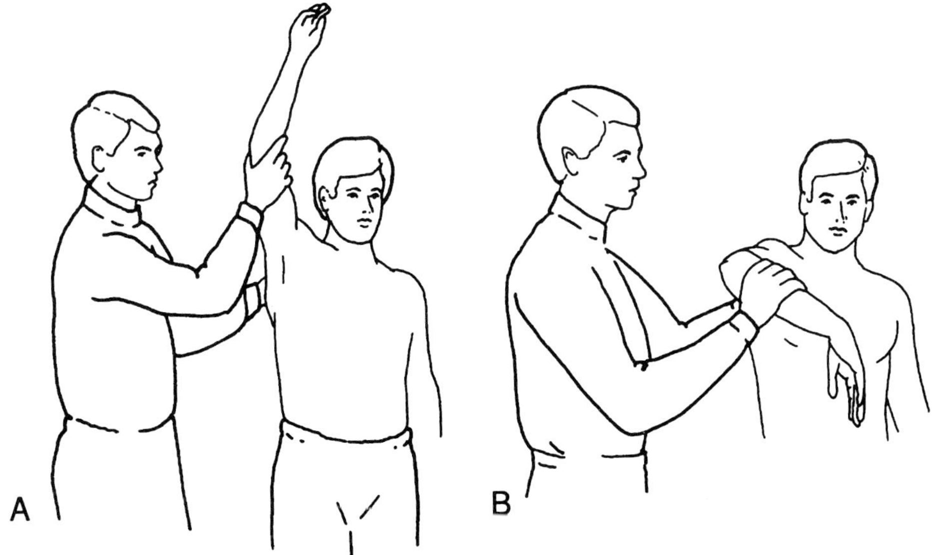

Figure 17.13.   A, full passive elevation impingement test will produce pain in rotator cuff disorders. B, with 90° abduction and forward flexion, the arm is internally and externally rotated, impinging a rotator cuff or bursal disorder against the coracoacromial ligament.

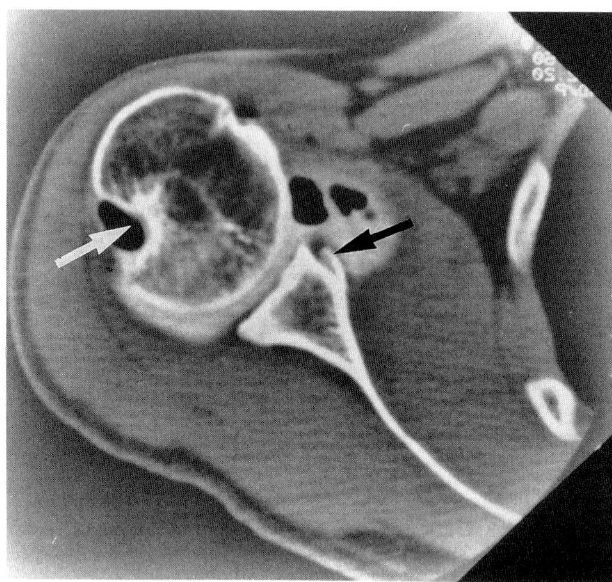

Figure 17.14.   Hill-Sachs and Bankart deformities demonstrated on a CT arthrogram. The anterior glenoid (*arrow*) shows both osseous and cartilaginous damage. A large Hill-Sachs fracture (*white arrow*) is present in the posterolateral humeral head.

dislocation will occur, but the patient will be very unhappy with the loss of so much abduction and external rotation. Despite the fact that you have cured the dislocation, you have a poor result. The object of the surgical exercise for recurrent anterior dislocations is to restore stability but, at the same time, maintain mobility.

There are basically four common procedures performed for recurrence.

1. The Bankart repair (1). This is by far the most popular approach (Fig. 17.15).
2. Variations of the Bankart repair. Numerous authors have suggested various methods, such as staples (Du Toit) (5), tendons (Gallie) (2), and screws to fix the anterior scapular structures to the front of the glenoid. By and large, these procedures are no longer used (11).
3. Capsulorrhaphies. From the original Putti-Platt (12) (Fig. 17.16) to Magnusson-Stack (4) (Fig. 17.17) or more recent modifications, capsulorrhaphies are frequently used. Often, they are combined with the Bankart repair.
4. Bone blocks. The most commonly recognized of these procedures is the Eden-Hybbinette block (Fig. 17.18).

There are a number of miscellaneous procedures, such as humeral and glenoid osteotomies that are rarely used.

Postoperative Course

Postoperatively, patients are immobilized for up to three weeks; they then start an exercise program similar to that for acute traumatic dislocations. The postoperative exercise program is every bit as important as the surgery and is outlined in the Appendix.

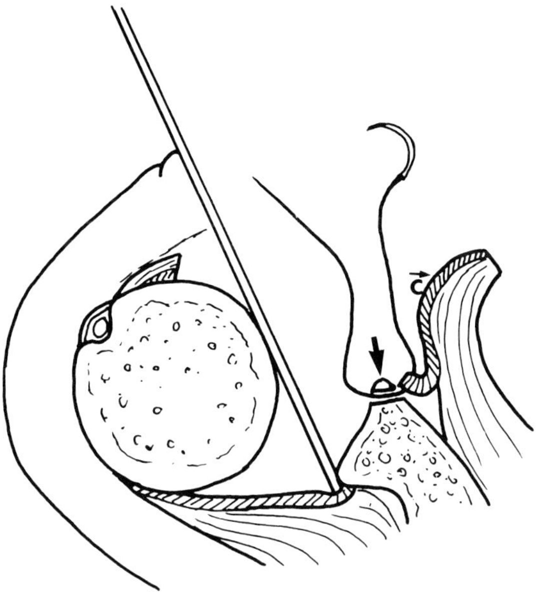

Figure 17.15.   Bankart procedure of suturing the anterior capsule (*c*) to the glenoid rim (*arrow*).

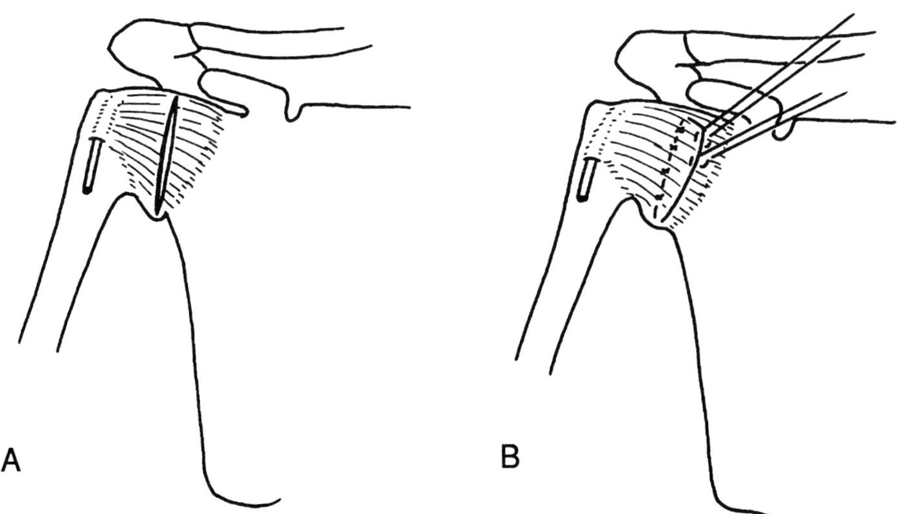

Figure 17.16.   Putti-Platt repair—the capsule and subscapularis are divided (**A**) and shortened by a "double-breasted suit" suture (**B**).

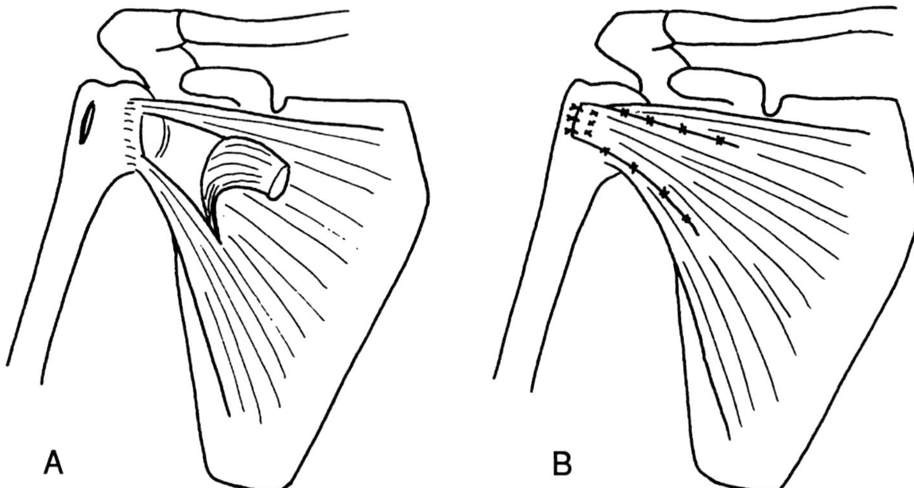

Figure 17.17.   Magnusson-Stack procedure. Transfer of the subscapularis tendon (**A**) from the lesser tuberosity, across the biceps tendon to the greater tuberosity (**B**).

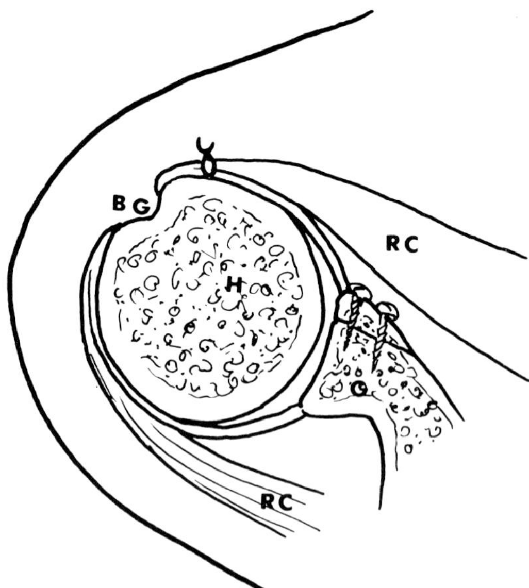

Figure 17.18.   Eden-Hybbinette procedure using a bone graft (held with two screws) from the iliac crest to extend the anterior glenoid labrum and repair the anterior capsular defect. (*H* = humeral head, *G* = glenoid, *RC* = rotator cuff, *BG* = bicipital groove.)

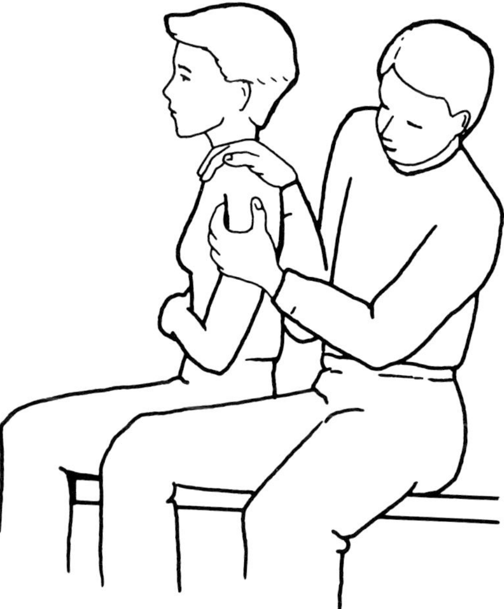

Figure 17.19. In this position with the patient relaxed, the humeral head can be subluxated both anteriorly and posteriorly.

Chronic Unrecognized Anterior Dislocation

A dislocation present beyond a few days is considered chronic and unrecognized. This usually occurs because the patient fails to seek medical care until that time (unlike patients with missed posterior dislocations).

Up to six weeks after dislocation, there is a chance that the shoulder can be reduced. Better to do your chronics under general anesthesia, and have the patient prepared for an open anterior approach if the closed reduction fails.

In the older patient (60 and up), it is often prudent simply to leave the chronic shoulder dislocated and ask the patient to accept limitations.

Atraumatic Voluntary Dislocations—Multidirectional Instability (MDI)

This condition is relatively common and is mentioned to remind you that an anterior dislocation from minor trauma may be more than what you see! Sometimes, these patients have multidirectional instability—they have anterior, interior, and posterior dislocation. If you're not careful, you will miss this history.

Usually, patients are female and the shoulder symptoms started spontaneously at a young age (early teens). Minimal to no trauma is required to produce the dislocation, and often the patient can voluntarily demonstrate the point. Spontaneous reduction occurs, and there is very little discomfort in the shoulder after the episode.

On examination, these patients are generally loose-jointed, and the shoulder itself can be subluxated or dislocated in all directions (Fig. 17.19). Thus the term multidirectional instability.

Rarely do these patients respond to surgery. They are best handled with an exercise program designed to strengthen the shoulder girdle muscles. Some sur-

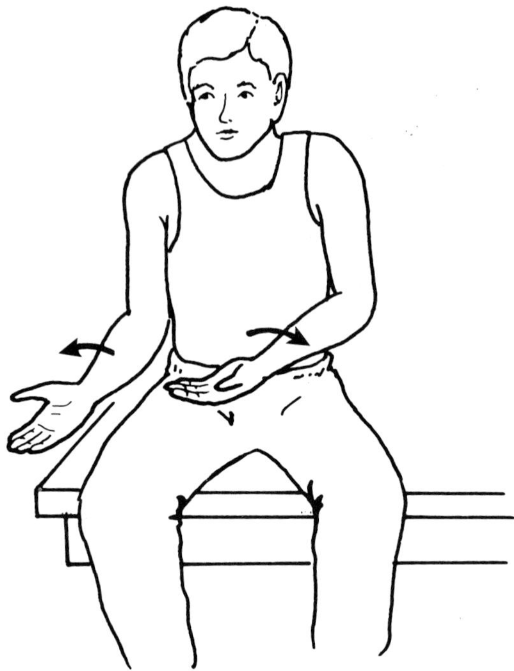

Figure 17.20.   If there is no external rotation of the shoulder joint after an injury, you have a posterior dislocation (until proven otherwise).

geons stress the possibility of underlying emotional disorders contributing to MDI and recommend appropriate counselling.

Acute Traumatic Posterior Dislocation

Incidence

Two percent of shoulder dislocations are posterior. Fifty percent will be missed on presentation. This is an uncommon diagnosis, commonly missed!

Presentation

The patient presents the "arm in the sling" position, has a poor exam, and has equally poor x-rays.

How Not to Miss a Posterior Dislocation

The presenting situation is often unusual, such as an intoxicated patient falling on the outstretched hand or an epileptic patient post-seizure. If you don't examine the immobilized shoulder, you will miss the dislocation.

Live by another rule: if an injured shoulder has 0° external rotation, a posterior shoulder dislocation is assumed to be present until ruled out on x-ray (Fig. 17.20). Loss of external rotation is also the most significant finding in the frozen shoulder—a condition far more frequent than posterior dislocation.

X-ray

Do the same views as for anterior dislocations (Fig. 17.21), and if you are still not satisfied, do a CT scan.

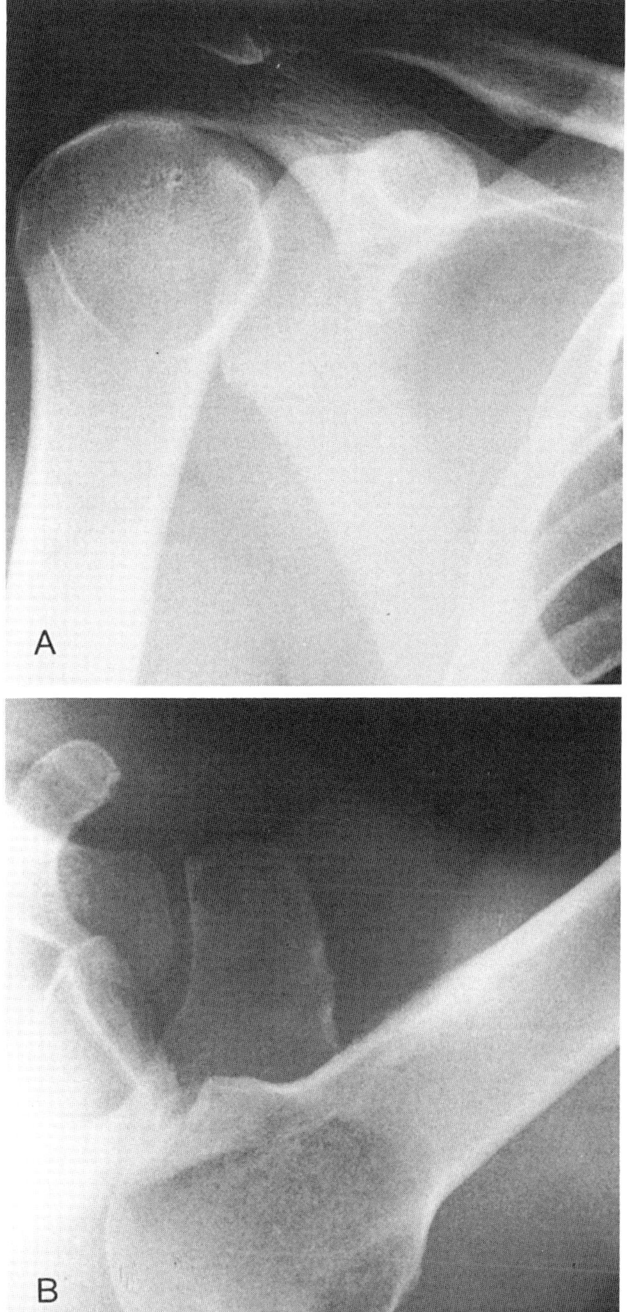

Figure 17.21.   **A,** AP of posterior dislocation. Something doesn't look right—you have a full AP of the greater tuberosity, which is said to look like a "full moon" humeral head. **B,** axillary view in the same patient. Note the humeral head posterior to the glenoid.

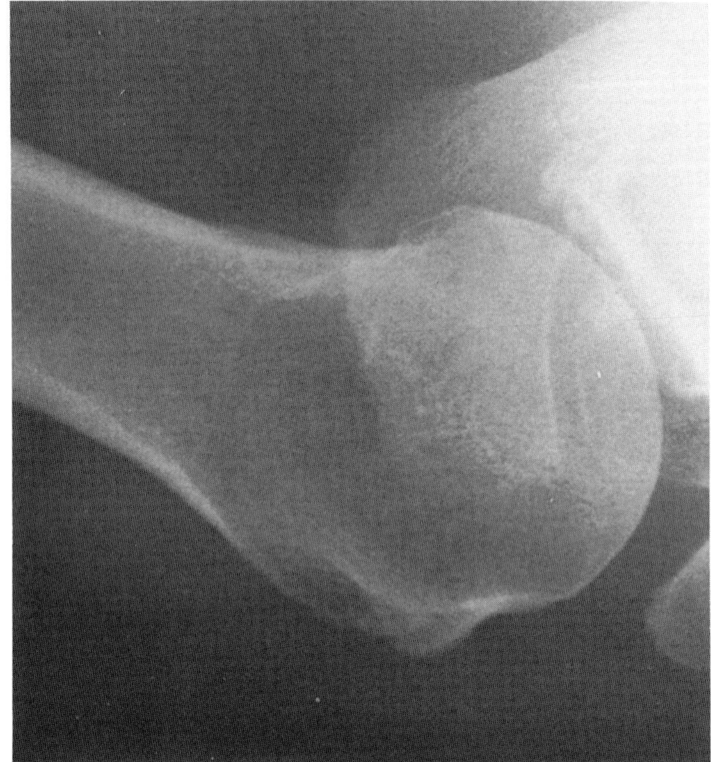

Figure 17.22.   Post-reduction of Figure 17.21*B*. Note perfect alignment between humeral head and glenoid.

Treatment

First, be sure you are not missing an atraumatic voluntary dislocation. Second, rule out complications, such as fracture of the humeral head or lesser tuberosity. Next, proceed as you would for an anterior dislocation, sedating the patient and using traction and manipulation for reduction (Fig. 17.22). Finally, be ready to quickly move to general anesthesia—posterior dislocations are more difficult to reduce than anterior dislocations. Don't struggle; put the patient to sleep. Even then, be prepared to open the shoulder anteriorly for an irreducible dislocation (8). If you note a humeral head fracture on the prereduction x-ray, the patient will probably require an open reduction.

Immobilization.   Post-reduction immobilization extends to three weeks and is shown in Figure 17.23 as the "handshake" position.

Complications of Acute Posterior Dislocation

Aside from a missed diagnosis, complications such as rotator cuff tears and neurovascular compromise are less frequent in posterior dislocations.

Chronic Unrecognized Posterior Dislocation

Posterior shoulder dislocations are initially missed as often as they are diagnosed. Don't you be the one to do the missing. If a patient has a shoulder injury

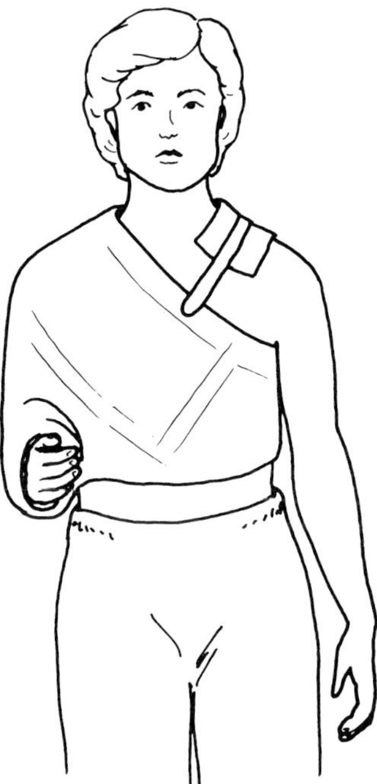

Figure 17.23.   The "handshake" position for immobilization of reduced posterior dislocation.

or pain, and cannot externally rotate, you have a posterior shoulder dislocation until proven otherwise.

A chronic posterior shoulder dislocation will almost never succumb to an attempt at closed reduction (8). If it is a young patient and a short history (less than a few months), an anterior open reduction will be required. An older patient with a longstanding posterior dislocation is best left in the dislocated position, except for the occasional patient who might respond to an arthroplasty.

Surgery for a chronic posterior dislocation is done anteriorly (8). Because of the distorted anatomy, key on the long head of biceps to guide you to the lesser tuberosity, from which the subscapularis can be taken down and the humeral head approached. If there is a large anterior (reverse) Hill-Sachs, the subscapularis should be sutured into the defect (8).

Postoperative Immobilization.   Quick mobilization to prevent stiffness is the order of the day after this operation.

Recurrent Posterior Dislocation

This is not a very common situation simply because of the sheer number of acute anterior dislocations compared to posterior dislocations (6).

When it does occur, simply back your way through the steps for recurrent anterior dislocations (3).

First, be sure of your diagnosis, and watch out for voluntary multidirectional instability. Next, take all your anterior operations and apply them posteriorly, that is, a posterior repair of the capsular and glenoid deficit, shortening the in-

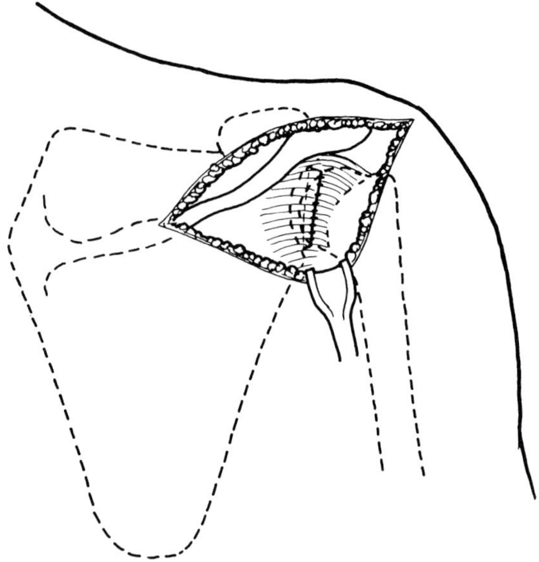

Figure 17.24.   The reverse Putti-Platt for recurrent posterior dislocations. The trapezius has been split and the rotator cuff (infraspinatus and supraspinatus, along with the joint capsule) has been "double-breasted" to effect a shortening.

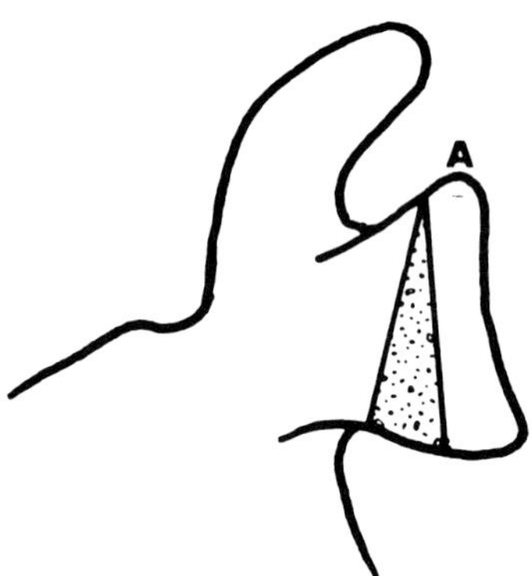

Figure 17.25.   An opening-wedge glenoid osteotomy for recurrent posterior dislocations. A capsular and tendon reefing can also be done (*A* = anterior).

fraspinatus (13) (Fig. 17.24). Glenoid osteotomies are more frequently used for posterior recurrent dislocation (Fig. 17.25).

Pseudosubluxation

After injury or stroke (especially in the older patient) muscle weakness allows the humeral head to subluxate inferiorly (Fig. 17.26). The unsupported shoulder of an early post-stroke patient is especially prone to this condition. Prevention, time, and early strengthening exercises are the method of management.

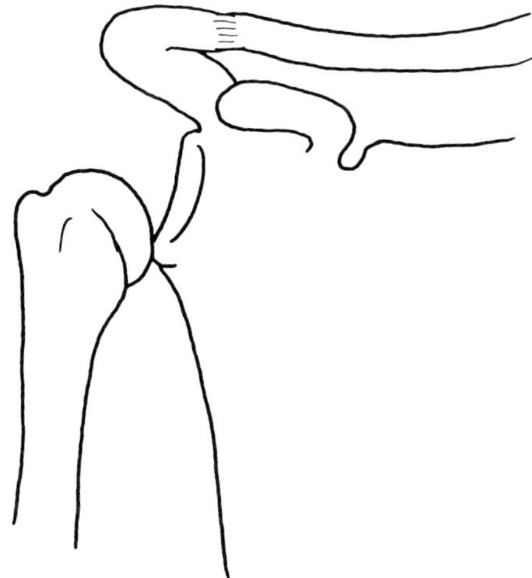

Figure 17.26.

REFERENCES

1. Bankart ASB: The pathology and treatment of recurrent dislocations of the shoulder joint. Br J Surg 26:23–29 (1938).
2. Bateman JE: Gallie technique for repair of recurrent dislocation of the shoulder. Surg Clin North Am 43:1655–1662 (1963).
3. Boyd HB and Sisk TD: Recurrent posterior dislocation of the shoulder. J Bone Joint Surg 54A: 779–786 (1972).
4. De Palma AF: Factors influencing the choice of a modified Magnusson procedure for recurrent anterior dislocation of the shoulder—with a note on technique. Surg Clin North Am 43:1631–1634 (1963).
5. Du Toit GT and Raux D: Recurrent dislocation of the shoulder. A 24-year study of the Johannesburg stapling operation. J Bone Joint Surg 38A:1–12 (1956).
6. English E and Macnab I: Recurrent posterior dislocation of the shoulder. Can J Surg 17:147–151 (1974).
7. Hill HA and Sachs MD: The grooved defect of the humeral head. A frequently unrecognized complication of dislocation of the shoulder joint. Radiology 35:690–700 (1940).
8. McLaughlin HL: Locked posterior subluxation of the shoulder—diagnosis and treatment. Surg Clin North Am 43:1621–1622 (1963).
9. Mosley HF: The basic lesions of recurrent anterior dislocation. Surg Clin North Am 43:1631–1634 (1963).
10. Neviaser JS: The treatment of old unreduced dislocations of the shoulder. Surg Clin North Am 43:1671–1678 (1963).
11. O'Driscoll SW and Evans DC: The Du Toit staple capsulorrhaphy for recurrent anterior dislocation of shoulder. Paper presented at American Shoulder and Elbow Surgeons, Atlanta (1988).
12. Osmond-Clarke H: Habitual dislocation of the shoulder. The Putti-Platt operation. J Bone Joint Surg 30B:19–25 (1948).
13. Rowe CR and Yee LK: A posterior approach to the shoulder joint. J Bone Joint Surg 26A:580–584 (1944).
14. Rowe CR and Zarins B: Recurrent transient subluxation of the shoulder. J Bone Joint Surg 63A: 863–872 (1981).

18

Injuries to the Shoulder Region

"Old bones are brittle."

—Anonymous

INTRODUCTION

The traumatic injuries we will discuss in this chapter include the common fractures:

- Clavicle
- Proximal humerus
- Scapula

Chapter 17 described shoulder dislocations, excluding traumatic disorders of the acromioclavicular and sternoclavicular joints.

Fractures of the Clavicle

The main function of the clavicle is to hold the shoulder girdle away from the body so that its muscles maintain their maximum leverage (1). In acting as a strut, it is an important cosmetic structure between the neck and the shoulder. Don't put an attention-grabbing surgical scar on it, especially in women who wish to wear low-cut dresses. In addition, the clavicle and its underlying subclavius muscle serve as protection for the neurovascular bundle as it exits the neck and chest to enter the arm (Fig. 18.1).

The clavicle is most likely injured by a fall on the shoulder (6), and it is least likely injured by a fall on the outstretched hand, or by a direct blow with an object like a hockey stick. The fracture usually lies at the junction of the medial two-thirds and lateral one-third of the shaft (Fig. 18.2*B*). The breaking of the passive strutting action of the clavicle, with the addition of muscle action, results in the shoulder girdle and lateral clavicular fragment lying in a downward and medial position, with the medial portion of the shaft resting posteriorly upward (Fig. 18.3). To relieve some of the pain, children will adopt a "torticollis" position (Fig. 18.2*A*).

The fracture most often occurs in children, but is not infrequent in the adult weekend athlete (5). Patients hold the arm in a sling-like position (Fig. 18.4), with an obvious deformity and tenderness along the shaft of the clavicle. A sharp spike on the medial fragment may dent the skin or, on rare occasion, even perforate the skin—an occurrence usually prevented by the platysma muscle.

The fracture is best demonstrated by an x-ray taken with the tube angled 30° upward (Fig. 18.2).

390

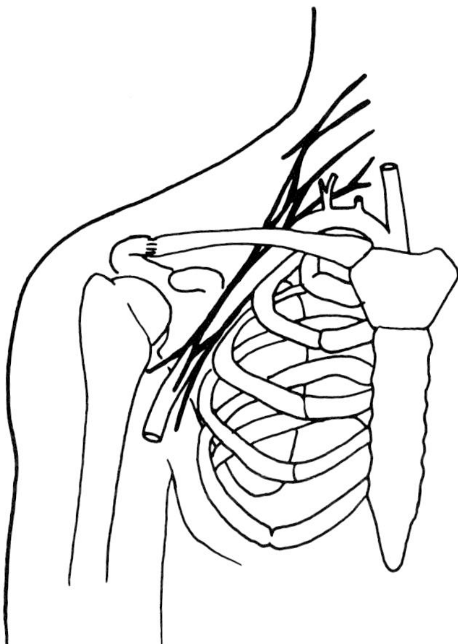

Figure 18.1.   The clavicle and its underlying subclavius muscle (not shown here) protect the brachial plexus and major vessels as they exit the neck to enter the arm.

A fractured clavicle is usually a straightforward diagnosis, with no associated complications; it is easily treated conservatively, and leads to union in 99% of cases. This fracture is a "piece of cake." On rare occasions, fracture fragments will damage the neurovascular bundle—always examine the upper extremity for integrity of the vascular and neurological systems. The subclavius muscle protects these important structures (Fig. 18.1). Even rarer still is a pneumothorax from a fracture fragment puncturing the apex of the lung.

Reduction is achieved passively by returning the shoulder to its strutted position away from the chest wall. This is best achieved by having the patient lie down and instructing him or her to actively pull the shoulder into the military position of attention. If you are going to use a figure-of-eight bandage (Fig. 18.5) to maintain the reduction, apply it firmly in this position, and then sit the patient up to tighten the bandage.

The figure-of-eight bandage is reserved for adults and older children who can be cautioned about its constriction on the neurovascular bundle. It is important to teach them to increase the military position of attention to relieve some of that pressure. Children under six won't tolerate the figure-of-eight, and they don't need it because their fractures do not displace (greenstick fractures). Even if they do displace their fracture and heal with a bump, bone remodeling will deal with the problem. Finally, see if you can keep a young child in a sling for more than a few days! The older child (6–12 years) is best treated in a sling for two to four weeks. As mentioned, adolescents and adults should try to tolerate the figure-of-eight bandage for four to six weeks. Sometimes, it becomes such a problem to wear that you need to switch the patient to a sling. The adult should also start early range-of-movement exercises in the bandage—active external rotation and abduction to 90°, three or four times a day.

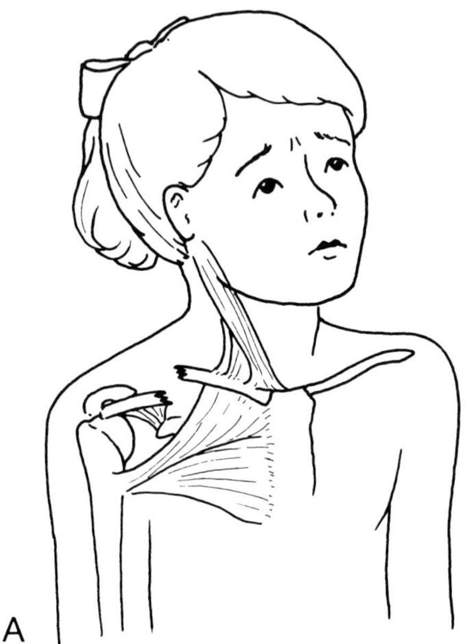

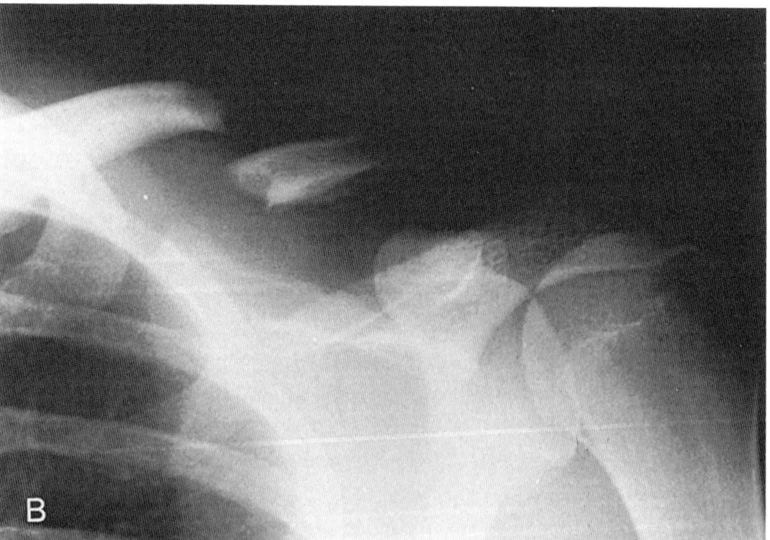

Figure 18.2.   **A,** typical location of a fractured clavicle on schematic. Note the "torticollis" position of the head. **B,** x-ray of a fractured clavicle.

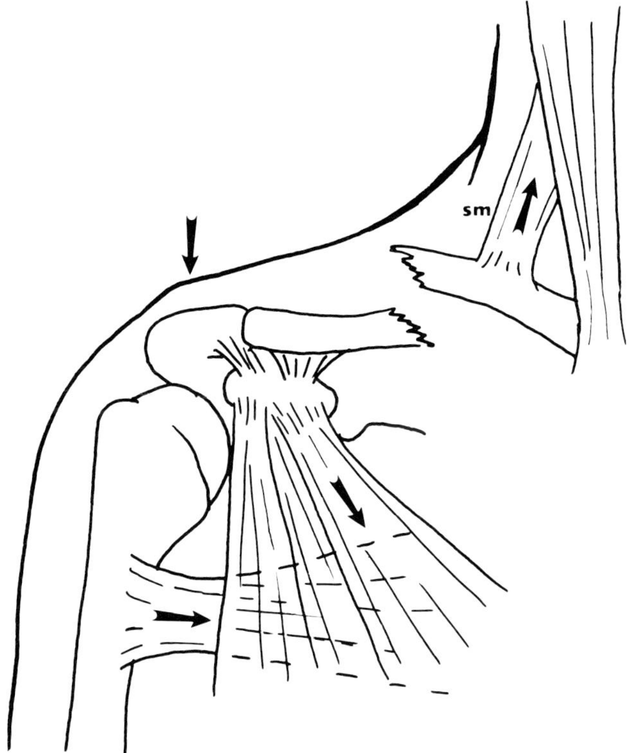

Figure 18.3.   Muscles that pull on a fractured clavicle:
1. Sternomastoid (*sm*) pulls the proximal fragment superiorly.
2. Pectoralis muscles pull the shoulder and distal clavicle fragment medially downward.

It is rare for complications and nonunion to occur, so don't get too aggressive with this fracture. If there is neurovascular damage or a painful nonunion, operative intervention with the application of a dynamic compression plate and bone grafting (Fig. 18.6) is indicated. Because the clavicle is such a subcutaneous and prominent bone, the plates and screws are obvious after healing, and usually have to be removed.

Fractures of the Proximal Humerus

The simplest way to understand these fractures is to see the proximal humerus as four parts (Fig. 18.7):

1. Head of the humerus
2. Shaft of the humerus
3. Greater tuberosity
4. Lesser tuberosity

Next, understand the muscles pulling on and displacing these fragments once injury separates them (Fig. 18.8).

To appreciate the complications of these fractures, review the blood supply to the humeral head (Fig. 11.13). If it is disrupted by fracture, avascular necrosis of the humeral head is a logical event. The close proximity of the brachial plexus,

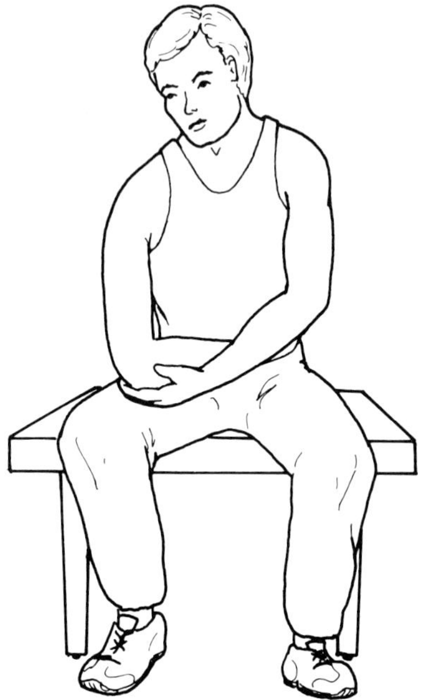

Figure 18.4.   The "sling position" as the patient appears in emergency—the same schematic as shown for the dislocated shoulder (Fig. 17.3).

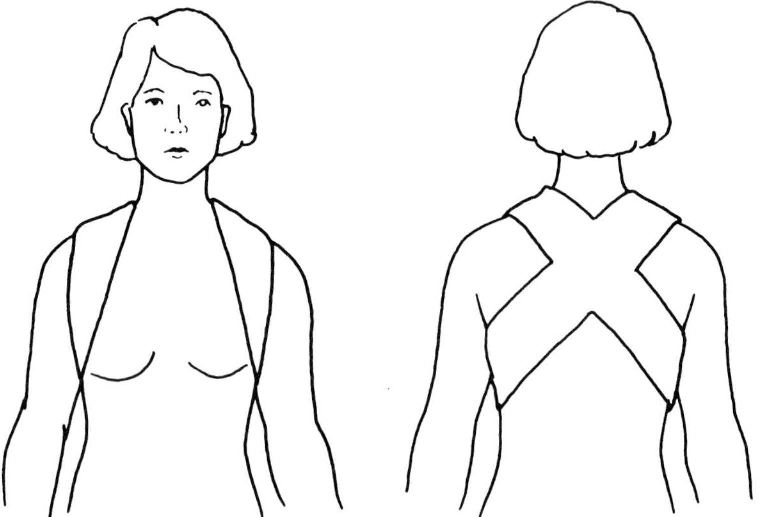

Figure 18.5.   A figure-of-eight bandage used to treat a fractured clavicle.

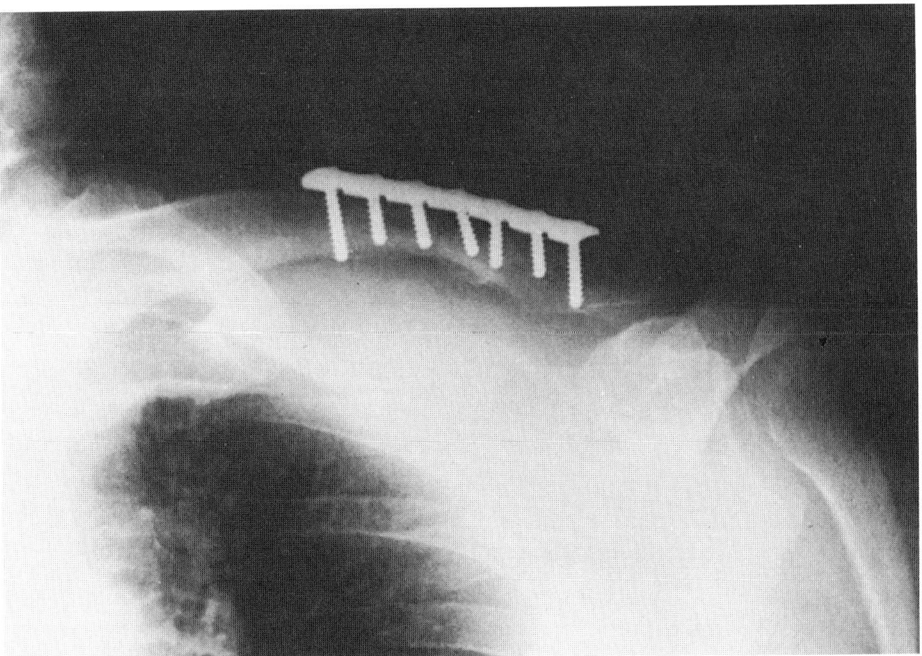

Figure 18.6.   Rarely is open reduction and fixation of a fractured clavicle indicated.

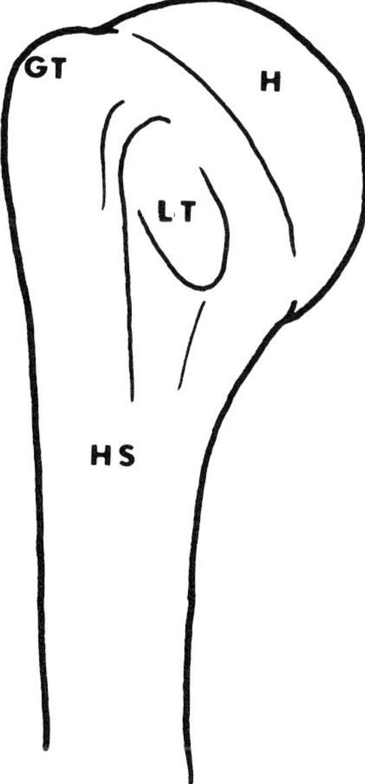

Figure 18.7.   The proximal humerus has four parts: 1. Humeral head (*H*). 2. Humeral shaft (*HS*). 3. Greater tuberosity (*GT*). 4. Lesser tuberosity (*LT*).

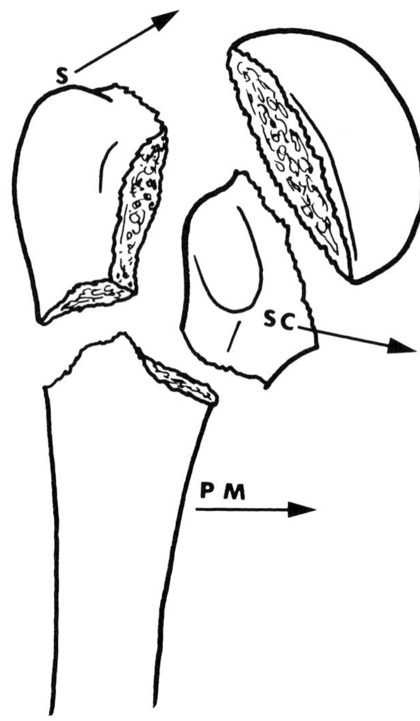

Figure 18.8.   The muscles that pull on the four parts: 1. Humeral head—none. 2. Humeral shaft—pectoralis major (*PM*). 3. Greater tuberosity—infraspinatus, supraspinatus (*S*). 4. Lesser tuberosity—subscapularis (*SC*).

especially its terminal axillary nerve (Fig. 11.12), is also vulnerable to injury from being impaled on the fracture fragments.

Classification

Neer (2) has developed the most commonly used classification of these fractures (Fig. 18.9). The classification is based on:

1. Codman's four parts to the proximal humerus (Fig. 18.7).
2. Nondisplacement or displacement—displacement is considered to be 1 cm or more.
3. Angulation (45° or more is considered angulation).
4. Dislocation of the humeral head from the glenoid.
5. Splitting of the humeral head.

It is important to appreciate that Neer's classification (2, 3) applies to displaced or angulated fragments. If there is a simple hairline fracture of the greater tuberosity without angulation or displacement (Fig. 18.10), treatment does not need Neer's classification but rather a sling and binder (Fig. 18.11). When these patients become comfortable, start a ROM exercise program (10–14 days). Some of Neer's displacement patterns are subtle or hidden, and very good x-rays are required to adequately see a clear picture of what is happening. This is very true for dislocations of the humeral head, especially those in which the humeral head lies posteriorly. For accurate depiction of the degree of splitting of the humeral head, a CT scan is the investigation of choice.

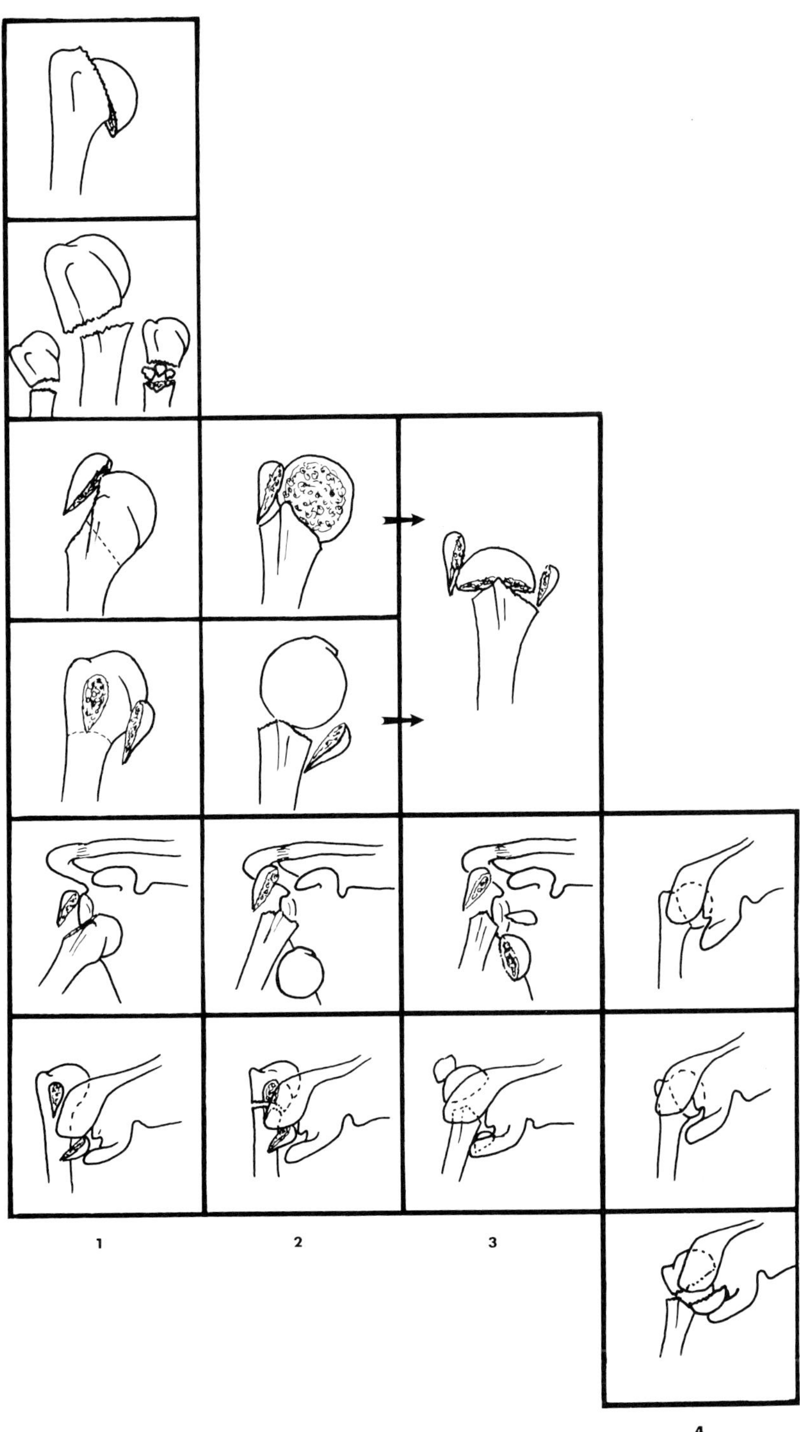

Figure 18.9.   Neer's classification of shoulder fractures that are angulated or displaced. *Column 1*, two-part fractures; *Column 2*, three-part fractures; *Column 3*, four-part fractures; *Column 4*, fracture-dislocations. Adapted from Neer (2).

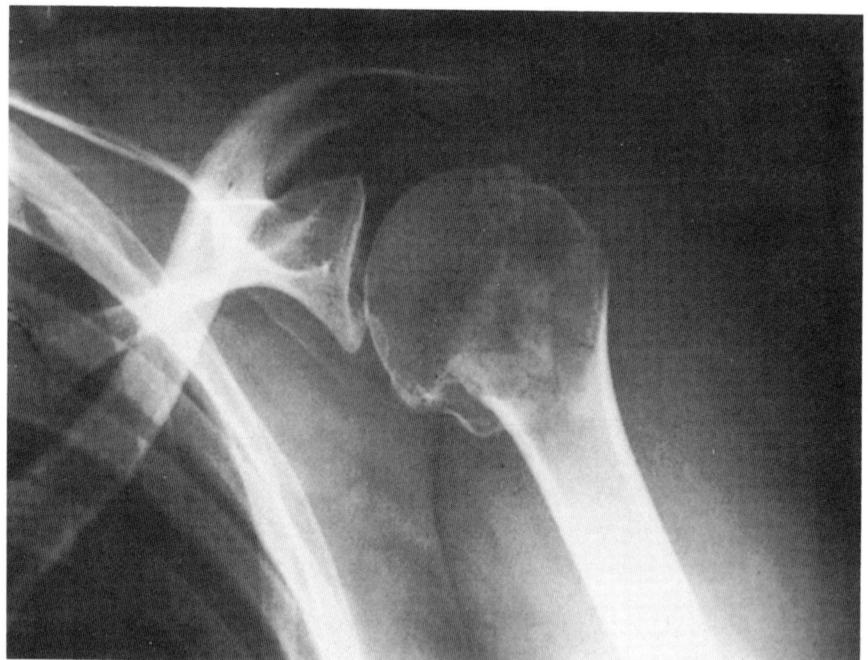

Figure 18.10. A simple undisplaced surgical neck fracture that is not covered by Neer's classification.

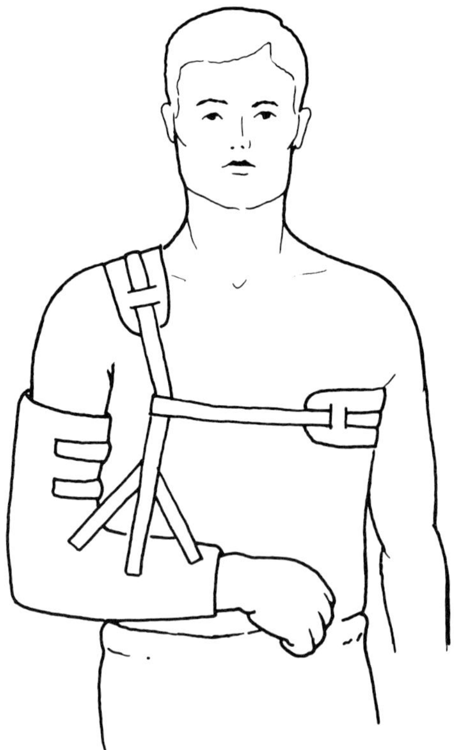

Figure 18.11. An example of a sling and binder for proximal humeral injuries.

Incidence and Mechanism of Injury

Proximal humeral fractures will constitute about 5% of all fractures seen in emergency. They most often occur in the older female patient, who more than likely has osteoporotic bone. The most common mechanism of injury is a fall on the outstretched hand.

Clinical Presentation

It is hard to miss a fracture of the proximal humerus. The patient comes to the emergency department with a story of having fallen and complains of the instant onset of shoulder pain. Appropriate x-rays will reveal the fracture pattern.

Common Fracture Patterns and Their Treatment

Undisplaced Fractures

Fortunately, most fractures (80%) will be undisplaced (Fig. 18.10) and can be immobilized in a sling and binder, to be followed by early pendulum exercise mobilization at one to two weeks.

Two-Part Surgical Neck Fractures

Most of these fractures are impacted and can be treated in the same way as undisplaced fractures. A fracture that is not impacted with a displaced humeral shaft (Fig. 18.12) will require closed reduction before the sling and binder are applied. Closed reduction followed by redisplacement requires rereduction and percutaneous pinning (4).

Two-Part Greater Tuberosity Fractures

Displaced greater tuberosity fractures are the result of direct blows to the lateral aspect of the shoulder, a common skiing injury (Fig. 18.13). In the older patient, they may occur in conjunction with an anterior dislocation of the shoulder joint. Obviously, shoulder dislocations should be reduced. Most displaced tuberosity fragments require open reduction, and anatomical reduction and stabilization of the fragment with heavy-duty suture. If a tear of the rotator cuff is present, it will also require repair.

Three-Part Fractures

The third part of this fracture is most often the greater tuberosity, but it may be the lesser tuberosity. These fractures are very unstable and require open reduction and internal fixation (Fig. 18.14). In some older patients with severe osteoporosis, a humeral head prosthesis is a much better choice.

Four-Part Fractures

Almost all of these fractures (Fig. 18.15) will be treated with excision of the humeral head and replacement with a Neer prosthesis (Fig. 18.19). In doing so, you must securely fasten the tuberosities to each other, to the humeral shaft, and to the prosthesis—with heavy duty nonabsorbable suture. Poor bone stock may require that the prosthesis be cemented into the humeral shaft.

Four-Part Fracture-Dislocations

These fractures (Fig. 18.9) are treated in the same way as four-part nondislocated fractures.

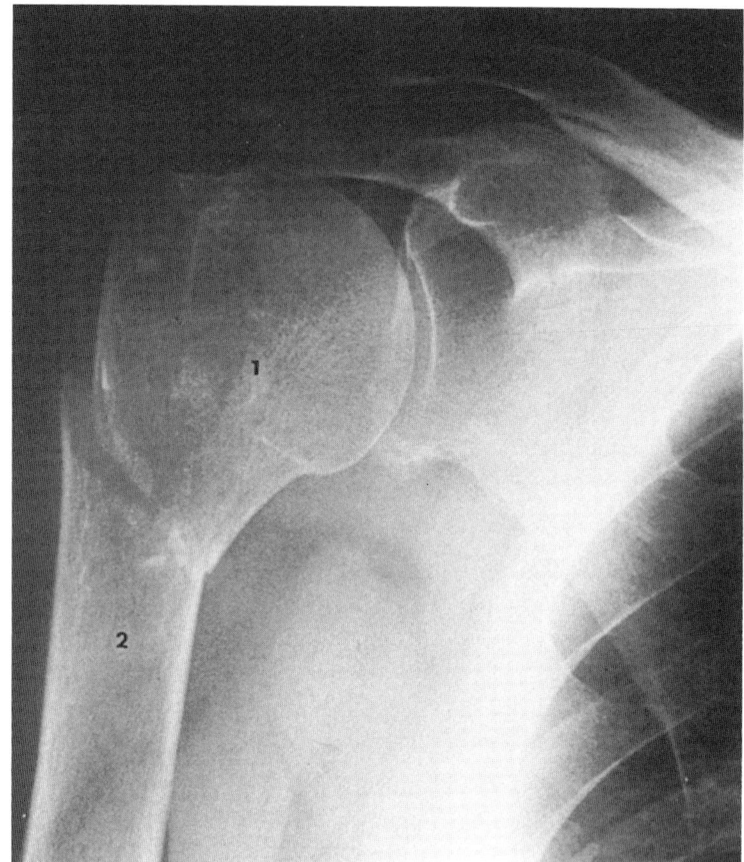

Figure 18.12.   A two-part (humeral head and shaft) proximal humeral fracture.

Head-Splitting Fractures

Small fragments fractured off the humeral head can usually be treated conservatively. Involvement of 50% or more of the humeral head requires surgical intervention and usually a prosthetic replacement. Rarely is a reduction with internal fixation successful.

Postoperative Rehabilitation

Neer has described a three-phase system of exercise rehabilitation that starts with passive-assistive exercises, graduating to active-resistive and stretching exercises. The third and longest phase in the rehabilitation program is an advanced stretching and strengthening exercise program. The first phase should start 7–10 days postoperatively. Inadequate rehabilitation will result in a painful, stiff shoulder and a very unhappy patient.

Scapular Fractures

Of the three areas of fracture (humerus, clavicle, and scapula), scapular fractures are the least common. They are usually caused by direct blows and

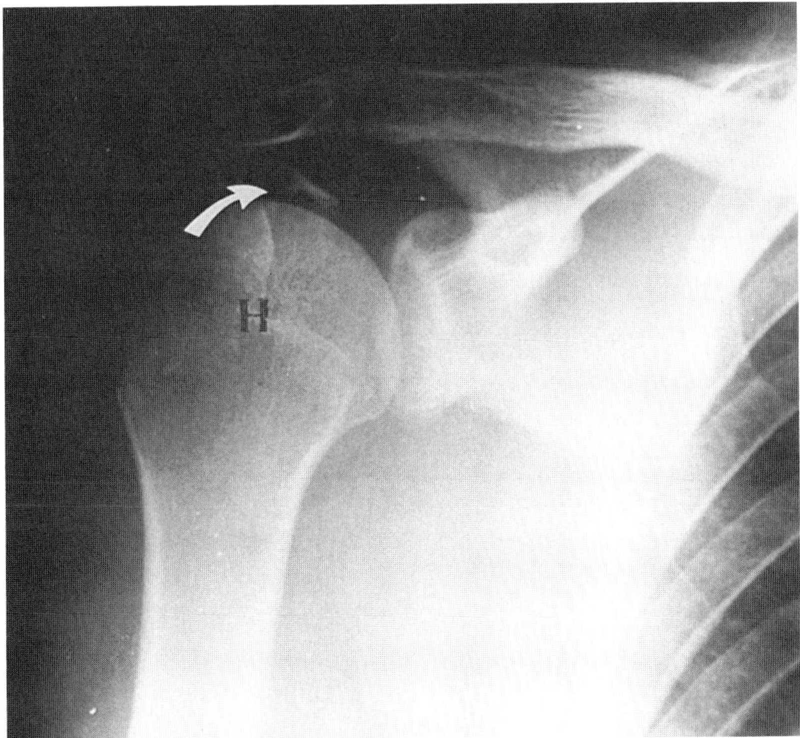

Figure 18.13.   A two-part greater tuberosity fracture: greater tuberosity (*arrow*); rest of proximal humerus (*H*).

are rarely associated with complications, but they do cause severe pain. Often, there are remote associated injuries to the thorax and skull, which are more important treatment determinants. Management of the scapular fracture alone is by sling immobilization until the patient is comfortable. Institution of active exercises begins as soon as possible (10–14 days) to maintain shoulder function.

On rare occasions, a scapular fracture will involve a large portion of the glenoid articular surface, which serves as the only indication for open reduction and internal fixation.

Acromioclavicular Joint

A frequent injury to the shoulder complex is to the acromioclavicular joint. A lateral blow to the tip of the shoulder, such as a fall on the deltoid region, is the usual mechanism of injury. All patients exhibit pain and swelling over the a-c joint.

The strains and separations have been divided into six categories (Fig. 18.16), based on weighted films (Fig. 18.17):

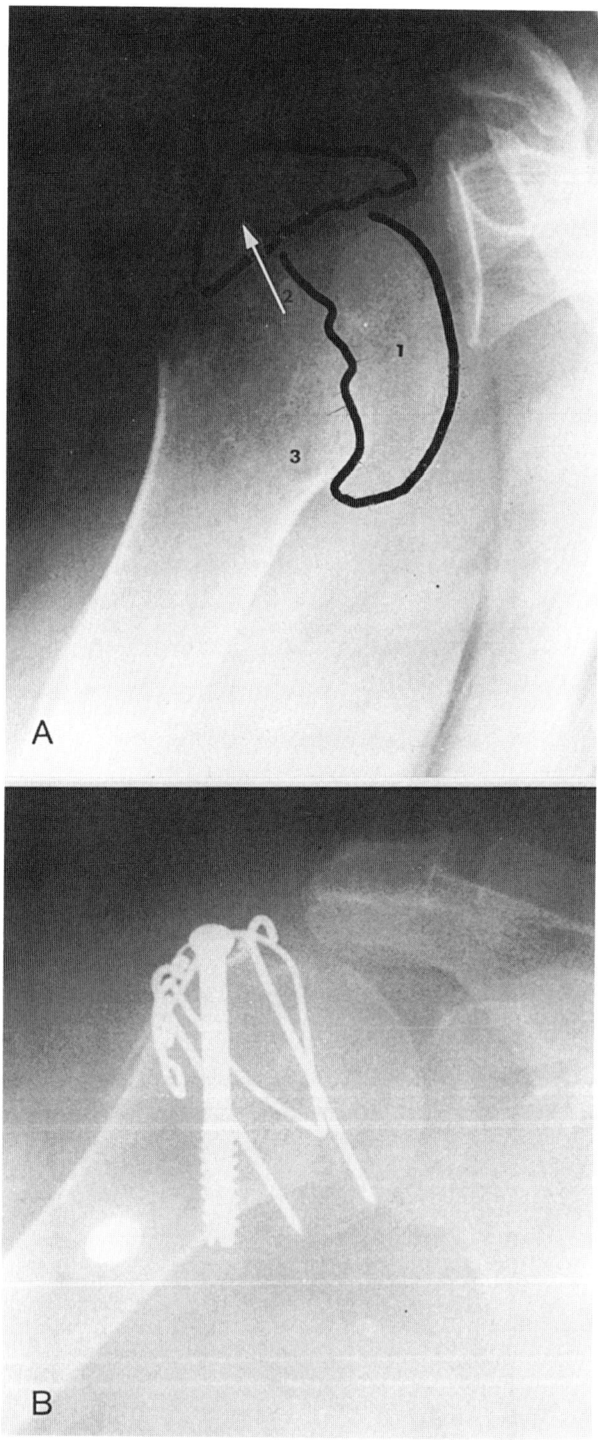

Figure 18.14.   **A**, three-part proximal humeral fracture: (*1*) head, (*2*) greater tuberosity, and (*3*) shaft. **B**, open reduction and internal fixation of three-part fracture.

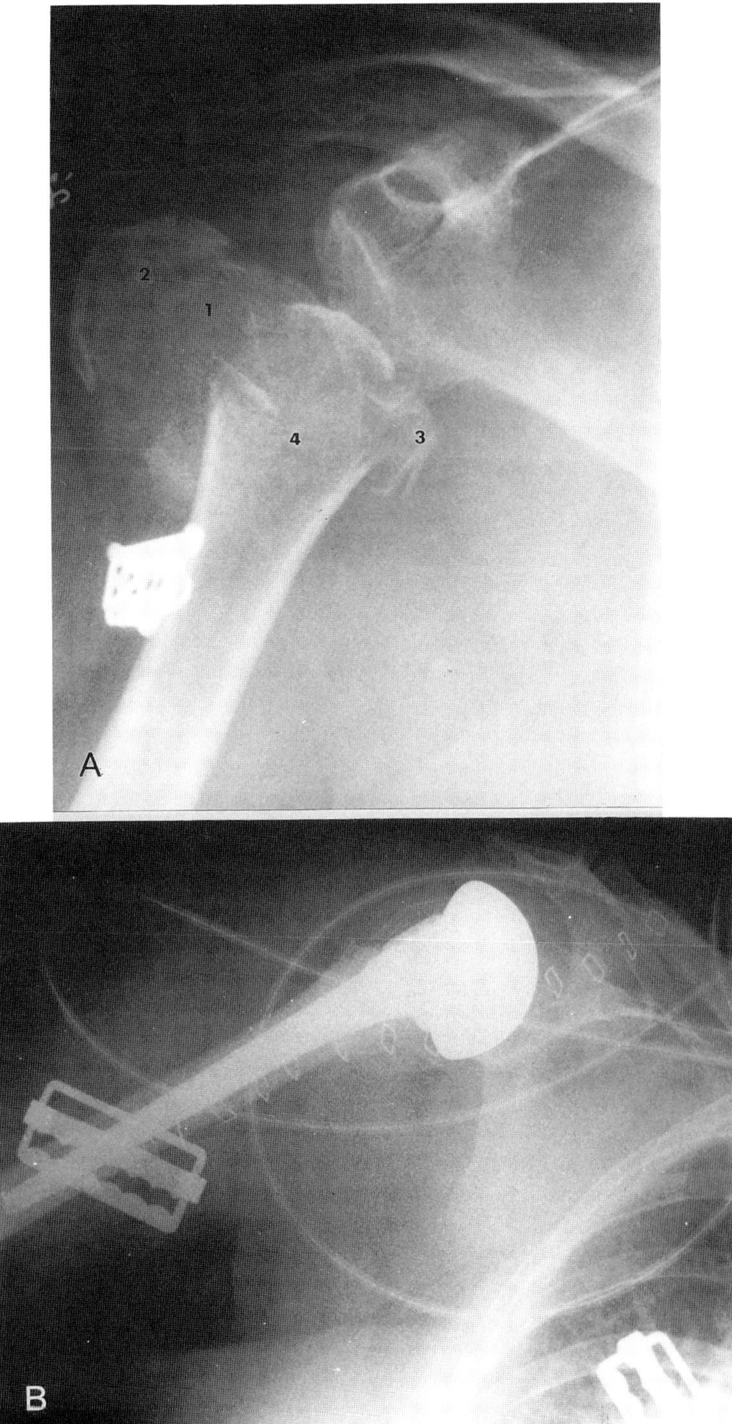

Figure 18.15.   A, four-part fracture: (*1*) humeral head, (*2*) greater tuberosity, (*3*) lesser tuberosity, and (*4*) shaft. *B,* Neer humeral prosthetic replacement for fracture in *A*.

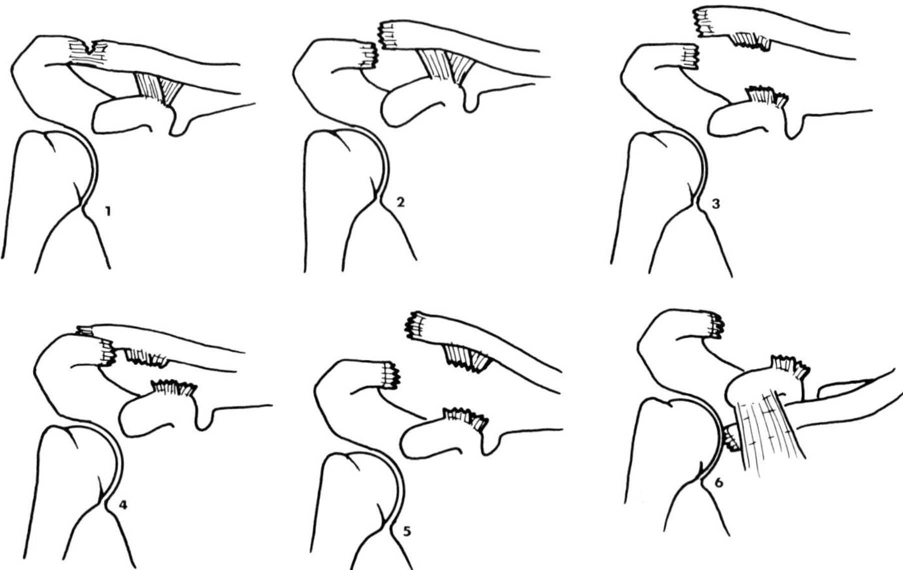

Figure 18.16.   The six categories of a-c strains and separations (see text for description).

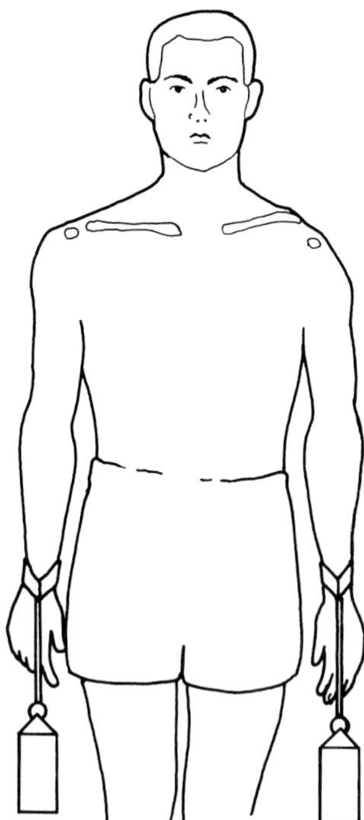

Figure 18.17.   The method of taking weighted films to show degree of separation of a-c joint.

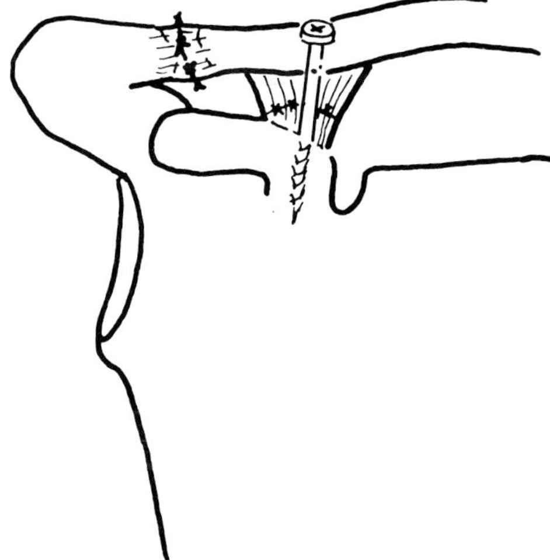

Figure 18.18.   A repair of a separated a-c joint with a lag screw across the coracoclavicular joint.

1. Sprain only—no clavicular displacement
2. Clavicular displacement less than the width of the clavicle
3. Clavicular displacement more than the width of the clavicle
4. Wide displacement of the a-c joint with posterior displacement of the clavicle
5. Very wide displacement of the clavicle, which is superior
6. Inferior clavicular displacement under the acromion

Types 1–3 are heated conservatively in a sling and binder until the patient is comfortable (5–10 days), then a mobilization, strengthening program is started. Types 4–6 require surgical intervention using threaded pins across the a-c joint (old method) or a screw to reconstruct the coracoclavicular ligament (preferred method) (Fig. 18.18).

Postoperative mobilization is begun early, and the hardware is removed at six to eight weeks to prevent breakage.

Chronic a-c joint problems may lead to arthritic degeneration of the joint. The associated pain and limited movement (loss of full abduction and adduction) can be resolved with excision of the outer .5 in. of the clavicle (Mumford procedure).

Sternoclavicular Joint

This joint may be dislocated anteriorly with major shoulder trauma. Rarely does the proximal end of the clavicle dislocate posteriorly and medially, but if it does it can cause life-threatening injury to the major vessels and/or the trachea.

The joint can be reduced by extension of the glenohumeral joint, holding the arms in position postoperatively with a figure-of-eight bandage. Use of pins to transfix the clavicle to the sternum is not indicated, because of the potential for migration into forbidden territory (the mediastinum).

REFERENCES

1. Codman EA: The Shoulder: Rupture of the Supraspinatus Tendon and Other Lesions in or About The Subacromial Bursa. Thomas Todd Co., Boston (1934).
2. Neer CS: Displaced proximal humeral fractures. Part 1. Classification and evaluation. J Bone Joint Surg 52A:1077–1089 (1970).
3. Neer CS: Displaced proximal humeral fractures. Part 2. Treatment of the three-part and four-part displacement. J Bone Joint Surg 52A:1090–1103 (1970).
4. Rush LV: Atlas of Rush Pin Techniques. Beviron Co., Meridian, MI (1959).
5. Sankarankutty M and Turner BW: Fractures of the clavicle. Injury 7:101–106 (1975).
6. Stanley D, Towbridge EA, and Norris SH: The mechanism of clavicular fracture. J Bone Joint Surg 70B:461–464 (1988).

19

The Shoulder in Sports

*"Cease, reverend Fathers! from those youthful Sports
Retire, before unfinish'd Feats betray Your slacken'd
Nerves."*
—John Armstrong

INTRODUCTION

There is no truer test of a clinician's ability than sports medicine. It is a constant struggle that pulls in many directions, but centers around such issues as:

- What motivates an individual to produce at 100% of function and will that motivation continue?
- During rehabilitation, the athlete often concludes that, if a little exercise is good, a lot must be even better. This can undo a carefully crafted progressive exercise program or skillfully completed surgery.
- In spite of specific task-related injuries, any athlete can suffer from any affliction, for example, shoulder pain from a C4-C5 cervical disc herniation.
- So many potentially negative professionals are involved in the care of the athlete—from the club owner or coach who wants continuous performance, to the therapist who has the latest modality or new twist to an exercise, to the surgeon who thinks aggressive surgical techniques will return an individual to a high level of competitive athletic function.

The most important aspect of keeping or recovering athletic function is a comprehensive team approach from the physician, surgeon, and therapist (9). Programs must be designed to maximize individual potential—physically and emotionally—and to prevent and minimize sports-induced injury, and institute aggressive conservative treatment when injury intervenes.

Shoulder-Specific Biomechanics

The shoulder was designed to be mobile, not stable. The relationship between the glenoid labrum and humeral head is so shallow that there is virtually no bony stability, as there is in the hip joint. As the most mobile joint in the body, it relies heavily on soft tissue restraints for stability. These restraints are either passive (ligaments and capsule) (Fig. 11.10) or active muscular, such as the rotator cuff and deltoid muscles (Figs. 11.2 and 11.3).

The most studied activity of the shoulder is throwing (2, 10, 15), an activity common to baseball, football, swimming, tennis, gymnastics, and track events such as javelin. This mechanism can be simplified into three basic activities: (1) wind-up and cocking, (2) acceleration, and (3) follow through (Fig. 19.1). Add to

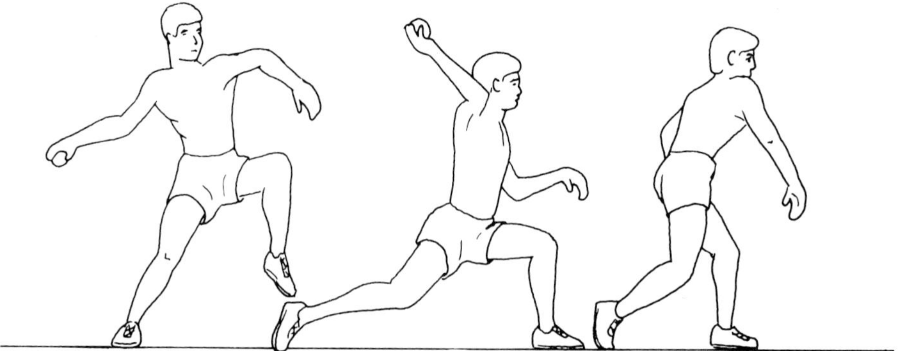

Figure 19.1. The three basic phases of the throwing mechanism: 1. Wind-up and cocking. 2. Acceleration. 3. Follow through.

this the necessity to "cock" the body by twisting the trunk and a leg, and you have an intricate sporting activity.

It is proposed that passive and active stabilizers act in concert to affect movement. Jobe (10) has further subdivided the active stabilizers into (1) the rotator cuff, and (2) the scapular muscles (e.g., deltoid and rotators). An imbalance in one mechanism can result in injury in another trying to compensate (8). The example he uses most often is the weak passive capsular restrainers constantly reinjured by an overactive compensating scapular muscle group. As a result, the passive restraints are further damaged and the active muscular components fatigue in failure. The result is shoulder mechanics imbalance and further injury to the rotator cuff.

Sport-Specific Shoulder Syndromes

Remember that any athlete can suffer from any routine shoulder problem covered in other chapters and any multitude of causes of referred shoulder pain. Be especially aware of the torn rotator cuff (Chapter 14). Don't get so focused on sport-specific conditions that you miss other problems.

Sport specific injuries are classified as:

1. Overuse
2. Impingement
3. Instabilities
4. Combinations of the above

Assessment

Every assessment of every problem in medicine starts with a good history and physical examination. Note the nature of the chief complaint. Is it pain or weakness in its various forms (e.g., apprehension, fatigue)? When does it occur in the task? Is it constant or does it only appear during warmup, sport-specific, or after activity?

Start with a routine physical examination that includes general observation of the shoulder for wasting and deformity, palpation for tenderness, and a range-of-movement assessment. When examining the individual, try to simulate the sport-specific task and analyze the movement in detail.

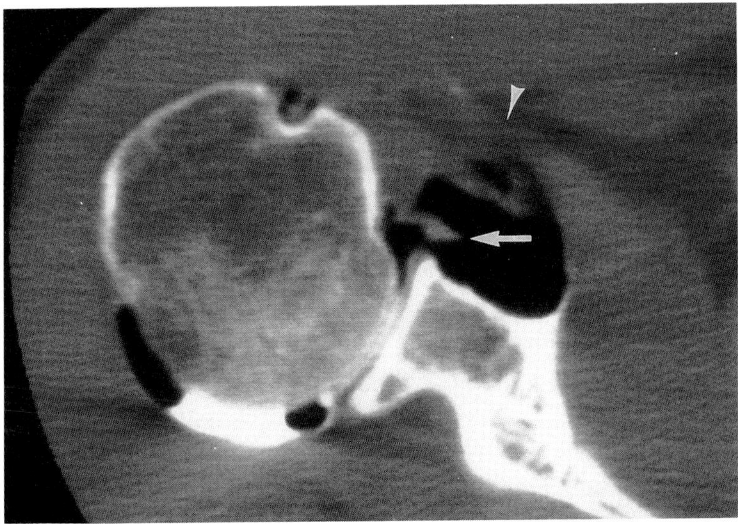

Figure 19.2.   Section through the mid-glenoid. The labrum is totally detached (*arrow*). The sub-scapularis tendon appears attenuated and irregular (*arrowhead*).

With an adequate history and physical exam, the diagnosis will be at hand in over 80% of athletes. Obviously, a routine shoulder x-ray needs to be done. Occasionally, CT scan is useful in detecting bony abnormalities such as a Bankart lesion (Fig. 19.2). MRI is becoming very useful for the assessment of what is most often a soft tissue injury (Fig. 19.3).

Overuse Syndrome

Repetitive microtrauma occurs at a rate that exceeds the body's ability to recover. The symptom is aching discomfort, accumulating with activity and lingering after sport (8, 13).

The minimal pathology is usually in the capsular restraints and the rotator cuff in the form of mild edema and inflammation. It is of such a low level that nothing will be seen on plain x-ray or MRI.

Treatment is two-phased. In the first brief phase, the athlete is rested for hours or days until the discomfort subsides. General fitness must be maintained during this phase. Recovery may be hastened with modalities such as ice and NSAIDs.

The second retraining phase, instituted as quickly as sustained comfort occurs, is centered around general warm up (7), specific stretching, and muscle strengthening exercises (see Appendix). At this juncture, modalities can be switched to deep heating, such as ultrasound and/or diathermy. Rarely, if ever, is surgery indicated.

Impingement

Shoulder mechanics require that there be adequate space between the humeral head and acromion for the rotator cuff and bursa (Fig. 19.4). By increasing

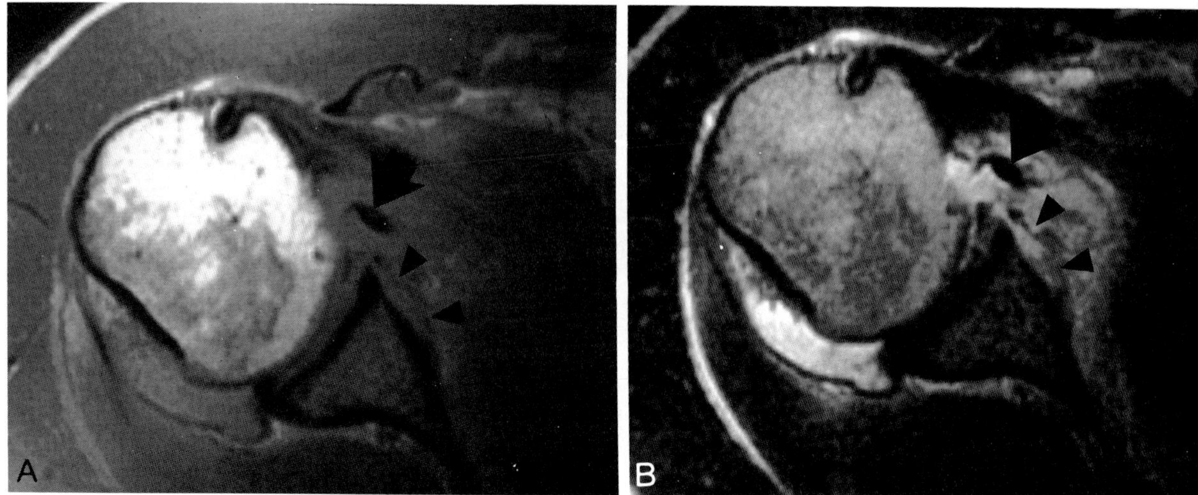

Figure 19.3.   Bankart lesion. Axial double-echo images (A = SE 1500/15, B = 1500/80). The anterior labrum (*arrow*) is detached from the bony glenoid. A portion of the anterior capsule (*arrowheads*) is seen floating in the large effusion. Note edema in subscapularis muscle along its scapular border.

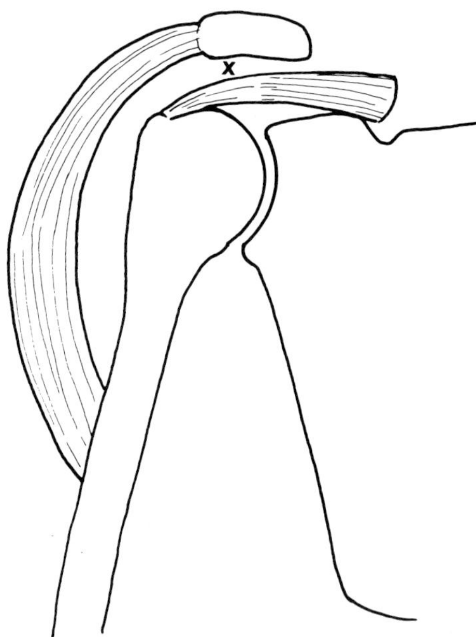

Figure 19.4.   "*X*" marks the area between humeral head and acromion occupied by the subacromial bursa.

the contents (bursitis and/or tendinitis) or decreasing the space (acromioclavicular osteophytes), impingement occurs (5, 14). Some see this as a logical step up from continuing overuse symptoms.

Neer (14) has pointed out that impingement occurs most often in the flexed position of abduction. He has focused on pathology in the anterior acromial region, including the acromioclavicular joint and the coracoacromial arch. In its end

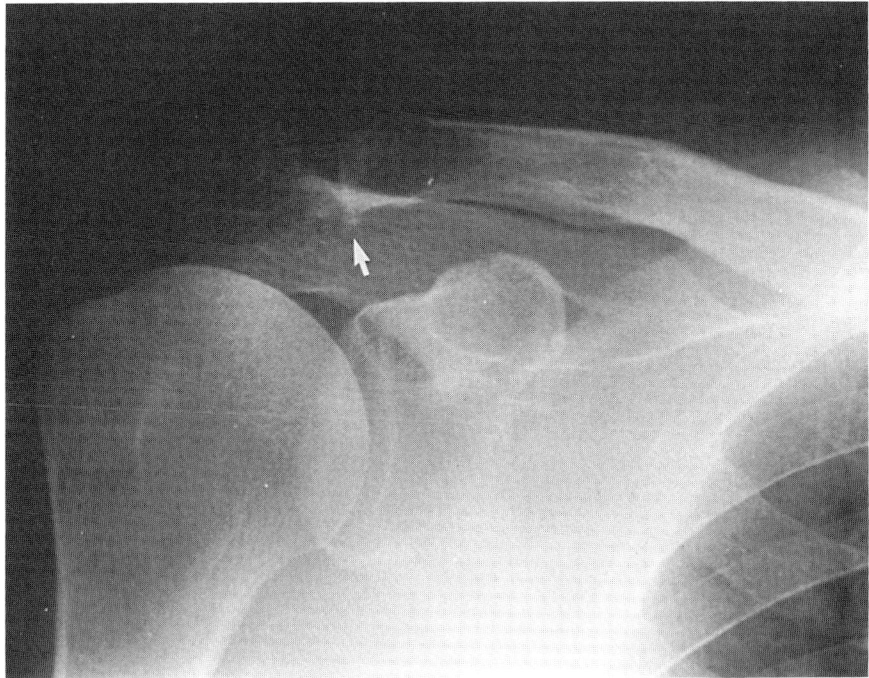

Figure 19.5.   Osteophyte on the undersurface of the a-c joint (*arrow*).

stage, acromioclavicular osteophytes appear (Fig. 19.5) and rotator cuff tears occur (Fig. 19.6).

Examination will reveal tenderness over the greater tuberosity and a painful arc. A positive impingement test will be elicited (Fig. 19.7). The presence of a rotator cuff tear in turn, will produce a weakness of flexion, abduction, and external rotation. MRI or arthrography will verify whether a tear is present (Fig. 14.15).

Jobe (9) has stressed that anterior subluxation has a high likelihood of being part of the impingement syndrome. The drawer sign will elicit this sensation in the skilled examiner's hand (Fig. 19.8).

Treatment of the impingement syndrome should start conservatively. Begin with rest, drugs, and modalities designed to reduce inflammation. The occasional use of intra-articular steroids may be considered; repetitive use of steroids will eventually ruin a joint and/or its tendons. Conservative care should continue for three months, and if there is no improvement look for subacromial osteophytes (plain x-ray) or a rotator cuff tear (MRI or arthrography). If definitive pathology is present, surgery is indicated to decompress the anterior acromial space (osteophytectomy and resection of the coracoacromial ligament) (12, 19). If needed, a rotator cuff repair is included (18). Some surgeons prefer to do this arthroscopically, which is acceptable in skilled hands but a fruitless exercise for the uninitiated (1, 16).

Always watch for subluxation as a possible associated lesion. If no definitive lesion is found, continue conservative care in the form of flexibility-specific strengthening exercises and general body conditioning. Exercises should be com-

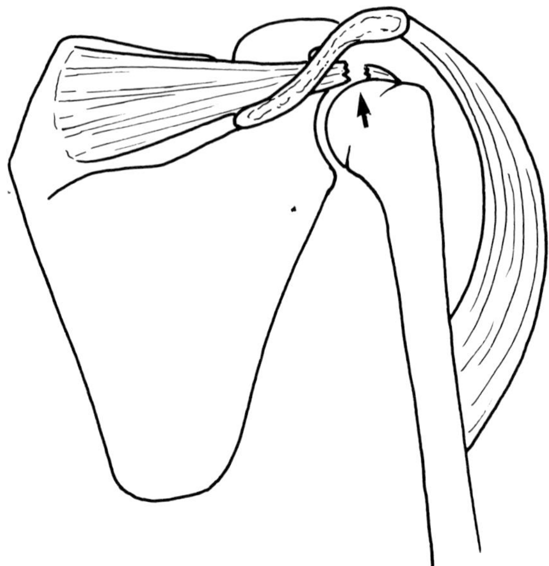

Figure 19.6. Rotator cuff tear (*arrow*).

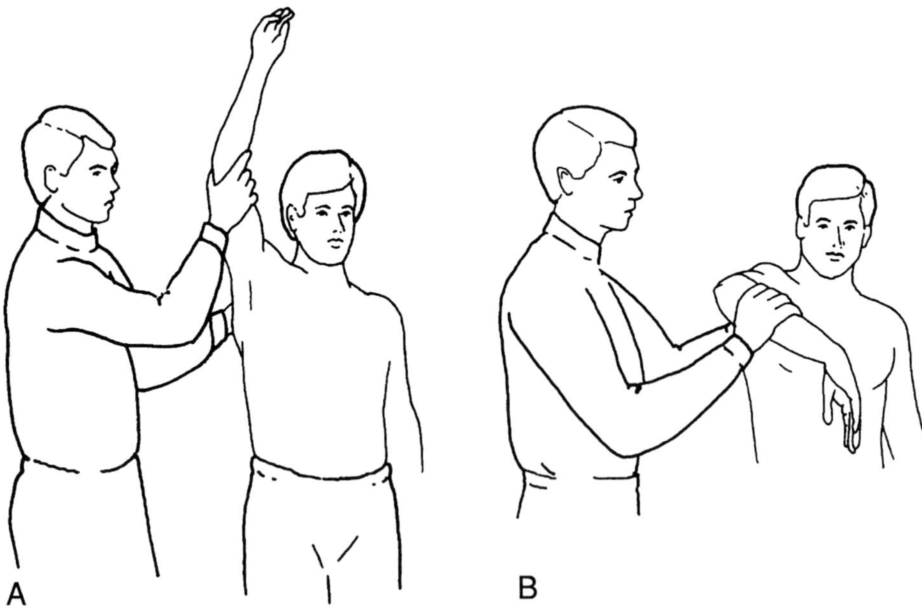

Figure 19.7. Two impingement tests: Full passive abduction (**A**). Elevation (flexion and abduction), during which the shoulder is rotated (**B**). If an impingement syndrome is present, one or both of these tests will reproduce pain.

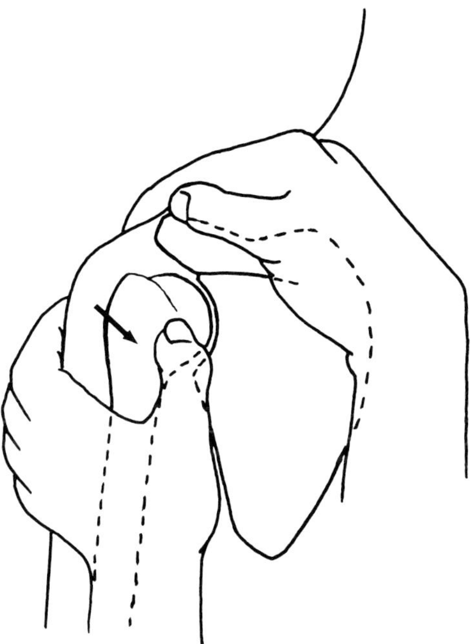

Figure 19.8.   The positive drawer sign. With the patient relaxed, the shoulder can be subluxated anteriorly.

pleted in a position below 90° of abduction and away from extension. Exercises such as bench presses and pushups take the shoulder into this range of aggravating motion, and should be avoided.

Instability

Jobe (8) contends that failure of treatment of sports-related shoulder problems is most often due to unrecognized anterior instability. Posterior instability is a rare phenomenon in the normally structured individual, but may be part of multidirectional instability in the loose-jointed individual. Jobe stresses the distinction between laxity due to injury to the anterior joint restraints (ligaments, capsule, and labrum) and instability due to ligamentous laxity in individuals with loose joints.

Instability is most often associated with dull aching discomfort during throwing and weakness at the end of the activity. The apprehension sign and the relocation test, or drawer sign, should be positive (3).

Treatment is obviously conservative in the form of strengthening exercises. Stretching exercises that stress the anterior joint capsular structures (extension) are excluded from the program. As always, modalities are useful; intra-articular steroids are useless.

Surgical intervention should exclude any procedure that limits external rotation in the throwing arm (4, 6, 11, 17). Jobe recommends the capsulorrhaphy as shown in (Fig. 19.9). Other surgical procedures for dislocation/subluxation of the shoulder joint have been discussed in Chapter 17.

Postoperative care is just as crucial as the surgical procedure. Postoperative immobilization extends for two weeks. The brace may be removed for shoulder adduc-

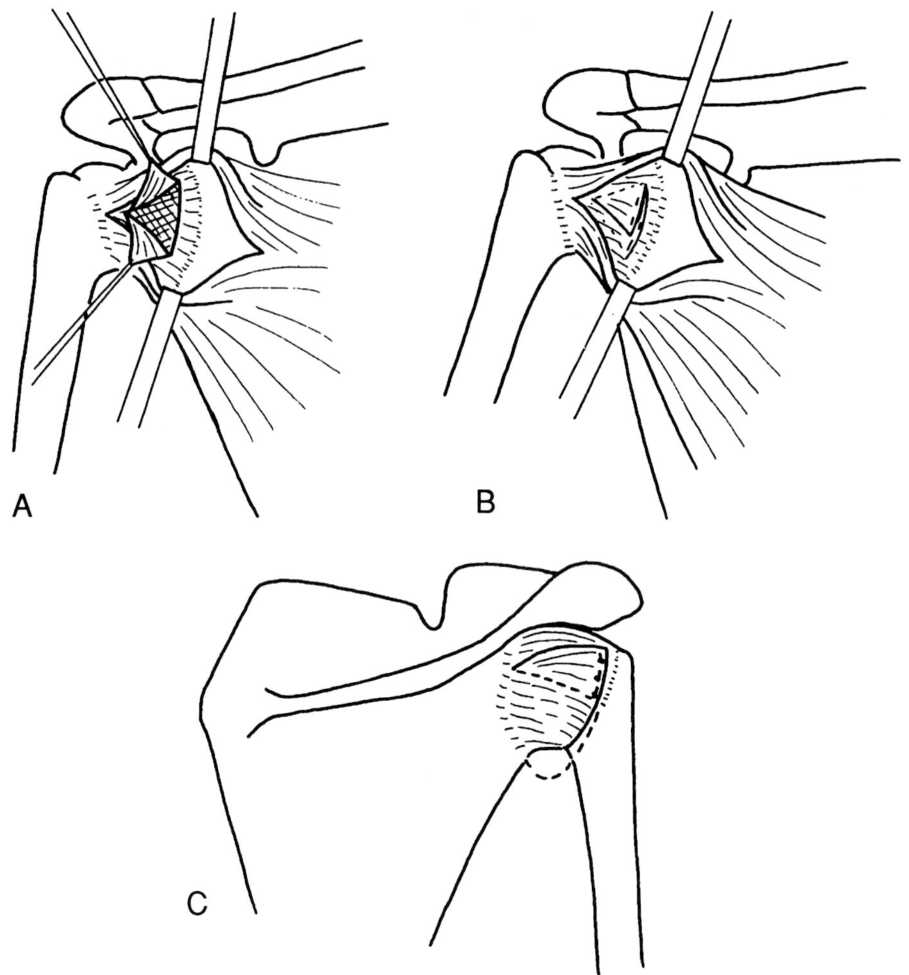

Figure 19.9.   Capsulorrhaphy as recommended by Jobe: The capsular incision (after splitting subscapularis) (**A**). The overlap or "double-breasted suit" of the capsule (**B**). The completed suturing (**C**).

tion and passive external rotation, and active elbow flexion and extension. Two weeks after surgery, the brace is removed for continuing gentle range-of-movement and isometric exercises. One month after surgery the shoulder should passively go to 90° of abduction, and strengthening exercises are begun. These will extend up to four months postoperatively before throwing activity begins. A graduated throwing program takes two to six months to get the athlete back to a functioning level.

Injuries to the Acromioclavicular and Sternoclavicular Joints

Both injuries may occur in the athlete, especially a-c joint subluxations and dislocations. They are discussed in Chapter 18.

CONCLUSION

Management of the sports-related shoulder problem has rewards and frustrations for both the athlete and the supervising physician or therapist. Falling into the aggressive surgical mode in the face of frustration more often than not fails to return the athlete to high-level performance. Stay the conservative road.

REFERENCES

1. Andrews JR, Carson WG, and Ortega K: Arthroscopy of the shoulder: technique and normal anatomy. Am J Sports Med 12:1–7 (1984).
2. Atwater AE: Biomechanics of overarm throwing movements and of throwing injuries. Exerc Sport Sci Rev 7:43–85 (1979).
3. Collins HR and Wilde AH: Shoulder instability in athletics. Orthop Clin North Am 4:759–774 (1973).
4. Cook FF and Tibone JE: The Mumford procedure in athletes—an objective analysis of function. Am J Sports Med 16:97–100 (1988).
5. Hawkins RJ and Kennedy JC: Impingement syndrome in athletes. Am J Sports Med 8:151–158 (1980).
6. Helfet AJ: Coracoid transplantation for recurring dislocation of the shoulder. J Bone Joint Surg 40B:198–202 (1958).
7. Jobe FW: Physiology of warm-ups and exercise. West J Med 133:427–428 (1980).
8. Jobe FW and Jobe CM: Painful athletic injuries of the shoulder. Clin Orthop 173:117–124 (1983).
9. Jobe FW and Moynes DR: Delineation of diagnostic criteria and rehabilitation program for rotator cuff injuries. Am J Sports Med 10:336–339 (1982).
10. Jobe FW, Moynes DR, Tibone JE, and Perry J: An EMG analysis of the shoulder in throwing and pitching. A second report. Am J Sports Med 12:218–220 (1984).
11. Lombardo SJ, Kerlan RK, Jobe FW, Carter VS, Blazina ME, and Shields CL Jr: The modified Bristow procedure for recurrent dislocation of the shoulder. J Bone Joint Surg 58A:256–261 (1976).
12. Neer CS: Anterior acromioplasty for the chronic impingement syndrome in the shoulder. J Bone Joint Surg 54A:41–50 (1972).
13. Neer CS: The shoulder in sports. Orthop Clin North Am 8:583–591 (1977).
14. Neer CS: Impingement lesions. Clin Orthop 173:70–77 (1983).
15. Perry J: Anatomy and biomechanics of the shoulder in throwing, swimming, gymnastics and tennis. Symposium on injuries to the shoulder in the athlete. Clin Sports Med 2:247–270 (1983).
16. Rockwood CA: Editorial: Shoulder arthroscopy. J Bone Joint Surg 70A:639–640 (1988).
17. Rowe CR, Patel D, and Southmayd WW: The Bankart procedure, a long-term end result study. J Bone Joint Surg 60A:1–16 (1986).
18. Tibone JE, Elrod B, Jobe FW, Kerlan RK, Carter VS, Shields CL, Lonbardo SJ, and Yocum L: Surgical treatment of tears of the rotator cuff in athletes. J Bone Joint Surg 68A;887–891 (1986).
19. Tibone JE, Jobe FW, Kerlan RK, Carter VS, Shields CL, Lombardo SJ, and Yocum LA: Shoulder impingement syndrome in athletes treated by anterior acromioplasty. Clin Orthop 188:134–140 (1985).

20

Tumors Around the Shoulder Joint

"Surgery does the ideal thing—it separates the patient from his disease. It puts the patient back to bed and the disease in a bottle."

—Logan Clendening

INTRODUCTION

When you consider that only 4,500 shoulder tumors occur in the United States per year (3), your chances of seeing such a patient are minuscule. But read on just in case!

Trends

Enneking (4, 5, 6) of the University of Florida (Gainesville) has been the guru of tumor surgery in the United States over the past two decades. Along with Dahlin (2, 3) and Mankin (7, 8) in the United States and Campanacci (1) in Italy, they have set trends in tumor surgery that are unparalleled. But these trends are waiting the test of time before they become established scientific principles in the management of tumors in the shoulder region and in other musculoskeletal tissues.

Anatomy

Tumors of the shoulder joint will affect the humerus (70%), scapula (20%), and clavicle (10%). Their frequency ranks third (tumors about the hip and pelvis rank first, followed by tumors of the distal femur).

Compartments

Theoretically, a number of shoulder compartments have been described (4). They include the deltoid, glenohumeral joint, posterior scapular (supra and infraspinatus regions), anterior scapular, anterior, lateral and posterior humeral region, and anterior pectoral region. In staging tumors, these compartments become very important determinants of treatment avenues.

Contents of Axilla

The final significant anatomical detail of shoulder region tumors is that they occur in close proximity to the axillary artery and the brachial plexus. Invasion of either one precludes any of the limb salvage procedures about to be described. For these patients, amputation becomes the only viable alternative.

416

Table 20.1.   Staging of Shoulder Tumors

Grade: G_0—benign
$\quad\quad\quad$ G_1—low-grade malignancy
$\quad\quad\quad$ G_2—high-grade malignancy
Local Extent: T_0—benign contained within tumor capsule
$\quad\quad\quad\quad\quad$ T_1—contained within compartment of origin
$\quad\quad\quad\quad\quad$ T_2—spread to a second compartment
Presence of Metastases: M_0—no metastases
$\quad\quad\quad\quad\quad\quad\quad\quad$ M_1—metastases

Table 20.2.   Enneking's Staging of Malignant Tumors

	Grade	Local Extent
IA	Low-grade (G_1)	Intracompartmental (T_1)
IB	G_1	T_2
IIA	G_2	T_1
IIB	G_2	T_2
III	Any grade or site with metastases	

Surgical Principles

Tumors about the shoulder are connective tissue in origin (sarcomas); unlike carcinomas, surgery is a more definitive ablation step than chemotherapy or radiation, although any combination of the three modalities is often used.

Surgery for sarcomas about the shoulder include limb salvage or amputation, depending on staging of the tumor (6). Staging systems (Table 20.1) are built on the surgical grade of the tumor (G), the local extent of the tumor (T), and whether or not metastases are present (M). Most benign tumors are G_0, T_0, or M_0—although a few benign tumors about to be described are locally aggressive.

Enneking (6) has proposed a system of classifying malignant tumors (Table 20.2). Tumors that are low-grade malignancy (usually chondrosarcomas) and confined to one compartment with no metastases are staged as G_1, T_1, and M_0. The worst staging (III) is any malignancy, within or beyond a single compartment with distant metastases (e.g., G_2, T_2, M_1).

With appropriate staging, a surgical treatment decision can be made. The lower grade malignancies, confined to one compartment with no metastases, can be treated with limb salvage. Limb salvage is usually followed by some form of reconstruction (bone graft, arthroplasty, or arthrodesis). Care must be exercised to get a wide enough margin around the tumor so that local recurrence is prevented (Table 20.3).

Any tumor that invades the brachial plexus and/or axillary vessels cannot be treated with limb salvage; if indications based on favorable metastatic grading allow, amputation is the surgical choice for these patients. Distant metastases usually, but not always, preclude limb salvage or amputation surgery. Adjunctive radiation and chemotherapy are also used extensively in the management of musculoskeletal tumors. The use of surgery, chemotherapy, and radiation is such a skilled decision that a whole new subspecialty—orthopaedic oncology—has developed to deal with the various subtleties.

Table 20.3.   Surgical Margins

Surgical Margin	Surgical Procedure	Results
Intralesional	Piecemeal debulking or curettage	Leaves microscopic tumor
Marginal	Excision of tumor and pseudocapsule through reactive zone	Leaves microscopic tumor
Wide	Excision of tumor, pseudocapsule, reactive zone, and a cuff of normal tissue	Risk of leaving microscopic tumor
Radical	Extracompartmental procedure removes tumor, pseudocapsule, reactive zone, and entire compartment	Minimal risk of residual microscopic tumor

From Enneking WF, Spanier SS, and Goodman MA: A system for the surgical staging of musculoskeletal sarcoma. Clin Orthop 153:105–120 (1980).

If limb salvage is the surgical decision, reconstruction is accomplished by bone grafting (5, 7), artificial joints (arthroplasty), or fusion. How successful reconstruction of the shoulder joint will be rests largely on the functioning capacity of the deltoid and rotator cuff. Absence of both functioning units precludes the use of any arthroplasty approach. Amputation is rarely followed by sustained use of an upper extremity prosthesis.

Clinical

Patients with tumors about the shoulder have rest or nighttime (nonmechanical) pain rather than pain aggravated by activity (mechanical pain). Considering that a frozen shoulder may present the same symptoms and will occur a thousand times more often than a shoulder tumor, it is easy to understand the usual delay in diagnosis with tumors about the shoulder.

Later in the disease process, local tenderness will appear, and later still, you may be able to palpate a mass and/or tissue induration.

Investigation

Plain x-rays are the single most valuable tool in the diagnosis of musculoskeletal tumors. Using age, location of the tumor, and its plain x-ray appearance, 90% of tumor diagnoses are usually evident. Plain x-rays are read as to the tumor's location, margin, and density. Figure 20.1 shows the value of determining the location of tumors; for example, osteosarcoma is the commonest malignancy located in the humeral metaphysis, and Ewing's sarcoma is the commonest tumor of the humeral diaphysis. Next, examine the margin of the lesion; is it sclerotic (usually a benign or slow-growing tumor) or is the margin blurred (usually more aggressive tumor) (Fig. 20.2)? In addition to determining the type of margin, note what the tumor is doing to the cortex (Fig. 20.2*B*). The final observation is based on the density of the tumor. Is it making bone (osteoblastic), destroying bone (osteolytic), or laying down cartilage (Fig. 20.3)?

Bone scanning is the next most useful investigation, revealing the extent of bony involvement as measured by deposit of isotopes in regenerating bone. The occasional skip lesion will also be picked up on bone scan, as well as multiple metastatic deposits. Blood chemistries yield mostly nonspecific information.

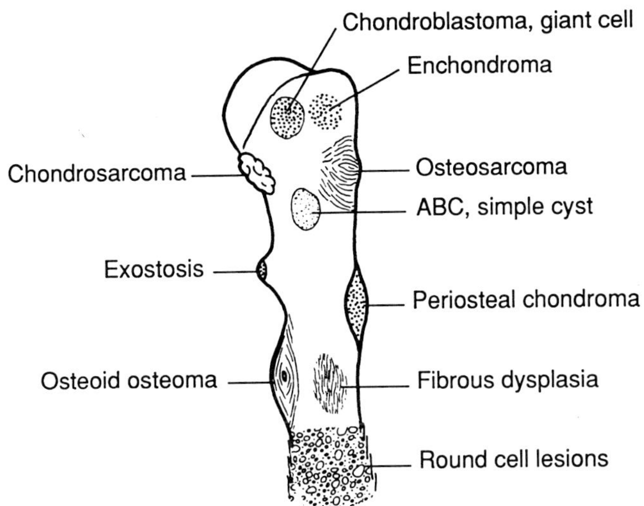

Figure 20.1.   The location of the tumor in the proximal humerus will help decide the "nature of the beast" (from Enneking [4]).

Other investigation, such as CT, MRI, and arteriography are used more for staging and surgical planning than diagnosis. Lung CT is the best investigative tool for detecting metastases.

Biopsy

The final step in the diagnosis of any tumor is the examination of tumor tissue. Biopsy, for tumors about the shoulder, has to be carefully planned so as not to interfere with limb salvage (8). It is especially tragic to convert a unicompartmental neoplasm to second compartment contamination by a poorly planned biopsy. By and large, biopsies of any malignancy should be done by the surgeon who is going to do the definitive surgical procedure. In today's world, that is usually an orthopaedic oncologist.

Biopsy can be needle, incisional, or excisional. Needle biopsy often yields too little tissue for examination. If you are certain you are dealing with a benign lesion, excisional biopsy is the usual and customary approach. Incisional biopsy for all suspected malignancies is regarded by most oncologists as the best method. For proximal humerus tumors, excisional biopsies are done through the anterior deltoid muscle.

Differential Diagnosis of Shoulder Tumors

Once plain x-rays and blood studies are completed, it is usually obvious that you are dealing with a bone tumor rather than a rotator cuff arthropathy, infection (Fig. 16.3), or miscellaneous conditions, such as fibrous dysplasia or Paget's disease (Fig. 20.4).

General Statements about Incidence

The most common primary malignancy about the shoulder is multiple myeloma (Fig. 20.5). Still, multiple myeloma is a distant second to the most common malignancy, metastatic carcinoma. Metastatic carcinoma of the proximal hu-

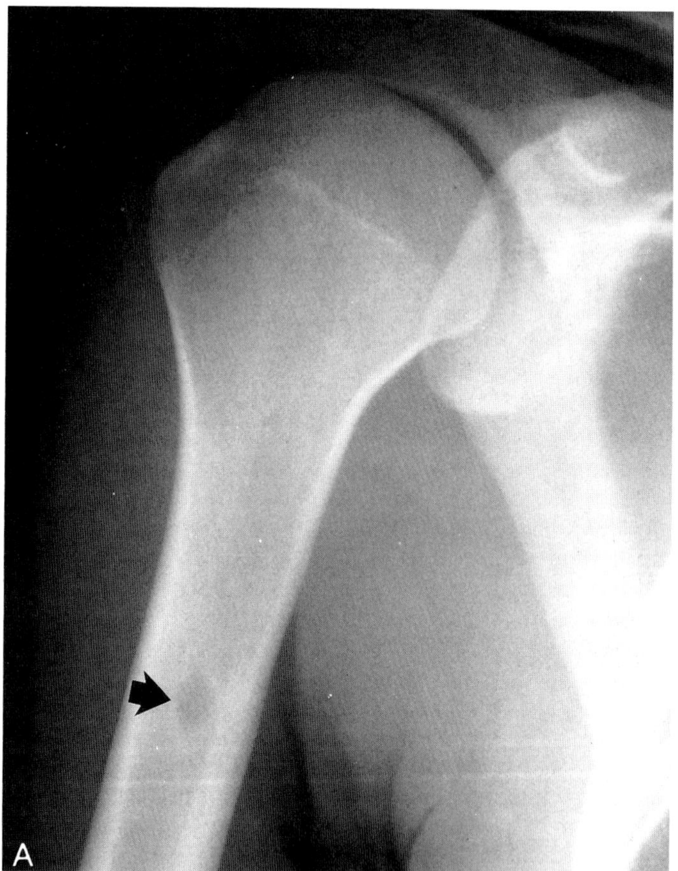

Figure 20.2.   **A,** sclerotic margin in a slowly growing osteoid osteoma.

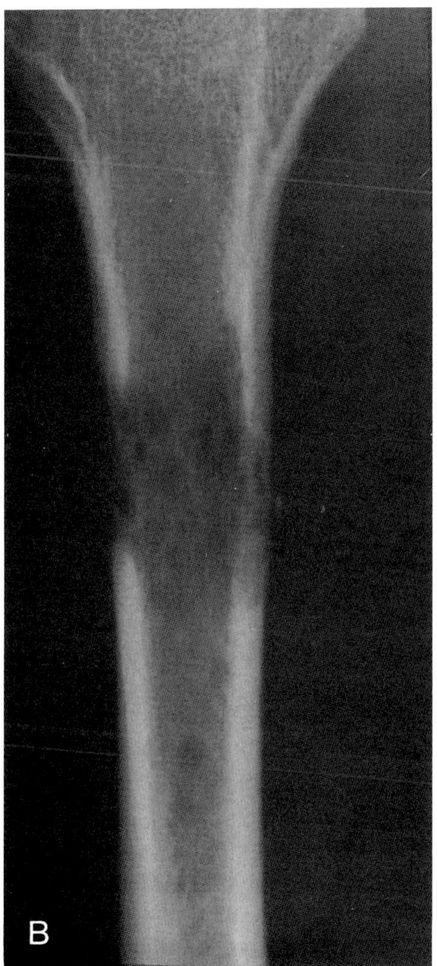

Figure 20.2. B, moth-eaten margin of a metastatic breast carcinoma. Also note the loss of cortical integrity—obviously a malignant lesion of bone.

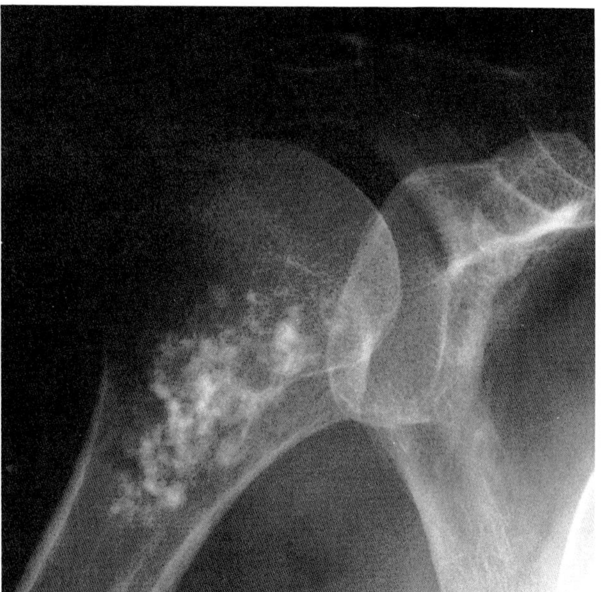

Figure 20.3.   Figure 20.2*B* is considered an osteolytic-type lesion. This enchondroma shows the fluffy increased density typical for cartilage.

merus usually seeds from kidney (renal cell), lung, breast, or prostate (Fig. 20.2*B*).

Excluding multiple myeloma, the most common malignancies in the adolescent are osteosarcoma and Ewing's sarcoma. When benign and malignant tumors are lumped together, cartilage tumors are the most common proximal humerus lesions. The two most common benign tumors around the shoulder are the unicameral bone cyst and the chondroblastoma. Table 20.4 lists the common tumors around the shoulder joint.

Specific Tumors Around the Shoulder

Benign Cartilage Tumors

Osteochondroma.   This is the most common benign tumor to appear about the shoulder (Fig. 20.6). They may be single or multiple (Ollier's disease) and have a typical appearance. Most are treated by a marginal excision through the false capsule.

Chondroblastoma (Codman's tumor).   Chondroblastoma is a benign cartilage tumor of the endosteal surface of the epiphysis in children (Fig. 20.7). Treatment is by extensive intralesional curettage and careful bone grafting to prevent collapse of the cartilaginous joint surface.

Enchondroma.   This is a perfectly benign lesion that can be observed over time (Fig. 20.3).

Benign Osseous Tumors

Osteoid Osteoma.   These are rare tumors that occur in the proximal humerus or glenoid. Typically, they produce night pain dramatically relieved by aspirin. They are hard to see on plain x-ray (Fig. 20.8), but light up on bone scan. A CT is needed to see the nidus and surrounding sclerosis. Treatment is by surgical excision of the nidus. Finding the lesion at operation can sometimes be very difficult and careful preoperative localization is necessary.

Osteoblastoma.   This is the big brother of osteoid osteoma—a large radiolucent center surrounded by sclerosis. Often the lesion will expand the cortex.

Miscellaneous Neoplasms of the Proximal Humerus

Simple Bone Cyst.   These occur in children between the age of 4 and 12. When adjacent to the epiphysis, they are considered active (Fig. 20.9). Eventually, if unhealed, they will migrate away from the epiphysis into the diaphysis and become latent. They are most often confused with aneurysmal bone cysts. Because they may lead to a pathological fracture, treatment is by aspiration and steroid injection and is successful 50% of the time. If unsuccessful, it may be repeated, or curettage and bone grafting can be tried. In spite of these efforts, some of these cysts will persist and all you can do is "nurse" the child towards maturity, when the cyst will become latent.

Aneurysmal Bone Cyst (ABC) and Nonossifying Fibroma (NOF).   ABC and NOF are lucent expansile tumors that are healed by curettage and bone graft.

Giant Cell Tumor.   Most (60%–70%) of giant cell tumors occur in the distal femur. A few occur in the spine and 10% occur in the proximal humerus (Fig. 20.10). Treatment for the less aggressive lesion is curettage, freezing, and bone

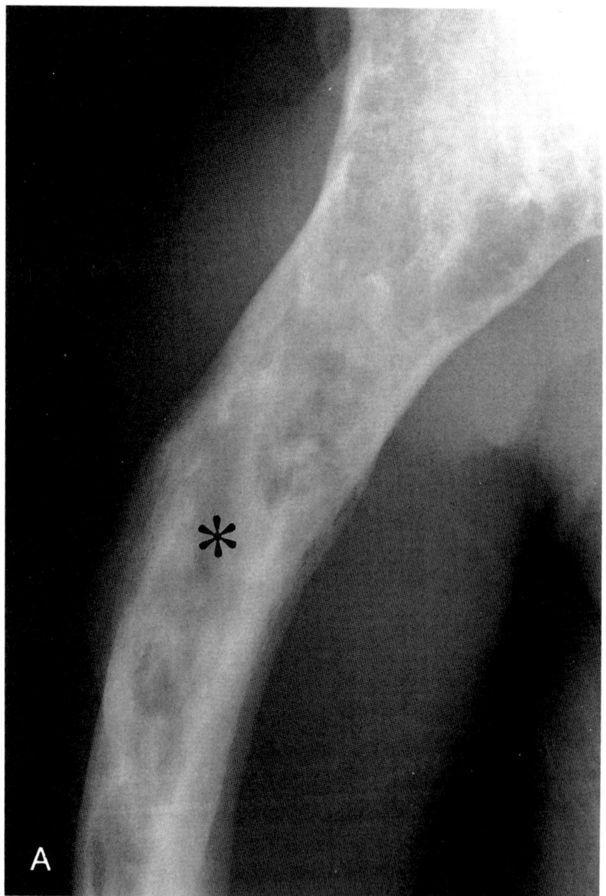

Figure 20.4.   A, the "ground glass" appearance (*) of fibrous dysplasia.

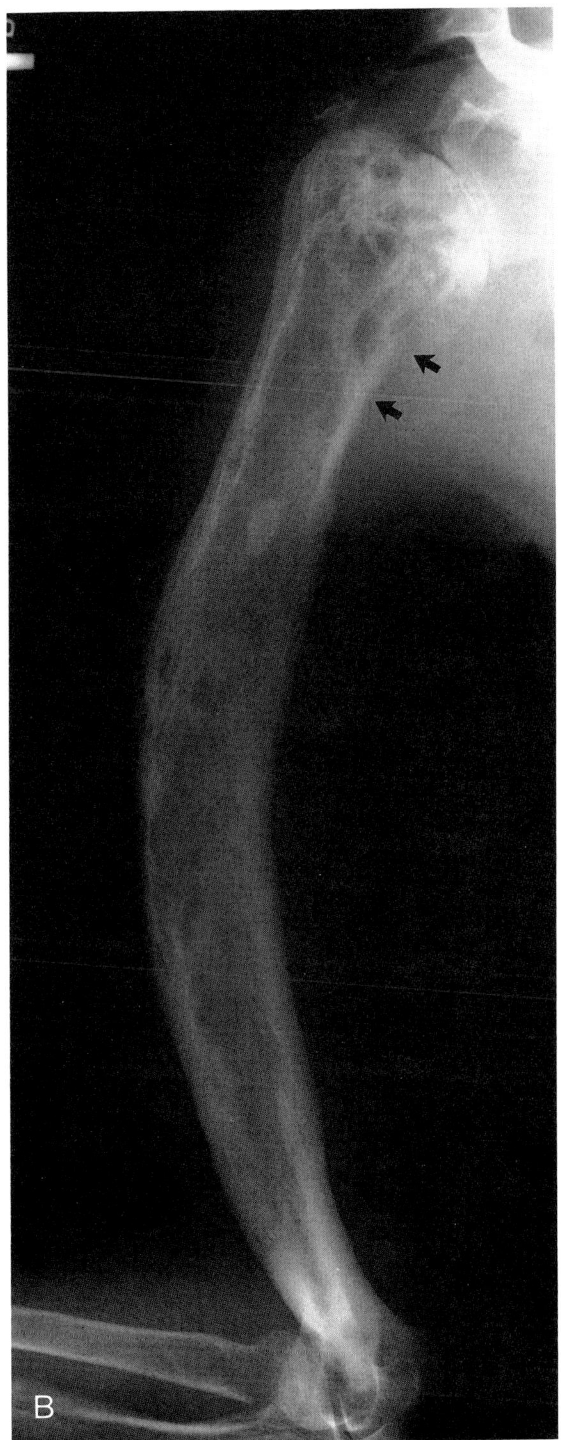

Figure 20.4.   B, Paget's disease of the entire humerus, with widening and bowing of the humeral shaft. Note the cortical resorption (*arrows*) that may be the first indication of sarcomatous degeneration.

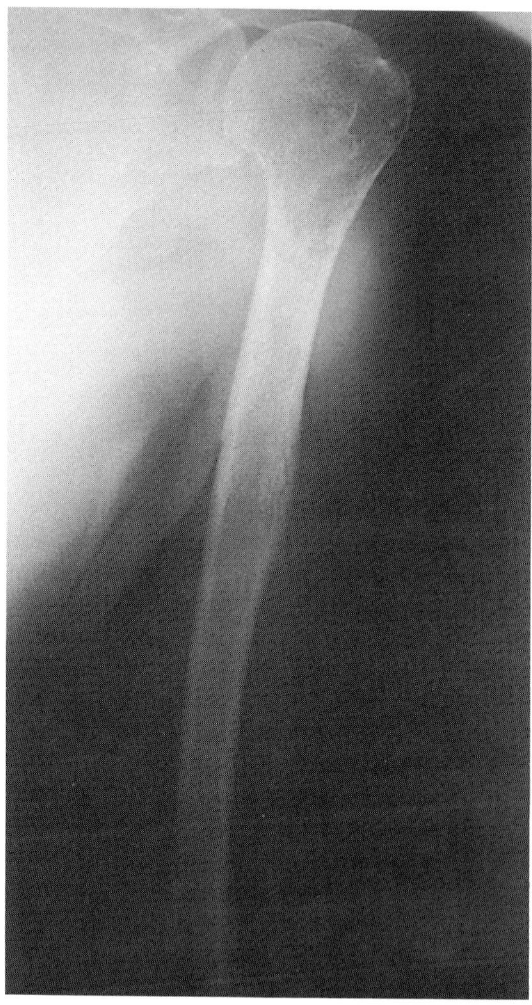

Figure 20.5.   Multiple myeloma. The changes are subtle but note the osteoporosis of the humeral head and the irregular scalloped margin in the metaphysis.

*Table 20.4.   Common Neoplasms of the Shoulder**

	Benign	Malignant
Cartilaginous	Chondroblastoma Enchondroma Osteochondroma (exostosis)	Chondrosarcoma
Osseous	Osteoid osteoma Osteoblastoma	Osteosarcoma
Reticuloendothelial	0	Multiple myeloma Ewing's sarcoma
Miscellaneous	Simple bone cyst Aneurysmal bone cyst Nonossifying fibroma Giant cell tumor	

*Don't be mislead by the word "common"; overall, these are rare occurrences in clinical practice, unless you are in a major tertiary tumor referral center.

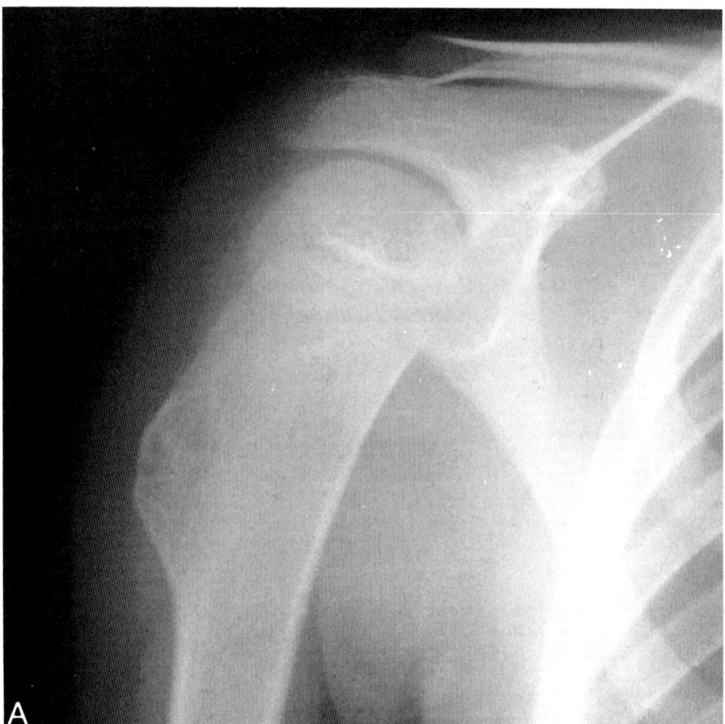

Figure 20.6.   **A,** osteochondroma of the humerus in a child.

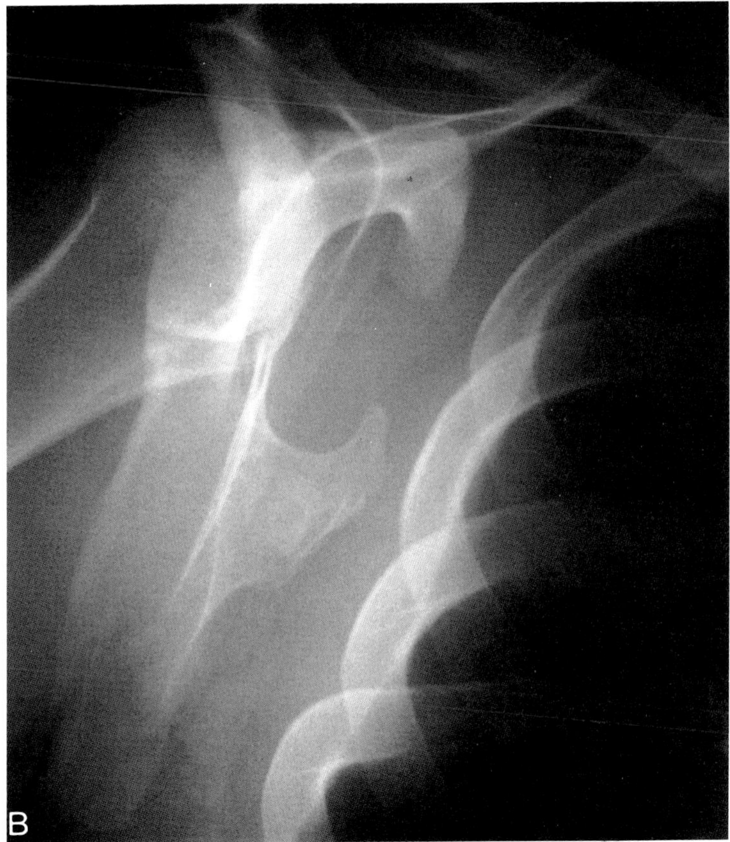

Figure 20.6.   B, osteochondroma of the scapula in an adult.

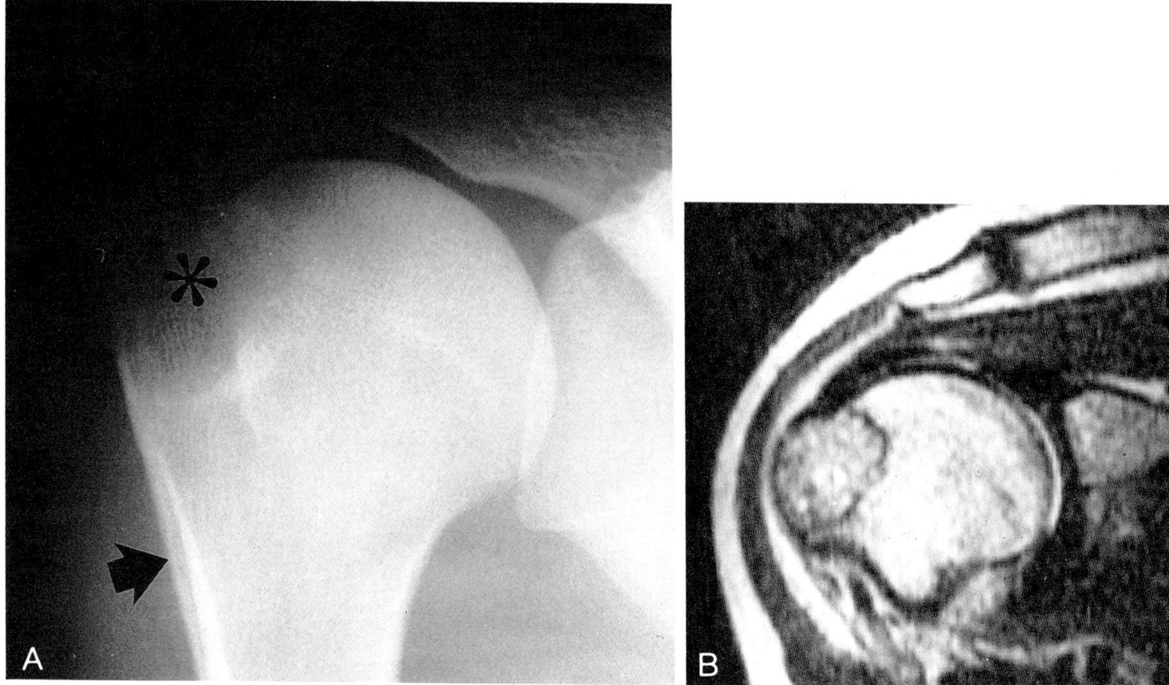

Figure 20.7.   Chondroblastoma (**A**). Plain x-ray reveals a lytic lesion (*) with sclerotic rim (this a benign lesion) and periosteal new bone (*arrow*). T2 MRI of the same lesion (**B**).

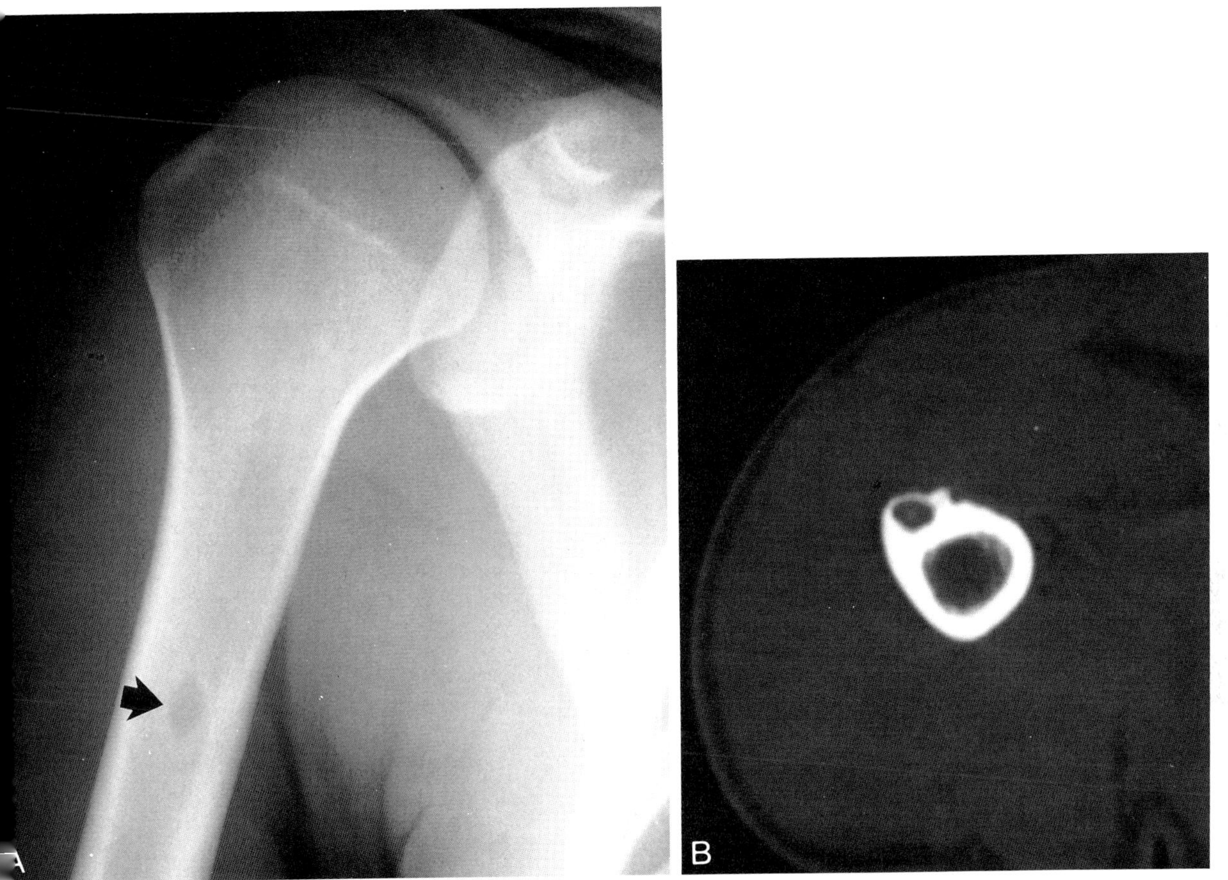

Figure 20.8.   An osteoid osteoma on plain x-ray (**A**) and CT (**B**).

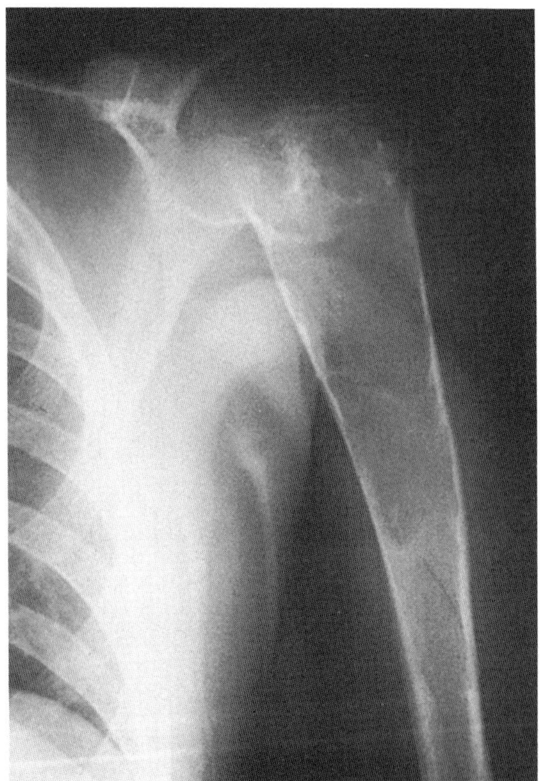

Figure 20.9.   Simple bone cyst—note the bubbly lytic lesion.

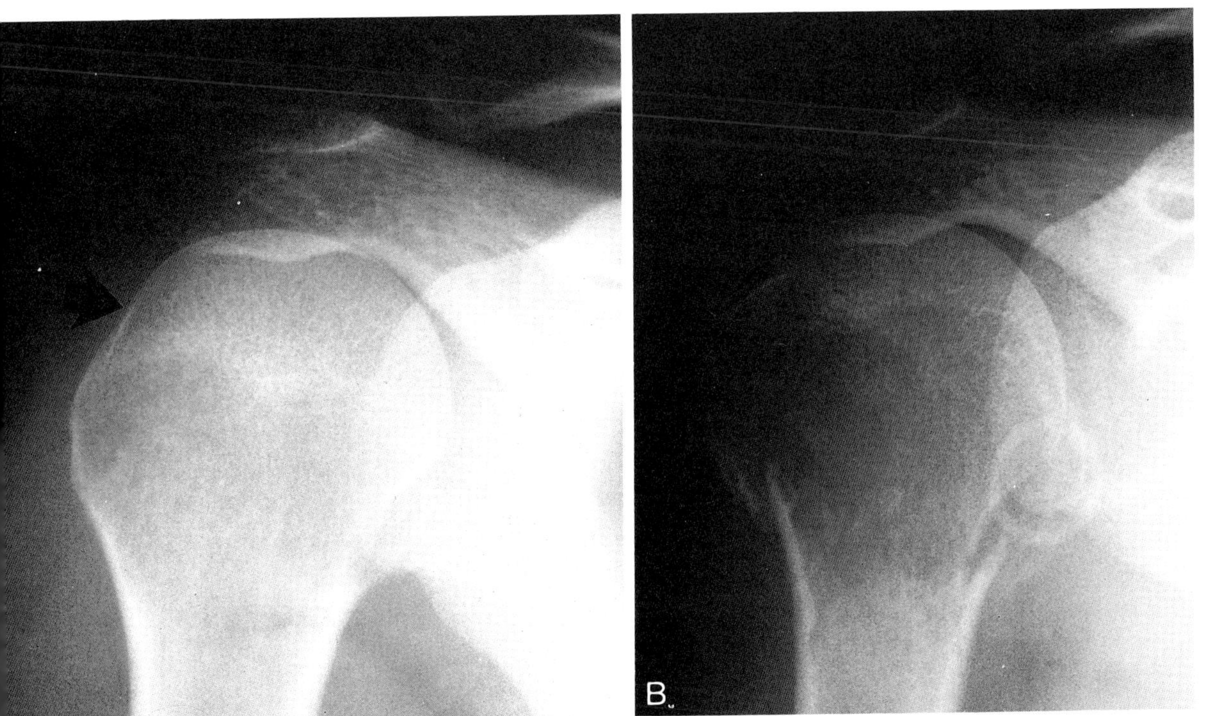

Figure 20.10.   Giant cell tumor of the humeral head with pathological fracture. **A,** early. **B,** later (after tumor was missed in **A**).

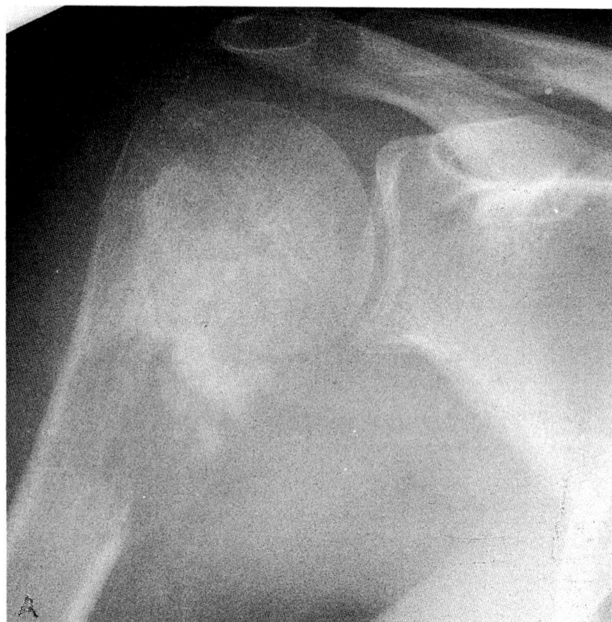

Figure 20.11.   Osteogenic sarcoma in adolescent. Note the gross destruction of the cortex and the permeative invasion of the proximal humerus.

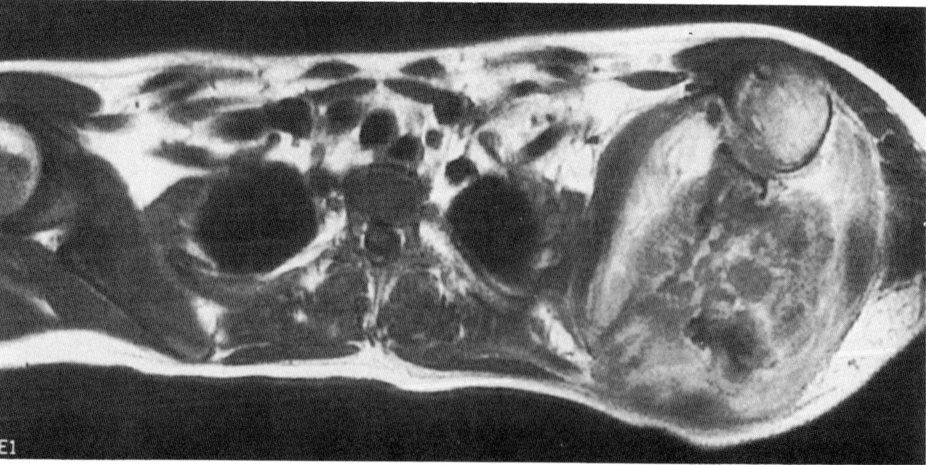

Figure 20.12.   Ewing's sarcoma of the left scapula. Note the huge soft tissue mass replacing the scapula.

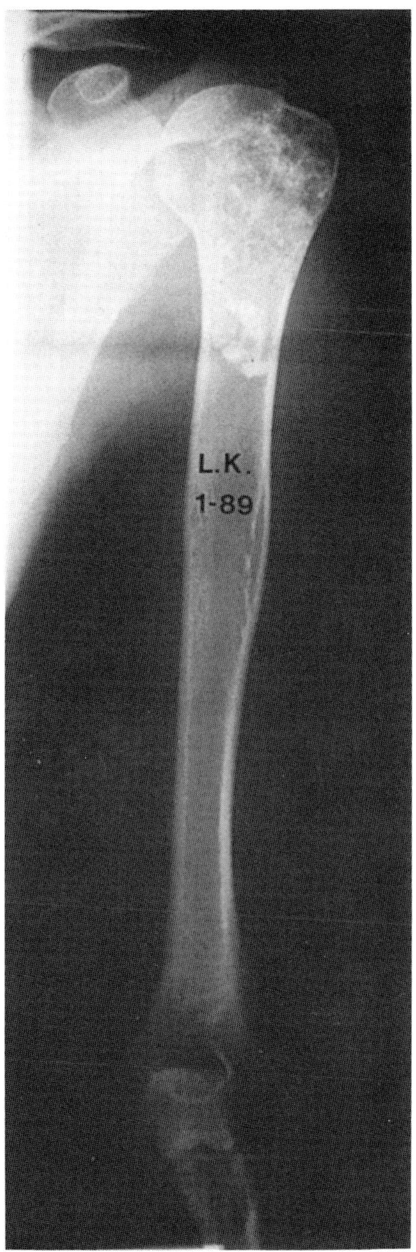

Figure 20.13.   A chondrosarcoma of the proximal humerus. Note the calcification (like enchondroma) but associated cortical thinning.

grafting. Limb salvage (marginal excision) surgery is the choice for the more aggressive lesions.

Malignant Neoplasms of the Shoulder Region

The three most common primary malignancies (excluding multiple myeloma) of the shoulder, in order of incidence, are osteosarcoma, Ewing's sarcoma, and chondrosarcoma.

Osteosarcoma.   This is an aggressive malignant tumor of adolescents. It presents as rest pain in the shoulder region. It has a typical x-ray appearance (Fig. 20.11). It is treated by a combination of preoperative and postoperative chemotherapy with intervening surgery, either limb salvage or amputation (1).

Ewing's Sarcoma.   Ewing's sarcoma is an aggressive marrow cell tumor that leaves a distinct picture in the diaphysis (Fig. 20.12). Treatment is a combination of chemotherapy and radiation therapy. Large proximal humerus or scapular lesions can then be surgically excised.

Chondrosarcoma (Fig. 20.13).   Of the three, this is the least aggressive tumor. Chemotherapy and radiation therapy offer no role in treatment; definitive treatment is by wide surgical excision (limb salvage) and reconstruction.

Multiple Myeloma.   This is the most common adult primary malignant tumor of bone (Fig. 20.5). It affects the proximal humerus in 5%–10% of cases. Diagnosis and treatment rarely include surgery, except for pathological fracture (see Chapter 9 for discussion of multiple myeloma).

CONCLUSION

Let us emphasize again, these tumors are rare and you will probably miss the first one you see. Do you accept the challenge?

REFERENCES

1. Campanacci M, Bacci G, Bertoni F, Picci P, Minutillo A, and Franceschi C: The treatment of osteosarcoma of the extremities: twenty years experience at the Isituto Ortepedico Rizzoli. Cancer 48:1569–1581 (1981).
2. Dahlin DC: Bone Tumors: General Aspects and Data on 6,221 Cases. Charles C. Thomas, Springfield, IL (1978).
3. Dahlin DC: Editorial: Malignant bone tumors: improvement in prognosis. Mayo Clin Proc 63:414 (1988).
4. Enneking WF: Modified system for functional evaluation of surgical management of musculoskeletal tumors from limb salvage. In: Musculoskeletal Oncology. Ed: Enneking WF. Churchill Livingstone, New York (1987).
5. Enneking WF, Eady JL, and Burchardt H: Autogenous cortical bone grafts in the reconstruction of segmental skeletal defects. J Bone Joint Surg 62A:1039–1058 (1980).
6. Enneking WF, Spanier SS, and Goodman MA: A system for the surgical staging of musculoskeletal sarcoma. Clin Orthop 153:106–120 (1980).
7. Mankin HJ, Gebhardt MC, and Tomford WW: The use of frozen cadaveric allografts in the management of patients with bone tumors of the extremities. Orthop Clin North Am 18:275–289 (1987).
8. Mankin HJ, Lange TA, and Spanier SS: The hazards of biopsy in patients with malignant primary bone and soft tissue tumors. J Bone Joint Surg 64A:1121–1127 (1982).

21

Differential Diagnosis of Neck Ache and Shoulder Pain

"Choose your specialist and you chose your disease."
—Anonymous

It is hoped that we have developed this book along logical lines. For each major group of lesions, we have described the anatomy, the pathologic processes that may occur, the pathogenesis of the characteristic symptoms, and the treatment.

Unfortunately, in practice, clinical pathology is rarely so clear-cut. Although we state in the preface that the most common source of cervicobrachial pain by far is cervical disc degeneration or rotator cuff tendinitis, it is very important to tie the two sections of the book together with a discussion on differential diagnosis that will include some unusual sources of arm pain. In Table 21.1 we include a list of the multitude of conditions that may occur as pain in the neck, shoulder, or arm. This list has only been included to remind clinicians that they must ask themselves in every instance: "I wonder what dreadful things are going on to give this patient such persistent pain in the neck and/or arm?" Included in this awesome list are a number of lesions that may be overlooked unless the physician is aware that they may occasionally occur as pain in the neck and/or arm.

You will notice that the classification is based on anatomical regions primarily and etiologies secondarily. This is a more workable approach than either the primary etiological approach or the use of symptoms to classify conditions.

GENERAL PRINCIPLES OF DIFFERENTIAL DIAGNOSIS

As we get older, we degenerate our joints. How fast this happens depends on a number of factors, the most important being genetic code. Also important is general wear and tear. Considering the tremendous range of movement in the neck and shoulder, and the number of times in a day one or another of the regions is "doing its thing," it is not surprising that 10% of the population will complain of pain in the neck and/or shoulder in any one month. Fortunately, they do not all run to the doctor, but accept this as part of everyday life. If the pain persists or becomes severe, these individuals will show up in your office. In at least 90% of the cases, you will recognize the problem as cervical disc disease or as a shoulder disorder. You will do so by using the following principles:

1. The history is your most important part of the assessment (17). Talk to your patients; ask them to show you where the symptom (pain) is located and how it radiates. Figure 21.1 is a summary of pain location for various problems.

439

Table 21.1.   Classification of Causes of Symptoms About the Neck and Shoulder

I. INTRACEREBRAL AND INTRASPINAL CONDITIONS
  1. Proximal to Disc
     a. Generalized disorders
        • Cerebrovascular accident (CVA)
        • Multiple sclerosis
        • Amyotrophic lateral sclerosis
        • Guillian-Barre
     b. Localized disorders
        • Tumors
        1. Extradural—primary or metastatic bone
        2. Intradural/extramedullary
           • Meningioma
           • Neurofibroma
        3. Intradural/intramedullary
           • Syringomyelia
           • Ependymoma
           • Glioma
  2. Disc/Vertebral Level
     a. Mechanical neck pain
        • Soft tissue (muscle spasm)
        • Bone/disc
           • Effects of trauma causing fracture, dislocation, or subluxation
           • Degenerative disc disease
     b. Nonmechanical neck pain
        • Inflammatory (ankylosing spondylitis and rheumatoid arthritis)
        • Infection of disc or vertebral body
        • Tumors of skeleton
        • Metabolic conditions (osteopenias)
     c. Mechanical neck/arm pain
        • Herniated nucleus pulposus
        • Osteophyte radicular
        • Osteophyte myelopathic
II. EXTRASPINAL CONDITIONS
  1. Neurological
     a. Proximal neurological entrapments or irritations
        • Greater occipital nerve (C_2) entrapment
        • Thoracic outlet syndrome (TOS)
        • Reflex sympathetic dystrophy
        • Pancoast tumor
        • Conditions affecting long thoracic nerve and suprascapular nerve
        • Brachial neuritis
        • Brachial plexopathy
     b. Distal neurological entrapments
        • Medial nerve
        • Ulnar nerve
        • Radial nerve
     c. Intrinsic peripheral nerve lesions
        • Neuropathies of diabetes
        • Herpes Zoster
  2. Shoulder Conditions
     a. Synovial articulations of the shoulder joint complex
        1. Trauma
           • Traumatic bursitis or synovitis
           • Subluxations
           • Dislocations

Table 21.1.—(Continued)

- Acute
- Recurrent
- Chronic

2. Inflammations
   - Rheumatoid arthritis and other arthritides
3. Infections
   - Acute pyogenic
   - Chronic pyogenic
   - Granulomatous (TB)
4. Neoplasm
   - Villonodular synovitis
   - Synovial osteochondromatosis
5. Degenerative changes
   - Osteoarthritis
   - Hemophilic arthritis
6. Vascular
   - Avascular necrosis humeral head
   - Postradiation necrosis
7. Metabolic
   - Gout
   - Ochronosis
   - Hemosiderosis

b. Tendinous and capsular lesions
   1. Subacromial bursitis
   2. Rotator cuff tendinitis
   3. Calcific tendinitis
   4. Diffuse capsulitis (frozen shoulder)
   5. Subacromial impingement syndromes
   6. Rotator cuff tears
   7. Bicipital tendinitis
   8. Recurrent dislocation of the biceps tendon
   9. Shoulder-hand syndrome

c. Osseous lesions
   1. Trauma
      - Untreated "minor" fractures
   2. Infection
   3. Neoplasm
      - Benign
      - Malignant
      - Primary
      - Metastatic
   4. Metabolic
      - Rickets
      - Scurvy

d. Muscular lesions
   1. Polymyositis
   2. Contracture of deltoid (post-injection)
   3. Polymyalgia rheumatica
   4. Muscular dystrophies

III. MISCELLANEOUS CONDITIONS
   1. Psychogenic Pain Syndromes
   2. Referred Pain
      - Abdominal
      - Thoracic
   3. Raynaud's Disease

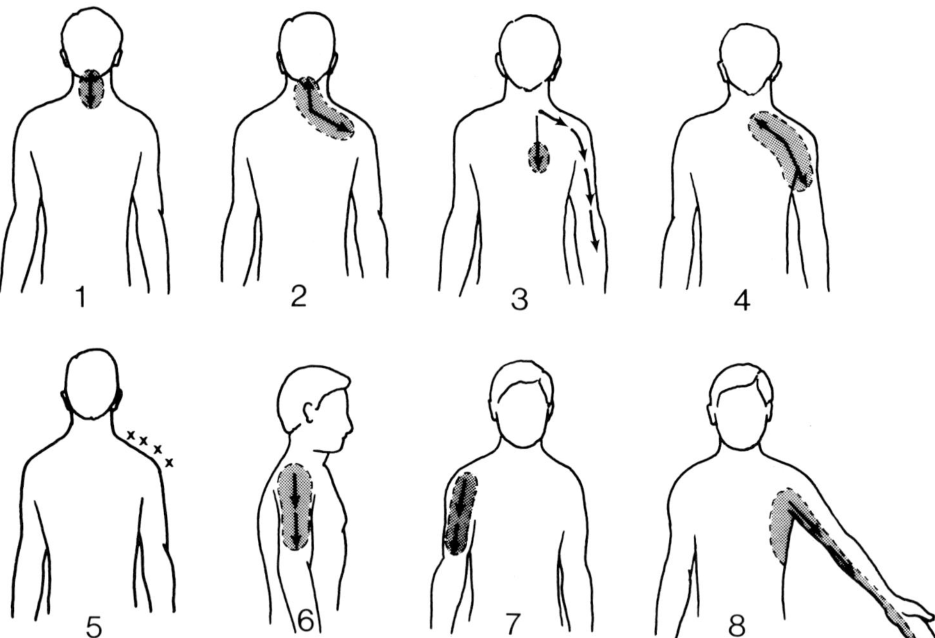

Figure 21.1.   Summary of pain locations: (*1*) axial neck, (*2*) neck and referred shoulder, (*3*) radicular arm and parascapular pain in cervical disc, (*4*) shoulder with some proximal posterior shoulder radiation, (*5*) a-c joint referral into side of neck, (*6*) classic location for shoulder pain, (*7*) biceps and some other shoulder pains, and (*8*) lower brachial plexus involvement (e.g., thoracic outlet syndrome, Pancoast tumor).

2. If the predominant symptom is not pain, watch out! You may be dealing with any one of the neurological diagnoses listed in Table 21.1 (e.g., the presenting symptom in ALS is weakness). It is very unusual for a cervical root encroachment to present weakness or paresthesias as the leading complaint (10).

3. If the predominant symptom is not mechanical pain, watch out! Cervical disc degeneration with or without neurological involvement and shoulder problems, such as rotator cuff lesions, all have aggravation of symptoms by mechanical activity. Pain at rest, that wakes the patient at night, is a red flag; look for tumors, infections, and other unusual diagnoses in Table 21.1.

   Sometimes, cervical disc disease is so acute that the patient cannot find a comfortable position to sleep in, except sitting in a chair. It is classic for a patient with a frozen shoulder to constantly wake with pain. But in both conditions, daily activities significantly increase pain. This represents the mechanical component of the symptoms, and you should not be mislead by the nighttime complaints. On the other hand, a patient who complains about a steadily increasing inability to sleep, with not too much additional aggravation of pain with activities of daily living, is suspect for such problems as tumors and infections.

4. When comparing neck problems with shoulder conditions, the shoulder usually presents more significant mechanical aggravation of symptoms. That is, movement of a painful shoulder most often produces sudden episodes of pain

followed by lingering discomfort. Neck conditions are aggravated by neck movement but not nearly to the extent as the shoulder.

5. Neck problems will commonly have referral of discomfort to both shoulders, whereas intrinsic shoulder problems rarely present a bilateral complaint.
6. The symptom pattern in the shoulder is usually pain but may also include stiffness and instability, symptoms not seen in cervical disc disease. The absence of sensory symptoms and signs in shoulder disorders also helps to distinguish shoulder problems from neck problems.
7. Intrinsic shoulder disorders are aggravated by shoulder movement on history and passive ROM testing during examination (6). Neck problems are aggravated by neck movement and passive ROM testing.
8. Tenderness to palpation, if done carefully and without force, will help localize disorders to the neck or shoulder.

Problems with the Principles!

Now that you have some basic principles, let us make life more difficult by stating:

1. It is not uncommon to have coexisting neck and shoulder problems. The classic is cervical disc disease leading to a frozen shoulder (2, 9). A Pancoast tumor may occur as a frozen shoulder. This is so unlike lumbar disc disease, where it is unusual to have concurrent symptomatic back and hip problems. Furthermore, the location of pain in the shoulder, referred from the neck, can be located over the deltoid (C5 root), exactly where primary shoulder conditions can cause pain localization. In the lumbar spine, referred "hip" pain is buttock in location, an unusual location for pain in primary hip disease. The presence of groin pain almost always signifies a primary hip disorder, and buttock discomfort points to a primary low back problem.
2. Watch out for the double crush (Fig. 21.2). This is most commonly cervical disc disease and carpal tunnel syndrome (14). If you meet this situation, with decreased nerve conduction velocities at the wrist, always treat the carpal tunnel syndrome primarily, especially if surgery is being considered.
3. Cervical myelopathy manifests itself as LMNL in the arm (pain, weakness, and paraesthesias), UMNL in the arm (clumsiness of hand movements), and UMNL in the legs (stiff, unsteady gait) (21). UMNL in the legs may be the presenting complaint and may appear on the surface to be just like lumbar spinal canal stenosis. Neurological exam will reveal a pyramidal tract lesion in the upper and lower extremities to alert you to the neck as the source of troubles. But if the CSM complaint is predominantly lower extremity, and the patient has associated lumbar spinal canal stenosis (so-called tandem stenosis) (7)—and you forget to examine the upper extremities—you will miss the cervical myelopathic lesion.
4. Neurological (radicular) lesions associated with cervical disc disease are not of the same clear-cut pattern as in lumbar disc disease. Chronic irritive (noncompressive) lesions without neurological signs are more common in the neck compared to the higher frequency of acute compressive radicular lesions with neurological signs in the lower extremity. Asking a patient to draw a road map of the location of leg pain and doing a neurological exam will almost al-

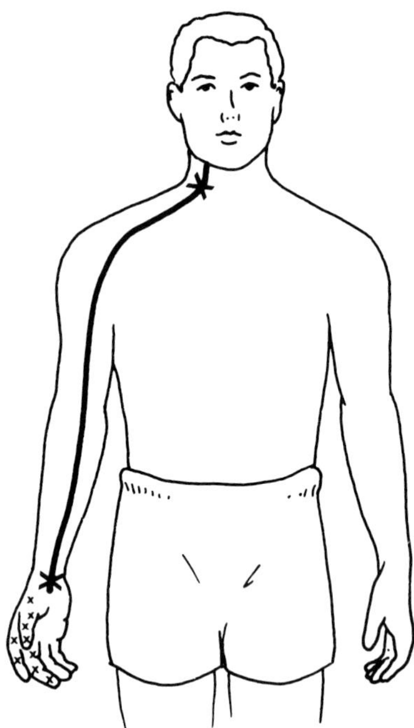

Figure 21.2.   The "double crush" of C6 fibers, proximal in the neck and distal in the carpal tunnel.

ways yield an anatomical level of lumbar root involvement. In cervical disc disease, the distribution for C6 and C7 root involvement is almost identical, and neurological exam often will not determine the anatomical level. You are then left with MRI or CT/myelography to determine the anatomical level. (Note that ordering an MRI or CT/myelogram in cervical disc disease is considered by most surgeons to be a giant step towards operative intervention).

5. Referral patterns in a-c joint conditions and C5 cervical root lesion can be very confusing (Fig. 21.1).

Differential Diagnostic Conditions

It is impossible to give a complete description of each of these conditions—that would be another text. But highlights of some of these problems will be presented, and references in this text will be given for other conditions previously discussed.

Intracerebral and Intraspinal Conditions

Cerebrovascular Accident (CVA).   Post-stroke patients may end up with shoulder subluxation as a result of the weakness of shoulder girdle muscles. The condition can be very painful and is especially resistant to slings and therapy.

Multiple Sclerosis (MS).   MS may occur with predominant spinal cord involvement that includes radiating arm pain. The association of other neurological symptoms, a neurological exam (multiple roots) and MRI (Fig. 21.3) will help diagnose MS.

Amyotrophic Lateral Sclerosis (ALS).   ALS occurs in the fourth to sixth decade, the same age group as cervical disc disease. It occurs as a spontaneous

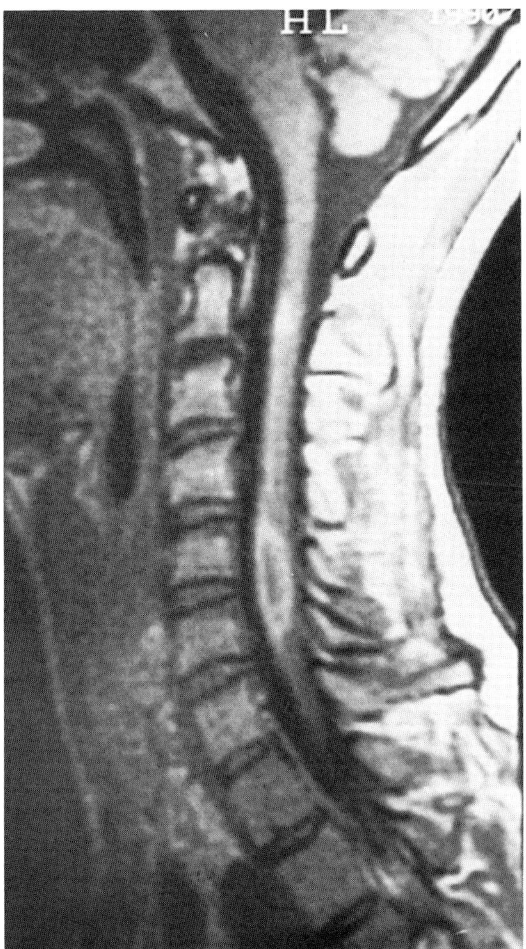

Figure 21.3. MRI in multiple sclerosis with plaques on spinal cord behind C2 and C5-C6.

painless weakness, atrophy, and fasciculations about both shoulders, usually asymmetric in degree. There are no associated sensory symptoms or signs. Electromyographic examination of the upper and lower limbs will be positive (increased duration of motor unit potentials). Sometimes these patients end up with a diagnostic CT/myelogram. Don't get trapped by a false-positive exam, because surgery will rarely make a difference to these patients.

Guillain-Barre (Acute Idiopathic Polyneuritis). This is an ascending paralysis and paraesthetic condition of peripheral nerves that affects the lower, followed by the upper, extremities. It may be subtle in its presentation, but most often is florid and obvious. Motor paresis is much more significant than sensory changes. There are no UMNL findings (pyramidal signs). Cerebral spinal fluid exam will show increased protein content without increase in cells.

Localized Tumors. Refer to Chapter 9 for a complete description of these tumors. Mentioned only briefly in that chapter is a syrinx of the cervical cord (Fig. 9.20). This is a central cord cyst, spanning a variable number of segments, that may be congenital, idiopathic, or posttraumatic. It presents arm and sometimes facial pain, especially at night when the syrinx fills with CSF. As the syrinx enlarges, there is less pain and a greater neurological deficit, especially a loss in thermal sensation. The neurological picture is not unlike CSM with LMNL and UMNL changes in the arms, and UMNL changes (spastic gait) in the legs.

Disc/Vertebral Level Conditions

Mechanical Neck Pain (see Chapters 3 and 7).
Nonmechanical Neck Pain (see Chapters 8 and 9).
Mechanical Neck/Arm Pain (see Chapters 3 and 7).

Extraspinal Conditions

Proximal Neurological Entrapments

Greater Occipital Nerve (C2) Entrapment.   The most proximal and enigmatic of the entrapments in this group is that of the greater occipital nerve. It is a branch of the cervical plexus that travels through some very complex muscular anatomy. Its entrapment produces headache over the occiput/parietal region without lower neck ache or radiating arm pain. Its assessment becomes part of the differential diagnosis of headache, which is well beyond the scope of this book.

There is no certain method of diagnosis and even less certain surgical cure. Management is almost always conservative.

Thoracic Outlet Syndrome (TOS).   The thoracic outlet syndromes tend to be a voguish diagnosis (16, 20). Popular in the 1950s and denigrated in the 1960s, these syndromes may be assuming their rightful place as true but uncommon sources of pain in the arm. Until recently, they have been overdiagnosed far too often by nonneurologically trained physicians and surgeons.

Before describing the clinical manifestations of the thoracic outlet syndromes, it is important to remind ourselves of the origins and insertions of the troublesome muscles in this region, their fascial coverage, and their relationship to the emerging neurovascular bundles. The significant muscles are the scalene muscles, which are attached to the first rib, the subclavius muscle running from the first rib to the undersurface of the clavicle, and the pectoralis minor running from the chest wall to the coracoid process (Fig. 21.4).

The muscles are encased in the neck by the deep cervical fascia, which splits below the clavicle to envelop the subclavius. Distal to the subclavius, the deep cervical fascia forms the clavipectoral fascia, which again splits to enclose the pectoralis minor. There is a thickened portion of the clavipectoral fascia, the so-called costocoracoid ligament, which holds the subclavian artery and vein firmly against the first rib (Fig. 21.5).

The brachial plexus and subclavian artery in the root of the neck emerge between the anterior and middle scalene muscles, with the subclavian vein lying anterior to the scalenus anterior. The neurovascular bundle then passes between the first rib and the clavicle and courses under the pectoralis minor to reach the axilla. The lower cord of the brachial plexus is closely apposed to the first rib (Fig. 21.6). Discomfort arises as a result of compression of the neurovascular bundle against a normal or abnormal first rib, with the symptoms produced by impairment of vascular flow, irritation of a cord of the brachial plexus, or a com-

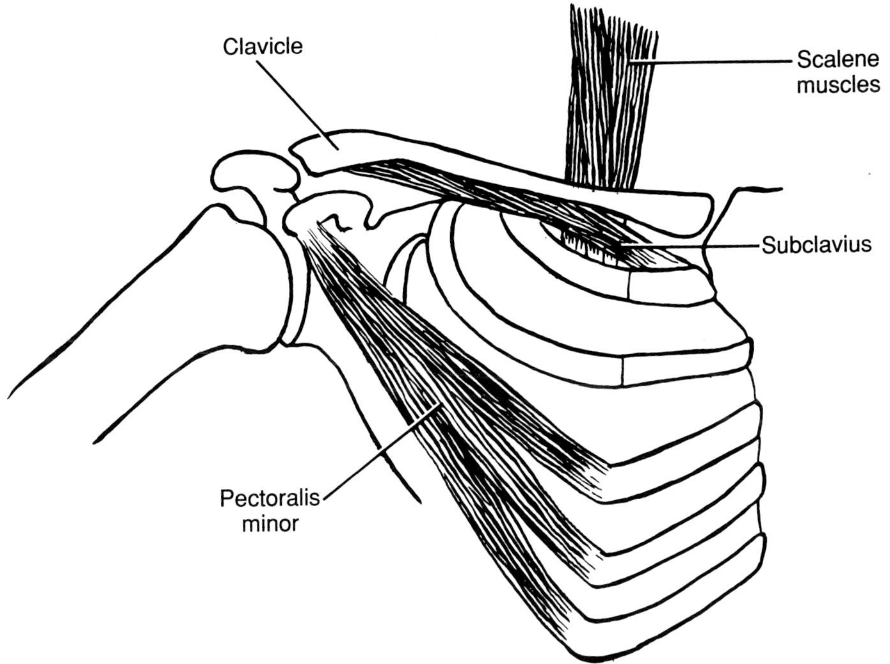

Figure 21.4. The important muscle groups in understanding TOS.

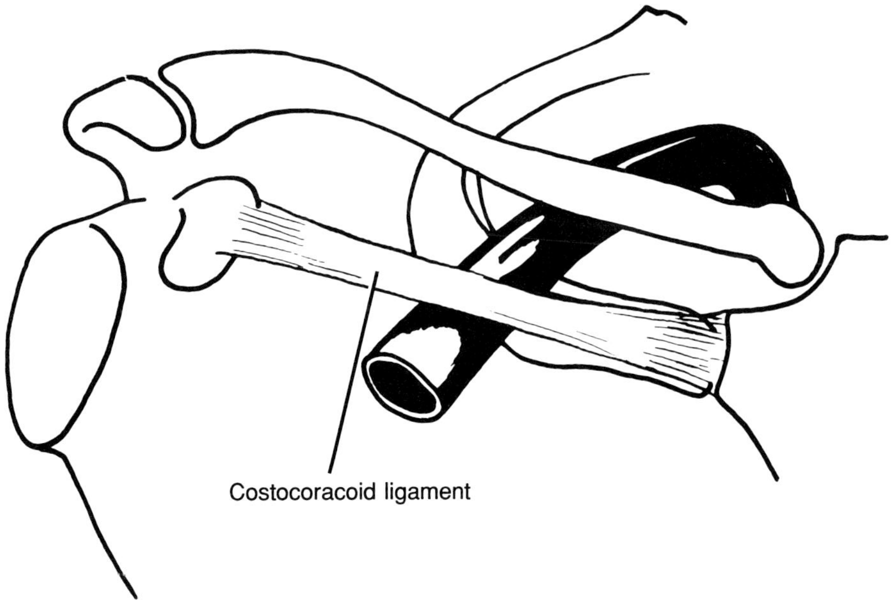

Figure 21.5. The costocoracoid ligament.

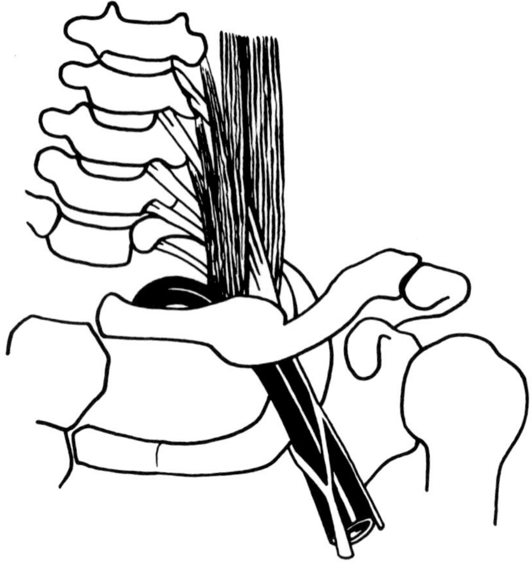

Figure 21.6.   The relationship of the brachial plexus and vessels to the first rib.

bination of these factors (3). Patients complain of pain in the arm, which may extend to the fingers. It is interesting to note that although patients with cervical root irritation commonly experience paresthesia in the hand and fingers, it is unusual for them to complain of pain extending below the wrist. This is one symptom that distinguishes the thoracic outlet syndromes from cervical root irritation (12).

Numbness involving the ring and little fingers is common, and patients may also note a strange disturbance of sensation in the palm. Quite commonly, they state that they are awakened in the middle of the night with a numb hand, which they tend to shake in order to "get the circulation back." In many, the symptoms are most noticeable on arising. During the day, prolonged activity may precipitate or aggravate the symptoms. The aggravating activity does not have to be arduous. For example, a patient in her late fifties may state that for some time she has experienced a dull, nagging ache in the right arm, associated on occasion with paresthesia involving the ring and little fingers. Although she is conscious of her discomforts, they do not vary much with normal daily household activities. However, if she performs a repetitive activity, such as sewing, knitting, or ironing, the pain gradually intensifies so that she has to stop. The story is characteristic and is reminiscent of the well-recognized intermittent vascular claudication found in the lower extremities with impaired peripheral circulation. The analogy is obvious. Patients with a thoracic outlet syndrome may tell the story of what may best be described as "claudicant pain," aggravated to an unbearable degree by continued muscular activity.

One could readily imagine that if such patients were forced to walk on their hands, they would give a history identical to that given by patients with intermittent claudication in their lower extremities, namely, that they could walk on their hands for one block, but the arm pain would gradually increase in severity and prevent them from continuing this bizarre activity. The impor-

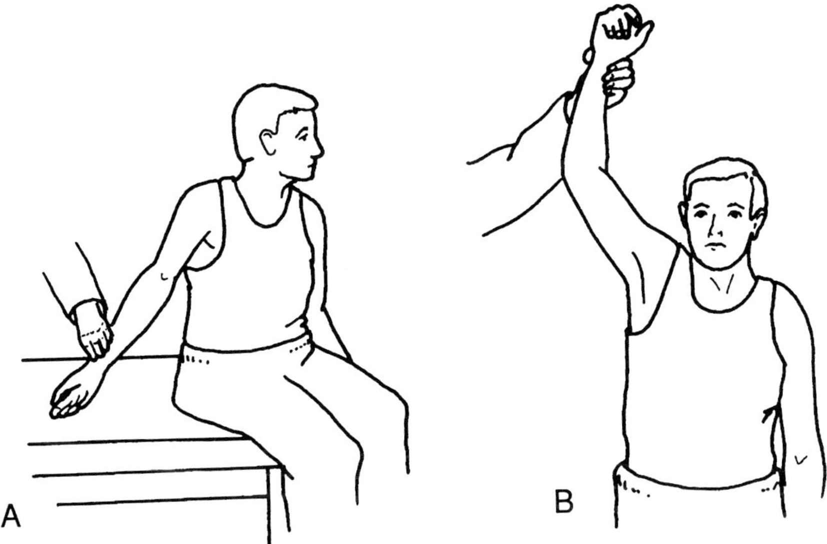

Figure 21.7.   Two ways of doing the test of Adson: **A,** the correct way, with the arm extended and the head turned in the opposite direction. A positive test includes obliteration of the radial pulse and reproduction of neurological symptoms. **B,** a popular way of putting the shoulder into abduction and external rotation.

tance of this observation lies in the assessment of the cause of the complaints. Obviously, it is of vital importance to evaluate the blood flow to the upper extremity by careful clinical assessment of the pulses and overlying bruits prior to any physical activity and, again, after repetitive activity of sufficient degree to produce symptoms.

On physical examination, the lower cord of the brachial plexus is the most affected, with the potential for atrophy and weakness of the thenars (C8 fibers in the median nerve) and a sensory loss in ulnar nerve distribution. Vasomotor changes may be evident if the condition is far advanced. They may only become evident with the aggravation tests of Adson (Fig. 21.7). When doing these tests, be aware that it is not uncommon for normal patients to obliterate their pulses in these maneuvers. The test should only be considered positive when the pulse is obliterated and the patient's symptoms are reproduced.

Simple noninvasive techniques, such as recording the radial artery pressure by Doppler ultrasound examination, will indicate whether more detailed investigation by arteriography should be carried out. Claudicant pain in the upper extremity is probably much more common than has previously been recognized. It is easy for the clinician to attribute an increase in forearm pain following knitting and ironing to a distaste for these activities rather than to any significant physiological change in the limb. Some patients may notice coldness, weakness, and discoloration in the hands. Raynaud's syndrome may be present (15). Rarely, vascular obstruction may be of sufficient severity to cause ulceration or even gangrene of the fingers. These conditions usually arise as the result of embolization of the distal digital or palmar artery, often from a traumatic arteritis at the site of the compression of the subclavian

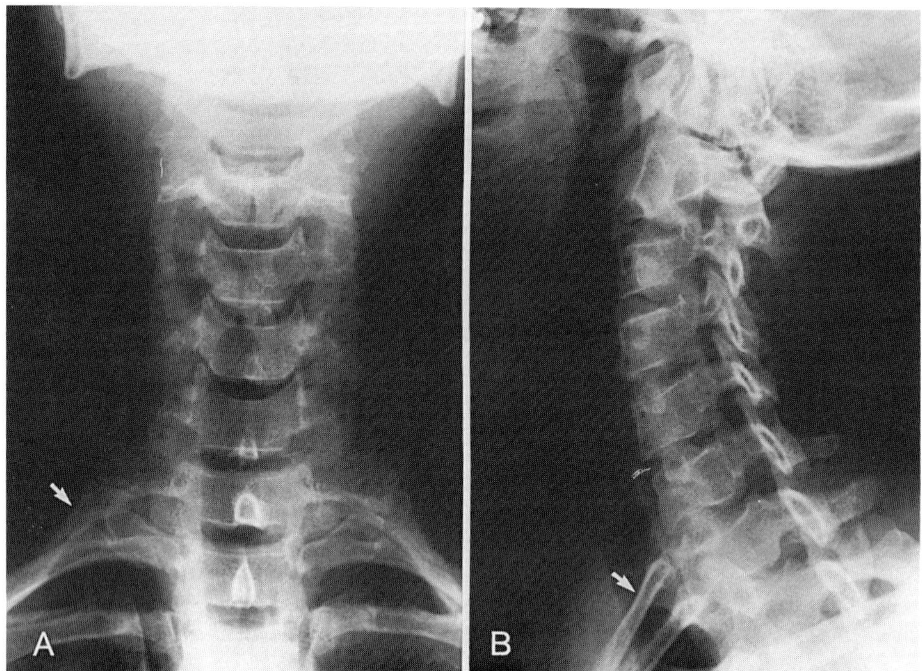

Figure 21.8.   **A,** cervical rib on AP (*arrow*). **B,** oblique in same patient (*arrow* points to cervical rib).

artery between the first rib and the clavicle. Occasionally, a subclavian aneurysm may form distal to the obstruction and provide a potent source of embolism and subsequent Raynaud's syndrome.

Obstruction to the blood flow in the subclavian vessels may lead to ischemic changes in the peripheral nerves and the production of what may best be termed an interstitial neuritis. The significance of this observation lies in the fact that, when pressure on the subclavian artery has been overcome, the neuritic pain, or whatever you want to call it, may intensify for a while and may persist for several months. Occasionally, the symptoms are those of venous obstruction: edema, cyanosis, and dilatation of the superficial veins, especially those around the shoulder. The symptoms, which may be intermittent, result from subclavian or axillary vein thrombosis. The diagnosis demands venography, with the arm abducted, and if confirmed, operative intervention is indicated to decompress the thoracic outlet.

Now let us consider the various thoracic outlet syndromes according to the anatomical abnormalities responsible for them. The normal smooth course of the neurovascular bundle passing between the scalenes and over the first rib may be jeopardized by several variants. A large cervical rib (1), or even a dense fibrous band on the tip of a rudimentary cervical rib, passing downward and anteriorly towards the first thoracic rib, may compress the neurovascular bundle (Fig. 21.8). Even an enlarged transverse process of the seventh cervical vertebra may produce an angulation of the emerging vessels.

Anomalies such as this were the first recognized sources of these symptom complexes. With increasing operative experience, it became obvious that the

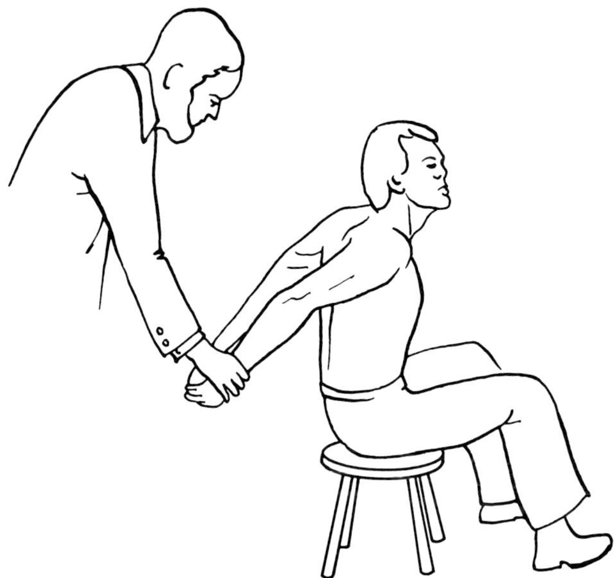

Figure 21.9.   Test designed to aggravate symptoms of costoclavicular compression (and it will aggravate patient if done too vigorously!).

scalene muscles showed considerable variation in their points of insertion into the first rib, and could compromise the neurovascular bundle either by direct pressure or by abnormally elevating the first rib. Adson's test (1) is designed to stretch the muscles, thereby elevating the first rib and compressing the neurovascular bundle. The anterior scalene muscle arises from the transverse processes of the third, fourth, fifth, and sixth cervical vertebrae. They are put under passive tension when the patient's head is turned toward the side of the pain, that is, when the cervical transverse processes are pointing posteriorly. Further tension can be applied by extending the neck in this position and at the same time flexing it laterally, that is, pushing the head toward the pain-free upper extremity.

This increased passive tension on the scalene muscle elevates the first rib, pressing it against the brachial artery. The elevation of the first rib will increase if the patient now takes a deep breath, further compressing the neurovascular bundles. As the vessels and brachial plexus pass under the clavicle, they also become subject to compression between the first rib and the clavicle. This is the so-called costoclavicular syndrome, which may result from a malunion of a fracture of the clavicle, an exostosis of the first rib, or a congenital abnormality of the first rib producing buckling.

Patients suffering from costoclavicular compression will experience an exacerbation of their symptoms if the shoulders are pulled downward and backward in the so-called military position, particularly if traction is applied at the same time to the arms with the glenohumeral joint held in extension. This manipulation approximates the clavicles against the first rib (Fig. 21.9).

It must be remembered that although this maneuver will cause dampening of the radial pulse in most patients, by itself a change in the volume of the radial pulse is not of significance. The important finding is the reproduction of the clinically experienced pain.

After the neurovascular bundle has escaped this hazard, it must pass over the rib cage, under the tendon of the pectoralis minor. In the pectoralis minor syndrome or, as it is sometimes called, the hyperabduction syndrome, the neurovascular bundle strapped against the chest wall by the pectoralis minor may be kinked around the coracoid process when maintaining the shoulder in the fully abducted extended position (Fig. 21.7B). Characteristically, these patients will experience paresthesia in their arms as they put their hands behind their heads and push their elbows backward, thereby abducting and hyperextending the glenohumeral joint.

The majority of patients suffering from thoracic outlet syndromes are middle-aged. When considering treatment, we must continually ask ourselves: "Why does a congenital lesion remain quiescent for four decades before symptoms develop?" The most commonly accepted explanation is that the symptoms arise as the result of postural changes, that is, the middle-aged slump. The important role played by postural changes is shown by the many patients who are significantly helped by postural reeducation, with particular attention given to overcoming a cervicodorsal angulation and atony of the trapezii.

Conservative treatment should always be your first line of attack. Simply reassuring the patient and recommending changes in activities of daily living will control most cases. If they do not, step up to rest in a sling and exercise therapy to improve posture and reverse drooping of the shoulder.

Indications for surgical intervention can be considered relative or absolute. Persistence of paresthesia and pain of sufficient severity to influence the patient's ability to work or to enjoy leisure hours may at times constitute a significant disability, but this must be considered a relative indication. Absolute indications for surgical intervention arise when there is irrefutable objective evidence of interference with the vascularity of the limb, that is, venous thrombosis or arterial aneurysm and/or emboli, or when there is evidence of impairment of peripheral nerve conduction.

Wilbourne (19) has divided TOS into true neurological TOS and disputed neurological TOS. True N-TOS will reveal slowed median sensory involvement and just the reverse for the ulnar nerve. EMG examination of the thenars will most likely reveal chronic MUP changes (increased amplitude and duration with decreased recruitment) and occasionally active axonal loss (fibrillation potentials) in the median nerve. Disputed-TOS will have no NCT or EMG abnormalities. Wilbourne (19, 20) described this as a disease of the thoracic surgical community, overdiagnosed and overtreated, with no scientific consensus as to diagnostic criteria or treatment methods.

If symptoms persist in spite of conservative care and if a cervical rib is present, excision often leads to a good result. In the hyperabduction syndrome, the insertion of the pectoralis minor should be divided, but now we enter an area of controversy. The simplest mode of decompression of all the other thoracic outlet syndromes, and the method advocated by the nonneurological surgical community, is removal of the first rib through an axillary approach.

Reflex Sympathetic Dystrophy (11).   Variously described as the shoulder-hand syndrome, causalgia, and Sudeck's atrophy, this is a relatively uncommon condition. This is fortunate, because it is so resistant to treatment. It most commonly occurs after illness (e.g., myocardial infarction) or injury (to the shoulder, elbow, or hand). The presentation is of a painful stiff shoulder, advancing to a generalized, diffuse painfully stiff upper extremity. Associated findings are swelling and vasomotor problems in the hand, which may advance to smooth shiny skin and atrophic nail changes. This end stage may include diffuse osseous demineralization on x-ray of any of the affected extremity bones.

Although the condition is thought to be due to sympathetic overactivity, patients also display a wide range of behavioral changes: depression, anxiety, and social withdrawal. Whether this is a primary cause or secondary response is not apparent.

The diagnosis is made by noting the history of the precipitating event, the collection of symptoms and signs, the absence of any aggravation of symptoms by neck movement, and the absence of specific neurological changes. All three phases of the bone scan will be positive, including the blood pooling stage (Phase 1). See Chapter 9 for a discussion of the three phases of bone scanning.

The condition is very resistant to treatment and requires a very sympathetic doctor and therapist. Various physical therapy modalities, such as ice and heat, and specific hand exercises, are needed long term. Various combinations of oral medications, such as NSAIDs, sympathetic blockers, and antidepressants are used. A stellate ganglion block may break the vicious circle and make all of the above treatment modalities more effective. Miscellaneous treatment with acupuncture and TENS have been claimed to be effective.

Apical Syndromes.   Patients with lesions of the first rib or apical (Pancoast) tumors may have pain in the shoulder and radiation down the arm; they may mimic a thoracic outlet syndrome. Usually, the telltale sign on clinical examination is the presence of Horner's syndrome (Fig. 21.10). Any neurological findings will be confined to the C8-T1 distribution unless the tumor is well-advanced and has invaded wider fields.

Intermediate Nerve Entrapment Syndromes.

Dorsal Scapular Nerve.   The dorsal scapular nerve arises from the upper trunk of the brachial plexus (C5) and passes almost immediately through the body of the scalenus medius muscle. It is at this point of entry into the scalenus medius that the nerve may be kinked and held rigidly. As a result, there is no safety factor of movement necessary for the smooth gliding of the nerve associated with forward movements of the shoulder. A tight nerve attempting to move in tight muscles may result in a neuropathy.

The dorsal scapular nerve is a motor nerve supplying the rhomboids (Fig. 21.11). Initially, the patient complains of unilateral rhomboid pain. Later, if the patient persists in normal activities, he or she is plagued by "spasms" in the rhomboids, sometimes visible to the examiner. Still later, the patient experiences a subjective weakness of the shoulder associated with pain radiating down the arm and tenderness over the involved rhomboid muscle. On clinical examination, the pain is aggravated by turning the head towards the affected extremity

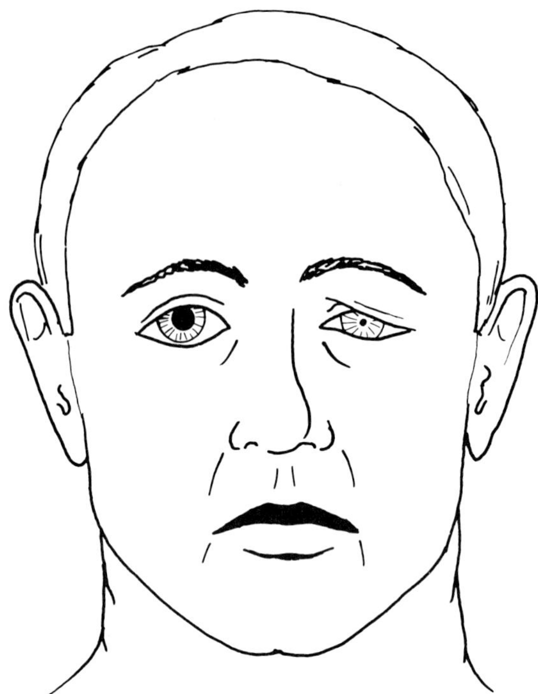

Figure 21.10.   Horner's Syndrome—interruption of the cervical sympathetic chain by a Pancoast tumor will produce miosis (example on the *left*), pseudoptosis, enophthalmus, ipsilateral vessel dilation, and anhidrosis.

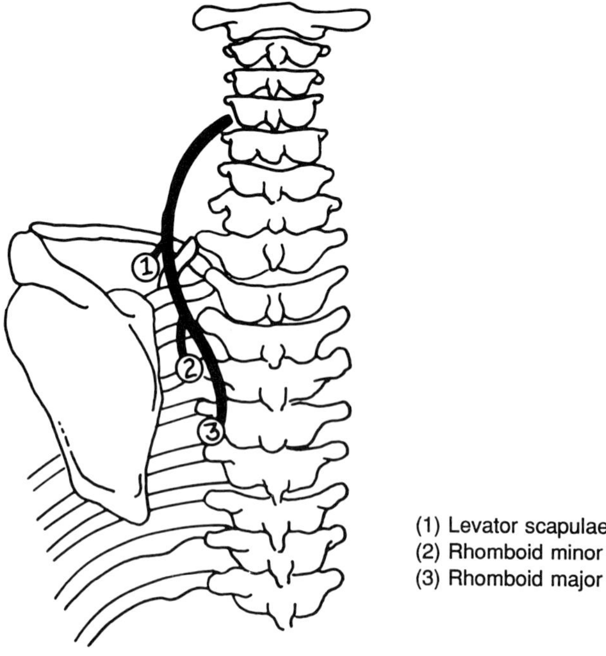

Figure 21.11.   The dorsal scapular nerve and its muscular supply.

and by lateral flexion of the neck in the opposite direction. The scalenus medius muscle is stretched by these movements. Patients demonstrate local tenderness and may state that they get relief from their symptoms by placing their hands on top of their heads.

It is easy to forget that entrapment of a dorsal scapular nerve may also be a component of a complex syndrome associated with an acceleration-extension injury of the neck, the so-called whiplash injury. A traction strain is more likely to occur if, at the moment of impact when the vehicle is struck from the rear, the passenger's head is fully rotated. The symptoms would develop on the side to which the chin was rotated at the moment of injury.

The majority of patients respond to physical therapy designed to build up the strength of the shoulder girdle muscles. In some patients, however, the symptoms persist and, if denervation potentials can be demonstrated on electromyography, surgical decompression is indicated.

Long Thoracic Nerve of Bell (3).   The long thoracic nerve of Bell innervates the serratus anterior. It arises from the fifth, sixth, and seventh cervical roots. The roots from C5 and C6 enter the scalenus medius, where they unite to form a common trunk. This trunk is later joined at the lateral border of the scalenus medius by the C7 roots.

Loss of function of the serratus anterior causes a much more noticeable winging of the scapula than rhomboid deficiency (Fig. 12.4).

Paralysis of the long thoracic nerve of Bell (3) at one time was called "hod carrier's palsy." This referred to bricklayers, whose job at the time involved carrying several bricks in a small box or "hod," fixed to a long pole carried over the bricklayer's shoulder. It was felt that this pulled down on the first rib, stretching the scalenus medius and thereby producing a nerve entrapment.

Although hod carriers are no longer employed and other mechanisms must play a role, on balance, the so-called idiopathic paralysis of the long thoracic nerve of Bell is yet another manifestation of thoracic outlet syndromes, with the involved nerve roots being entrapped within the scalenus medius. Treatment is usually watchful waiting, in the hope that function will return.

Suprascapular Nerve Entrapment.   The suprascapular nerve is derived from the upper trunk of the brachial plexus (C5 and C6). The nerve passes behind the plane of the brachial plexus to the upper border of the scapula, where it passes through the suprascapular notch under the transverse ligament (Fig. 21.12). It is a pure motor nerve and innervates the supra and infraspinatii muscles. Because it is a motor nerve, the pain associated with entrapment is deep and poorly localized.

Usually as the result of chronic athletic trauma (pitching, tennis), the nerve may become contused, swollen, and constrained within the suprascapular notch. The condition was first described by Kopell and Thompson (9) as the first stage in reflex inhibition of scapular movement, leading to the clinical syndrome of a frozen shoulder.

Suprascapular nerve lesions more commonly occur, however, in the reverse manner. The patient develops a frozen shoulder as the result of a diffuse rotator cuff tendinitis, and shoulder girdle movements are subsequently dependent almost entirely on the scapulothoracic glide. This results in excessive stretch in

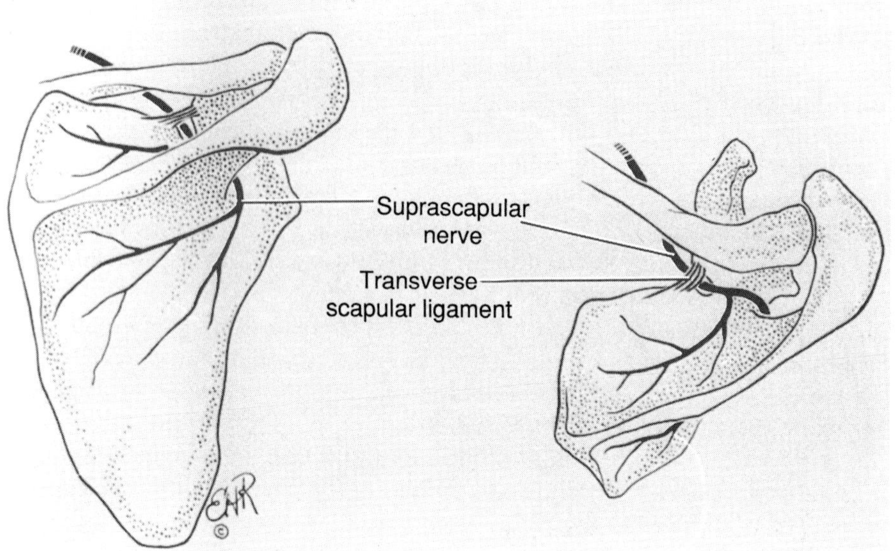

Figure 21.12. The suprascapular nerve passing under the transverse scapular ligament in the suprascapular notch.

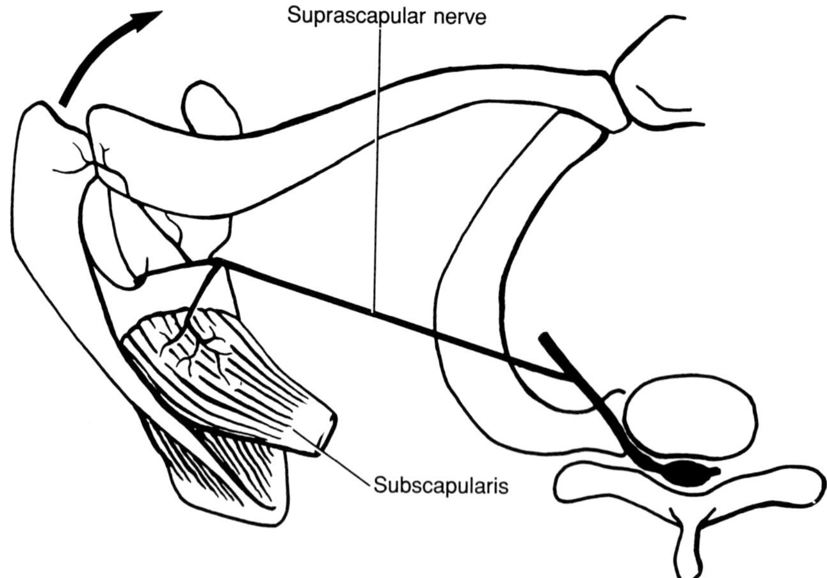

Figure 21.13.   Stretching of the suprascapular nerve.

the suprascapular nerve on forward flexion of the arm, especially if the nerve is trapped in the suprascapular notch (Fig. 21.13) (4).

Clinically, the patient will complain of severe pain in the affected shoulder, with the symptoms aggravated and perpetuated by activity. Characteristically, the spinatii will show gross atrophy and marked tenderness on pressure. Weakness is in abduction and external rotation of the shoulder joint.

There is no cutaneous sensory component to the suprascapular nerve and thus no sensory loss.

A similar clinical picture can, on occasion, involve a total rotator cuff tear, and it can also be seen in neurological disorders such as a syringomyelia and neuralgic amyotrophy. Before you can be certain of the diagnosis of suprascapular nerve entrapment, you must be able to block the pain with an injection of local anesthetic into the notch. Positive electromyography lends strong support to the diagnosis. If the diagnosis can be irrefutably established, then a neurolysis with division of the suprascapular ligament must be performed to reverse the clinical picture.

Brachial Neuritis.   Also known as neuralgic amyotrophy or Parsonage-Turner syndrome (18), it is one of the most painful conditions to affect the shoulder. It is thought to be a viral infection of motor nerves, and is almost always of sudden and profound onset. Just as suddenly, the pain disappears in days or weeks, and the shoulder is left weak and atrophied. Obviously, multiple roots are involved on motor exam; no sensory changes occur. Rapid development of weakness and wasting distinguishes the clinical picture from a rotator cuff lesion; characteristic involvement of the deltoid distinguishes it from a suprascapular nerve entrapment; complete lack of sensor changes distinguishes it from a root or plexus lesion. The condition is more frequently found in men and may involve both shoulders.

EMG will show signs of neurogenic atrophy. Spontaneous recovery of varying degrees occur in spite of treatment.

Brachial Plexopathy.   Injury to the brachial plexus usually occurs as the result of high-velocity vehicle (motorcycle) accidents or surgical misadventure. Wilbourne (20) has seen plexopathies following TOS axillary decompressions in numbers equal to cases of true N-TOS. The clinical presentation ranges all the way from a partial stretch of a single root that recovers to multiple root avulsions or surgical injury, leaving arm flail with no hope of recovery. Complications, such as reflex sympathetic dystrophy are not uncommon. Fortunately, the injury is rare, because consequences can be devastating.

Distal Neurological Entrapments.

Radial Nerve Entrapment.   The origin of the extensor carpi radialis brevis presents a firm fibrous proximal border. After bifurcation, the deep branch of the radial nerve passes under this fibrous origin of the extensor carpi radialis brevis to reach the supinator, through which it passes (Fig. 21.14). The superficial branch courses down the forearm between the extensor carpi radialis brevis and the brachioradialis. Occasionally, however, the superficial branch may accompany the deep branch for a short distance and then pass through the muscle fibers of the extensor carpi radialis brevis.

The deep branch may become tethered as it passes under the falciform edge of the origin of the extensor carpi radialis brevis (4); rarely, the superficial branch may become constricted in an abnormal course lower down, through the muscle belly (8).

Most commonly, the deep branch is involved and pain is experienced locally on the radial side of the elbow and may radiate proximally and distally. Supination of the forearm or dorsiflexion of the wrist will intensify the pain. The most signif-

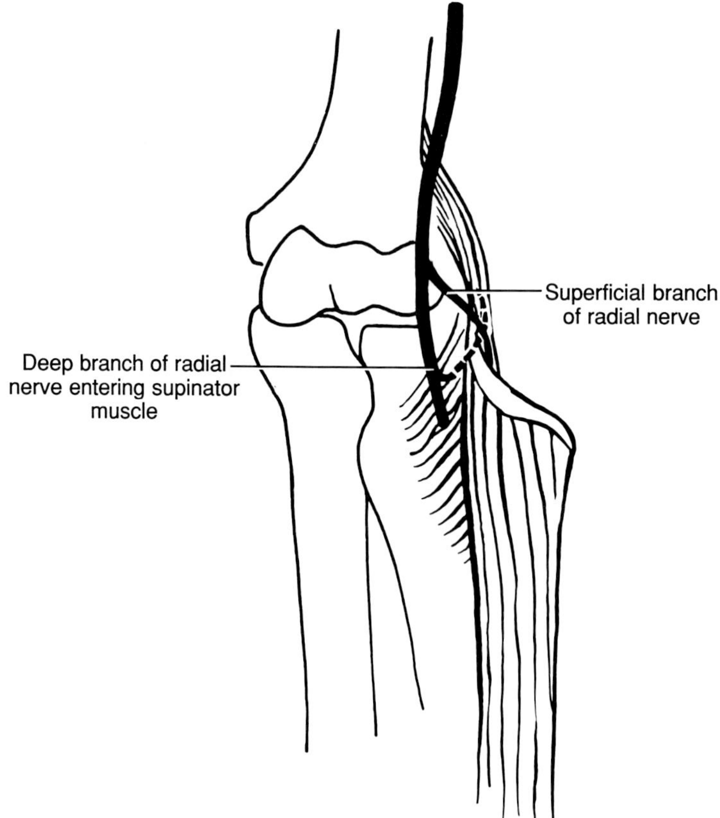

Figure 21.14.   The deep branch of the radial nerve passes under the fibrous origin of the extensor carpi radialis brevis (reflected) to enter the supinator.

icant diagnostic finding is reproduction of pain at the elbow on extending the middle finger against resistance. Longstanding lesions may result in paralysis of the long extensors of the fingers. An unusual feature of this paralysis is that the weakness may involve the fingers, individually and serially. The patient may describe and demonstrate difficulty in extending the index finger first, then a few weeks later the middle finger, and eventually all the extensors become involved if the lesion is untreated.

There are several lesions that produce pain and tenderness on the lateral aspect of the elbow. The presenting symptom of sixth cervical root irritation may be pain over the lateral aspect of the elbow and, on examination, there may be marked tenderness. The tenderness is over the muscle mass of the common extensors on the anterolateral aspect of the elbow joint, just distal to the radial head. The tenderness of the radial nerve entrapment syndrome is posterolateral and distal to the joint. The tenderness of "tennis elbow" is directly over the lateral epicondyle. The pain associated with tennis elbow is intensified by clenching the fist tightly and by resisted dorsiflexion of the wrist. The pain of entrapment of the deep branch of the radial nerve is intensified by supination of the forearm and by resisted extension of the middle finger.

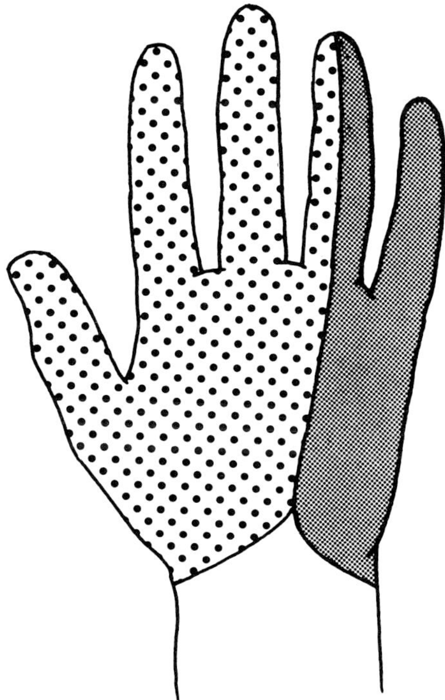

Figure 21.15.   Distribution of pain and paraesthesia in the median (*open dots*) and ulnar nerves (*closed dots*). The split of the ring finger may be variable.

Radial nerve palsy is distinguished from a C7 radiculopathy by the triceps weakness and flexor carpi radialis weakness produced by the latter. Both are absent in radial nerve entrapment in the supinator tunnel. In addition, radial nerve entrapment rarely has a sensory component, while C7 radiculopathy often has paraesthetic sensation and may have numbness in the third digit. Treatment of radial nerve entrapment often requires surgical release of the deep branch (posterior interosseous) of the radial nerve as it enters the supinator tunnel.

Ulnar Nerve Entrapment.   The ulnar nerve may be entrapped at the elbow or the wrist (Guyon's canal). Most frequently, the sight of compression is the elbow, secondary to fractures or other trauma. The symptoms include medial epicondylar pain and paraesthesia in the ulnar 1 1/2 fingers (Fig. 21.15). Weakness may be detected in the muscles innervated by the ulnar nerve distal to the elbow, that is, the flexor carpi ulnaris, the flexor digitorum profundus to the fourth and fifth fingers, the interossei, and the hypothenars. The sensory loss is over the ulnar 1 1/2 fingers.

The ulnar nerve is easily palpable in the epicondylar groove of the elbow and normally is sensitive to pressure. With a neuropathy, palpation may reveal that the nerve is thickened and unduly sensitive to pressure, including the easy reproduction of paraesthesia. Full flexion of the elbow may reproduce the clinically experienced symptoms. With recurrent dislocations, the nerve can be felt moving into the dislocation position on flexion of the elbow. The diagnosis can be readily confirmed by a nerve conduction study. Ulnar nerve neuropathy arising at the elbow generally requires surgical relief by subperiosteal excision of the medial epicondyle, which is preferable to the commonly preformed anterior transposition of the ulnar nerve.

The ulnar nerve may also be trapped at the wrist in Guyon's canal. The common pathology is a ganglion. Entrapment is of the superficial and deep branches of the ulnar nerve, except the sensory branch to the dorsal 1 1/2 fingers, which comes off proximally to Guyon's canal. This means that the loss of sensation will be on the volar aspect of the ulnar 1 1/2 fingers. Compression of the deep branch will produce weakness of the hypothenars, interossei, and adductor pollicis. The absence of neck ache and arm symptoms above the wrist distinguishes this condition from cervical disc disease.

Diagnosis is made with NCT and treatment is surgical release and excision of any compressing pathology, such as a ganglion.

Median Nerve Entrapment.   Symptoms may arise if the median nerve becomes tethered at the wrist or at the elbow (13). Median nerve compression at the wrist—carpal tunnel syndrome—is well known and tends to occur in females who use their wrists and hands for repetitive movement. Frequently, the presenting symptom is nighttime pain and, classically, numbness and tingling in the thumb, index finger, and middle finger (Fig. 21.15). All too often, the patient complains of whole-hand numbness, which is very confusing (5). Often, the pain spreads proximally, with the patient complaining of a diffuse aching involving the whole upper extremity; this is made worse with activity. The clinical picture in such instances may mimic a sixth cervical root lesion, especially because, in a root lesion, the arm pain is frequently associated with paresthesia involving the radial three digits. Further confusion occurs on examination when, as in carpal tunnel syndrome, the median nerve is tender at the wrist on direct pressure. Autonomic disturbances are quite common in carpal tunnel compression, with the patient complaining of blanching of the involved fingers on exposure to cold. This is rarely seen with root compression.

The main distinguishing feature on examination is that forced sustained dorsiflexion of the wrist will aggravate the symptoms produced by a sixth cervical root compression, but will rarely alter the symptoms in a carpal tunnel compression. Paresthesia in the hand is increased in carpal tunnel syndrome when the wrist is forcibly held palmar-flexed (Phelan's test) (14). Tapping the volar wrist (Tinel's sign), often reproduces the paraesthetic sensations. The diagnosis can be confirmed by sensory and motor nerve conduction studies across the wrist. Don't forget the double crush syndrome (Fig. 21.2) when evaluating carpal tunnel syndrome.

Greater difficulty in diagnosis may arise when median nerve compression occurs at the elbow in the so-called pronator syndrome. At the elbow, the median nerve passes between the ulnar and humeral head of the pronator teres before passing under the proximal edge of the flexor digitorum sublimis (Fig. 21.16). The nerve may become compressed between the proximal edge of the sublimis muscle and the pronator.

As with compression of the median nerve at the wrist, the patient may have pain in the forearm and paresthesia involving the radial three digits. There may be weakness of the thenar muscles and the more proximally innervated muscles of flexor pollicus longus and flexor digitorum profundus to the index finger. Ex-

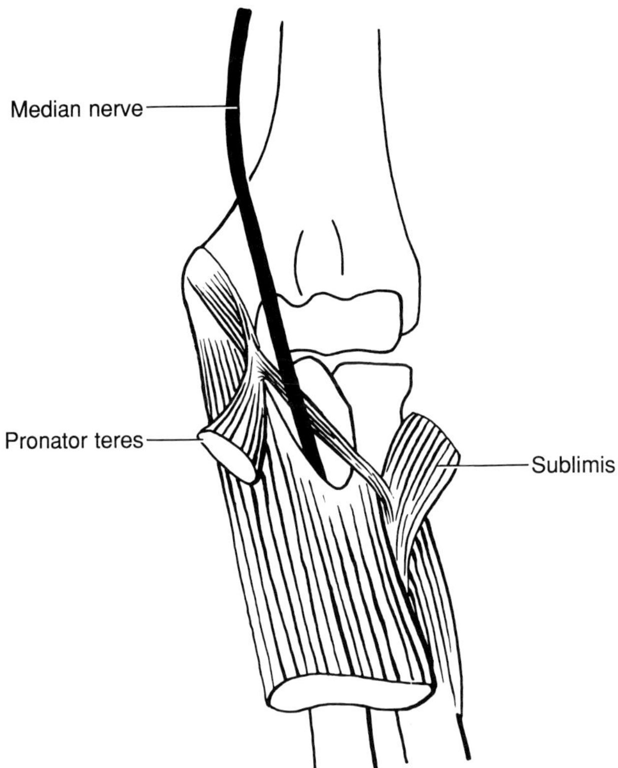

Figure 21.16. The median nerve may be entrapped by the fascial edge of the flexor digitorum sublimis.

amination frequently reveals diminution of appreciation of pinprick of the thumb, index finger, and middle finger, with occasional involvement of the radial side of the ring finger and the radial side of the palm. This signifies involvement of the superficial branch of the median nerve, which arises proximally to the transverse carpal ligament, and is not involved in carpal tunnel compression. The demonstration of diminution of sensory appreciation over the radial side of the palm suggests a more proximal nerve lesion, such as the pronator syndrome or, indeed, a C6 or C7 root compression.

Characteristically, with median nerve compression at the elbow patients will complain of increased pain in the forearm on pronation against resistance; direct pressure over the median nerve in the proximal portion of the forearm will reproduce the clinically experienced pain. Diagnosis is made with careful nerve conduction tests (NCT) and treatment, if documented electrically, is surgical release.

Intrinsic Peripheral Nerve Lesions.

Neuropathies.

Diabetic Neuropathy. There are many forms of neuropathies that complicate diabetes. Only three affect the extremities and, almost universally, there is much more involvement of the lower rather than the upper extremities.

Diabetic Sensory Neuropathy. This is the most common diabetic neuropathy, affecting the distal lower extremities. The symptoms are all sensory (numbness and tingling), affecting the distal legs and especially bothersome at night. Rarely are the arms affected.

Diabetic Mononeuropathy (Amyotrophy).   Not at all uncommon in the lower extremities, this condition affects the upper extremities rarely. The presentation is one of dramatic onset of unilateral radicular pain, not unlike sciatica. The distinguishing features in the lower extremities are the absence of back pain and a predilection for femoral nerve distribution, rather than for the sciatic nerve. As mentioned, the condition rarely affects the upper extremities.

Diabetic Plexus Neuropathy.   As with the above-mentioned neuropathies, this one rarely affects the upper extremities. The picture is one of a symmetrical, insidious onset of bilateral proximal leg weakness. Pain (especially back pain) is usually absent. There is never any bladder or bowel involvement. The paralysis may become profound and recovery, although slow, may also be profound.

Shingles (Herpes Zoster).   As the result of an acute viral infection of the spinal sensory ganglia, pain occurs in a radicular distribution, followed by a similarly distributed vesicular skin rash. If this occurs in a cervical radicular distribution and you see the patient before onset of the rash, you most often miss the diagnosis. Within a few weeks of onset (usually while the patient is in traction and a collar for the treatment of a cervical disc rupture!), the rash appears, making the diagnosis obvious. With time and antiviral drugs, the rash settles and the pain disappears. In some patients, chronic pain (postherpetic syndrome) persists as a troublesome problem.

Shoulder Conditions

Table 21.1 listed a host of shoulder problems causing pain in the region. These have all been discussed in Chapters 12–20, and you are referred to them for a complete discussion. A discussion of muscular problems about the shoulders follows.

Muscular Lesions.

Polymyositis.   This is an inflammatory myopathy in the category of autoimmune disease. It is frequently of insidious onset, occasionally of acute onset. Symptoms are progressive weakness of the limb girdle, trunk, and neck flexor muscles. Muscle pain may be associated, and if the changes are more pronounced around the neck and shoulders, the condition is easily confused with cervical disc disease having bilateral referred shoulder pain. Some patients have the typical skin changes of dermatomyositis.

Clinically detectable weakness distinguishes this condition from polymyalgia rheumatica. The diagnosis can be confirmed by muscle biopsy (showing muscle necrosis and repair), increased serum levels of muscle enzymes, and EMG changes (increased insertional activity and fibrillation potentials).

Polymyalgia/Rheumatica.   This is a disease of elderly patients who have symptoms of malaise, weight loss, and an increased ESR as part of a myalgic picture. The pain may be confined to the shoulder girdle region, but is more often diffuse.

The absence of weakness, with normal CPK enzymes and normal EMG exam, distinguish this problem from polymyositis.

Miscellaneous Conditions

Psychogenic (Nonorganic) Pain Syndromes.   It is our custom to address this issue early in any text on discussion of spinal problems. Simply because it is low on the list here, do not assume these syndromes are unimportant. In fact, they constitute a hard core of frustrating treatment problems, especially if you don't recognize the various syndromes. See Chapter 5 for a complete discussion.

Referred Pain.   Irritation of the phrenic nerve innervated diaphragm may produce pain over the tip of one shoulder. This irritation may be from a bleeding viscus or peritoneal infection. The reason for the shoulder pain is explained by complex neurosynaptic mechanisms in the cervical plexus that trigger the sensation of pain in the C4 cutaneous nerve distribution.

Similarly, cardiac conditions may produce shoulder discomfort, the classic example being the pain of myocardial infarction referred to the left jaw, shoulder, and arm.

Raynaud's Phenomenon (15).   Small vessel disease affecting the hands can produce bilateral discomfort that is very similar to cervical nerve root involvement. The absence of shoulder or neck pain and the absence of any increase in pain by postural changes helps to distinguish Raynaud's from cervical disc disease.

CONCLUSION

This chapter is an exhaustive list of the various conditions that produce symptoms about the neck and shoulder. Although most painful conditions in this region will be caused by cervical disc disease and soft tissue problems within the shoulder joint, it is best that you are aware of this bewildering list of conditions, because they may stump you. Good Luck.

REFERENCES

1. Adson AW and Caffey IR: Cervical rib. A new method of approach for relief of symptoms by division of the scalenus anterior. Ann Surg 85:839 (1927).
2. Bateman JE: Neurological painful conditions affecting the shoulder. Clin Orthop 162:44–54 (1989).
3. Bell C: On the nerves. Giving an account of some experiments on their structure and function which lead to a new arrangement of the system. Philos Trans R Soc Lond 3:398 (1821).
4. Caillet R: Neck and Arm Pain. FA Davis Co., Philadelphia (1964).
5. De Quervain F: Uber eine form von chronischer tendovaginitis. Cor Bl Schweize Arzte (Basel) 25:389 (1895).
6. English E and Macnab I: Recurrent posterior dislocation of the shoulder. Can J Surg 17:147–151 (1974).
7. Epstein NE, Epstein JA, Carras R, Vishnubhakat SM, and Hyman RA: Coexisting cervical and lumbar spinal stenosis: diagnosis and management. Neurosurgery 15:489–496 (1984).
8. Finkelstein H: Stenosing tendovaginitis at the radial styloid process. J Bone Joint Surg 12A:509–514 (1930).
9. Kopell IIP and Thompson WAL: Pain and the frozen shoulder. Surg Gynecol Obstet 109:92–96 (1959).
10. Lawrence J: Disc degeneration, its frequency and relationship to symptoms. Ann Rheum Dis 28:121–127 (1969)
11. Mandel S and Rothrock RW: Sympathetic dystrophies. Postgrad Med 87:213–218 (1990).
12. Pang D and Wessel HB: Thoracic outlet syndrome. Neurosurgery 22:105–121 (1988).
13. Phelan GS, Gardner WJ, and Lalonde AA: Neuropathy of the median nerve due to compression beneath the transverse carpal ligament. J Bone Joint Surg 32A:109–112 (1950).

14. Phelan GS and Kendrick JI: Compression of the median nerve in the carpal tunnel. JAMA 164: 524–527 (1957).
15. Raynaud AGM: De l'asphyxie locale et de la gangrène symétrique des extremités (thesis). Rignois, Paris (1862).
16. Roos DB: The thoracic outlet is underrated. Arch Neurol 47:327–328 (1990).
17. Spurling RG and Scoville WB: Lateral rupture of the cervical intervertebral discs. Surg Gynecol Obstet 78:350–356 (1944).
18. Tsairis P, Dyck PJ, and Mulder DW: Natural history of brachial plexus neuropathy. Arch Neurol 27:109–113 (1972).
19. Wilbourne AJ: Slowing across the thoracic outlet with thoracic outlet syndrome: fact or fiction. Neurology 34(Suppl):143–146 (1984).
20. Wilbourne AJ: The thoracic outlet syndrome is over diagnosed. Arch Neurol 47:328–330 (1990).
21. Wilkinson M: Cervical Spondylosis: Its Early Diagnosis and Treatment. WB Saunders, Philadelphia (1971).

APPENDIX

Exercise

"It is extremely difficult for a physician who puts too much trust in what he reads to form a proper decision from what he sees."

—Andrew Boorde

GENERAL STATEMENT

Exercise is the movement of specific body parts and/or the body generally, designed to improve local function and general aerobic fitness. Improved fitness is classified as a specific or general increase in muscular strength, joint mobility, joint or body posture, and endurance. Endurance not only includes muscle function, but also cardiorespiratory fitness.

General Exercises

These exercises include repetitive and rhythmic activities of all body parts. They are divided into low impact or high impact, depending on floor contact. If both feet are off the ground at any one time during the exercise, the activity is considered high impact (e.g., running). If one foot is on the ground through all phases of the activity, it is low-impact aerobics (e.g., walking). High-impact aerobics are not recommended for axial (spine) problems. Low-impact aerobics, such as brisk walking, cycling, swimming, and equipment exercises (e.g., Nordic Track) are excellent for general body fitness. They are useful for mild neck and shoulder problems, such as fibrositis, but have limited benefit for problems with moderate to severe neck or shoulder weakness or contracture.

For example, if you plan to prescribe low-impact aerobic stationary cycling, the American College of Sports Medicine (ACSM) (1) recommends:

- 15–60 minutes of exercise;
- 3–5 days/week;
- At 60%–90% of maximum heart rate reserve.

Maximum heart rate reserve (MHRR) is calculated as 220 − age. For a 55-year-old: MHRR = 220 − 55 = 165/minute; 60%–90% of that number is a pulse of 100–150/minute.

Ride the stationary cycle with the seat at the right height, allowing the knee 15° of flexion at the bottom of the pedal stroke. Keep the knees tracking in the natural position and the toes off the front end of the pedal. Ride with limited torque, but alternately raise and lower the resistance every three to five minutes during the ride.

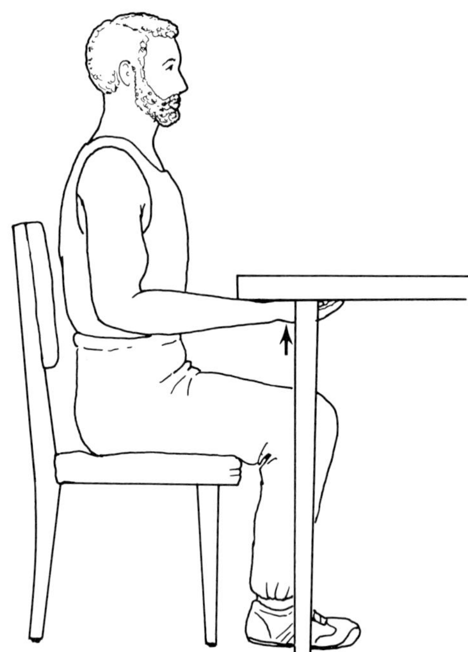

Figure A.1.   Isometric elbow flexion exercise. The elbow flexors (biceps and brachialis) are contracting against the resistance of the table, without the muscle fibers changing length. This is beneficial to shoulder function.

Specific Exercises

The benefits of general exercises cannot be transferred to specific problems of neck or shoulder muscle weakness and/or contracture. For these situations, you need to prescribe a more specific program directed at the local problem. Specific exercises can be classified as:

1. Strengthening
2. Range of movement
3. Stretching
4. Postural
5. Endurance
6. Relaxation

Strengthening Exercises

Specific muscle strengthening can be accomplished in three basic ways.

Isometric strengthening.   During this program, no joint movement occurs and no change in muscle length occurs. Rather, the joint is positioned and maximum contracture is made (Fig. A.1). The problem with this exercise program is that its strength improvement is localized to the muscle fibers being contracted and excludes other muscle fibers needed for recovery. The exercise also needs a Valsalva maneuver for completion, which can be detrimental to patients with cardiac (blood pressure) problems.

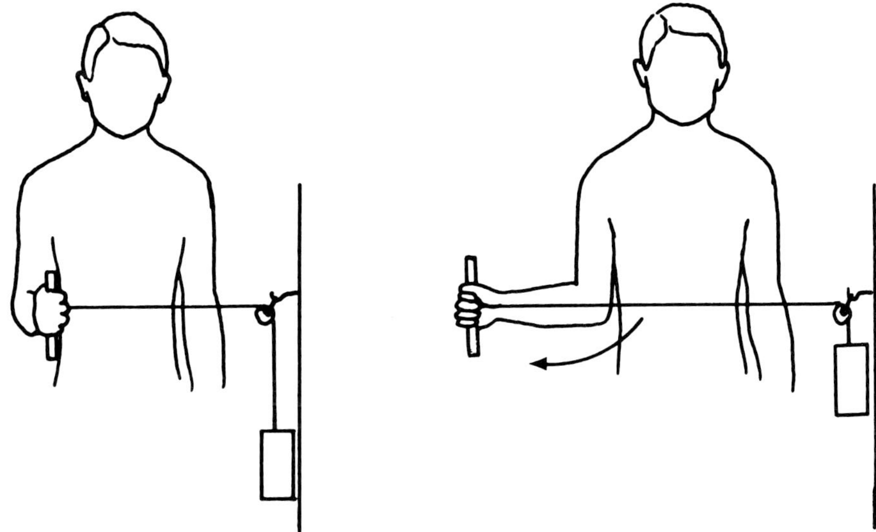

Figure A.2. Isotonic shoulder external rotator exercise. Taking the shoulder through the range of movement of external rotation against a weight.

Isometrics are limited to necks and shoulders that are very painful or immobilized (e.g., shoulder spica), and they usually serve as a beginning program. For the healthy body builder, they can be an important form of exercise.

Isotonic strengthening.   During this exercise effort (Fig. A.2), the joint is moved along with the muscle agonist. The exercise benefit is quantified according to the number of repetitions and the degree of resistance (weight). This form of exercise is the most useful for patients wishing to exercise at home under their own supervision.

Isokinetic strengthening.   Like isotonic exercises, joint and muscle movement occurs but the speed and resistance is constantly controlled (Fig. A.3). In a supervised program, this is the best way to rebuild muscle strength. Expensive equipment is needed for this exercise, usually requiring a physical therapy prescription.

Neck Strengthening Exercises

Figs. A.4 to A.8 are exercises for the neck. The exercises are each repeated at least six times.

Shoulder Strengthening Exercises

Figs. A.9 to A.24 are exercises for the shoulder. Repetitions and weights will vary with patient's age, sex, and limiting physical condition.

Range-of-Movement Exercises (Figs. A.25 to A.35 and Fig. A.43)

Range-of-movement (ROM) exercises are used to maintain joint mobility. If your patient has a stiff joint, it is often necessary to initiate ROM exercises before strengthening exercises. Some exercise therapists believe the ROM of a joint can be increased with strengthening exercises. Stretching exercises are also part of a program to increase ROM in a joint (see next section). When the

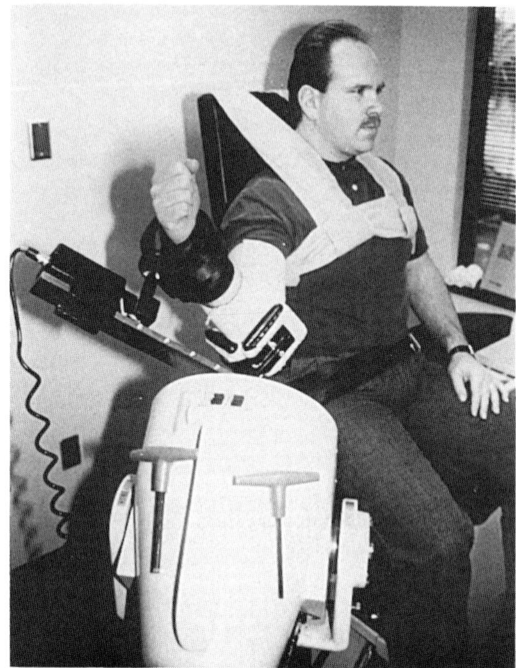

Figure A.3.   Isokinetic strengthening of the shoulder.

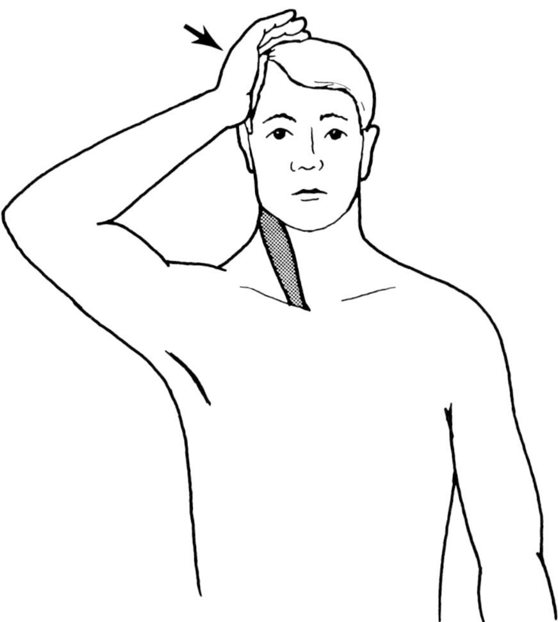

Figure A.4. Isometric neck strengthening, using the hand as resistance, forcing lateral flexion. If the neck is held in one position, the lateral flexors, including sternomastoid, are isometrically strengthened. By allowing lateral neck flexion (or rotation, which is the primary function of the sternomastoid), the exercise becomes isotonic.

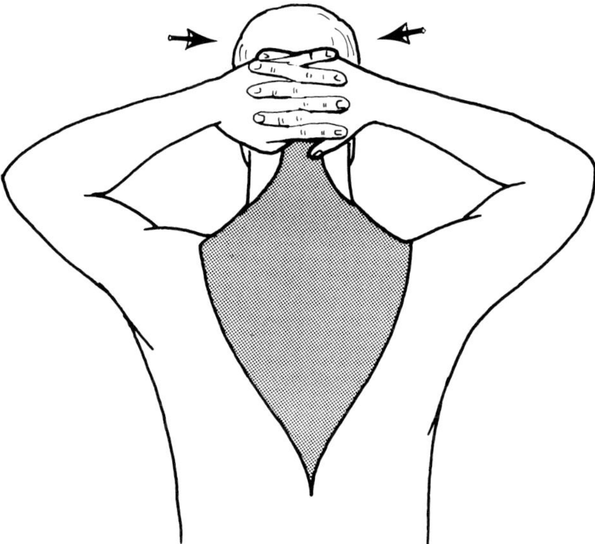

Figure A.5.   Isometric neck extensor and trapezius exercises.

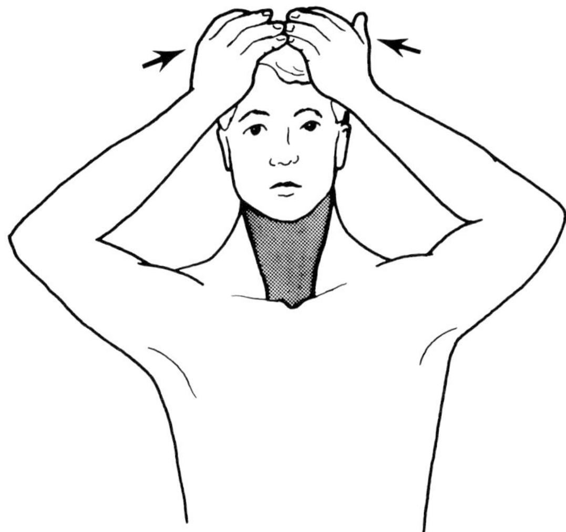

Figure A.6.   Isometric neck flexion exercises.

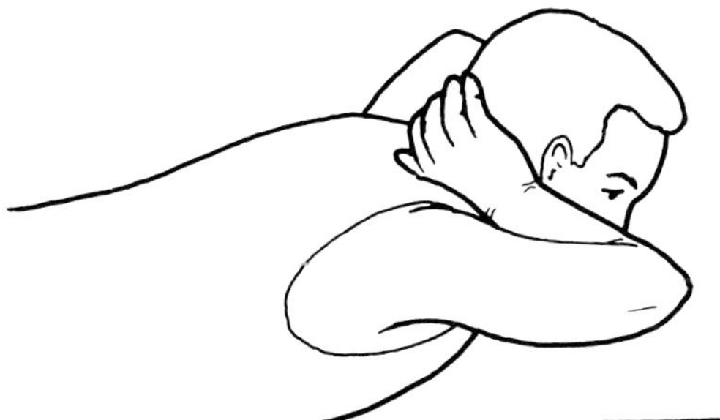

Figure A.7.   Isotonic neck extension (if the exercise is done through a range of neck extension, with resistance).

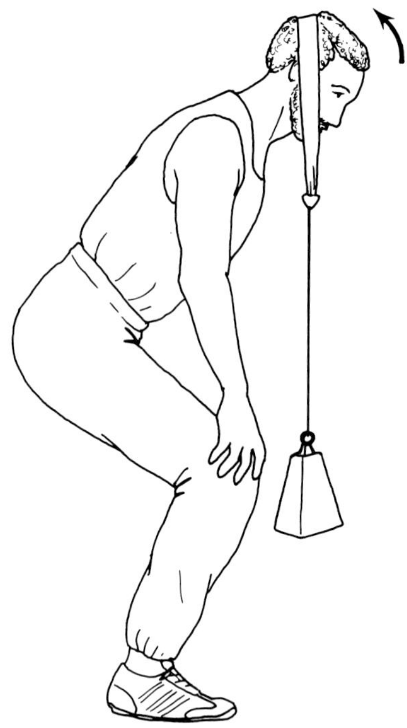

Figure A.8. A better way to do neck extension exercises, with a range of movement (isotonic) or without a range of movement (isometric).

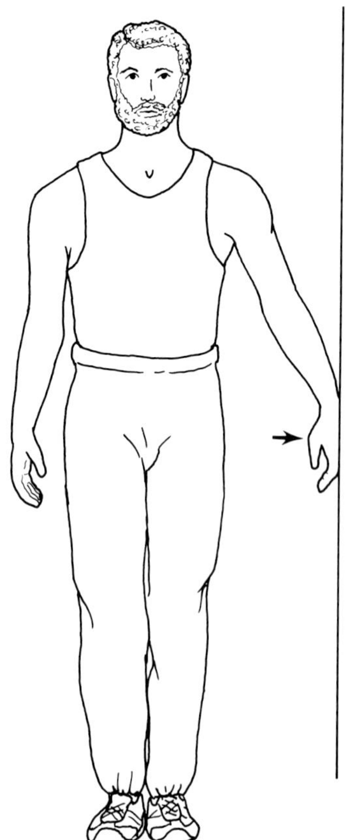

Figure A.9. Isometric shoulder abduction strengthening exercise.

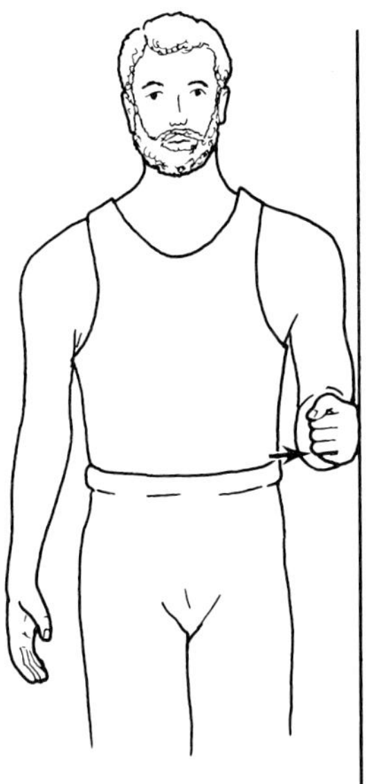

Figure A.10.   Isometric shoulder external rotators strengthening exercise.

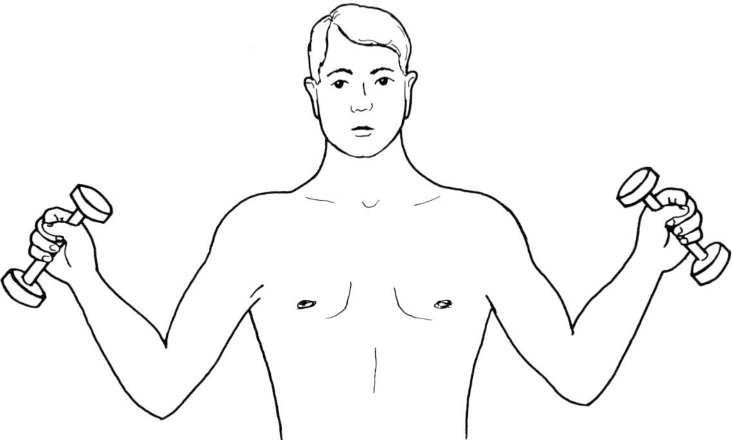

Figure A.11.   Isotonic shoulder strengthening exercises using free weights (2–5 lb for women, 2–10 lb for men). The exercise can be directed at one or all movements of shoulder abduction, flexion, extension and/or rotation.

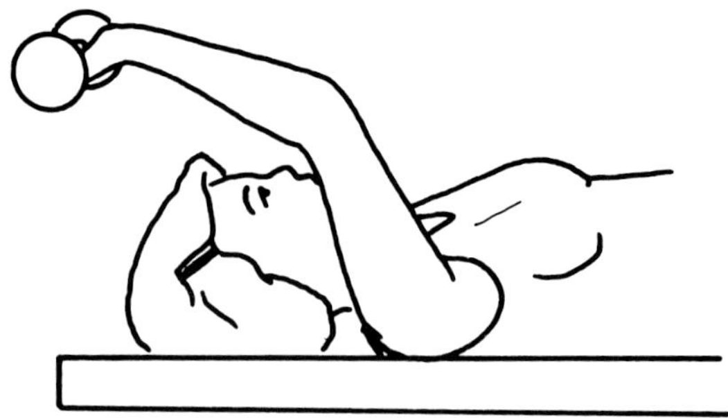

Figure A.12. Isotonic shoulder flexion/extension exercises with free weights. From the anatomical position the shoulder is flexed as far as possible, followed by extension.

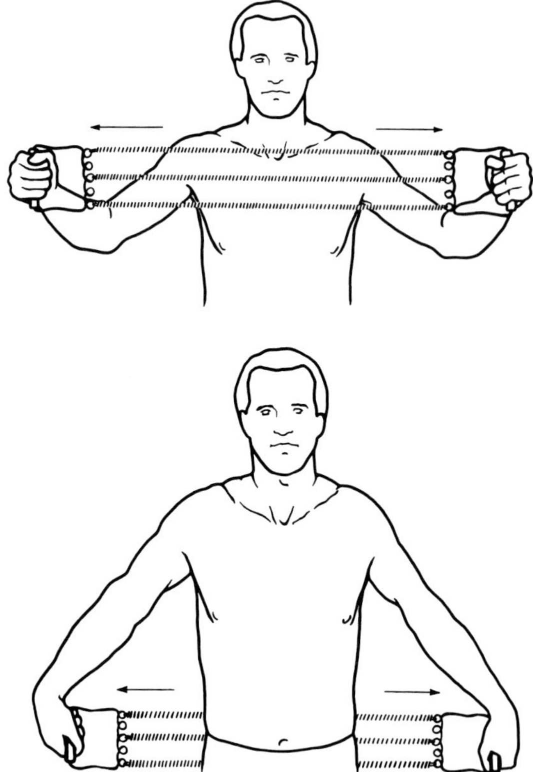

Figures A.13 and A.14. Isotonic shoulder exercises with springs instead of free weights.

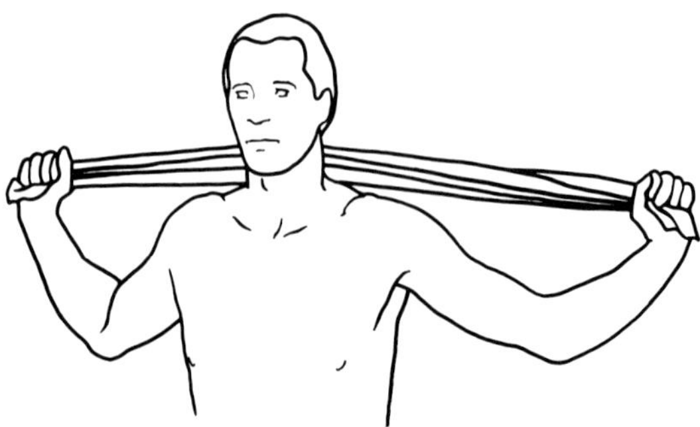

Figure A.15. Isotonic shoulder exercises with a flexible (rubber) theraband.

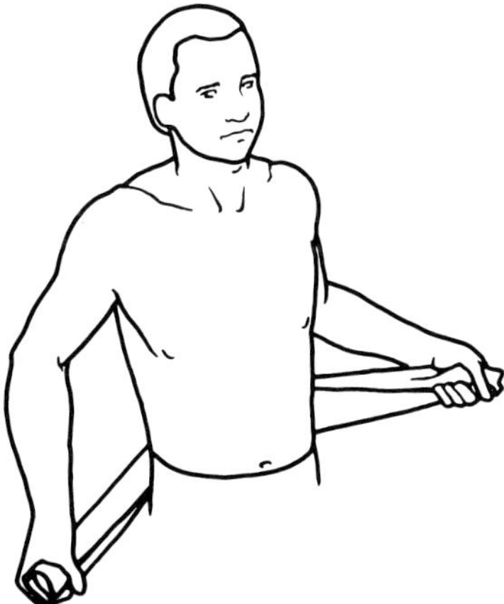

Figure A.16.   More isotonic shoulder exercises with the theraband.

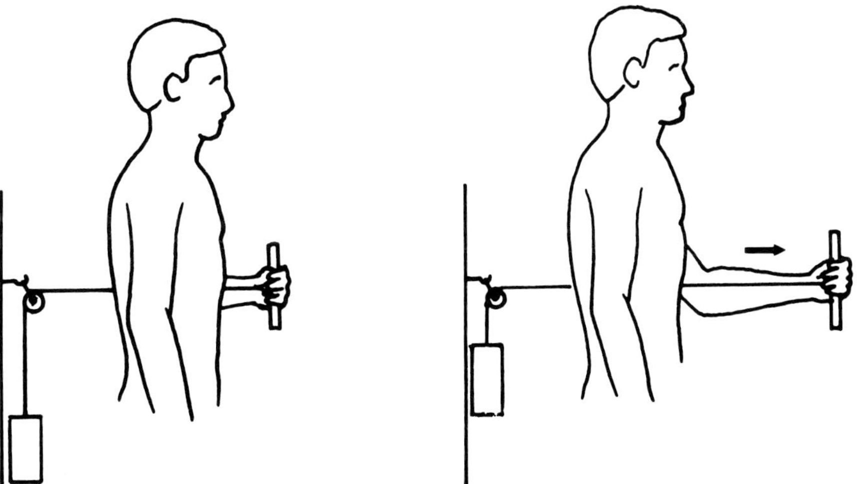

Figure A.17.   Isotonic shoulder flexion exercises.

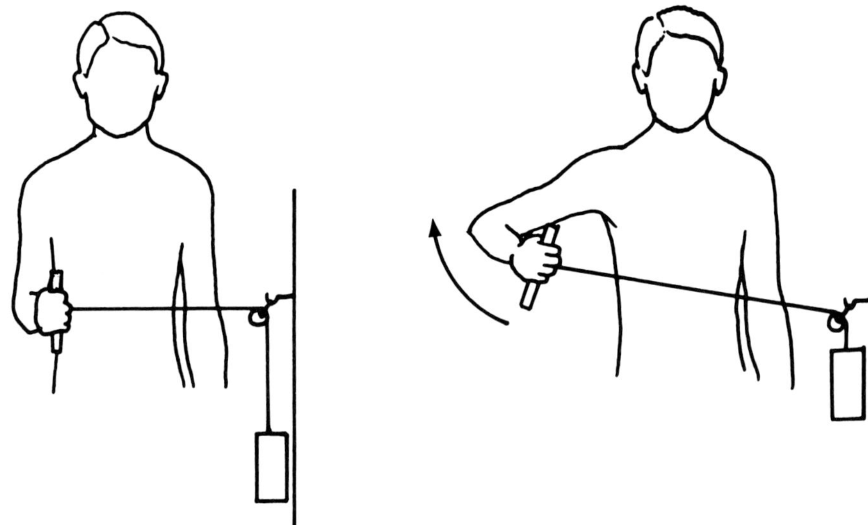

Figure A.18. Isotonic shoulder abduction exercises.

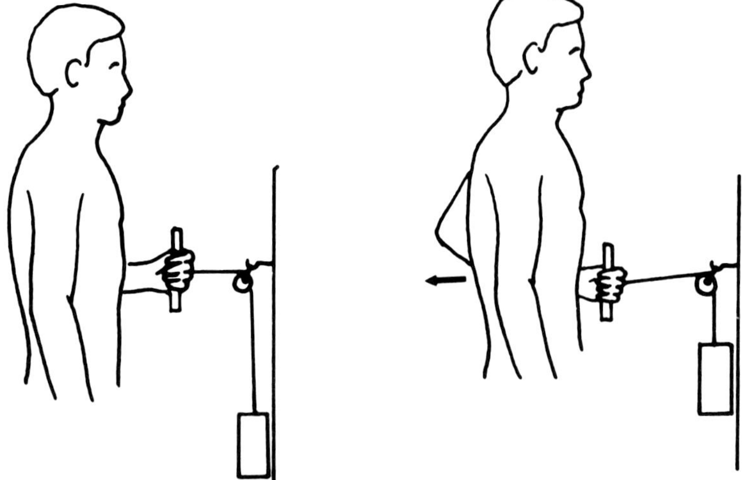

Figure A.19. Isotonic shoulder extension exercises.

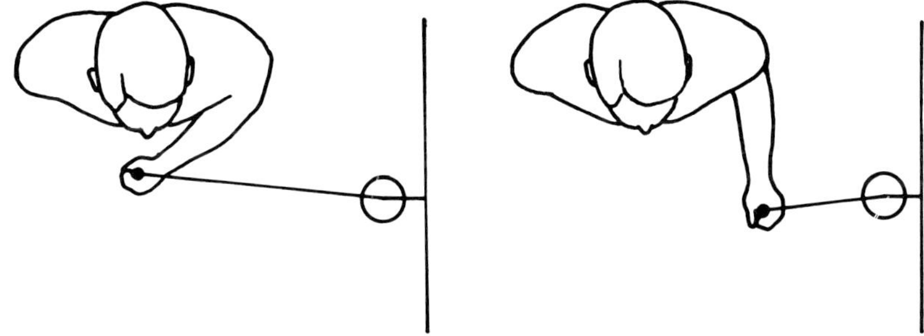

Figure A.20.   Isotonic shoulder internal rotation exercises.

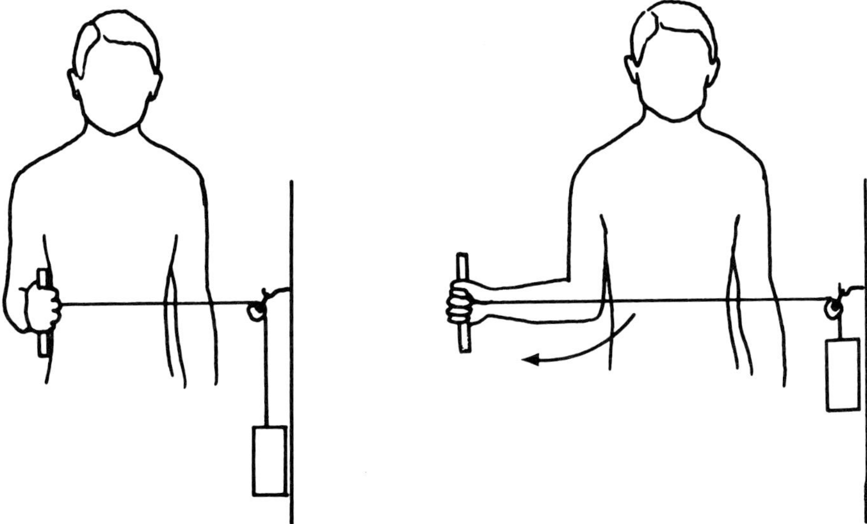

Figure A.21.   Isotonic shoulder external rotation exercises.

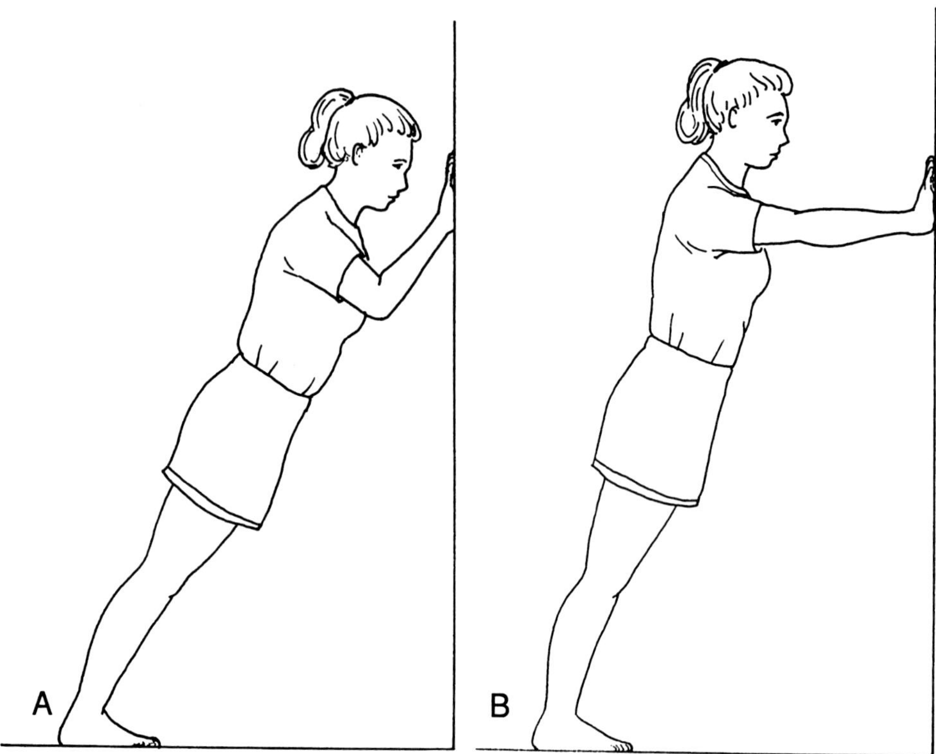

Figure A.22.   *A*, standing "'push-up" exercise for shoulder strengthening. *B*, next phase of the standing push-up.

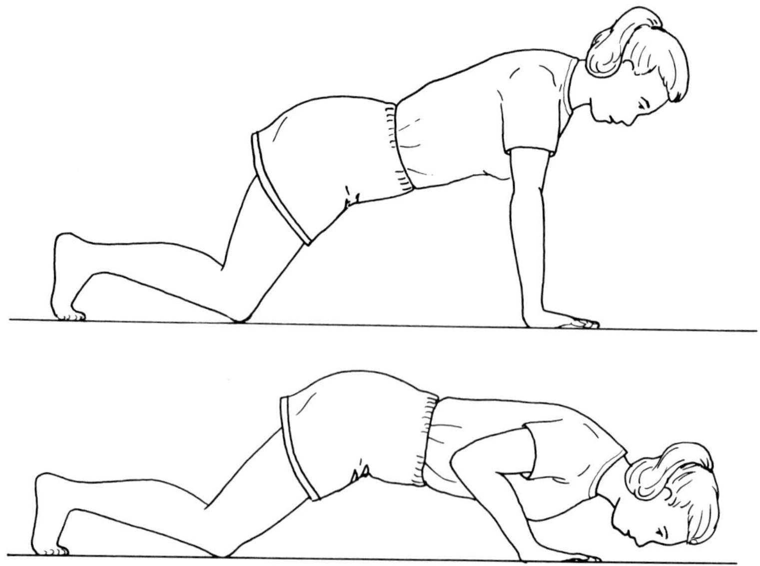

Figure A.23.   *Top*: next phase of an advancing push-up exercise. *Bottom*: beginning position for the trunk push-up exercise.

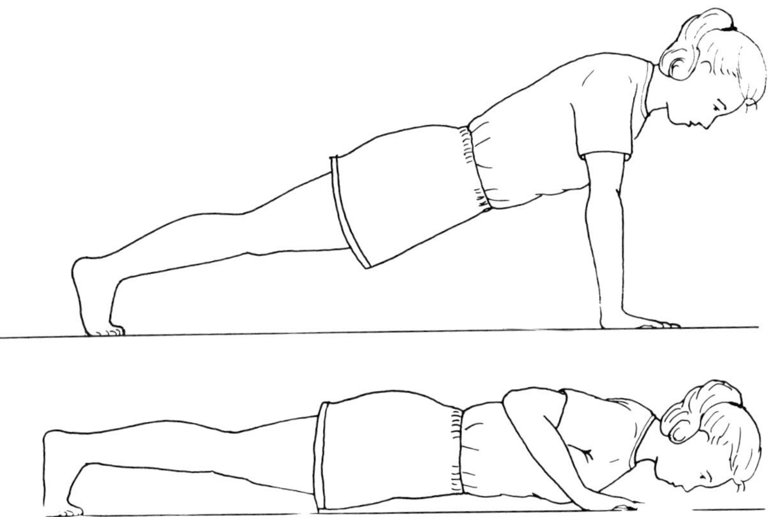

Figure A.24. *Top*: full push-up. *Bottom*: beginning position for a full push-up.

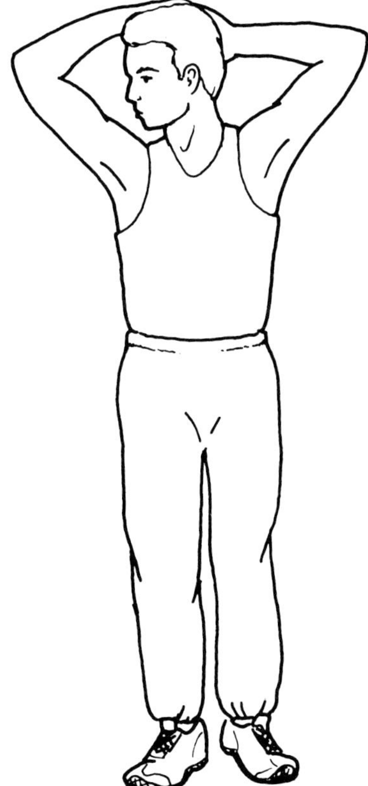

Figure A.25. Neck ROM exercise (rotation).

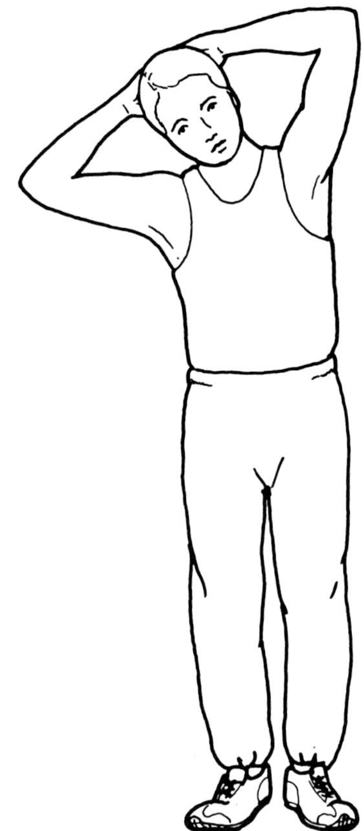

Figure A.26.   Neck ROM exercises (lateral flexion).

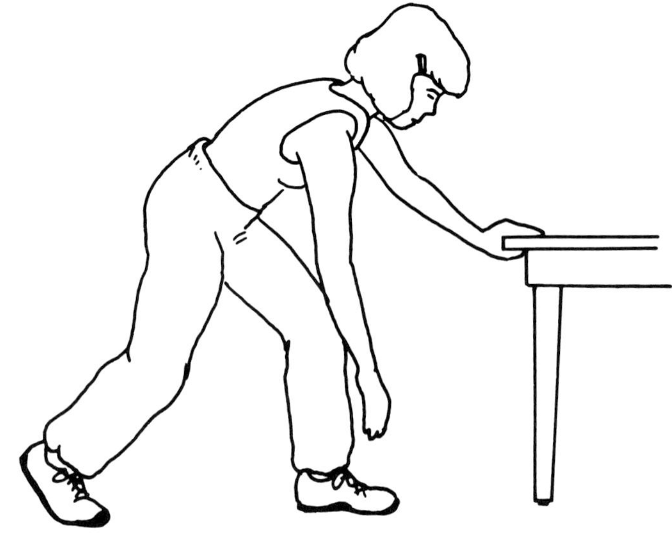

Figure A.27.   Granddaddy of all shoulder exercises: the pendulum exercise. The arm, hanging free, is passively rotated through a circumduction range of movement by moving the trunk.

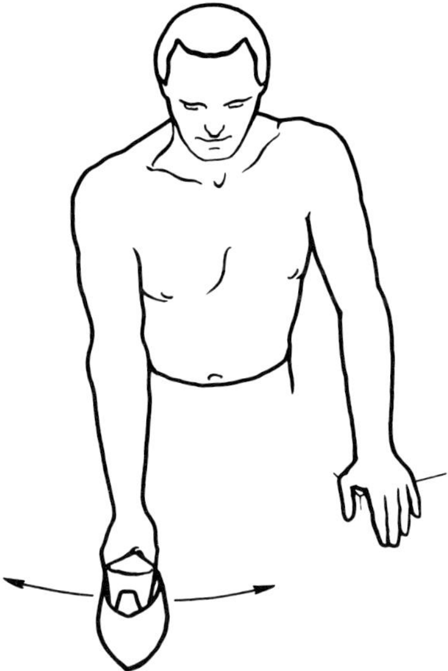

Figure A.28.   The pendulum exercise can be altered by placing a weight in the hand (an old iron), limiting the direction (in this figure, to abduction/adduction), and including a more active role for the shoulder muscles.

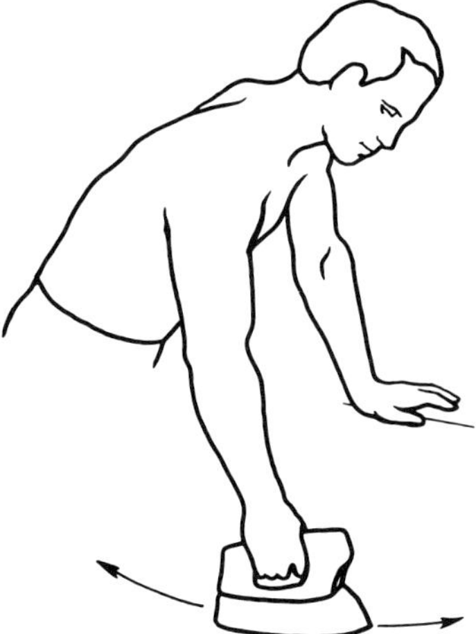

Figure A.29.   The pendulum exercise modified to flexion/extension.

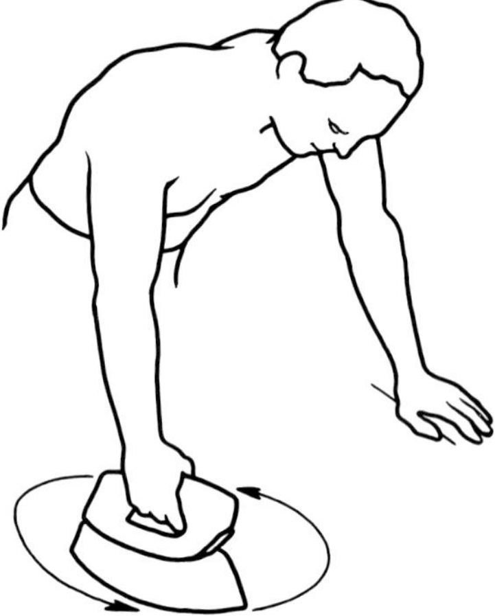

Figure A.30.   Circumduction with a hand weight as a passive or an active ROM exercise.

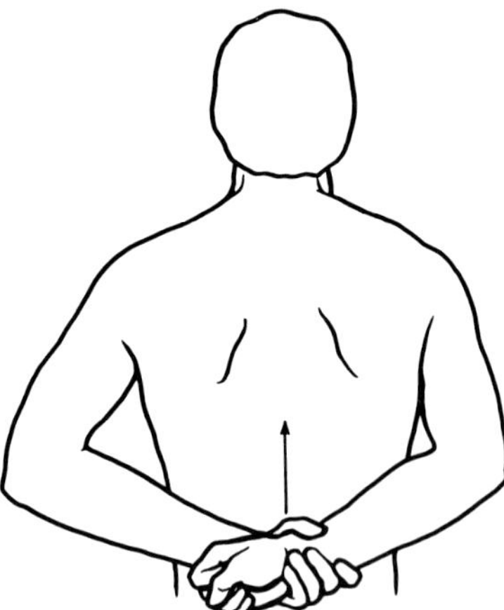

Figure A.31.   Internal rotation ROM exercise; the more passive the exercise and the more the opposite arm assists, the more the exercise becomes a stretching exercise.

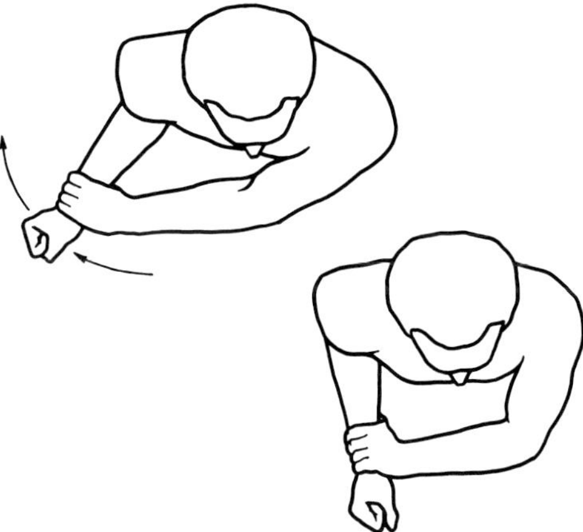

Figure A.32.   External rotation ROM or strengthening exercises.

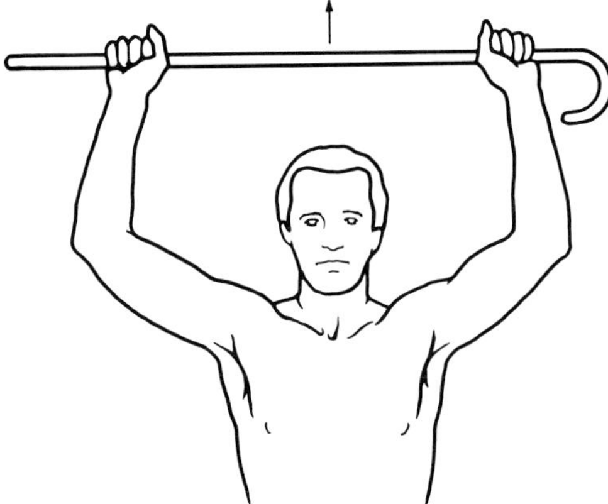

Figure A.33.   Abduction ROM for the shoulder using a walking stick. The advantage of the stiff cane is that the stronger and the more mobile joint can assist the weaker and/or stiffer opposite joint.

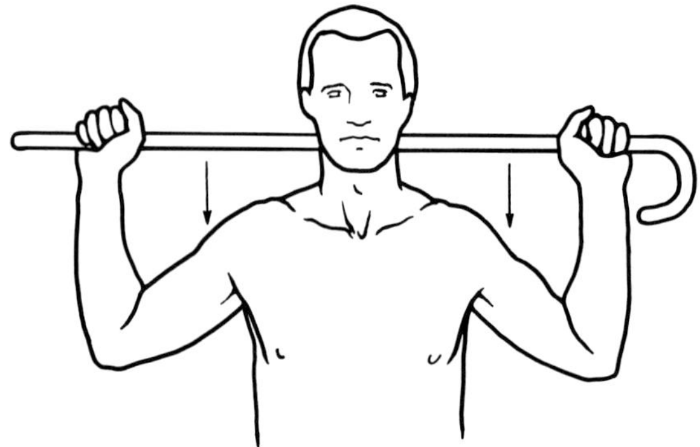

Figure A.34.   Shoulder flexion ROM exercises with the walking stick.

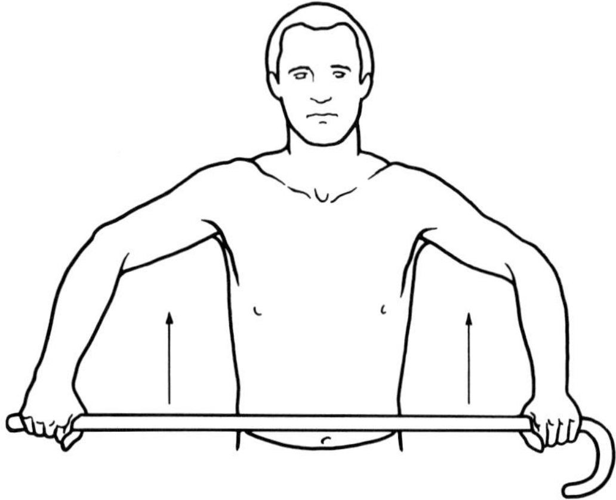

Figure A.35.   The lower ranges of shoulder abduction are being exercised.

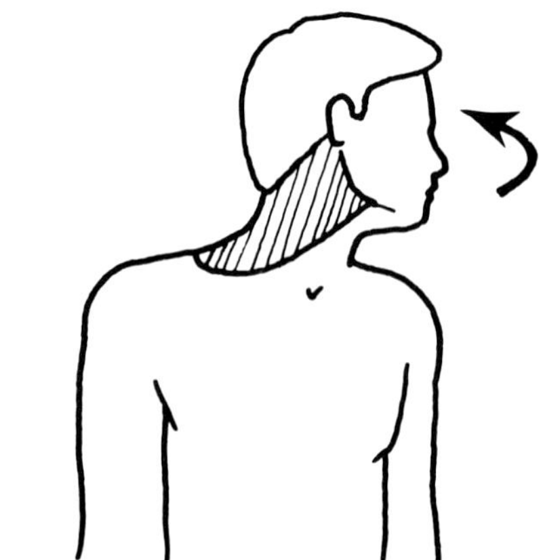

Figure A.36.   Neck stretching exercises—rotation.

various strengthening, ROM, and stretching exercise programs are considered together, it becomes obvious that there are as many different shoulder exercise programs as there are therapists! The important questions to answer in exercise therapy are:

1. What is the functional loss—strength, endurance, loss of ROM, stiffness, postural, etc.?
2. What exercise program works best for me to help the patient overcome the functional loss?

Stretching Exercises (Figs. A.36 to A.42)

Stretching exercises are closely related to ROM exercises. The difference is subtle, but ROM exercises imply that active muscle contraction is occurring to increase the ROM of the joint. Stretching exercises are a more passive group of exercises in which a therapist passively stretches a contracted muscle. The stretch is usually preceded by a modality, such as deep heat, on the theory that this leads to muscle relaxation and an easier stretch. The passive stretch is then done to elongate and relax the muscle. Gently done within the physiological ROM, these exercises can be considered a form of manipulation. They are used predominantly for myofascial pain syndromes (chronic neck pain), while ROM exercises are used more frequently for specific joint contractures.

Stretching exercises are also popular as part of a warm-up for a specific sporting event.

Postural Exercises

These exercises are used predominantly in the neck. They are used when habit, occupation, tension, or diffuse mild arthritis thrust the neck forward (Fig. A.44). This is the so-called position of attack (i.e., the cat) and is often a part of occupational neck strain and/or myofascial pain syndromes. Part of the problem is weak posterior neck muscles, allowing gravity to pull the head down and forward.

For these patients, it is necessary to point out the abnormal posture, train new posture, and add strengthening exercises for the weak muscle groups.

Endurance Exercises

These exercises are more specific for athletic training and are designed to increase ability to perform a specific task over a period of time. They include general aerobic fitness exercises and specific muscle exercise, starting with strength training that—through increasing repetitions without increase in resistance—builds endurance. These programs have limited use in immediate postoperative rehabilitation but are an essential part of late rehabilitation of the high-performance athlete.

Relaxation Exercises

Relaxation exercises are a hypnotic-type approach to the patient with muscle tension or myofascial pain. They are only useful in the patient who has insight into and acceptance of the reasons for the chronic neck pain.

They are most often done in classes and to the accompaniment of music. The patient is placed in a position of rest (usually lying down) and is given instruction

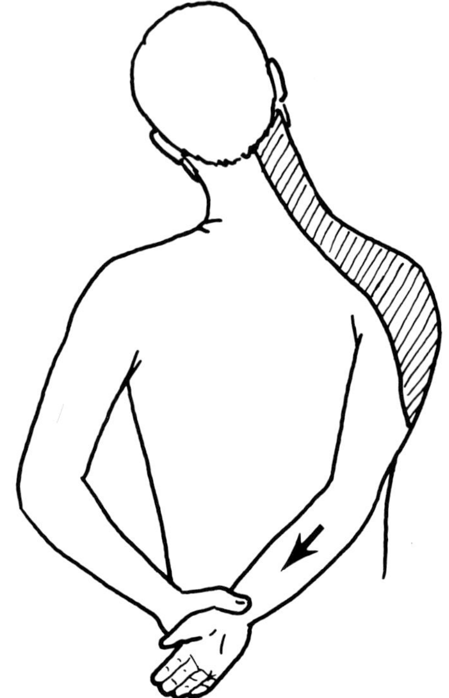

Figure A.37.   Neck stretching exercises—lateral flexion.

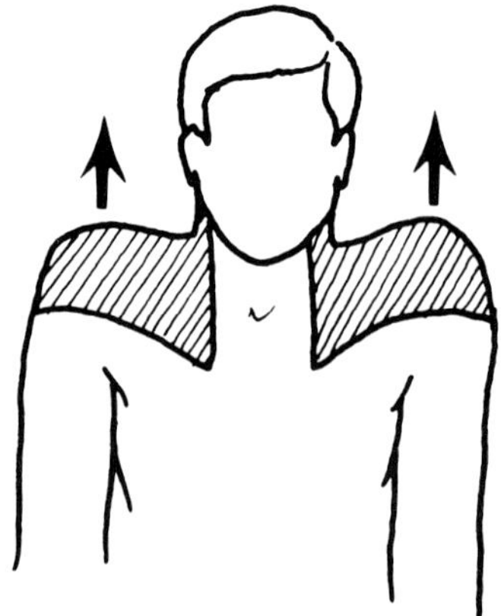

Figure A.38.   Neck stretching exercises. The *shaded muscles* (trapezii) are being stretched.

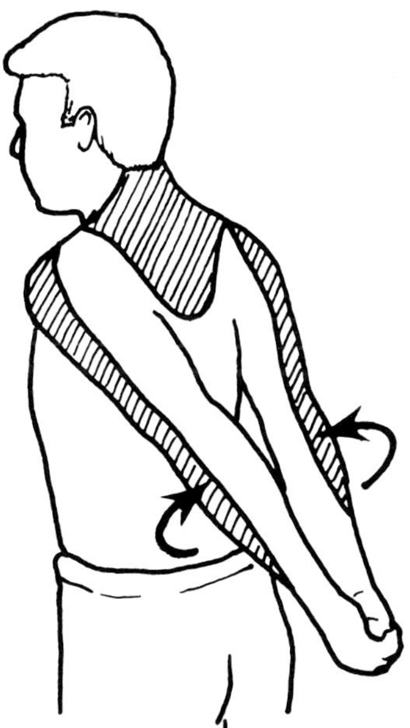

Figure A.39.   Shoulder and neck stretching exercises.

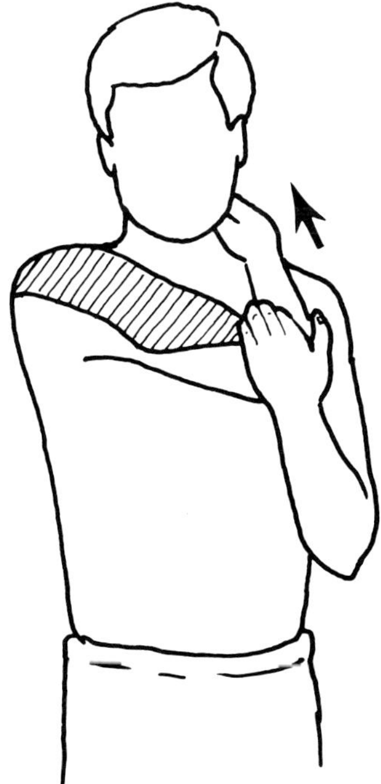

Figure A.40.   Shoulder extensor and abduction stretching exercises.

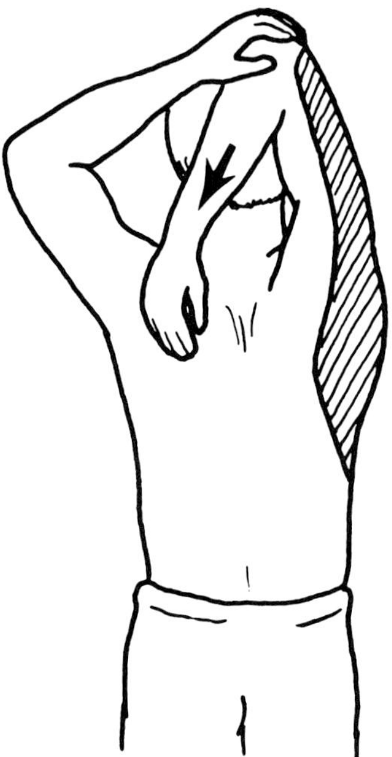

Figure A.41.   Shoulder adductor strengthening exercises.

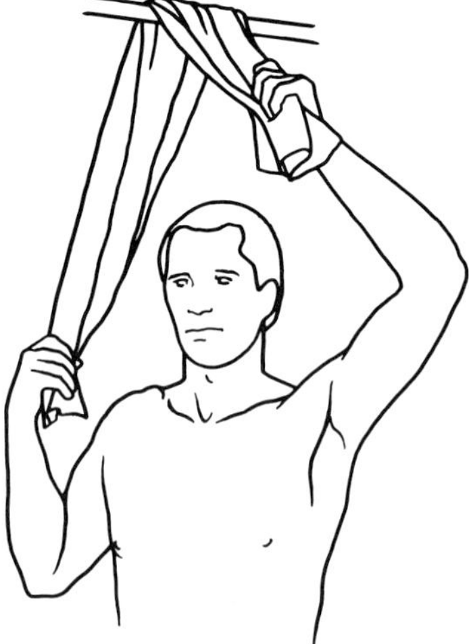

Figure A.42.   Method of stretching the shoulder using a towel strung over a shower bar. The strong mobile shoulder stretches the capsule and adductors of the shoulder.

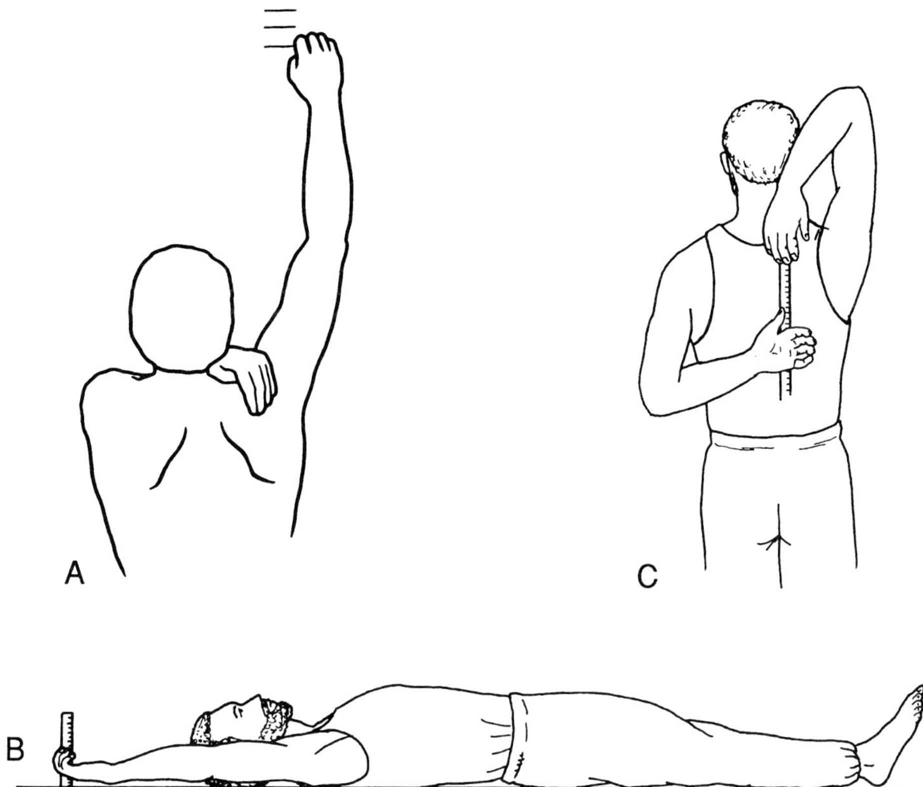

Figure A.43.   *A*, method by which the patient can record increasing shoulder elevation. *B*, the same recording in the supine position. By how many inches or centimeters does the hand miss coming down to the floor? *C*, recording internal rotation. The right hand holds the ruler to measure the left. Obviously the therapist has to read the measurement.

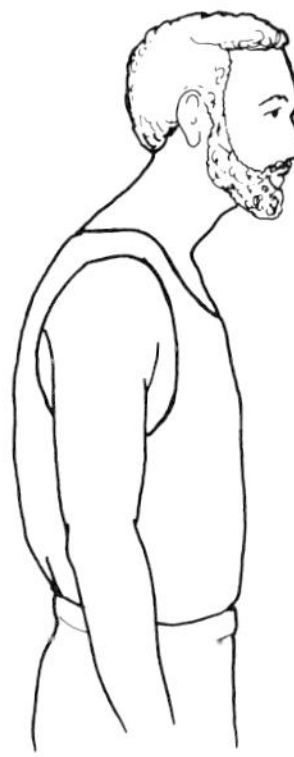

Figure A.44.   The tension neck syndrome with the neck held in the position of "attack."

in how to relax muscles, from distal to proximal (fingertips to neck). Some programs augment this approach with electromyographic biofeedback so the patient has the auditory sensation of relaxed muscles.

CONCLUSION

This exercise appendix is a very limited introduction to neck and shoulder exercises. It should be obvious, from the wide variety of exercise categories, that there are many different ways to exercise. Each exercise program must be tailored to the patient and is most effective when done under the direction of a therapist.

REFERENCE

1. American College of Sports Medicine: The recommended quantity and quality of exercise for developing and maintaining fitness in healthy adults. Sports Med Bull 13:1, 3–4 (1978).

INDEX

Page numbers followed by "f" denote figures; those followed by "t" denote tables.